Tactical Emergency Medicine

Tactical Emergency Medicine

EDITORS

RICHARD B. SCHWARTZ, MD, FACEP

Chairman and Associate Professor
Department of Emergency Medicine
Medical College of Georgia

LTC JOHN G. McMANUS, JR., MD, MCR, FACEP, FAAEM

Assistant Chief, Academic Affairs
EMS Fellowship Director
Department of Emergency Medicine, Brooke Army Medical Center, Fort Sam Houston, Texas
EMS Medical Director Fort Sam Houston and Camp Bullis Fire
Clinical Associate Professor Emergency Medicine University of Texas
Heath Science Center San Antonio

RAYMOND E. SWIENTON, MD, FACEP

Associate Professor, Emergency Medicine
Co-Director, Section of EMS, Disaster Medicine and Homeland Security
University of Texas Southwestern Medical Center at Dallas, Dallas, Texas

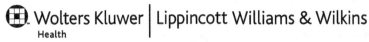

Wolters Kluwer | Lippincott Williams & Wilkins
Health
Philadelphia • Baltimore • New York • London
Buenos Aires • Hong Kong • Sydney • Tokyo

Acquisitions Editor: Frances R. DeStefano
Managing Editor: Nicole Dernoski
Project Manager: Jennifer Harper
Senior Manufacturing Manager: Benjamin Rivera
Marketing Manager: Angela Panetta
Design Coordinator: Holly Reid McLaughlin
Cover Designer: Carol Tippit Woolworth
Production Services: Aptara, Inc.

Printed in the USA

Library of Congress Cataloging-in-Publication Data

Tactical emergency medicine / [edited by] Richard B. Schwartz, John G. McManus Jr.,
Raymond Sweinton.
     p. ; cm,
   Includes bibliographical references and index.
   ISBN-13: 978-0-7817-7332-4 (alk. paper)
   ISBN-10: 0-7817-7332-6 (alk. paper)
   1. Emergency medicine.   2. Medicine, Military.   I. Schwartz, Richard B.
II. McManus, John G.   III. Sweinton, Raymond.
   [DNLM: 1. Emergency Medical Services—organization & administration.
2. Emergency Medical Technicians—education.   3. Emergency
Medicine—organization & administration.   4 Military Medicine—organization &
administration.   5. Wounds and Injuries—therapy. WX 215 T118 2008]
   RC86.7.T33   2008
   616.02'5—dc22

2007042791

Care has been taken to confirm the accuracy of the information presented and to
describe generally accepted practices. However, the authors, editors, and publisher are
not responsible for errors or omissions or for any consequences from application of
the information in this book and make no warranty, expressed or implied, with respect
to the currency, completeness, or accuracy of the contents of the publication.
Application of the information in a particular situation remains the professional
responsibility of the practitioner.

The authors, editors, and publisher have exerted every effort to ensure that drug
selection and dosage set forth in this text are in accordance with current
recommendations and practice at the time of publication. However, in view of ongoing
research, changes in government regulations, and the constant flow of information
relating to drug therapy and drug reactions, the reader is urged to check the package
insert for each drug for any change in indications and dosage and for added warnings
and precautions. This is particularly important when the recommended agent is a new
or infrequently employed drug.

Some drugs and medical devices presented in the publication have Food and Drug
Administration (FDA) clearance for limited use in restricted research settings. It is the
responsibility of the health care provider to ascertain the FDA status of each drug or
device planned for use in their clinical practice.

To purchase additional copies of this book, call our customer service department
at (800) 638-3030 or fax orders to (301) 223-2320. International customers should call
(301) 223-2300.

Visit Lippincott Williams & Wilkins on the Internet: at LWW.com. Lippincott
Williams & Wilkins customer service representatives are available from 8:30 am to
6 pm, EST.

10 9 8 7 6 5 4

To my family: my children Kyle and Kenzie for showing me what is important in life My wife Polly for her love and support My mother for her strength And my father who I never knew, but whom has been, an inspiration to me.

—Dr. Richard B. Schwartz

For all the gals who mentored me and kept me in line! Jessica, Carol, Deborah, Annemarie, Catherine, Marybeth, Carlin, Laura and Nutmeg! Also, to my former instructors: Dr. Len Dalton, Dr. Tom Davis, Dr. Thomas Fox, Dr. Mohamud Daya and Dr. Jerris Hedges. Finally, thanks Dad (John Sr.) for not sending me off to the orphanage!

—Dr. John G. McManus, Jr.

This book is dedicated to all who protect our citizens, defend our country, provide care to the ill and injured; placing themselves in harm's way to preserve our freedom and peace.

To my wife, Anne, and our children, Kyle and Heather, thank you for your love and support. To my father, now in eternal peace, and to my prayerful mother, thank you.

—Dr. Raymond E. Swienton

Special thanks to Carol Pogue and Sabrina Byrum for their assistance and dedication in the development of this textbook.

CONTENTS

CONTRIBUTORS

Bret T. Ackerman, DO, FACEP
Adjunct Associate Professor
Department of Military and Emergency Medicine
F. Edward Hebert School of Medicine
Uniformed Services University of Health Sciences
Bethesda, Maryland
Attending Emergency Physician
Department of Emergency Medicine
Womack Army Medical Center
Fort Bragg, North Carolina

Stephen Brock Blankenship, MD
Staff Physician
Deployment Medicine, Inc.
Department of Emergency Medicine
Wake Forest University Baptist Medical Center
Winston-Salem, North Carolina

James E. Brown, EMT-TP, MD
Associate Professor and Program Director
Integrated Residency in Emergency Medicine
Department of Emergency Medicine
Boonshoft School of Medicine
Wright State University
Dayton, Ohio

W. Thomas Burnett, MD
Medical Director
Division VI SWAT
Virginia State Police
Salem, Virginia
Associate Medical Director
Department of Emergency Medicine
Carilion Clinic
Roanoke, Virginia

Phillip Carmona, NREMT-P, RN
Burn Center
Vanderbilt University Medical Center
Nashville, Tennessee

Frank L. Christopher, MD
Associate Professor
Department of Military and Emergency Medicine
Uniformed Services University of the Health Sciences
Bethesda, Maryland
Commander 261st Medical Batallion
44th Medical Comand (Corps) (Airborne)
Fort Bragg, North Carolina

Timothy A. Coakley, MD, FAAEM, CDR, MC, USN, DMO
Deputy Force Surgeon
Navy Expedition Area Combat Command
Naval Amphibious Base, Little Creek
Norfolk, Virginia

Phillip L. Coule, MD, FAAEM
Associate Professor
Director, Center of Operational Medicine
Associate Professor
Department of Emergency Medicine
Medical College of Georgia
Augusta, Georgia

LTC Donald M. Crawford, DO
Chief, Emergency Medicine Service
Medical Dierctor, Teaching Faculty
Department of Emergency Medicine
Brooke Army Medical Center
San Antonio, Texas
Associate Professor
Department of Military and Emergency Medicine
Uniformed Services University of the Health Sciences
Bethesda, Maryland

John M. Croushorn, MD
Brigade Surgeon
Task Force 185 AVN
Operation Iraqi Freedom—OIF2
Clinical Director
Department of Emergency Medicine
Montclair Hospital
Birmingham, Alabama

Peter J. Cuenca, MD
Clinical Instructor
Department of Emergency Medicine
Brooke Army Medical Center
San Antonio, Texas

Robert A. DeLorenzo, MD
Associate Adjunct Professor
Department of Military and Emergency Medicine
Uniformed Services University of the Health Sciences
Bethesda, Maryland
Program Director
Department of Emergency Medicine
Brooke Army Medical Center
Fort Sam Houston, Texas

Karen A. Deeds

Robert W. Deeds, TX-TF I, FEMA
Canine Search Specialist

Jerry R. DeMaio

Robert Dickerson

Faith A. Dillard, MS, MD
Associate Director
Department of Emergency Services
Prince William Hospital
Manassas, Virginia

Alexander L. Eastman, MD
Senior Fellow in Government Emergency Medical
   Security Services
University of Texas Southwestern Medical Center
Surgeon
Department of Surgery
Parkland Memorial Hospital
Dallas, Texas

William P. Fabbri, MD, FACEP
Medical Officer
Feberal Bureau of Investigation

Raymond L. Fowler, MD, FACEP
Associate Professor Emergency Medicine
Deputy EMS Medical Director
Co-Section Chief for EMS, Disaster Medicine,
& Homeland Security
University of Texas Southwestern Medical Center

COL James Fudge, DVM
Chief Veterinarian Medicine
US Army Institute of Surgical Research
Fort Sam Houston, Texas

Robert T. Gerhardt, MD, MPH, FACEP
Research Director
SAUSHEC Emergency Medicine Residency Program
Aviation Medicine Consultant for Emergency Medicine
U.S. Army Aeromedical Center
Associate Professor of Military and Emergency Medicine
USUHS
Department of Emergency Medicine
San Antonio Uniformed Services Health
   Education Consortium
Brooke Army Medical Center
Fort Sam Houston, Texas

Mark E. Gebhart, MD, EMT-P, FAAEM
Assistant Professor
Director, Homeland Emergency Learning and Preparedness Center
Boonshoft School of Medicine
Department of Emergency Medicine
Wright State University
Attending Physician, Good Samaritan Hospital
Dayton, Ohio

Lt. Mark E. Gibbons, EMT-T/P
Maryland State Police
Baltimore, Maryland

COL James L. Greenstone, Ed.D, JD, DABECI, MSC
Deputy Commander
Medical Reserve Corps
Texas State Guard
Police Psychologist and Director of Psychological Services
Fort Worth,
Texas Police Department (Retired)
Fort Worth, Texas
Professor
Capella University
Harold Abel School of Psychology
Walden University
School of Health and Human Services
Master Peace Office, State of Texas

LTC Benjamin Harrison, MD, FAAEM, FACEP
Program Director
Madigan—University of Washington
Department of Emergency Medicine

Jeffrey D. Ho, MD
Assistant Professor
Faculty Physician
Department of Emergency Medicine
University of Minnesota
Minneapolis, Minnesota

Kermit D. Huebner, MD, FACEP
Assistant Clinical Instructor
Military and Emergency Medicine
Uniformed Services University of Health Sciences (USUHS)
Bethesda, Maryland
Chief, Education and Training, Operational Medicine
United States Army Medical Research Institute of Infectious
   Diseases (USAMRIID)
Fort Detrick, Maryland

Jeremy N. Johnson, DO
Resident
Department of Emergency Medicine
Madigan Army Medical Center
Tacoma, Washington

LTC Troy Johnson, MD
Deputy Commander for Clinical Services
Fort Drum, New York

Richard V. King, PhD
Associate Professor and Director of Education
and Research in EMS
Disaster Medicine, and Homeland Security, Health Care
Sciences and Emergency Medicine
University of Texas Southwestern Medical Center
Dallas, Texas

Kelly R. Klein, MD, FACEP
Assistant Professor
Department of Surgery
University of Texas Southwestern Medical Center at Dallas
Attending Physician
Department of Emergency Medicine
Parkland Hospital
Dallas, Texas

Douglas M. Kleiner, PhD, ATC, CSCS, EMT-T, FAGSM
President & CEO
Tactical Medics International
Jacksonville Beach, Florida

MAJ Brian Krakover, MD
Battalion Surgeon
82nd Airborne
Fort Bragg, North Carolina

Julio R. Lairet, DO, EMT-P, Maj(s), USAF, MC
EMS Fellow
Department of Emergency Medicine
Indiana University School of Medicine
Indianapolis, Indiana

Dorothy Lemecha, DO
Fellow in Government Emergency
Medical Security Services
Assistant EMS Medical Director
University of Texas Southwestern Medical Center

William F. Mastrianni, MA, EMT-P
Assistant Director, Chief of EMS Operations
Charleston County (SC) EMS
Team Commander, SC-1 DMAT
Adjunct Faculty, National Fire Academy

LTC Paul T. Mayer, MD
Director, Combat Medic Training
Ft. Sam Houston, Texas

LTC John G. McManus, Jr., MD, MCR, FACEP, FAAEM
Assistant Chief, Academic Affairs
EMS Fellowship Director
Department of Emergency Medicine
Brooke Army Medical Center
Fort Sam Houston, Texas
EMS Medical Director Fort Sam Houston and Camp Bullis Fire
Clinical Associate Professor Emergency Medicine University
of Texas
Heath Science Center San Antonio

Carl Menckhoff, MD
Associate Professor
Department of Emergency Medicine
Medical College of Georgia
Augusta, Georgia

Jeffery C. Metzger, MD
Assistant Professor of Emergency Medicine
Medical Director, Dallas Police Department
Deputy EMS Medical Director
University of Texas Southwestern Medical Center

Paul E. Moore, MS, NREMT, C-EM
Section on EMS, Disaster Medicine, & Homeland Security
University of Texas Southwestern Medical Center

Robert F. Mulry, RN, NREMT-P
Special Agent
Federal Bureau of Investigation

Andre M. Pennardt, MD
Adjunct Assistant Professor
Military and Emergency Medicine
Uniformed Services University of the Health Sciences
Bethesda, Maryland
Group Surgeon, 10th Special Forces Group (Airborne)
Fort Carson, Colorado

COL (ret) James A. Pfaff, MD
Faculty Emergency Medicine
San Antonio Uniformed Services Health Education Consortium

Jason R. Pickett, MD, EMT-P
Emergency Physician
Department of Emergency Medicine
Wright State University
Dayton, Ohio
Kettering Medical Center
Kettering, Ohio

Guillermo J. Pierluisi, MD, MPH
Chief, Department of Emergency Medicine
Flagler Hospital Inc.
St. Augustine, Florida

Michael W. Proctor, MD
Regional Director of Extramural Training
Center for Biosecurity and Public Health Preparedness
The University of Texas Health Science Center
Houston, Texas

Matthew Ratliff, EMT-P

LTC John Rayfield, MD
Attending Staff
Teaching Staff, Department of Emergency Medicine
San Antonio Uniformed Services Health
Education Consortium
Brooke Army Medical Center
San Antonio, Texas

John D. Schwartz, PhD
Associate Professor
Department of Fisheries and Wildlife
Michigan State University
E. Lansing, Michigan

Richard B. Schwartz, MD, FACEP
Chairman and Associate Professor
Department of Emergency Medicine
Medical College of Georgia

Officer Navin K. Sharma, BSN, RN, CEN, EMT-P
Clinical Instructor
Department of Emergency Medicine
Oregon Health Sciences University
Staff RN, Department of Emergency
Providence Portland Medical Center
Portland, Oregon
Police Officer—TEMS Team Leader
Special Operations—Tactical EMS
Vancouver Police Department
Vancouver, Washington

Greene Shepherd, PharmD
Clinical Associate Professor
College of Pharmacy
University of Georgia
Athens, Georgia
Associate Professor
Department of Emergency Medicine
Medical College of Georgia
Augusta, Georgia

Michael D. Shertz, MD, FACEP
Clinical Assistant Professor
Department of Emergency Medicine
Oregon Health Sciences University
Staff Physician, Department of Emergency Services
St. Vincent Medical Center
Portland, Oregon

Alexander M. Silverstein, JD, NREMT-P
Supervisory Special Agent
Federal Bureau of Investigation

Brian L. Springer, MD, EMT-T
Assistant Professor
Department of Emergency Medicine
Wright State University Boonshoft School of Medicine
Dayton, Ohio
Attending, Emergency Department
Kettering Sports Medicine
Kettering Medical Center
Kettering, Ohio

Raymond E. Swienton, MD, FACEP
Associate Professor, Emergency Medicine
Co-director, Section of EMS, Disaster Medicine and Homeland Security
University of Texas Southwestern Medical Center at Dallas
Dallas, Texas

Nelson Tang, MD, FACEP
Assistant Professor
Department of Emergency Medicine
The Johns Hopkins University
Director, Division of Special Operations
Johns Hopkins Medical Institution
Baltimore, Maryland

Paul J. Vecchio, BS, US Army Special Forces (retired)
Administrative Services Director
Center of Operational Medicine
Department of Emergency Medicine
Medical College of Georgia
Augusta, Georgia

Ian S. Wedmore, MD
Adjunct Assistant Professor
USUHS
Bethesda, Maryland
Emergency Medicine Consultant to the US Army Surgeon General
Madigan Army Medical Center
Tacoma, Washington

Eric S. Weinstein, MD
Department of Surgery
Section of Emergency Medicine
Yale University School of Medicine
New Haven, Connecticut
SC-1 DMAT
Summerville, South Carolina

Col. John M. Wightman, EMT-T/P, MD
Director, Critical Care Air Transport Teams
88th Medical Operations Squadron
Wright-Patterson Air Force Base, Ohio

Capt Annette Williams, MD
Faculty Emergency Medicine
San Antonio Uniformed Services Health Education Consortium

Justin B. Williams, MD
Assistant Professor
Staff Physician
Department of Emergency Medicine
San Antonio Uniformed Services Health Education Consortium

Scott E. Young, DO
Staff Physician
Department of Emergency Medicine
Darnall Army Medical Center
Fort Hood, Texas

Bradley N. Younggren, MD
Clinical Instructor
Internal Medicine
Division of Emergency Medicine
University of Washington
Seattle, Washington
Assistant Program Director
Department of Emergency Medicine
Madigan Army Medical Center
Fort Lewis, Washington

FOREWORD

During the last three decades, the concept of medical support for law enforcement special operations was born out of necessity, matured through the knowledge and experience of many civilian and military medical and tactical operators, and adopted nationally by most tactical teams and their agencies. It should be emphasized that tactical emergency medical support (TEMS), just like our emergency medical and trauma care systems, owes much of its inception and success to our military special operations experience, especially during war.

TEMS formally began in 1989 when then Lt. (Dr.) David Rasumoff* of the Los Angeles County Sheriff's Department (LASD) Emergency Services Detail (ESD) and Deputy Sheriff (Dr.) Richard Carmona of the Pima County, Arizona Sheriff's Department SWAT Team moderated the first formal law enforcement special operations (SWAT) medical support course.

Carmona, a former U.S. Army Special Forces medic and weapons specialist and a Deputy Sheriff and SWAT team leader, and Rasumoff, a long-time medical officer with LASD ESD, had become friends through the tactical community and had informally shared tactical and medical information over the years. This friendship and their perceived need to formalize and share their respective practices and experiences is what led to the first course and eventually the TEMS Program.

This first offering of a formal course attempting to define the role of medical support within law enforcement special operations was held in Los Angeles in 1989, was sponsored by the National Tactical Officers Association (NTOA), and would not have been possible without the leadership of Captain. (Ret.) John Kolman, a SWAT icon and the founder of the NTOA. This first course was well attended by military and police special operators and medics from across the country. The course and its participants began to lay the foundation for this newly emerging area of law enforcement special operations.

The first course offering was very successful and the demand for a second course was evident. The NTOA agreed to sponsor the second annual course and it was held in 1990 in Tucson, Arizona and cosponsored by the Pima County

Sheriff's Department. The attendance doubled, and it was clear that there was an unmet need in the tactical community. During this conference, Carmona and Rasumoff met Josh Vayer who was, then developing the Counter Narcotics Tactical Operations Medical Support Course, (CONTOMS). Vayer explained that the Uniformed Services University of the Health Sciences (USUHS), was developing the CONTOMS course to medically support law enforcement tactical operations and the course content Carmona and Rasumoff had developed could be complementary to CONTOMS material. Vayer offered Carmona and Rasumoff an opportunity to join the CONTOMS faculty and teach with them. Rasumoff and Carmona had been doing their courses on a "shoestring" budget and CONTOMS was federally funded, so this was an easy decision. Carmona and Rasumoff contributed their slides and teaching materials to CONTOMS and began teaching the CONTOMS 5-day course while developing and teaching a 2-day NTOA TEMS course.

In 1990, John Kolman invited Carmona and Rasumoff to begin writing a regular TEMS column in *The Tactical Edge*, the journal of the NTOA. This column was named "Inside the Perimeter," and continues today. It should be noted that the term *TEMS* was first developed and used by Carmona in one of the early articles published in 1990 in *The Tactical Edge*.

Another irony here is that the ideas and information that laid the foundation for TEMS by Carmona and Rasumoff were really not new ideas but rather adaptation and modification of military special operations medical support. And in an interesting twist of fate, Carmona had learned that Vayer's commander at USUHS was Col. (Ret.) Craig Llewelyn, an iconic Special Forces surgeon who had trained Carmona and many others as Special Forces medics many years earlier! As we traversed the 1980's and 1990's and entered the new millennium, the field of TEMS grew, attracted new talent, and began to more clearly define standards of practice. During this time in the 1990s, the International TEMS Association began and many other individuals and organizations, such as H&K, began to offer TEMS training. Today, TEMS is a standard of care for special operations teams in the United States as well as some foreign nations. TEMS remains a dynamic, ever-evolving medical area. As new science and practice develops and as new threats and challenges face our special operations teams, TEMS is continually modified and reintegrated to serve the best interests of our citizens and operators.

---

*Deceased

This textbook, *Tactical Emergency Medicine*, whose contributors are composed of medical operators with both military and civilian law enforcement training and experience, synthesizes the needed multi-disciplinary knowledge of TEMS, from prevention to care.

Depending on the environment in which the medical operator practices TEMS, the rules of engagement will be different, but the basic philosophy and approach, whether military or civilian, of keeping your team healthy, preventing illness and injury, and treating the injured, will be the same.

This textbook provides a wealth of diverse cumulative TEMS-related information and may serve as reference for all TEMS providers.

Richard Carmona, MD, MPH, FACS
17th Surgeon General of the United States

Tactical Concepts

Section Editor: BRET T. ACKERMAN

Chapter 1

Team Composition and Basic Capabilities and Equipment

Alexander L. Eastman, Navin K. Sharma and Kermit D. Huebner

OBJECTIVES

After reading this section, the reader will be able to:

1. Understand the various structures of functioning tactical emergency medical support (TEMS) units.
2. Discuss the capabilities of TEMS providers and the advantages and disadvantages of the use of various medical providers in the support of TEMS operations.
3. Understand the controversies over arming TEMS providers.

Tactical Emergency Medical Support (TEMS) unit compositions vary across the country according to a number of factors. These include the different laws and codes of the respective jurisdiction, available resources, and command structure preference to name a few. Types of unit compositions currently in existence in the United States within law enforcement agencies are as follows:

1. Internal
   a. Law enforcement (LE)-based TEMS units
2. External
   a. Fire-based TEMS units
   b. Private emergency medical services (EMS)-based units
   c. Hospital-based units

INTERNAL UNITS

Internal Law Enforcement-based TEMS

This model is comprised of full-time law enforcement officers (LEOs) with formalized medical training. The medical certification of these individuals runs from emergency medical technician (EMT)-basic to licensed physicians depending on the jurisdiction, the "LEO-medics" agency involved, and the needs of the tactical team.

Washington state's first advanced life support (ALS) level LEO-based regional TEMS unit instituted by the Vancouver, Washington police department is one such example (1). The unit officially called the South West Washington Regional TEMS Unit attached to the regional SWAT team is comprised primarily of full-time commissioned police officers with collateral TEMS duties. This unit recently expanded its scope of practice to include other high-risk specialty police units, such as the Civil Disturbance Unit (riot squad) and the Explosive Ordinance Disposal Unit (bomb squad). Additionally, members of this unit are utilized by the police department during recruitment physical agility tests; they also conduct department-wide emergency medical aid in-services.

EXTERNAL UNITS

Fire-based TEMS

This model comprises EMS providers in systems where the EMS system is fire-based. Again, the level of provider in this system can vary from EMT-basic to EMT-paramedic. On some teams, tactical medics go through formal police academy training becoming certified peace officers and in others, these medics are provided tactical training, but not to the level of peace officer certification. Either way, familiarity with SWAT operations, tactics, and the wide array of equipment and weapons are essential.

Issues, advantages, and disadvantages related to fire-based TEMS teams are discussed in further detail subsequently.

Private or Third-service EMS-based TEMS

Some EMS systems are so-called "third systems" (i.e., they are governmental systems, but not fire- or police-based, and some are a private entities). In these jurisdictions, TEMS providers are composed of EMS personnel who work primarily for this third service provider. This is common in many Canadian units, and also is modeled well by the Austin, Texas, tactical medics. The primary function of members of these organizations remains the provision of civilian EMS care, but a select group is trained further in tactical EMS.

Hospital-based TEMS

This model is increasing in popularity primarily among many academic based institutions. In this model, many of the TEMS providers are physicians. Often the TEMS support will include resident physicians in training who will later be medical program director's (MPDs) for TEMS units. This model will also incorporate other medical providers.

ISSUES RELATED TO TEMS COMPOSITIONS

Law Enforcement Status

There are two distinct issues that should be considered in the composition of the TEMS element: What, if any, law en-

forcement status should unit members have and what level of medical provider is best? There are successful TEMS programs across the United States with diverse compositions. What works best in one location may not work well in another location. Each choice must be considered in a cost-benefit analysis specific to that jurisdiction.

Some teams require all of their TEMS providers to be fully sworn officers who are qualified first as tactical team members and second as medics. This approach has several benefits: (i) having a team member as the TEMS provider instills confidence in other team members and meets operational security requirements; (ii) the medic can provide his/her own security when not caring for a patient; and (iii) the medic has arrest and custodial authority, which can be very useful when caring for a prisoner. On the other hand, medical support of the team then becomes a collateral duty; continuing education and skills maintenance in both the tactical and medical arenas may become burdensome and the available manpower for this type of assignment is usually very limited. "Role confusion" (defined as individuals not knowing if they are functioning as a medic or an operator) is often cited as a disadvantage of this model. This theoretical concern appears to be perpetuated by anecdote, but has not been documented in the literature and ignores the reality that TEMS must consider both the medical and tactical situation and the medical situation together. All of these problems can be overcome in individual circumstances with adequate training and command leadership. Despite the apparent advantages of an internal system, the majority of TEMS teams in the United States remain external systems (2).

Many teams have opted to utilize fire/rescue/EMS personnel as TEMS providers. The advantage of this is that the medical support of the team is their primary function, and they are not distracted by other duties. Generally, tactical team members will have greater confidence in their medical skills compared to classroom-trained EMTs who are police officers first and have limited practical patient care experience. Continuing education and skills maintenance are also easier to achieve. It also seems that the manning for this kind of assignment is more readily available. However, in most situations, these providers have no arrest powers and will require an officer in attendance if they are treating a prisoner. In most situations, they also require the team to provide for their security at all times and represent an operational security risk if careful screening and background investigations are not accomplished before making them part of the unit. Their relative lack of tactical skills can be remedied with rigorous training and most team commanders consider it easier to train a medic in tactics than to train a tactical officer in medicine.

A few tactical teams continue to rely on "standby" coverage of their operations by conventional fire/rescue/EMS. Although this is probably the easiest type of coverage to accomplish, it delays the delivery of care to the patient and is a grossly inadequate model for addressing tactical operational medical support. TEMS is much more than EMS in a less permissive environment. It encompasses a special set of decision-making skills, clinical knowledge, and the integration of operational and medical processes. As inferred earlier from military data, the opportunities for successful intervention in the management of casualties are greatest in the first few minutes after wounding. Any plan that delays arrival of the medical provider at the patient's side, such as having conventional EMS on standby, will have a deleterious effect on the outcome and should be avoided whenever possible.

Law enforcement status is one important factor to consider when designing your TEMS system. Although having providers with arrest powers is beneficial, it is not essential. Many outstanding programs are running in the United States today—some use sworn officers as medics and some do not. The confidence team members have in their medical providers is probably related more to a positive experience working together over time than to any other factor. Regardless of which configuration you select as the best fit for your program, it is important to remember the "one person—one job rule." On any given mission, a single individual tasked with the duties of more than one position (e.g., medic and point man) will perform neither as well as if he had only one job. This does not preclude team members from cross-training for a variety of roles. In fact, cross-training for multiple functions is one hallmark of a military special operations medic, but the scope of an individual's responsibility on a specific operation should be limited to that which can be successfully accomplished by a single individual.

Medical Provider Skill Level

The medical qualifications of TEMS unit members can vary from EMT-basic to physician, and arguments can be made for each level. Again, each choice must be considered in a cost-benefit analysis specific to the individual jurisdiction. Members with basic EMT training have the requisite familiarity with the prehospital environment and often work closely with law enforcement personnel on a daily basis. They are readily available at a modest cost, can maintain their skills and certifications with minimal clinical opportunities, and have adequate skills to provide lifesaving interventions during care under fire (basic airway maintenance, hemorrhage control, and rapid extraction). The down side is their limited scope of practice, their inability to initiate advanced interventions, their requirement for medical control, and their limited ability to liaison with the medical community.

Paramedics, likewise, have the necessary field training and familiarity with the prehospital environment. They have an appropriate range of skills for the TEMS setting and are generally available in most communities at rea-

sonable cost. Like EMTs, paramedics require medical control and, therefore, their independent decision-making on the scene of a tactical incident, where communications may be problematic due to tactical circumstances, is limited. They also require clinical opportunities to maintain skills and certification and continuing medical education begins to compete with operational training at this level, although proficiency in both skill sets is achievable in a well-managed program. Although registered nurses may possibly have a broader scope of practice than paramedics and are likely to do a good job as a liaison with the hospital community, most lack experience in prehospital care. They also require medical control and are more costly than paramedics. Historically, nurses have not been heavily involved in TEMS.

Increasingly, physicians have become active TEMS responders, in addition to serving as TEMS medical directors. Several emergency medicine residency programs offer training in TEMS to their residents. These residents often go on and function as MPDs for TEMS units after graduation. They present the advantages of a broad scope of practice, as well as the status to function most effectively as a liaison with the local medical community. They obviously do not require medical control and can independently provide a full range of skills and interventions on the scene. However, most physicians have limited experience in prehospital care. They are the most costly provider to retain and may have limited availability for no-notice emergency response due to their clinical commitments. Furthermore, many physicians are unaccustomed to functioning in a support role where there may be more important priorities than the delivery of medicine.

Armed versus Unarmed Tactical Medics

This is probably the most controversial issue in TEMS. However, this issue should not derail the planning/formation of your tactical medical team. There are excellent programs that arm their medics and excellent programs that do not. Obviously, those programs that utilize sworn officers as their medics do not face this controversy.

The primary argument for arming medics is that TEMS providers should not be placed in circumstances where they cannot protect themselves or their patients. The military routinely arms its medics, and they have a duty to defend their patients, even though they are noncombatants. Medics who are able to provide basic self-protection will be able to move more independently within the crisis site at the incident commander's discretion. If the TEMS provider must be "protected" by other team members, the team's capability may be degraded. The armed tactical medic can function with the team in the hot zone as an effective team member who serves as the commander's expert in medical matters. Legal authority and proper training to carry a firearm may also provide a limited amount of off-duty protection for the TEMS operator. Perpetrators rarely take the time or interest to distinguish between tactical officers and medics. To them, everyone represents authority and several cases of coincidental encounters and stalking of tactical medics have occurred. Although personal protection is only one small piece of the countermeasures to this risk, it is generally more practical if arming authority exists. According to a 1999 survey by Smock, et al., 67% of tactical physicians are armed when working with the tactical team.

Armed TEMS providers must have statutory authority to carry a firearm and should be trained and tested to the same standard as the law enforcement officers they support. Training should address the applicable use of force policies, defensive tactics, fire control practices, and weapons retention skills. In fact, providers should train to an additional standard in weapons retention, because this type of patient care is likely to place them in positions of vulnerability that they may not routinely face. Additionally, armed providers must train with the tactical team on a regular basis to build the trust and confidence of the team. The 1999 Smock survey of tactical physicians indicated each physician spent an average of 78 hours per year training with the tactical team. Without the commitment to regular and intensive training, the armed TEMS program faces great difficulties.

Arguments against arming TEMS providers include the possibility that this may create "role confusion" and that the TEMS provider will be more concerned with tactical objectives rather than the medical care of casualties. As stated earlier, this is not a strong argument as the TEMS provider must consider the tactical situation along with the medical situation. However, a single TEMS provider cannot provide his own security in the warm zone while caring for a patient. He will still be relying on the team to establish a safe perimeter within which he can work. Tactical medicine should never be confused as a back door route to tactical team membership and personnel who are motivated by this objective should be identified and excluded from the tactical medical unit.

Although unarmed medics may not be able to defend themselves or their patients as well, and may become an operational liability during high threat circumstances, they have several advantages. There is no need for increased training; no potential threat to fire control and team liability may be lessened. Perhaps most important, the arming issue is a political "red flag" that may attract controversy that will not be weathered well by a start-up program. TEMS program proponents must weigh the costs and benefits of even raising this issue early in the program's development and make a decision to proceed in the context of their particular circumstances.

TEMS units have identified a number of mechanisms for arming providers. The most obvious method is to utilize medics who are also sworn officers. This system functions well and allows the provider full law enforcement authority, although the level of medical skill tends to be more basic than that provided by other programs. Many jurisdictions have reserve or auxiliary sheriff/police officer programs that provide the opportunity for part-time status as a fully sworn officer. Alternatively, the laws of some jurisdictions permit every citizen to carry a weapon if the appropriate licenses or permits are obtained. TEMS elements planning to use this approach should ensure that their members' training and testing exceeds that required of citizens and meets the same standard as the officers they support. However, it should be noted that the statutory authority permitting citizens to carry firearms does not confer law enforcement authority and training for medics armed via this mechanism should reflect this difference. For example, where a sworn officer has a duty to affect a legal arrest and may use reasonable force in doing so, the citizen does not have the same duty and use of force may be restricted to self-defense. In a few locales, the senior law enforcement officer has the legal authority to grant permission for any individual to carry a firearm. Although this may cover the statutory requirement, it does not address the training requirement and should not be used as a mechanism for arming tactical medical personnel without a comprehensive training standard.

Many smaller tactical teams do not have the support or the resources to train and maintain the firearms qualifications of TEMS providers. It is simpler and more practical to have TEMS providers function in the cold zone and only enter the warm or hot zones under the protection of the tactical team. Both the armed and unarmed approaches have advantages and disadvantages, and the individual team must make their own decision based on their state laws, mission, and team composition.

TEMS UNIT CAPABILITIES

The capability of a TEMS unit depends on its composition and structure. As mentioned previously, the capability will vary based upon if the team is an internal or external team and the resources available. The following is a generalized list of capabilities that should be considered for and effective TEMS team:

1. Formulating medical threat assessments (MTAs) prior to mission for SWAT (and other high-risk unit) commanders and team leaders.
2. Serving as a medical safety officer for the tactical team during training and call outs.
3. Providing "care under fire" within inner and outer perimeter areas of mission.
4. Providing medical intelligence to the command post during active tactical negotiations (i.e., "medicine across the barricade").
5. Briefing SWAT (and other high-risk unit) commanders and team leaders on medical evacuation plans.

6. Coordinating medical evacuation procedures with local EMS and air medical evacuation units.
7. Providing "buddy-aid" medical emergency survival training to tactical team members.
8. Completing after action reports. In case of casualties, a written medical report should be completed and turned in to the MPD.
9. Proactive monitoring of tactical personnel by conducting bi-annual pre- and poststress vital sign checks, including annual 12-lead electrocardiograms (EKGs).
10. Maintaining current emergency data cards on all tactical personnel.
11. Maintaining an emergency supply of prescriptive medications used by tactical members.
12. Being readily accessible to tactical members and their immediately families for medical advice.

EQUIPMENT

Equipment setup to support TEMS operations is situation and deployment specific. Unlike in the civilian EMS world where large quantities of a wide variety of gear are carried and readily available, in the TEMS world one has to be more conservative due to space limitations and operational issues. However, having said that, efficient TEMS systems should have full ALS level equipment at their disposal as situations demand.

For example, a mission to a remote rural target would require more self-sustaining ALS equipment needs versus an urban assault where civilian EMS is readily available as a "staged" asset.

Many versatile setups exist amongst various TEMS Units. Mission tested and proven equipment setups by some agencies are described here:

1. Individual first-aid kit (IFAK). This is a first aid kit that every operator should carry in a standardized location. It should contain basic airway equipment (nasopharyngeal airway), hemorrhage control equipment (tourniquet, hemostatic agent (Hemcon), dressings), chest seal's, and other equipment as directed by state law and MPD.
2. TEMS vest for rapid deployment or tactical leg bag (entry bag). This is typically worn over the provider's ballistic protection as displayed in the subsequent photograph by members on the Vancouver police department's TEMS unit. Contents are limited to hemorrhage control devices, one 500 cc Normasol IV set up, chest decompression equipment, and rapid airway management equipment. Additionally, an over-the-shoulder rapid extraction device is carried by each element within the TEMS unit. This type of setup allows the provider to operate with maximum agility and rapidly treat life threatening trauma, while still affording level-IIIA ballister protection. Although the use of

a vest allows for easy availability of equipment, some TEMS operators feel that the vest can be bulky and difficult to utilize. The use of a tactical leg bag is a very acceptable alternative, and there are many good products on the market.
3. Medic aid bag. Additionally each medic should have an aid bag that is packed specifically with the provider's medical skill level in mind. This is often not brought into the hot zone during the initial assault, but is immediately available in the event there are casualties and can be brought forward.
4. Other specialty equipment:
    a. High-threat extraction equipment should be considered. The ability to rapidly extract a casualty from a high-threat environment may make the difference between life and death. The use of "drag lines" is highly encouraged. Many of these products are commercially available from companies such as North American Rescue Products.
    b. Remote ALS bag. TEMS units respond to missions in remote areas where little or no civilian backup exists. Additionally, there have been situations where even though civilian EMS was readily available, access to them was precluded by the situation at hand.

A case-in-point was during a 1999 standoff with an armed subject in an urban high-density residential area. Although most neighbors were evacuated, an elderly couple with significant medical history (recent cardiac bypass, brittle diabetic, chronic obstructive pulmonary disease, congestive heart failure, both on home oxygen, and wheel chair bound) had to shelter in place. Should they have needed emergent medical attention due to a precipitating cardiac or respiratory event, the staged fire and EMS units could not have responded. The Vancouver police department TEMS was the closest, and only, available medical asset that could respond. This situation necessitated the availability of rapid ALS- and advanced cardiac life support (ACLS)-level care to the couple without jeopardizing civilian EMS personnel. The Vancouver police department TEMS filled that gap and accomplished the mission.

Several such situations have occurred nationwide, thereby prompting TEMS programs to incorporate ALS/ACLS-level care among its ranks and rethink some of the more traditional TEMS training and equipment needs. The incorporation of oxygen cylinders into these packs needs considered with regard to the potential risks and benefits (Figs. 1.1 and 1.2). Although the oxygen may play a vital role, it presents an explosive risk if struck by a high-velocity projectile. For this reason, oxygen should be kept in the cold zone and not be brought forward unless necessary or the situation allows.

Example stocking of a remote ALS pack:

■ Advanced airway kit
■ Controlled drug box (secure)

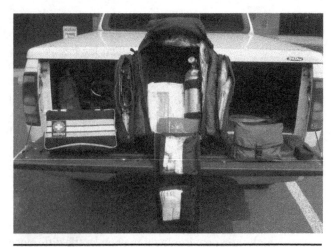

FIGURE 1.1. An example of a rapidly deployable, self-contained, remote ALS pack.

- Automatic external defibrillator (AED) with cardiac monitor screen
- IV start kits (two 1,000 cc setups)
- ACLS drug kit
- ALS drug kit (non-ACLS)
- Over-the-counter medicine kit

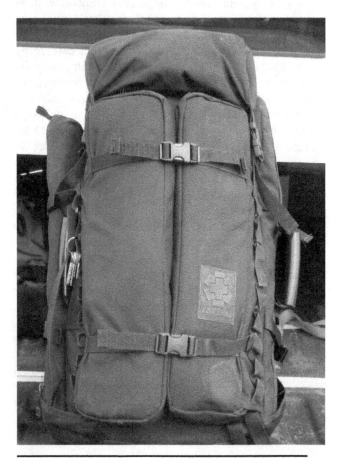

FIGURE 1.2. Example of a TEMS remote ALS rescue pack.

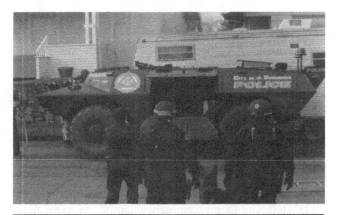

FIGURE 1.3. Vancouver, Washington Police Officer-Tactical Medics and K9 ready to load out on the V-150 for a SWAT mission.

- Major trauma kit
- Minor trauma kit
- Emergency obstetrics kit
- Extraction litter
- Basic life support (BLS) kit
- Glaucometer
- Pulse oximeter
- C-collar
- Sharps container
- Global positioning system (GPS)

   c. SWAT-TEMS rescue rig.

Many armored "rescue" vehicles exist with various teams. However, most are tactically designed units to support SWAT operations rather than a TEMS-specific mission and do not provide for an optimum medical treatment platform. Figure 1.3 illustrates one such vehicle, the "V-150," which is ballistically protected to stop 0.223 caliber rifle rounds that the Vancouver TEMS unit has access to.

Another option that is available in many jurisdictions is the acquisition of surplus military ambulances that can be retrofitted and designed to better serve as a medical treatment platform. This type of unit can respond with other SWAT hardware to the SWAT command post and stay there as a resource for the TEMS officers in the hot zone or inside the perimeter. This type of vehicle becomes extremely valuable in remote or rural missions where conventional EMS backup is not readily available or in urban situations, which would preclude non-LE personnel from entering. The drawback to such a setup is the obvious lack of external armor; therefore, internal adaptations are necessary. Covering the main oxygen tank with ballistic protection and the use of ballistic panels on the inside of the box are some examples and can be achieved relatively inexpensively.

   d. Sick call kit (suture supplies, medical prescriptions, etc.).

Units that have TEMS physicians or mid-level practitioners should have a "physician-specific" kit. This comes in handy when operating in environments where access to definitive care is significantly delayed. Medical supplies to support minor illness should be included in this kit. Access to such specialized kits that may contain sterile suture kits, controlled substances, and prescriptive instruments, for example, must be easy and stored with appropriate security if they are to be secured outside the direct control of the physician (e.g., in the SWAT command van or the TEMS rescue rig).

e. Medivac rescue kit.

Agencies that operate in remote sites should strongly consider making a pack with the following items:

1. Handheld GPS.
2. Smoke grenades for daytime landing zone (LZ) ops.
3. Flares for nighttime LZ ops.
4. High-energy food bars and hydration supplies.
5. Spare batteries for cell phones, chargers, etc.
6. Emergency space blankets.

SPECIAL CONSIDERATIONS

TEMS and Trauma

Some in tactical EMS are of the belief that TEMS units should equip (and train) themselves primarily for trauma. Furthermore, this perception is also harbored by some in civilian EMS and the fire service, thereby limiting the development of TEMS units to their fullest potential in some jurisdictions. Experience has shown that units must be prepared for more than just trauma. The TEMS provider must be trained to manage a broad spectrum of conditions and not just trauma.

TEMS Primarily Treats Adults

TEMS units typically train with SWAT teams on a multitude of "officer-down" scenarios. This type of specialized training is what gives the TEMS provider the ability and the edge to operate inside the perimeter. Although this may usually be the norm, all it takes is one situation involving this special population of infants, children, pregnant women, and the elderly who are placed in harms way to result in a bad outcome for the TEMS providers and the agency they represent. This is a common "lesson learned"

from operations, but is often not considered in the MTA for a mission.

The Need for Advanced Electronics

Another commonly debated issue is that of advanced electronic monitoring devices. Some believe the TEMS theater has little or no place for cardiac monitors, pulse oximeters, and portable 12-lead machines, such as the Life Pack 12 and glucometers.

However, others who have had firsthand experiences in major incidents, such as the WTO riots in Seattle, remote site operations, and long standoff urban assaults where conventional EMS can not be accessed believe otherwise. Whatever the case, the ultimate decision to include such equipment as readily available inventory on a mission will depend upon the TEMS unit's defined mission goals and objectives.

An example of the later is the Vancouver (WA) police TEMS unit. Mission experience has driven this unit to become a self-sustained ALS Unit. Having their TEMS rescue unit as their "medical treatment platform and supply base" on all missions, affords the unit the ability to readily access specific ALS gear as needed. This strategy mirrors that of SWAT, the bomb squad, and the CDT units where they bring along their respective "resource vehicles" to mission command posts.

In summary, unlike military operations, LE operations have to contend with treating citizens and suspects. Often these are nontraumatic cases. LE units will encounter the presence of infants and children at, or close to, target locations. Pregnant women at target locations have posed unexpected challenges. Fragile elderly are being seen with increasing frequency inside many target locations. The complicating factor is that in many such cases the threat assessment and intelligence provide no forewarning of the presence of this population segment within the targets.

Experience has hence shown that maintaining a rapidly deployable pediatric/obstetric kit is not unrealistic and is actually prudent to include. A rapidly deployable full ALS treatment kit with ACLS pharmacy should be given strong consideration.

REFERENCES

1. Sharma NK. Vancouver police deploy SWAT-tactical EMS. *The Tactical Edge.* 2000;18:35–38.
2. Carmona RH. The history and evolution of tactical emergency medical support and its impact on public safety. *Top Emerg Med.* 2003;25: 277–281.

Military Tactical Operations

Andre M. Pennardt

OBJECTIVES

After reading this section, the reader will be able to:
1. Describe tactical movement techniques for small and large elements.
2. Discuss the differences between civilian and military tactical movements.
3. Describe movement techniques while "under fire."
4. Discuss offensive and defensive postures.

TACTICAL MOVEMENT

Compared to civilian tactical team movement, military tactical movement may frequently involve greater distances, greater variation in the type of terrain traveled, and larger numbers of personnel. In addition, whereas civilian tactical movements typically are conducted in proximity to a known hostile force, military tactical movements may include travel in areas where enemy contact is not expected. Fire teams and squads are rough military equivalents for small civilian tactical teams; platoons and companies are progressively larger groups. Combat casualty care is generally provided by medics at platoon and company levels, whereas self- or buddy aid, combat lifesavers, or other first responders are the means of initial treatment at team and squad levels. Casualties are transported from small elements to collection points established by larger units (e.g., platoon or company) when mission requirements permit to facilitate casualty stabilization and monitoring by medics and preparation for evacuation. Compared to civilian operations, the time to definitive treatment and evacuation during military operations is usually longer due to the latter's focus on mission completion as the highest priority and greater distances involved.

In order to achieve protection from hostile fire when moving, routes are selected that place cover between soldiers and the areas where the enemy is known or suspected to be. The use of terrain features, such as ravines, gullies, hills, wooded areas, and walls, reduces the risk of the enemy seeing the troops and directing effective fire against them. Open areas and hilltops or ridges, which may silhouette soldiers against the sky, must be avoided whenever possible. During movement soldiers must be able to see their fire team leader. The squad leader must be able

to see his fire team leaders. The platoon leader should be able to see his lead fire team leader.

INDIVIDUAL MOVEMENT UNDER FIRE

Individual soldiers typically use one of three movement techniques when receiving enemy fire or while under enemy observation: the low crawl, the high crawl, and the rush. The low crawl provides the lowest silhouette and is used to cross terrain where the concealment is very low and enemy fire or observation prevents the soldier from getting up. It is the slowest of the three individual movement techniques. The body is kept flat against the ground during the low crawl. The weapon is grasped at the upper sling-swivel with the firing hand, while the front hand guard rests on the forearm keeping the muzzle off the ground and the weapon butt drags on the ground. In order to move, the arms are pushed forward and the firing side leg is pulled forward. The soldier then pulls himself forward with his arms while pushing with the other leg. This sequence is repeated until the danger area is completely crossed.

The high crawl permits faster movement than the low crawl while still providing a low silhouette. This technique is used when there is good concealment, but enemy fire or observation prevents the soldier from getting up. The body is kept off the ground and rests on the forearms and lower legs. The weapon is cradled in the arms keeping the muzzle off the ground. The knees are kept well behind the buttocks to ensure that the body stays low. The soldier alternately advances his right elbow and left knee, followed by the left elbow and right knee, in order to move forward.

The rush is the fastest way to move from one position to another and should last from 3 to 5 seconds. While the rushes must be kept short to keep enemy personnel from tracking the soldier, he must not stop and hit the ground in the open simply because 5 seconds have elapsed. The goal of each rush is to move to the next covered and concealed position via the best route. The soldier slowly raises his head and picks the next position and route and then slowly lowers his head again. He draws the arms into the body keeping the elbows in, pulls his right leg forward, raises the body by straightening the arms, and then gets up quickly and runs to the next position. At the conclusion of the rush the soldier plants both his feet, drops to his knees while at the same time sliding a hand to the weapon butt, drops forward breaking the fall with the butt, and goes to a prone firing position. If a soldier has been firing from one position for some time, the enemy may have spotted him and may be awaiting his coming up from behind cover. By rolling or crawling a short distance from his position before beginning a rush, the soldier may be able to fool an enemy who is aiming at the original location and waiting for him to rise.

SMALL TEAM MOVEMENT

Fire teams use the wedge as the basic formation when moving (Fig. 2.1). The wedge provides easy control of team members, good flexibility and security, and allows immediate fires in all directions. Although the interval between soldiers in the wedge formation is normally 10 meters, the wedge can expand or contract depending on terrain, visibility, and other factors. When rough terrain or poor visibility make control of the wedge difficult, the normal interval is reduced so that all team members can still see their leader and team leaders can still see their squad leader. As control becomes easier, the wedge expands again to improve security. Severely restrictive terrain results in contraction of the edges of the wedge to the point of forming the single file formation (Fig. 2.2). The file provides easier control than the wedge, but is less flexible and secure. Although the file allows immediate fires to the flanks, it masks most fires to the rear.

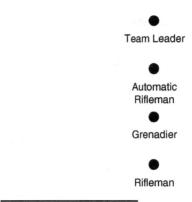

FIGURE 2.2. Fire team file.

Squads utilize three standard formations for movement: column, line, and file. The squad column is the most common squad formation (Fig. 2.3). The column provides good dispersion laterally and in depth, while simultaneously maintaining control and maneuver capability. The lead fire team is the base fire team allowing the trail fire team to act as a maneuver element to flank the enemy upon contact. The rifleman in the trail fire team provides rear security when the squad moves independently or as the rear element of a platoon.

The squad line is designed to provide maximum firepower to the front (Fig. 2.4). This formation provides limited maneuver capability, because both fire teams are committed. It is more difficult to control than the column and provides little security to the flanks and rear. The characteristics of the squad file are the same as that of fire team file, except for the difference in size. The squad file is similarly

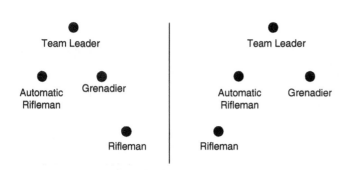

FIGURE 2.1. Fire team wedge.

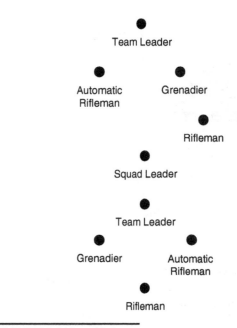

FIGURE 2.3. Squad column.

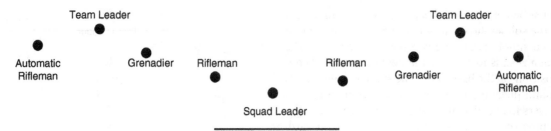

FIGURE 2.4. Squad line.

used when restrictive terrain prevents a more dispersed or expanded formation. Control can be increased by placing the squad leader at the front of the squad file and a team leader at the rear of the formation.

There are three movement techniques that may be used by squads: traveling, traveling overwatch, and bounding overwatch. Leaders decide which technique to use based on the likelihood of enemy contact and the need for speed. Movement techniques are not fixed formations, but rather refer to the distances between soldiers, teams, and squads that vary based on mission, enemy, terrain, visibility, and any other factors affecting control. Each technique is associated with different ease of control, personnel dispersion, speed of movement, and relative security, and can be used with any formation.

Traveling is utilized when enemy contact is not likely. It offers the greatest speed, but the least security, especially forward. During traveling the distance between

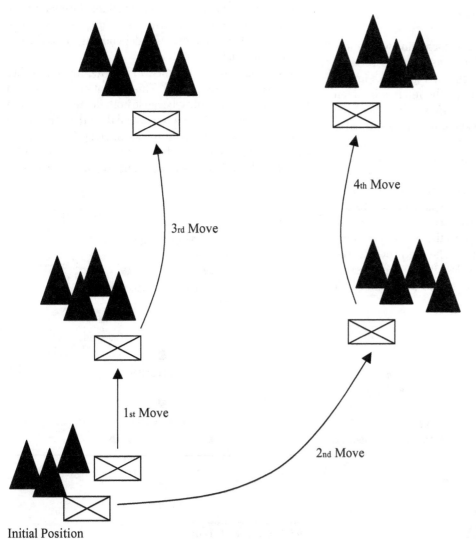

FIGURE 2.5. Squad successive bounds.

individual soldiers would typically be 10 meters and 20 meters between fire teams. Traveling overwatch is the basic squad movement technique and used when enemy contact is possible. It provides less control and slower speed, but more security, than traveling. Distances between individual soldiers increase to approximately 20 meters and 50 meters between fire teams. The lead fire team is far enough ahead to detect or engage the enemy before the opposing force can engage the remainder of the squad, but close enough to still be supported with small arms fire from the trail fire team.

Bounding overwatch is used when enemy contact is expected. While it provides the most control, dispersion, and security of the three movement techniques, it is also the slowest. Although the distance between individual soldiers remains roughly 20 meters, the distance between fire teams will vary with the terrain and other operational conditions. One fire team moves forward (bounds), while the other team overwatches from a position that can cover the route by fire. If the bounding team is engaged, the overwatch team provides supporting fires and movement. The length of a bound can vary with terrain, visibility, and required control, but must remain within the supporting range of the overwatch team. Teams can bound successively (Fig. 2.5) or alternately (Fig. 2.6). Successive bounds

provide more control, but alternate bounds can be executed faster. The alternate bounds method may be used when the overwatch team can observe the bounding team pass to its flank and advance to a new position. The team moves as a team if there is good cover; otherwise soldiers move individually or in pairs by short rushes from cover to cover or by crawling.

Prior to a bound, the leader is required to give the following information to his subordinates: direction of the enemy location if known, current and next positions of the overwatch element, route of the bounding element, actions to be taken at the completion of the bound, and the means of providing follow-on orders to the elements.

LARGE TEAM MOVEMENT

There are a variety of platoon formations including platoon column, line (with squads in line or in column), vee, wedge, and file. Each is associated with different characteristics of control, flexibility, fire capabilities and restrictions, and movement speed. As with small team formations, the leader chooses a platoon formation based on his analysis of the mission, enemy, terrain, troops, and time available (METT-T).

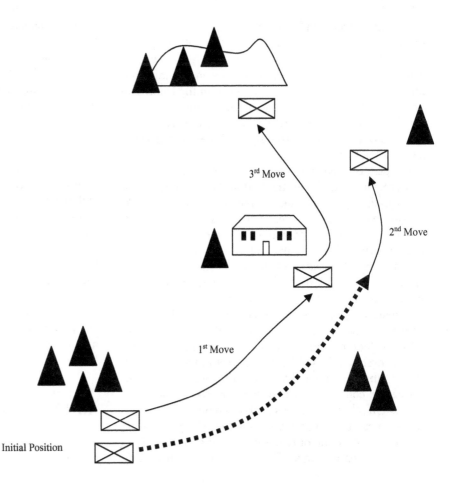

FIGURE 2.6. Squad alternating bounds.

The platoon column is the primary movement formation for the platoon. It provides good control for maneuver, speed, and dispersion laterally and in depth. It allows a high volume of fire to the flanks, but only limited firepower to the front and rear. The three squads normally found in a platoon are each arranged in column (Fig. 2.3) as lead, center, and trail squads. The lead squad is the base squad allowing the other elements to maneuver in the event of enemy contact. The platoon leader usually is located with the lead squad for maximum control and keeps any attached weapons elements and fire support officer near him to rapidly employ them upon contact. The platoon medic is typically located with the trail squad.

The platoon line with squads on line is a formation that allows the delivery of maximum fire to the front, but is difficult to control and slow to move. All elements are on line resulting in a larger version of the formation in Figure 2.4. Fire to the flanks and rear is very limited. The platoon line with squads in column consists of a left flank, center, and right flank squad; each squad is in column (Fig. 2.3). This formation may be used when the platoon leader does not want to deploy all personnel on line so that the squads can react to unexpected contact. Although this formation is easier to control and can move more rapidly than the platoon line with squads on line, it is harder to control and has less speed than the platoon column.

The platoon vee is characterized by two forward squads, one of which is on each flank. The third squad is in the rear where it can either overwatch or trail the other squads. This formation is difficult to control and relatively slow in movement. It may be used when the enemy information is vague, but contact is expected from the front. The vee allows an immediate heavy volume of fire to the front and flanks and provides the flexibility of the rear squad for maneuver. One of the front squads is designated as the platoon's base squad.

The platoon wedge is essentially the reverse of the platoon vee. One squad is in the lead and designated as the base squad, while a rear squad is positioned on each flank. The two rear squads can overwatch or trail the lead squad. Although still difficult to control and move, the platoon wedge provides better control and speed than the vee. This formation may be used when the enemy situation is vague and contact is not expected. If contact is made by the lead squad, the platoon leader has two squads available to maneuver against the enemy. The platoon wedge allows a heavy volume of fire to the front and flanks.

The platoon file has the same characteristics as the fire team and squad files (Fig. 2.2). This formation is used when visibility is poor due to terrain, vegetation, light, or weather conditions. The distance between soldiers is less than in other formations to allow communications by passing messages up and down the file. The platoon file may be set up in one of two ways. The first method is to have three separate squad files follow one another using

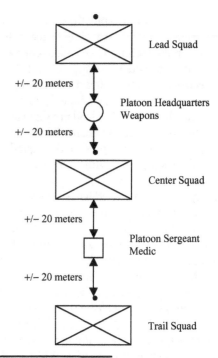

FIGURE 2.7. Platoon traveling

one of the movement techniques. The alternate method is to have a single platoon file with fire teams acting as security elements at the front (point team) and on each flank.

The platoon may use any of the three movement techniques used by the squad: traveling, traveling overwatch, and bounding overwatch. Traveling is again only used when enemy contact is unlikely and speed is necessary (Fig. 2.7). Traveling overwatch is utilized when contact is possible, but speed is still needed. The lead squad uses travel overwatch, while the trailing squads use traveling. The distance between the lead squad and platoon headquarters, shown in Figure 2.7, increases to between 50 and 100 meters.

Bounding overwatch is the movement technique of choice when enemy contact is expected. Either successive or alternate bounds may be conducted. One squad bounds to a chosen forward position and then becomes the overwatching element unless contact is made en route. Another squad overwatches the bounding squad from covered positions from which it can see and suppress likely enemy positions. The third squad remains uncommitted and ready for employment as directed by the platoon leader.

ACTIONS AT DANGER AREAS

Danger areas are any places on a route that are likely to expose a moving unit to enemy observation or fire, including open areas, roads, villages, and streams. Efforts should be made to avoid danger areas; if a unit must cross, it does so with great caution and as rapidly as possible. The decision on how the unit will cross is based on the time available, unit size, danger area size, and amount of security that can be posted. Small units may cross all at once, in buddy teams, or one individual at a time. Larger units typically cross one element at a time. Prior to crossing a danger area, near- and far-side rally points are designated. The near side is secured toward both flanks and the rear. The far side is then reconnoitered and secured, followed by crossing of the danger area by the remainder of the unit.

OFFENSIVE AND DEFENSIVE POSTURES

Offense

Military offensive operations include movement to contact, attacks, raids, reconnaissance and security operations, and ambushes. They differ in a number of aspects from civilian tactical operations: the location of the enemy may be unknown, objectives may be behind enemy lines, objectives may be larger and better defended including the extensive use of obstacles, such as wires and minefields, friendly forces are subject to counterattack even after an objective has been secured, and ambushes may be used to destroy moving enemy forces.

Movement to contact is usually conducted when a unit lacks detailed information about the enemy. The goal is to identify enemy strengths and weaknesses upon contact and then generate combat power rapidly to overwhelm the opposing force. The smallest element possible should make contact so as to prevent enemy detection of other elements until they are in the assault. Contact should be maintained once gained in order to prevent the enemy from breaking away and regaining the initiative.

Attacks are offensive action characterized by movement supported by fire and may be hasty or deliberate. Hasty attacks are conducted with immediately available forces in order to maintain offensive momentum or take advantage of a vulnerable enemy situation. Normally there is not sufficient time for extensive preparation. Deliberate attacks on the other hand are carefully planned and coordinated when the enemy has a well-organized defense or when hasty attacks are not possible or have already failed. Medical support is more difficult for hasty attacks, because there is insufficient time to develop extensive casualty care and evacuation plans.

Raids are operations involving rapid penetration of enemy territory to secure information, create enemy confusion, or destroy the opponent's installations and support systems. Upon completion of the specific mission, a raid ends with a planned withdrawal back to friendly territory.

Casualty evacuation is frequently not tactically feasible until the completion of the raid and occurs as part of the overall final withdrawal of the force. Ambushes are surprise attacks from concealed positions on moving or temporarily halted enemy elements. They incorporate some of the advantages and characteristics of the defense into offensive operations.

In preparing to assault an objective, the unit deploys into its assault formation allowing the placement of the bulk of its firepower to the front. This occurs as the unit moves through the assault position, which is normally the last covered and concealed position before reaching the objective. As movement occurs onto the objective itself, the assault force must increase the volume and accuracy of its fires. Fire teams are assigned specific targets to keep the enemy suppressed allowing the rest of the unit to maneuver. There is more emphasis on suppression and less on maneuver as the assault element gets closer to the enemy. The intent is to have at least one fire team break into the enemy position while everyone else continues to use suppressing fire. Soldiers use proper individual movement techniques and fire teams retain their basic shallow wedge formation throughout the assault; the unit as a whole does not move on line to sweep the objective. The unit must consolidate and reorganize quickly once enemy resistance has ceased on the objective in order to prepare against a potential counterattack.

Defense

The intent of military defensive operations is to retain the initiative by forcing the enemy to react and preventing him from executing his own plan. The defense is planned to detect the enemy first without being found, hinder the attacking force's freedom of movement through the use of obstacles and fires, identify or create a weakness in the enemy's plan, and then maneuver to exploit that weakness through a swift and violent counterattack. This is in contrast to defensive postures for civilian tactical operations, which are typically designed to contain a hostile force rather than fix and destroy an attacking enemy.

Defensive positions are classified as primary, alternate, or supplementary. Primary positions provide the best means to achieve assigned missions. Alternate positions allow coverage of the same sector of fire as the primary positions and are occupied when the latter become untenable or unsuitable for task completion. Supplementary positions allow completion of task that cannot be accomplished from primary or alternate positions, such as covering additional enemy avenues of approach and protecting the flanks and rear of the unit. All positions should take advantage of natural cover and concealment as well as be improved through additional camouflage. Every position should be observed and supported by the fires of at least two other positions. Sectors of fire are used to assign responsibility and ensure distribution of fires across the front; they should always overlap with adjacent sectors to prevent the creation of dead zones not covered by fires. Engagement areas are designed to concentrate all available fires into a zone where leaders intend to kill the enemy. Engagement priorities are established to ensure key enemy targets are eliminated first. Fire patterns are created to establish relationships between specific weapons and targets to prevent multiple fires on the same target, which wastes ammunition and allows other targets to remain unengaged.

Types of defensive postures include defense in sector, perimeter defense, and defense on a reverse slope. The defense in sector maximizes the combat abilities of infantry forces by allowing units to fight throughout the depth of an assigned sector using dispersed small unit tactics. The platoon leader typically assigns sectors to individual squads in order to maximize freedom of action for each element. Squads conduct detailed reconnaissance of their sectors to identify likely enemy avenues of approach and potential positions, choke points, and kill zones. The platoon leader confirms initial and successive positions and incorporates them into his concept of defense by designating the sequence in which they will be occupied. Positions are prepared and improved as time permits. When security elements warn of an approaching enemy, squads prepare to engage him from their primary positions. Ambushes are initiated as the enemy enters a choke point or kill zone. Squads move to their next positions prior to becoming decisively engaged to repeat the same process. The goal is to force the enemy to exhaust himself by reacting to numerous ambushes and then massing friendly forces at a decisive point to conduct a violent counterattack along previously rehearsed routes to complete the enemy's destruction. Effective evacuation is extremely difficult during the defense in sector, because the diversion of resources to remove casualties from the battlefield will disrupt the smooth succession of ambushes and disengagement to move to new positions.

The primary advantage of a perimeter defense is that it permits the unit to defend against an attack from any direction. The outline trace of the unit is circular or triangular rather than linear. Squads are positioned to reduce the size of unoccupied areas between them. Because the bulk of forces are on the perimeter with a centrally located reserve, the major disadvantage of this type of defense is that combat power is not concentrated initially against an enemy avenue of approach. Casualty collection points can be established centrally with follow-on evacuation away from the enemy avenue of approach.

A platoon can also choose to organize a defense on the reverse slope of a hill or ridge that is masked from direct enemy fire and observation. The lack of enemy observation increases freedom of movement in the position, makes incoming indirect fire less effective, and improves the likelihood of surprising the attacking force. The crest must be controlled through the use of fire by forward squads. An overwatch element may be placed on the forward slope of the next high ground to protect the flanks and rear of forward positions, reinforce their fires, and cover their withdrawal as long as such a position is within supporting distance. Because the lack of observation works both ways, observation points must be placed well forward of the crest to prevent the enemy from suddenly appearing at close range without sufficient warning. Other disadvantages of this type of defense include relatively short fields of fire, the inability to cover obstacles on the forward slope with direct fire, and the potential difficulty associated with withdrawing under pressure if the enemy gains the crest and assaults down the hill.

MISSION CONSIDERATIONS VERSUS MEDICAL CARE

Civilian tactical operations tend to place great emphasis on the safety of tactical personnel and innocent bystanders or victims, such as hostages. On the other hand, mission success for military tactical operations tends to be defined by achievement of key objectives, such as the capture of vital terrain, destruction of enemy facilities, or death or capture of important enemy personnel. Although both types of tactical operations naturally seek to minimize "friendly" casualties, military operations are more likely to be characterized by "acceptable" casualty rates as long as other objectives are achieved.

Medical personnel supporting military tactical operations must have a clear understanding of mission objectives and priorities. Although the immediate evacuation of serious casualties from the field to appropriate treatment facilities is always desirable from a medical perspective, this may not be feasible in the context of achieving overall mission success during a military operation. It is incumbent upon military commanders to anticipate casualties and develop planned courses of action in response to such events during each phase of an operation. For example, if an assault force sustains casualties during its infiltration to a target, a variety of courses of action are possible, each of which may affect the overall mission differently. Calling for and awaiting rotary wing evacuation may result in unacceptable time delays in reaching the target as well as reveal the location of the assault force to the enemy. Transporting casualties to the target may slow the movement of the assault force as well as delay definitive treatment possibly resulting in casualty death. Leaving the casualties behind with a medical provider and security element reduces the availability of medical support at the target itself and may reduce the number of assaulters below what is required for mission success.

Medical personnel must work closely with military commanders and planners to ensure that preparation for a mission includes the development of appropriate courses of action in response to the number and severity of casualties for each phase of an operation. In addition, they must be prepared to provide an accurate and rapid situational assessment of casualty condition and projected outcome to commanders so that the latter can make an informed decision on matters, such as evacuation versus continuing the mission during the actual operation. It is critical that military medical providers recognize that the disposition of casualties during a mission is a command decision, rather than a medical one. Commanders use medical recommendations as one of the factors in deciding on a course of action when casualties occur; however, it is their perceived need for success of a particular mission that will ultimately always prevail.

COVER, CONCEALMENT, AND CAMOUFLAGE

Cover and concealment are critical aspects of all military tactical operations including offense, defense, and movement. If the enemy can see a soldier, then he can hit him with his fire. Cover provides actual protection from bullets, fragments, and other forms of direct or indirect fire. Concealment on the other hand merely hides a soldier from enemy observation, thereby making him more difficult to hit. It does not protect him from enemy fire. In contrast to civilian tactical operations, which are primarily concerned with protection from direct small arms fire, military tactical operations must also consider the likelihood of indirect fire, such as artillery or mortars, and more powerful direct fire weapons, such as rocket propelled grenades, when selecting appropriate cover. Cover and concealment are extremely important during military casualty care operations, because effective treatment cannot be provided in their absence. Any attempts by a medic to administer care in the open will likely draw enemy fire and only result in an additional casualty. Every effort must be made to safely and rapidly move a casualty into effective cover as soon as possible.

Both cover and concealment can be natural or manmade. Natural forms of cover include such things as trees, logs, stumps, ravines, and hollows. Manmade cover includes such things as walls, trenches, fighting positions, rubble, and craters. All of these offer varying degrees of protection against both direct and indirect enemy fire. Natural concealment may include bushes, tall grass, smaller trees, and shadows, whereas manmade concealment includes such things as camouflage uniforms and netting and natural materials that have been moved from their original locations. A key aspect to manmade concealment is that it must blend into the natural concealment provided by the surrounding terrain.

Light, noise, and movement discipline, as well as the use of camouflage, all contribute to concealment during tactical operations. Light discipline consists of restricting the use of lights during periods of darkness, including not walking around with headlamps or flashlights on, not smoking in the open, and not using vehicle headlights. Similarly, shine, such as reflected light from a windshield or watch crystal, must be avoided during daylight hours. Because at least a limited light source is often required to administer treatment at night, the medic must ensure that such light use is kept to a minimum and shielded from direct enemy observation to prevent detection of his location. Noise discipline involves taking action to deflect sounds generated by unit operations away from the enemy and, whenever possible, using soundless means of communications, such as arm-and-hand signals. Casualties who are frightened or in pain may tend to neglect noise discipline. Medics should anticipate this and be prepared to quiet casualties through reassurance and pain control measures. Movement discipline includes staying low and not moving within fighting positions unless absolutely necessary in the defense and not utilizing routes that lack cover and concealment in the offense.

Camouflage is anything used to keep the enemy from recognizing soldiers, their equipment, and their position. Both natural and manmade material can be used to blend with your surroundings. Camouflage should be changed and improved often. The time between changes and improvements depends on a variety of factors including weather and the material used. Natural camouflage may die, fade, or otherwise lose its effectiveness. Similarly, manmade camouflage may fade or wear off. Failure to correct these conditions may result in a diminished blending with one's surroundings and increase the likelihood of enemy detection. The use of camouflage tends to be more important in military than civilian tactical operations in part due to their generally longer duration, which increases the need for remaining hidden from enemy detection.

In order to maximize the effectiveness of camouflage, a soldier must first study the terrain and vegetation of the area. Unnatural shapes, such as helmets and bodies, must be broken up. Colors for uniforms, skin, and equipment are chosen that do not contrast with the surroundings. Personnel, vehicles, and equipment should be dispersed over a wide area if possible, because it is easier for the enemy to detect them when bunched together. All unnecessary movement must be avoided, because motion draws the attention of the eye and negates the effectiveness of camouflage. Positions should not be built in open areas or where the enemy expects to find them, but rather in places like the side of a hill and away from road junctions or lone buildings.

RAPID ARMORED AND VEHICLE RESCUE

Rapid armored and vehicle rescue are more likely to be utilized during civilian tactical operations than military ones. Although infantry forces may often operate in conjunction with armored vehicles, normal doctrine does not include the use of these vehicles to perform rescue operations of casualties. It is, however, feasible to use a Bradley fighting vehicle, uparmored high-mobility multipurpose wheeled vehicle (HMMWV), or similar vehicle to establish immediate cover from small arms fire for an exposed casualty. Effective use of suppressive fires against enemy forces is critical to any subsequent successful extraction of the casualty inside the vehicle or using ground personnel.

SUGGESTED READINGS

Urban Operations. Washington, DC: Dept of the Army [HQ]; June 2003. Field Manual 3-06.

Medical Platoon Leader's Handbook. Washington, DC: Dept of the Army [HQ]; December 18, 2003. Field Manual 4-02.4.

The Mechanized Infantry Platoon and Squad (APC). Washington, DC: Dept of the Army [HQ]; March 15, 1985. Field Manual 7-7.

Infantry Rifle Platoon and Squad. Washington, DC: Dept of the Army [HQ]; March 1, 2001. Field Manual 7-8.

The Infantry Rifle Company. Washington, DC: Dept of the Army [HQ]; October 31, 2000. Field Manual 7-10.

Camouflage, Concealment, and Decoys. Washington, DC: Dept of the Army [HQ]; August 30, 1999. Field Manual 20-3.

Combat Skills of the Soldier. Washington, DC: Dept of the Army [HQ]; August 3, 1984. Field Manual 21-75.

Soldier's Manual and Trainer's Guide MOS 11B Infantry Skill Level 1. Washington, DC: Dept of the Army [HQ]; August 6, 2004. STP-11B1-SM-TG.

Chapter 3

Infiltration/Exfiltration

John M. Croushorn

OBJECTIVES

After reading this section, the reader will be able to:

1. Describe the methods of infiltration and exfiltration used by special operations units.
2. Understand the physiology in airborne operations.
3. Be able to describe the fast rope insertion and extraction system, formally known as the special procedure insertion and extraction system, FRIES/SPIES methods.
4. Discuss the risks of ground infiltrations by foot and the advantage of tactical and nontactical vehicles.
5. Be familiar with diving operations to include open- and closed-circuit diving.
6. Describe the Combat Rubber Raiding Craft and its use in infiltration and exfiltration.
7. Understand the types of injuries encountered during waterborne infiltration and exfiltration.
8. Discuss the ways to mitigate the risk of the previously mentioned operations.

HISTORICAL PERSPECTIVE

"When you're on the march, act the way you would if you was sneaking up on a deer. See the enemy first."
—Third Order from Rogers' Rules of Ranging

Inherent in special operations is the ability for units to control and leverage resources against their opponents. An important aspect of this strategy is the movement to and from an objective expeditiously and in such a way to maximize the elements of surprise and tactical advantage. This is important both from a strategic as well as tactical perspective. Special operations units practice infiltration and exfiltration as integral components of their mission capability. Movement in force by air, ground, and waterborne assets are often utilized to this end. It is important for the tactical medicine provider to be aware of these infiltration and exfiltration techniques to adequately preplan for potential health risks to unit members as well as advising commanders on safety and risk mitigation.

Within the military, infiltration and exfiltration techniques are part of the basic building blocks that all special operation forces hone. Airborne training is prerequisite for involvement operationally. Small boat operations and

helicopter insertion is considered basic in the operators fund of knowledge. More advanced techniques, such as self-contained underwater breathing apparatus (SCUBA) training and Military Free Fall, are taught to teams based on their operational assignments. Additionally, advanced field trade craft in approaching targets by ground is taught in courses, such as the Special Operation Target Interdiction Course (SOTIC). Among law enforcement special operations units, certain methods may never be employed given their resources and their operational environment. However, responsibilities of law enforcement special operations teams continue to expand with the growing realities of the global war on terrorism and homeland defense.

METHODS

Air Infiltration

Air infiltration has classically been divided into parachute and nonparachute methods. Conventional airborne operations utilize static line techniques from fixed wing or rotary wing aircraft at altitudes that are safe for normal human physiology. Military free fall parachute operations that begin at higher altitudes, such as high altitude low opening (HALO) or high altitude high opening (HAHO), provide greater tactical advantage at the cost of increased risks. The nonparachute methods include the use of delivery by aircraft to a landing zone and the use of helicopters in tactical placement of forces without touching down in a landing zone.

Parachute Infiltration

Static line airborne operations in the military use the T-10B or MCI-1B parachute systems. The T-10B is a non-steerable parachute used for large unit deployment. The MCI-1B is more maneuverable and used in smaller unit operations with accompanying higher risks due to increased maneuverability. These jumps take place at altitudes below 10,000 feet, most occurring between 500 to 2,000 feet. Sea level to 10,000 feet is considered the physiologic zone. The healthy human is well adapted to this zone and can function without physiologic support. The only significant problem relating to altitude encountered in this zone is ventilation of the middle ear. Ventilation of the middle ear can be facilitated with the Valsalva maneuver (1).

Injuries occur in both training and tactical operations. However, until recently, not much was known about actual operational casualty and attrition rates. A comprehensive study of casualty, attrition, and surgery rates for recent combat airborne operations revealed an overall casualty rate 12%. Injuries resulting in the soldier being unable to continue the mission were much lower at 4.7% and serious injuries requiring surgical intervention was 1.7%. The majority of the injuries, (68.7%), were lower extremity injuries (2).

High-altitude techniques require special training and an operational assignment to units that conduct this specialized mission. The MC-5 ram-air parachute system (RAPS) is utilized in the Military Freefall Parachutist School for parachute operations between 10,000 feet and 25,000 feet. They are more maneuverable than the static line parachutes and afford a greater degree of control and capability for insertion of special operation forces.

Man is not physiologically equipped for survival at high altitudes. The dangers inherent in high-altitude parachuting are hypoxia, hyperventilation, and trapped gas disorders. As altitude increases, barometric pressure decreases and even the ascent to begin parachute operations can affect the body adversely. For high-altitude parachuting, supportive equipment is used to mitigate these risks.

Above 10,000 feet, physiologic support is needed; this is the beginning of the physiologic deficient zone. The first physiologic problem encountered is hypoxia. Symptoms of hypoxia include loss of color vision, anxiety, and mental confusion. Symptoms can vary from person to person. Because of this, it is necessary that operators receive training in an altitude chamber to recognize their hypoxia symptoms and how to use appropriate protective equipment. To mitigate this danger, an oxygen mask is worn with a regulator controlling the concentration of inspired oxygen. Positive pressure support is not a necessity until altitudes above 30,000 feet (1).

Above 18,000 feet, altitude decompression sickness (DCS) can occur. Active pressurization and nitrogen "wash out" can prevent this. Without pressurization, the operator can minimize the chance of DCS by prebreathing and continuing on 100% oxygen. This breathing of 100% oxygen washes the inert gas nitrogen from the lungs and creates a gradient to "off gas" nitrogen from the blood stream and reduces the chances of decompression sickness. Several factors affect the development of DCS. These include: minimal prebreathing period, rapid change in altitude, prolonged exposure to altitude, and increased pressure environments (i.e., SCUBA diving) prior to operations at altitude.

Above 33,000 feet, breathing 100% oxygen no longer prevents hypoxia. Therefore, to prevent hypoxia above 33,000 feet, oxygen will need to be delivered by positive pressure breathing (1).

Nonparachute Air Techniques

Fixed wing and rotary wing infiltration/exfiltration can be utilized to transport teams directly onto landing zones for disembarkation or retrieval operations. This direct method of utilizing air transportation is useful for units that have heavy equipment needs, the ability to operate out of remote landing sites or secure staging areas, and sites that can accommodate helicopter or fixed wing landing. Air infiltration is rapid and resources can remain on station for extraction or close air support (whether direct fire or surveillance). Special operations forces utilize a range of aircraft from large helicopter platforms, such as the MH-47E "Chinook" and MH-53 "Pave Low," to the small MH-6 "Little Birds" whose narrow rotor disk allows it to operate in many confined spaces that traditional troop carrying helicopters cannot operate. Additionally, the helicopter platform allows for infiltration/exfiltration where physical landing of the aircraft is not possible or detrimental to the operation.

Air rappel and fast rope insertion involve the use of transient static helicopter positioning and disembarkation from that platform to the ground. Air rappel is useful when the termination point of the rappel is not on the ground (i.e., window, platform above ground). The rappel provides added control at the sacrifice of time disconnecting from the rope. The fast rope insertion and extraction system (FRIES), use a large braided rope to provide increased surface area for resistance and control of descent. The system evolved from the special procedure insertion and extraction system (SPIES), McGuire and STABO rigs developed during Vietnam. For insertion, personnel grasp the rope, exit the aircraft, and make a hasty descent to the ground by gripping the rope with their hands and feet. Operators then simply let go of the rope and continue on their mission. The system also incorporates attachment points on the rope for the extraction of personnel. Operators wear a harness and connect to integral rings in the rope leaving their arms and hands free to continue to use weapons and other equipment during the extraction.

Danger in this system of insertion is the lack of safety restraint, which is sacrificed for the commodity of speed. Proper training and weight discipline help to mitigate this risk. Appropriately trained crew chiefs and rope masters can eliminate rope length and aircraft height disparity during operations. One well referenced incident of fast rope injury occurred during the black hawk down incident in Mogadishu, Somalia.

"The first casualty occurred when the Rangers fast roped in. Ranger Blackburn lost his grip and fell from the fast rope—seventy five feet (other reports indicate a fall of about forty feet), three stories, to the ground. He landed on his back. 'He was hurt real bad,' remembered one of the Rangers who saw him. 'Internal bleeding, head trauma, busted his right leg and hip'" (3). Eighteen-year-old Private Todd Blackburn was unconscious and bleeding from the nose and ears (3).

"According to one knowledgeable source, Ranger Blackburn had a closed head injury with a Glasgow coma score of approximately 6, a skull fracture, multiple rib fractures, fractures of the femur and humerus and he had a retroperitoneal hematoma. Reportedly he had no evidence of internal bleeding and was hemodynamically very stable, in the field, at the casualty collection point, and at the 46th Combat Support Hospital" (3).

This accident was affected by weight discipline and a lack of training and was a result of evasive action taken by the MH-60 he was riding on. Fast rope insertion is an expedient way of delivery of forces that is used by many units around the world and with the proper training can be executed safely. Emphasis on training should be reinforced by the tactical medical provider. This is the most significant risk modifier.

Land Infiltration/Exfiltration

Open terrain and urban environments where special operations missions are executed require operators to eventually have "boots on the ground." Planning for these operations incorporate land based infiltration and exfiltration whether by choice or contingency. Operators need to be familiar with global positioning system (GPS) navigation down to basic techniques using a compass and a map, neither of which requires batteries. Navigation and tactical movement are skills practiced thoroughly by even basic military and law enforcement teams. When there is move-

ment by foot, the tactical medicine provider should be aware of the stress placed upon operators. Physical conditioning is a good preventative measure; however, mission planning should include an assessment of weight distribution, terrain to be covered, and other physiologic stressors. Rest-work cycles as well as rest-travel cycles should be anticipated to meet the unit's goals. Carrying equipment for a raid, assault, or ambush may be very different from that required to set up a hide sight to observe a target for 5 days in a remote location. Environmental conditions, such as weather, temperature, and altitude, also factor into risk assessment. The use of land-based vehicles, when appropriate, facilitates infiltration and exfiltration regardless of conditions.

Armored vehicles can provide some protection from small arms and other ballistic threats. This is valued in the law enforcement and military special operations. Tactical vehicles may incorporate armor and enhanced surveillance equipment to reduce risk to operators. Law enforcement utilizes these vehicles to create routes of ingress on property protected by simple barrier fences and to provide a safe method of travel with active shooter scenarios.

Additionally, these vehicles provide an advantage during ingress with the capability to carry equipment and weapons as well as enhancing mobility. Certain communications, advanced medical capability, and heavy weapon augmentation are difficult to provide without vehicle support. The ability to preposition support assets is essential in contingency planning with every infiltration and exfiltration as well as during mission execution.

In urban settings, deception may be utilized by using indigenous vehicles. Some law enforcement SWAT operators still refer to the "bread truck" for infiltration and exfiltration. Chosen for its size and adaptability, it was ideal for carrying a SWAT team inconspicuously to an operation. This feign is still used today in disguising vehicles as nonlaw enforcement vehicles. With current advances in technology, these nontactical vehicles (NTVs) can be outfitted with advanced communications, as well as navigation and surveillance equipment, while taking full advantage of deceptive techniques.

Ground mobility vehicles (GMVs) are modified HUMMVs used by military special operations to extend operational capabilities. Various crew served weapons are utilized and a number of passenger configurations have been fielded. The GMVs have seen extensive use on deployments in Afghanistan and Iraq.

Waterborne Infiltration/Exfiltration

Underwater ingress and egress is another tool utilized by special operation forces. Within the military, Naval Special Warfare (NSW) is given responsibility for an extensive list of maritime operations that require specialized, more advanced diving skills. Other military and law enforcement special operations teams utilize these techniques primarily as a method of undetected infiltration and exfiltration.

SCUBA refers to open-circuit systems (this is what is commonly used for recreational diving), closed-circuit systems (i.e., MK 25 UBA or LAR-V Dräger Rebreathers), and semiclosed circuit systems (i.e., MK 16).

Open-circuit diving is the simplest method to get underwater and stay there long enough to do useful work. It may be used for any operation not requiring secrecy or when underwater detection capabilities are very limited (4). Open-circuit dives allow for greater depth than close-circuit systems, which are generally limited to 20 feet.

Closed-circuit diving operations involve the use of equipment that will recirculate expired gas and remove carbon dioxide. If properly used, these devices do not release gas bubbles that diminish the underwater signature of the divers and the presence of surface bubbles. Although the range and duration cannot approach that of open-circuit equipment, the advantage of stealth makes this system the primary operational dive apparatus used by special operations forces.

Surface swim techniques are apart of special operation waterborne operations. Distances beyond closed-circuit and open-circuit swims can be bridged with surface swim. Surface swim is also an integral exfiltration technique with or without small boat support. Physical conditioning and water conditions are factors that affect mission planning and execution as well as the risk of these operations.

Diving injuries can be divided into injuries during descent, injuries during ascent, and inspired gas disorders. Descent injuries are described as squeeze injuries because the descent into water involves the increase of pressure. Most of these injuries can be prevented by restricting divers from operations if they have an upper respiratory infection and are unable to clear sinus passages and eustachian tubes. Pressure equalization is required to prevent squeeze (Box 3.1).

▶ BOX 3.1. The Laws of Dysbarism

Boyle's Law: the volume of a gas varies inversely with the pressure. This law explains all the "squeeze" syndromes.

Henry's Law: the amount of gas dissolved in a liquid is proportional to the partial pressure of the gas in contact with liquid. Henry's law relates to nitrogen coming out of solution and forming bubbles in blood and body tissues. Decompression sickness is explained by this law.

Dalton's Law: as atmospheric pressure increases, the partial pressure of a gas increases. Nitrogen is a lipid-soluble gas which more easily in blood and tissues (due to its increased partial pressure) and causes an anesthetic, narcotizing effect. Nitrogen narcosis is explained by this law.

Injuries during ascent are related to the change from high pressure to low pressure and resultant overexpansion. This can also lead to pneumothorax as well as gas embolism. Prevention is focused on not holding one's breath on ascent. Decompression sickness (DCS) is also included in this category of injury. It is classically attributed to ascending too rapidly. DCS is also referred to as the Bends or Caisson disease. Recompression is the first line of treatment for DCS and is curative unless the central nervous system has incurred a permanent injury.

Inspired gas disorders are oxygen toxicity and nitrogen narcosis. Both of these disorders result in altered mental status that may prevent an operator from being able to complete their mission. It may also prevent them from completing simple tasks that are required to dive safely. The primary mitigation of this risk is the buddy system. If the diver's buddy recognizes signs of either of these disorders he helps the effected diver to surface safely.

Environmental injuries may also occur. Cold weather diving holds a greater risk to operators than exposure to cold weather on land. Water conducts heat 25 times faster than air. Because of its greater conductivity, water does not have to be extremely cold for it to adversely affect the diver's ability to conduct his mission (4). Dehydration is also a risk factor in operations given the decreased accessibility to potable water.

Water landing by small boat insertion provides advantage in speed and the ability to carry supplies and equipment to the point of debarkation. That may be the land or water given the tactical situation. Military special operations have simplified their reference to small boat operations as Combat Rubber Raiding Craft (CRRC) operations. "CRRCs are noncommissioned, inflatable rubber boats, powered by outboard motors and capable of limited independent operations (4)." The military primarily uses the Zodiac F-470 inflatable boat. Operators rehearse actions during small boat operations and their responsibilities during embarkation, traveling, and disembarking the boat.

Military kayaks, such as the Klepper Arius 2 or the American Long Haul Commando, provide a very low surface signature, increased load carrying capacity, speed, and stealth. They are utilized in waterborne insertion and exfiltration operations around the world and have been used in this way since World War II.

Helocasting or free drop from a helicopter into water is a combination of transport technique to accomplish waterborne insertion. Static line or free fall parachuting into water is also used for insertion. Aircraft provide an expedient and available resource to move personnel and equipment in and out of locations quickly. The CH/MH-47 Chinook or MH-53 Pave Low are used in "limp duck" missions to drop and recover CRRCs. UH/MH 60s can be utilized for "Kangaroo Duck" or "Rolled Duck" missions helocasting a CRRC and personnel. Fixed wing aircraft also have the capability of conducting "hard duck" operations to infiltrate CRRCs.

For appropriate care in waterborne operations, the medical provider should have specialized education in dive medicine. Individuals involved in these operations should undergo diving physicals on a regular basis to determine their initial and continued qualification to perform diving duties. The tactical medical provider should present during training ascents as well as pressure and oxygen testing. For many law enforcement units, this can be coordinated through local and experienced medical support.

In all waterborne techniques, the tactical medical provider should focus efforts on preplanning to anticipate hyperthermia, hypothermia, and dehydration risks as well as dive illness/injury mitigation when operations will include an underwater component. Fighter management for waterborne operations consists of surveillance for swimmer fatigue, repetitive diving, operational tempo in activities other than diving, and individual experience. Knowing the most appropriate route to care from embarkation to disembarkation as well as the procedures for extracting personnel to medical assets at any point in the mission is an essential task of the tactical medic. Other common problems encountered include seasickness, tendonitis, and repetitive motion injuries.

TAKE HOME POINTS

Special operation forces utilize techniques to infiltrate from the air, water and ground. Routine infilration/exfiltra-tion techniques involve increase risks that need mitigation. The tactical medical provider must be aware of these risks and understand the different ways to mitigate them. Of the infiltration techniques discussed, underwater techniques provide the greatest physical demands and risks. Proper preplanning, training, health surveillance, active participation by the tactical medical provider, and command emphasis on safety are the most important risk modifiers.

SUMMARY

As with most risk mitigation, standard preventative measures (i.e., protective equipment and standard operating procedures) as well as adequate training and rehearsals can minimize the chance of injury in these activities. There are, however, inherent risks in these operations that can dramatically affect the functionality of a team and the success of a mission.

REFERENCES

1. DeHart RL. *Fundamentals of Aerospace Medicine*. 2nd ed. Baltimore: Williams & Wilkins, 1996.
2. Kotwal RS, et al. Army Ranger casualty, attrition, and surgery rates for Airborne operations in Afganistan and Iraq. *Aviat Space Environ Med*. 2004;75:833–840.
3. Cloonan C. Special operations combat medic course: Mogadishu raid exercise. May 1999.
4. Special Forces Waterborne Operations. Department of the Army, Washington DC; August 2004. FM 3-05.212 (TC 31-25).

Chapter 4

Continuum of Force

Bret T. Ackerman and Jeffrey D. Ho

OBJECTIVES

After reading this section, the reader will be able to:

1. Describe the types of intermediate weapons available.
2. Understand the concept of nonlethal weapons and their role in the force continuum.
3. Understand the potential effects of these weapons on the human body.
4. Understand the concept of sudden, in-custody death syndrome (ICDS).

INTRODUCTION

The concept of the "force continuum" exists to explain the spectrum of available officer reactions to a subject's actions. The subject's actions can range from being completely compliant all the way up to the level of potentially lethal assault. Accordingly, an officer's perception and reaction to these actions can range from the lowest use of force (generally accepted as "officer presence" without contact to encourage or discourage certain types of behavior) all the way up to the level of deadly force (1). In between these two ends of the spectrum are many options, including empty hand control techniques and the use of intermediate weaponry. There are different models of force continuums used by various law enforcement agencies and each model has inherent advantages and disadvantages. A sample of a federal model is shown and is an example of typical information contained in the continuum, regardless of model type (Fig. 4.1).

Force continuums allow the operator to enter at any level of force deemed reasonably necessary to confront the situation at hand. It is not necessary to escalate from the lowest levels to get to the highest levels if what is needed is a high level of force to meet an officer's needs. However, it is also not mandatory that the officer stays at a high level of force if the situation calls for a lesser use of force. Essentially, force continuums are designed to be dynamic guides that allow the user to adapt to changing situations.

Within the force continuum lies the use and concept of nonlethal, intermediate weaponry. Intuitively, the term *nonlethal* leads one to believe that it is any weapon that cannot kill. This is misleading because even benign appearing objects, such as a clipboard or a ballpoint pen, can become lethal weapons given the right circumstances. However, the official definition, as set by the United States military for nonlethal weaponry, is one that is "explicitly designed and primarily employed so as to incapacitate personnel or material, while minimizing fatalities" (2). Certain intermediate weapons available to the modern law enforcement officer fall under the nonlethal category and may include weapons such as conducted electrical weapons, chemical irritants, and impact devices.

Intermediate Weapons

Electrical "stun" type devices are a unique, intermediate style of nonlethal weapon. Also known as conducted electrical weapons (CEWs), electromuscular disruption munitions (EMD) or electronic control devices (ECDs), they are more commonly referred to as a TASER. These weapons are also discussed in Chapter 5.

The most popular CEW in use today is the TASER model X26. It uses compressed nitrogen to fire two metallic darts up to a maximum of 35 feet with a predetermined angled rate of spread. It is capable of transmitting an electrical impulse through two cumulative inches of clothing or air space. When it makes adequate contact and the darts are of adequate separation, it causes involuntary contractions of the regional skeletal muscles which render the subject incapable of voluntary movement. If the darts are fired at very close range and do not achieve adequate separation, full muscular incapacitation may not be achieved and the device is then used to encourage certain behavior through pain compliance. Additionally, the TASER device has electrical contact points at its tip that are approximately

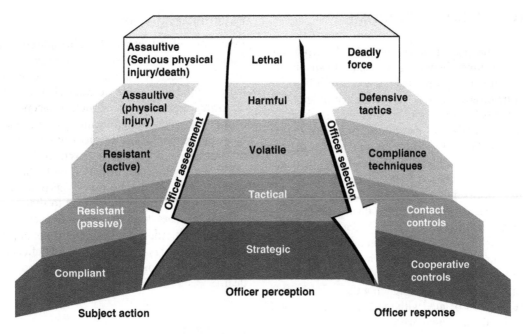

Source: Federal Law Enforcement Training Center, Department of Homeland Security.

FIGURE 4.1. Sample force continuum.

1.5 inches apart. These contact points may be touched to a subject during discharge of the weapon and are also considered a pain compliance technique as the separation is not adequate to cause a full, involuntary contraction of muscles. This technique is often referred to as a "drive stun" mode of operation.

It is beyond the scope of this chapter to fully discuss the engineering concepts that allow CEWs to be safe yet effective. Suffice it to say that CEWs utilize high voltage, but very low amperage electrical currents to disrupt normal nerve signals to skeletal muscles. Although this principle of weapon technology has been around for at least 30 years, it has recently improved to the point where it has gained the interest of law enforcement agencies. In doing so, this technology appears to be experiencing the controversial "growing pains" of societal acceptance.

Approximately 15 years ago, chemical irritants, such as pepper spray, were in the same position that TASER devices are today. At that time, chemical irritants entered the law enforcement market and were considered a useful tool for subject control, but critics feared that this new tool would worsen health problems (e.g., asthma) or even cause death (3). Given time, though, this concern was reduced through lab study and observational surveillance. Although chemical irritants were once blamed for in-custody deaths, they are now considered practical and necessary alternatives in use-of-force situations. It appears that CEWs are currently in the throes of a similar acceptance process.

A search of the literature reveals numerous studies, position papers, and review articles about both chemical irritants and CEWs. In fact, the CEW's continue to be studied by the manufacturer's, the military, academic institutions, international groups, and law enforcement agencies, making it, arguably, one of the most thoroughly researched piece of equipment found on a law enforcement officer's duty belt.

Fears of CEW use causing death usually center on theories of electrocution or induced arrhythmia. Because CEWs are more likely to be used on subjects who are actively resisting arrest or in agitated states, there are also theories that they may worsen underlying metabolic acidosis or cause death due to a delayed mechanism, such as induced rhabdomyolysis. These fears are often furthered by media inaccuracies that compare CEWs to electric chairs (4) or civil rights organizations and media stories that may confuse readers by stating conclusions that are not supported by factual data (5–7).

There are studies being performed daily on CEW's and the evidence is mounting against these weapons playing a role in sudden, custodial deaths. Currently, there are studies indicating a high degree of measurable safety margins regarding induction of cardiac arrhythmia, low risk of induced significant myocardial damage when used in typical control settings (the manufacturer of TASER devices reports that the majority of reported uses in the field are for 5-second exposures or less [8]), and no demonstration of induced hyperkalemia or worsening acidosis (9–12).

IN-CUSTODY DEATH SYNDROME

Sudden and unexpected in-custody death syndrome (ICDS) is an alarming phenomenon. It leads to suspicion, mistrust, and often inappropriate knee-jerk administrative decisions by involved agencies. The ICDS phenomenon following agitated behavior is not new and similar phenomena have been described in psychiatric literature dating back to the mid-1800s (13). The association with mental illness conditions, especially psychoses with paranoid features, was notable until the mid-1960s when development of traditional antipsychotic medication seemed to correlate with a decrease in these types of deaths (14). In the 1980s, it was noted that there was resurgence in these types of deaths. The rise in these cases has been hypothesized to be related to the introduction and growing popularity of the illicit stimulant cocaine in the street culture of America (15). Currently, we are still experiencing these deaths and they are also being associated with methamphetamine and other illicit stimulant/hallucinogen abuse on an increasing basis.

Over the years, there have been attempts to link ICDS with single causative factors such as use of chemical irritants (e.g., pepper spray), restraint and positional asphyxia, structural cardiac abnormalities, or use of illicit stimulant medication (3,15–26). Many of these links have been questioned, disproved, or found to be absent (27–33). This has generated more questions than answers in the search for a common cause. It is important to recognize that in our society, people tend to look for singular, proximate causes to adverse events and often confuse an action most proximate to the time of a death to be the cause of death. This leads people to disregard other factors that may be more remote in time, such as medical conditions or lifestyle abuse issues that may be causative. This is an error of logic and has been identified in previous literature (34).

There are several theories that have been advanced as to the etiology of the ICDS. Current theories include: underlying cardiovascular disease; psychiatric related; asphyxia; stimulant related; excited delirium/metabolic acidosis; weapon induced. These theories are not necessarily mutually exclusive and an ICDS patient may have more than one of these apply in a given situation.

Underlying Cardiovascular

It is well demonstrated that unexpected deaths occur due to underlying cardiovascular disease. This may take the form of congenital problems, such as hypertrophic obstructive cardiomyopathy, significant coronary artery disease, or lifestyle induced cardiomyopathies. All of these have been demonstrated to place the diseased subject at significant risk of sudden death, especially during physically exertional events, such as resisting arrest, fleeing, or during periods of agitation.

Psychiatrically Related

Psychiatric illness, especially schizophrenia with paranoid features, has been linked to sudden death. These deaths have been described in unmedicated subjects with underlying mental illness for decades (16). It is believed that abnormal dopamine and serotonin receptor relationships in the brain play a significant role in mental illness etiology. Most mental health medications work to alter this relationship and there is research to show that at death, there is a significant correlation with abnormal brain receptor anatomy in psychotic subjects that experienced sudden death, which is very similar to that seen in chronic cocaine abusers that also go on to experience sudden death (25,35). Additionally, many, if not all, mental health medications carry warnings for side effects that include cardiac arrhythmia, delirium, agitation, seizures, and death.

Asphyxia

There are several methods of proposed asphyxia induced sudden death. There have been reports of death following placement of prisoners and patients in a maximal restraint position (involving binding of hands behind the back, binding the ankles together, and connecting the hand and ankle restraints in the area of the subject's low back or buttock region) (21,24). However, despite moratoriums on not positioning people in this fashion, ICDs continued to occur. Significant laboratory evaluation of this positioning has also failed to demonstrate evidence of significant respiratory compromise (31,32). It has also been felt that placing persons in a prone position, especially if they are obese, causes suffocation. Simple prone positioning has not been shown in lab settings to restrict respiration (31,32). There is also evidence to the contrary that shows that prone positioning may also be beneficial to respiratory dynamics, especially in obese patients; however, some caution is needed in interpreting this data, because it was generated during subject anesthesia (36,37). It is unclear if prone positioning over an obstacle (such as on the floor board of the backseat with the vehicle drivetrain hump in the position of the subject's diaphragm) can create respiratory compromise and this should probably best be avoided. Another type of asphyxial event is hypothesized to occur with compression or "weight force" applied to a subject's thorax. In law enforcement work, this is most commonly seen in the "polyester pile" or "swarm" method of subduing a person where multiple officers take a person to the ground by swarming over the top of them. Published work indicates that weight up to 50 pounds can be accommodated without compromising a person's respiration (33). There have also been cases of persons asphyxiating when very heavy weight is applied to their thorax (such as when a car drops off a jack onto a person), but it is unclear how much weight is too much.

Until this issue is settled, this method of control should be used judiciously.

Stimulant Related

There are many references in the literature of ICDS being closely associated with illicit stimulant use/abuse as a factor, especially cocaine and methamphetamine with occasional PCP and ephedrine as well. There are several possible mechanisms proposed for this. First is the obvious acute toxicity of overdose, which is most notable in persons that conceal large amounts internally to avoid detection. In the nonconcealer, however, it is thought that acute use can produce a delirium psychosis condition (also known as excited or agitated delirium) as well as factors that may lead to profound metabolic acidosis (through hyperagitation, hypermetabolism, vasoconstriction, and hyperthermia). It is unclear why some persons undergo this condition and others do not and it is proposed that there may be a genetic predisposition to this (38). But there is demonstrable evidence that chronic abusers of these drugs undergo similar brain receptor changes that are seen in mental health patients and it is felt that this change is very closely related to acute, psychotic behavioral changes (25).

Excited Delirium/Metabolic Acidosis

This theory has gained recent popularity and the described features of excited delirium syndrome (EDS) include agitation, incoherence, hyperthermia, paranoia, inappropriate and often violent behavior, constant motion, and feats of incredible strength (15). This type of behavior appears to be closely associated with a higher risk of sudden, unexpected death (39). It is believed that precursors to this condition are chronic, illicit stimulant abuse, presence of certain mental health conditions, and also the use of certain mental health medications. It is thought that the state of EDS sets the stage for the subject to enter a metabolic acidosis condition and this can be profound at times (40). If left untreated, the subject will become acidotic to a point that is not compatible with life and experience a cardiorespiratory arrest. Critics of this concept believe that it is simply a theory of convenience to exonerate overzealous law enforcement officers who inadvertently kill people during the course of carrying out their job. However, the growing body of data seems to suggest commonality of these factors in persons who undergo the ICD process.

Weapon Induced

For the most part, specific weapons in an officer's armamentarium lead to very predictable results when applied to a subject. (e.g., striking a subject with an impact baton will lead to contusion and potential fracture and possibly even death if struck in certain areas). However, the introduction of conducted electrical weapons (CEWs) has produced controversy on whether or not these devices lead to ICDS events. The theories on how this is possible include instant arrhythmia/electrocution, respiratory compromise worsening an acidosis condition to delayed death from myocardial necrosis, or renal failure from rhabdomyolysis. There are animal and human studies available that do not demonstrate support for these theories under normal operating circumstances (11,12,14,41). In one animal study, a statistically insignificant rise in cardiac troponin was found but this remains controversial because the methodology included applications of CEWs in ways not normally found such as extremely prolonged durations of application (11). The duration of applications used in the study were not realistic when compared with one CEW manufacturer report that 67% of its reported field uses are 5 seconds or less (10). Additionally, preliminary data as reported by a CEW manufacturer do not support respiratory compromise during CEW application (41). Perhaps the most compelling data comes from a major CEW manufacturer itself, because it has recorded data on over 122,000 human volunteers with no reports of associated death (10).

In looking at the previously mentioned theories, it is apparent that there is no single, unifying cause of ICD. Some theories appear to have very good correlation and some do not. Additionally, several of the theories are interrelated with each other; this makes it difficult to pinpoint a uniform final common pathway leading to the ICDS process. Because this topic is gaining in research popularity, it is expected that the available body of knowledge in this area will increase greatly in the near future.

TAKE HOME POINTS

1. Conducted electrical weapons are becoming more popular with law enforcement agencies. All available data appears to support their high degree of effectiveness and safety.
2. Sudden, ICDS is a real and alarming phenomenon with several possible etiologies, many of them related. There is not necessarily a final common pathway that leads up to this but there is a clear association with certain underlying conditions and behaviors.

REFERENCES

1. US Government Accountability Office. *Report to the Chairman, Subcommittee on National Security, Emerging Threats and International Relations, Committee on Government Reform, House of Representatives. TASER Weapons: Use of Tasers by Selected Law Enforcement Agencies.* Washington: US Government Accountability Office; May, 2005. Report GAO-05-464. http://www.gao.gov/new.items/d05464.pdf. Published February 12, 2006.

2. Anonymous.*Department of Defense Directive 3000.3 Policy for Non-lethal Weapons*. Washington: US Dept of Defense; July 9, 1996. http://www.dtic.mil/whs/directives/corres/pdf/d30003_070996/d30003p.pdf. Published March 7, 2006.

3. American Civil Liberties Union of Southern California. Pepper spray update: more fatalities, more questions. *Pepper Spray Update*. June 1995. http://www.aclu-sc.org/attachments/p/Pepper_Spray_New_Questions.pdf. Published March 6, 2006.

4. Anonymous. Taser packs potent but brief punch of electricity. *USA Today*. June 3, 2005:A13.

5. Amnesty International. Excessive and lethal force? Amnesty International's concerns about deaths and ill-treatment involving police use of TASER's. *Amnesty International Library*. November 30, 2004. http://web.amnesty.org/library/index/engamr511392004. Published March 6, 2006.

6. Anglen R. 73 cases of death following stun gun use. *Arizona Republic*. October 12, 2004. http://www.azcentral.com/specials/special43/articles/0915taserlist16-ON.html. Published March 6, 2006.

7. Anglen R. Taser safety claim questioned. *Arizona Republic*. July 18, 2004. http://www.azcentral.com/specials/special43/articles/0718taser-main18.html. Published March 6, 2006.

8. Anonymous. TASER training video and information disk [computer program]. Version 13. Scottsdale, AZ: *TASER International*. April, 2006.

9. US Dept of Defense, Human Effects Center of Excellence. *Report on Human Effectiveness and Risk Characterization of Electromuscular Incapacitation Devices*. Washington: US Dept of Defense; October 18, 2004.

10. McDaniel WC, Stratbucker RA, Nerheim M, et al. Cardiac safety of neuromuscular incapacitating defensive devices. *PACE*. 2005;28: S284–S287.

11. Levine SD, Sloane C, Chan T, et al. Cardiac Monitoring of subjects exposed to the TASER. *Acad Emerg Med*. 2005;12 (suppl 1):71.

12. Ho JD, Miner JR, Lakireddy DR, et al. Cardiovascular and physiologic effects of conducted electrical weapon discharge in resting adults. *Acad Emerg Med*. 2006;13:589–595.

13. Bell L. On a form of disease resembling some advanced stages of mania and fever, but so contradistinguished from any ordinary observed or described combination of symptoms as to render it probable that it may be overlooked and hitherto unrecorded malady. *Am J Insanity*. 1849;6:97–127.

14. Di Maio TG, Di Maio VJM. Excited Delirium Syndrome Cause of Death and Prevention. 1st ed. Boca Raton: Taylor & Francis Group; 2006.

15. Eckart RE, SL Scoville, CL Campbell, et al. Sudden death in young adults: a 25-year review of autopsies in military recruits. *Ann Int Med*. 2004;141:829–835.

16. Stratton SJ, Rogers C, Brickett K, et al. Factors associated with sudden death of individuals requiring restraint for excited delirium. *Am J Emerg Med*. 2001;21:187–191.

17. Maron BJ, Roberts WC, Epstein SE. Sudden death in hypertrophic cardiomyopathy: a profile of 78 patients. *Circulation*. 1982;65:1388–1394.

18. Ross DL. Factors associated with excited delirium deaths in police custody. *Mod Pathol*. 1998;11:1127–1137.

19. Reay DT, Fligner CL, Stilwell AD, et al. Positional asphyxia during law enforcement transport. *Am J Forensic Med Pathol*. 1992;13:90–97.

20. O'Halloran RL, Lewman LV. Restraint asphyxia in excited delirium. *Am J Forensic Med Pathol*. 1993;13:289–295.

21. O'Halloran RL, Frank JG. Restraint asphyxia. *Am J Forensic Med Pathol*. 2000;21:420–422.

22. O'Halloran RL, Frank JG. Asphyxial death during prone restraint revisited: a report of 21 cases. *Am J Forensic Med Pathol*. 2000;21: 39–52.

23. Wetli CV, Mash D, Karch SB. Cocaine-associated agitated delirium and the neuroleptic malignant syndrome. *Am J Emerg Med*. 1996;14:425–428.

24. Karch SB, Stephens BG. Drug abusers who die during arrest or in custody. *J R Soc Med*. 1999;92:110–113.

25. Pestaner JP, Southall PE. Sudden death during arrest and phencyclidine intoxication. *Am J Forensic Med Pathol*. 2003;24:119–122.

26. Ruttenber AJ, Lawler-Heavner J, Yin M, et al. Fatal excited delirium following cocaine use: epidemiologic findings provide new evidence for mechanisms of cocaine toxicity. *J Forensic Sci*. 1997;42: 25–31.

27. US Dept of Justice, Office of Justice Programs, National Institute of Justice. The effective ness and safety of pepper spray. *Research for Practice*. November 1, 2005:1–14. http://www.ncjrs.gov/pdffiles1/nij/195739.pdf. Published November 1, 2005.

28. Chan TC, Vilke GM, Clausen J, et al. The effect of oleoresin capsicum "pepper" spray inhalation on respiratory function. *J Forensic Sci*. 2002;47:299–304.

29. Chan TC, Vilke GM, Neuman T, et al. Restraint position and positional asphyxia. *Ann Emerg Med*. 1998;32:116–118.

30. Chan TC, Vilke GM, Neuman T. Reexamination of custody restraint position and positional asphyxia. *Am J Forensic Med Pathol*. 1998;19:201–205.

31. Chan TC, Neuman T, Clausen J, et al. Weight force during prone restraint and respiratory function. *Am J Forensic Med Pathol*. 2004;25:185–189.

32. Kornblum RN, Reddy SK. Effects of the TASER in fatalities involving police confrontation. *J Forensic Sci*. 1992;37:956–958

33. Glatter K, Karch SB. Positional asphyxia: inadequate oxygen, or inadequate theory? *Forensic Sci Int*. 2004;141:201–202.

34. Farnham FR, Kennedy HG. Acute excited states and sudden death: much journalism, little evidence. *Br Med J*. 1997;315:1107–1108.

35. Mash DC. Dopamine transport function is elevated in cocaine users. *J Neurochemistry*. 2002;81:292–300.

36. Pelosi P, Croci M, Calappi E, et al. Prone positioning improves pulmonary function in obese patients during general anesthesia. *Anesth Analg*. 1996;83:578–583.

37. Blanc L, Mancebo A, Perez M, et al. Short-term effects of prone position in critically ill patients with acute respiratory distress syndrome. *Intensive Care Med*. 1997;23:1033–1039.

38. Mash DC. Neuropharmacology of cocaine excited delirium. Paper presented at: The 33rd Annual FL Medical Examiners Educational Conference; August 11, 2006; Jupiter, Florida.

39. Ho JD, Reardon RF, Heegaard WG. Deaths in police custody: an 8 month surveillance study. *Annals Emerg Med*. 2005;46 (suppl): S94.

40. Hick JL, Smith SW, Lynch MT. Metabolic acidosis in restraint-associated cardiac arrest: a case series. *Acad Emerg Med*. 1999;6:239–243.

41. Anonymous. Human test subjects were able to breathe within normal limits during a 15-second exposure. *TASER International*. September 22, 2005. http://phx.corporate-ir.net/phoenix.zhtml?c=129937&p=irol-newsArticle&ID=759721&highlight-. Published March 12, 2006.

Chapter 5

Specialty Munitions

Jeffery C. Metzger and Alexander L. Eastman

OBJECTIVES

After reading this section, the reader will be able to:

1. Describe "continuum of force" and gaining compliance.
2. List specialty munitions used to gain compliance.
3. Understand the risks and benefits of specialty munitions.

INTRODUCTION

Police officers often have to bring uncooperative subjects into compliance with their instructions. Historically, arrest and control tactics focused on hand-to-hand methods, such as joint locks and takedowns, and impact weapons, such as clubs, batons, and sticks. Because of the officer's ethical and legal responsibility to use the least force possible to effects arrests, as well as the movement toward safer, more palatable hands-off techniques, several tools have been developed to assist the officer in bringing suspects under control.

Initially described as *nonlethal* or *less-than-lethal* munitions, early experience showed that if used in a manner in which they were not designed for they could inflict serious and even fatal injuries. Now termed *specialty munitions* or *specialty weapons* by most users, these tools are designed to bridge the gap in the force continuum between hands-on force and lethal force. They provide a method to temporarily incapacitate a subject from a distance offering a measure of protection for the officer, while typically not causing mortal damage to the suspect. They come in a variety of modalities with each having unique attributes and injury patterns.

Induction of Compliance

The act of one human being exerting his will over another against their will and in the face of active resistance is never pleasant to watch. Countless examples exist of adverse public reactions when these incidents have been witnessed or broadcast. Although unpleasant, the officer's ultimate goal in using force is to bring the sometimes violent, uncooperative suspect into compliance. To understand specialty weapons, their effects, and potential

consequences, tactical emergency medical service (TEMS) providers must understand the principles officer's use to gain suspect compliance. Traditionally, force continuums have relied on a stepwise escalation of these techniques to guide the use of force.

Psychological compliance is always the first level of force use in bringing a subject under control. This relies on a number of factors. First, the officer's appearance, demeanor, and presence of his uniform often are enough to gain control of the situation. Forceful commands and "verbal judo" techniques often initiate a psychological response in the suspect to submit and follow the officer's instructions.

Pain compliance is the mainstay of most force techniques and is the principle that most specialty munitions are based upon. There are a number of systems and techniques, ranging from soft, empty-handed takedowns and joint locks, to hard, impact weapons. By the infliction of pain on the subject, an officer is able to gain control and exert his will after suspect submission.

A more recent development and a subset of the principle of pain compliance that has generated a tremendous amount of interest of late is that of "mechanical compliance." Devices like conducted energy weapons (CEWs) that cause electromuscular disruption and incapacitation of voluntary skeletal muscle are an example of this type of compliance induction.

Last, when all other options have failed or when presented with a significant threat, the ultimate action to gain suspect control is the application of deadly force. Deadly force confrontations, often thought of as the use of an officer's firearm, can also be resolved with knives, choke holds, and a number of other techniques taught in officer survival courses. Advocates of specialty weapons often point to a reduction in deadly force confrontations in jurisdictions that have progressive specialty weapon programs.

Impact Munitions

One of the first impact munitions developed was the "bean bag," a ballistic canvas filled with small pellets or sand that was fired from a standard 12-gauge shotgun. These "bean-bag" rounds have a relatively large mass (40 g) and travel at a high velocity (300 fps), which together impart a significant amount of kinetic energy to whatever they strike. When the projectile strikes a surface with the flat side of the bag, injuries tend to be blunt in nature (i.e., splenic rupture, pneumothorax, subcapsular liver hematoma). However, when it strikes skin with the corner, it can penetrate the surface and cause significant damage. There are several reports of penetrating and blunt injuries after bean bag use (1–5). To decrease penetrating injuries, manufactures began making the bean bag with a softer cotton or nylon canvas. One disadvantage to the bean bag is its poor aerodynamic properties, which decreases it's accuracy at longer ranges. To improve its aerodynamics, manufacturers began making a drag stabilized bean bag that is essentially a bean bag with one or more strips of canvas on one end that stabilizes the projectile during flight. This improves the effective range by approx 5 to 10 yards and eliminates corners seen with the square bag, decreasing the chance of penetration. Bean bags have also been developed that can be fired from a 37 mm or 40 mm launcher.

Another type of impact munition is the "rubber bullet." These also come in a variety of shapes and sizes as well as delivery methods. Options fired from a launcher or shotgun include round rubbers balls of varying sizes (typically 0.30 to 0.60 inches) and numbers that can disperse and hit a broader target. They spread their cumulative kinetic energy to a larger surface area which may decrease the chance of penetration. Despite this, many studies have reported severe blunt and penetrating injuries from this type of weapon (6–12). There are also larger fin stabilized rounds that have improved aerodynamics and a longer effective range. Finally, there are rubber baton rounds, designed to be fired from a 37- or 40-mm launcher, which carry more mass than rubber balls and typically come in singles or triplets (13). Most of the rubber bullets, fin stabilized rounds, and rubber batons are meant to be fired low on the body or skip fired (aimed at the ground and skipped up into the target) to increase dispersion and decrease the risk of injury. A variation of the rubber bullet is the hand thrown grenade that fragments into small rubber pieces dispersed in a 360-degree pattern. This device may be useful for crowd control situations or deployment into a room where direct target acquisition is not feasible, and these have also been combined with chemical irritants to increase pain and thus increase compliance.

A variation on the rubber impact weapons, "wood baton" rounds are much harder and have an increased risk of inflicting damage if used improperly. They are also designed to be skip fired, which spreads them out making the injury pattern broader and also slows them down to decrease the chance of injury. Some jurisdictions have limited their use to defeat windows and obstacles rather than use to gain suspect control.

Newer impact devices have been developed using foam that can be spin stabilized, which allows for greater control at distances. The density of foam can be altered to find the best compromise between stopping power and lethality.

They are typically designed to be fired at large muscle groups, such as the legs or buttocks, which may lead to simple hematomas or bruising but rarely cause significant injury. Certainly, if they penetrate the skin they can cause deeper injuries to blood vessels, nerves, or other organs. If they hit a hard surface, such as bone, they may cause fractures and can cause blunt abdominal injury if fired into the abdomen. They can also cause significant injuries if they hit sensitive structures, such as the head, neck, or genitalia. Any person hit with an impact device needs to be evaluated for obvious penetrating injuries but occult blunt injury must be strongly considered as well. If there is any doubt, they should be transported to a medical facility where they can undergo diagnostic studies or observation for unapparent injuries.

ELECTROMUSCULAR DISRUPTION MUNITIONS

Electromuscular disruption (EMD) munitions (also known as conducted electrical weapons) use a very high voltage, low amperage electrical current to incapacitate a person based both on pain compliance and mechanical compliance. Modified types of EMDs include contact weapons, such as batons, in which contact with electrodes on the end of the device causes the shock, as well as distance weapons in which two electrodes are fired from the end of the weapon and can travel up to 35 feet and deliver the charge from a distance. EMD devices cause tetanic contractions in the skeletal muscles between the electrodes, removing most if not all voluntary control of those muscles. This loss of control is part of its effectiveness but it is also associated with a great deal of pain during the shock. Serious injuries with EMD devices are rare. The actual amount of electrical energy delivered is quite low. Although the voltage delivered can be up to 50,000 volts, the amperage is very low, giving a total wattage of 7 to 26 watts. Standard monophasic cardiac defibrillators operate at 50 to 360 joules, whereas the energy delivered by the most powerful EMD devices is around 1 to 2 joules per pulse.

Despite this low amount of energy delivered, there have been several instances where deaths have occurred after

▶ **TABLE 5.1.** Summary of Electrical Characteristics of Various Conducted Energy Weapons.

Electromuscular Disruption	Pulse Rate	Voltage	Current	Energy (into load)
Taser X26E	19	50,000	2.1 mA	0.07 J
Taser M26	15–20	50,000	3.6 mA	0.50 J
Stinger	20–22	7,000	56 mA	0.02 J
LEA MP1 Stun Pistol	20	7,150	34.7 mA	0.08 J

Data obtained from Taser. www.taser.com/law/download/specs.htm. Accessed May 1, 2006; Stinger Systems. Stinger Systems. www.stingersystems.com/Docs/Stinger_Specs.pdf. Accessed May 1, 2006; Law Enforcement Associates Inc. LEA Stun Gun. www.leacorp.com/lesslethal.asp. Accessed May 1, 2006.

the use of EMD devices. Advocates of EMD devices have shown that these deaths, while temporally close to the use of these devices, share characteristics with other "in-custody deaths." Most deaths in the literature have been attributed to a medical state described as "excited delirium," the combination of an altered sensorium and the use of stimulants such as cocaine, which seems to significantly increase the risk of death in police custody. There is currently strong debate about the role of EMD devices in these deaths. Several studies have examined the physiological effects of these devices with no conclusive data linking these weapons to the reported deaths (14,15). Further studies must be done to determine the exact cause of death in these patients and the safety of EMD devices in this population (Table 5.1).

Although death and significant electrical injuries are rare after the use of EMDs, a number of other injuries must be considered and anticipated after the deployment of an EMD device, especially those that use fired probes. For example, products from Taser International, the most popular model presently used in U.S. law enforcement, use a probe that resembles the barb of a standard Eagle Claw #8 fishhook. The probes are approximately 0.3 to 0.5 inches long and have a barbed tip to help them stay in place after deployment. They can cause severe injuries if they strike a sensitive location such as the eye (16). If a probe is imbedded near an eye or major blood vessel or anywhere in the neck, groin, or female breast, it should be stabilized in place and the person transported to the nearest medical center for evaluation and possible surgical removal. Otherwise, the probe can be removed by tightening the surrounding skin with one hand and by pulling the probe straight out in a swift, smooth motion with the other hand. The wound should be cleaned and bandaged. The probes should be inspected to confirm they are intact and then secured in a sharps container and given to the appropriate authority for evidence. Other injuries must also be considered.

When a person is standing and has an EMD device used on them, they may fall and sustain other injuries. They should be evaluated and treated as any other fall from standing. Pregnant women must be immediately evaluated at a medical center as miscarriage has been reported following EMD device use (17). Certainly, any person who appears to be exhibiting signs of excited delirium (e.g., bizarre or aggressive behavior, shouting, paranoia, panic, hallucinations) or who complains of chest pain, shortness of breath, or severe headache needs to be evaluated by a medical professional.

CHEMICAL MUNITIONS

Chemical munitions have been in use for over 2,000 years. Currently there are only a few options routinely used and available in law enforcement operations. The most widely used chemical munitions are 2-chlorobenzalmalononitrile (CS), chloroacetophenone (CN), and oleoresin capsicum or "pepper spray" (OC). Although their specific characteristics are different, all of these chemical agents are designed to achieve suspect compliance through significant pain compliance.

CN is a lacrimator that causes profuse tearing associated with blepharospasm and irritation. It also causes painful irritation to other mucous membranes, such as the nose and respiratory tract, as well as exposed skin. As with other agents, CN causes profuse rhinorrhea, sneezing, hypersalivation, chest tightness, dyspnea, and nausea. The effects of CN occur within seconds of exposure and can produce significant psychological effects including panic and confusion. CN use has dramatically decreased over the last decade due to increasing concerns about its safety profile.

CS was developed later and is becoming much more popular due to its increased potency and decreased toxicity over CN. Known colloquially as "tear gas," CS is actually a solid at room temperature and usually dispersed as a fine powder. CS is primarily an irritator, and although it also causes eye irritation and blepharospasm, it can often be overcome by a determined individual. The onset of skin and respiratory symptoms, however, can be more intense with CS than CN and also occurs within seconds of exposure.

OC is an inflammatory agent with similar effects to CS and CN. It is derived from the plant-based chemical capsaicin found in chili plants. It is usually in a liquid form and although its effects also begin within seconds of exposure, they persist longer, up to 45 to 60 minutes.

Deaths have been reported from each of these agents. Aside from their intended short-term irritating effects, they have been shown to produce other adverse outcomes. Direct eye injury, respiratory compromise, contact dermatitis, and burns have been reported; however, these are all rare (18–29). People exposed to these chemicals should be treated like any other chemical exposure. Effective treatment is fresh air, preferably with a slight breeze to vaporize and disperse the chemical. Washing the chemical off with water can cause increased symptoms initially as the agent is solubilized but can effectively remove the agent from the body surface and shorten the duration of effect.

Several solutions have been described to help ameliorate the effects of chemical agents. A solution of water and 5% sodium bisulfite may be effective against powder agents, because the alkalinity of the solution increases solubility but is often not needed if a sufficient supply of water is available. A chemical decontaminant Diphoterine has been shown to be effective in immediately decontaminating soldiers voluntarily exposed to CS and has also been shown to prevent its ocular and dermal effects if applied prior to exposure (30). For oily products, such as OC, anecdotal reports indicate that a mixture of water, sugar, and baby shampoo may be effective. The baby shampoo and sugar act as an emulsifier to help rid the exposed surface of the chemical agent.

If a suspect exposed to one of these chemicals must be transported to a medical facility, they should be at least grossly decontaminated and their clothing removed if possible prior to arrival to the facility. Several instances of medical personnel getting contaminated after transport have occurred.

Prior to deployment of these chemicals, a risk assessment must be done to assure safety of the team as well as bystanders in surrounding areas. TEMS providers may be asked by team commanders to render an opinion regarding the potential adverse effects of chemical agents. Consideration must be given to wind speed and direction to avoid spread of the gas to areas, such as nursing homes, daycares, and schools, as well as areas where team members may be staged without proper protective equipment (31).

CONCLUSIONS

The use of pain to induce compliance of an aggressive or violent suspect is as old as policing itself. Recently, specialty munitions have been developed as part of the force armamentarium to increase the safety of tactical operators and to decrease risk of injury to suspects. When used properly, the risks of injury are lower than lethal means, such as firearms, but they may cause serious and even fatal injury. TEMS providers must anticipate and search for these injuries when appropriate.

REFERENCES

1. Charles A, Asensio J, Forno W, et al. Penetrating bean bag injury: intrathoracic complication of a nonlethal weapon. *J Trauma*. 2002;53(5):997–1000.
2. Grange JT, Kozak R, Gonzalez J. Penetrating injury from a less-lethal bean bag gun. *J Trauma*. 2002;52:576–578.
3. de Brito D, Challoner KR, Sehgal A, et al. The injury pattern of a new law enforcement weapon: the police bean bag. *Ann Emerg Med*. 2001;38:383–390.
4. Olivas T, Jones B, Canulla M. Abdominal wall penetration by a police "bean bag." *Am Surg*. 2001;67:407–409.
5. Suyama J, Panagos PD, Sztajnkrycer MD, et al. Injury patterns related to use of less-lethal weapons during a period of civil unrest. *J Emerg Med*. 2003;25:219–227.
6. Kalebi A, Olumbe AK. Death following rubber bullet wounds to the chest: case report. *East Afr Med J*. 2005;82:382–384.
7. Petrov SV, Bogdanov AS, Utochkin AA, et al. Blunt non-penetrating wounds to the chest and abdomen with non-standard injuring shells [Article in Russian]. *Vestn Khir Im I I Grek*. 2004;163:60–61.
8. Lavy T, Asleh SA. Ocular rubber bullet injuries. *Eye*. 2003;17:821–824.
9. Mahajna A, Aboud N, Harbaji I, et al. Blunt and penetrating injuries caused by rubber bullets during the Israeli-Arab conflict in October, 2000: a retrospective study. *Lancet*. 2002;359:1795–1800.
10. Roux FE, Mejdoubi M. Potential neurosurgical damage of rubber bullets. Analysis of 2 pediatric cases. *Neurochirurgie*. 2001;47:576–579.
11. Balouris CA. Rubber and plastic bullet eye injuries in Palestine. *Lancet*. 1990;335:415.
12. Cohen MA. Plastic bullet injuries of the face and jaws. *S Afr Med J*. 1985;68:849–852.
13. Chute DJ, Smialek JE. Injury patterns in a plastic (AR-1) baton fatality. *Am J Forensic Med Pathol*. 1998;19:226–229.
14. Ho JD, Miner JR, Lakireddy DR, et al. Cardiovascular and physiologic effects of conducted electrical weapon discharge in resting adults. *Acad Emerg Med*. 2006; In press.
15. Jauchem JR, Sherry CJ, Fines DA, et al. Acidosis, lactate, electrolytes, muscle enzymes, and other factors in the blood of Sus scrofa following repeated TASER((R)) exposures. *Forensic Sci Int*. 2005; In press.
16. Ng W, Chehade M. Taser penetrating ocular injury. *Am J Ophthalmol*. 2005;139:713–715.
17. Mehl LE. Electrical injury from Tasering and miscarriage. *Acta Obstet Gynecol Scand*. 1992;71:118–123.
18. Leyland M. CS gas injury to the eye. *Eye*. 1997;11:428–429.
19. Gundorova RA, Khotim VE, Makarov PV, et al. Eye lesions from the contents of tear gas canisters and treatment methods. *Vestn Oftalmol*. 1996;112:55–56.
20. Thomas RJ, Smith PA, Rascona DA, et al. Acute pulmonary effects from o-chlorobenzylidenemalonitrile "tear gas": a unique exposure outcome unmasked by strenuous exercise after a military training event. *Mil Med*. 2002;167:136–139.
21. Varma S, Holt PJ. Severe cutaneous reaction to CS gas. *Clin Exp Dermatol*. 2001;26:248–250.
22. Bayeux-Dunglas MC, Deparis P, Touati MA, et al. Occupational asthma in a teacher after repeated exposure to tear gas. *Rev Mal Respir*. 1999;16:558–559.
23. Worthington E, Nee PA. CS exposure–clinical effects and management. *J Accid Emerg Med*. 1999;16:168–170.
24. Treudler R, Tebbe B, Blume-Peytavi U, et al. Occupational contact dermatitis due to 2-chloracetophenone tear gas. *Br J Dermatol*. 1999;140:531–534.
25. Sommer S, Wilkinson SM. Exposure-pattern dermatitis due to CS gas. *Contact Dermatitis*. 1999;40:46–47.
26. Vaca FE, Myers JH, Langdorf M. Delayed pulmonary edema and bronchospasm after accidental lacrimator exposure. *Am J Emerg Med*. 1996;14:402–405.

27. Anderson PJ, Lau GS, Taylor WR, et al. Acute effects of the potent lacrimator o-chlorobenzylidene malononitrile (CS) tear gas. *Hum Exp Toxicol*. 1996;15:461–465.

28. Zekri AM, King WW, Yeung R, et al. Acute mass burns caused by o-chlorobenzylidene malononitrile (CS) tear gas. *Burns*. 1995;21:586–589.

29. Hu H, Christiani D. Reactive airways dysfunction after exposure to teargas. *Lancet*. 1992;339:1535.

30. Viala B, Blomet J, Mathieu L, et al. Prevention of CS "tear gas" eye and skin effects and active decontamination with Diphoterine: preliminary studies in 5 French Gendarmes. *J Emerg Med*. 2005;29:5–8.

31. Horton DK, Burgess P, Rossiter S, et al. Secondary contamination of emergency department personnel from o-chlorobenzylidene malononitrile exposure, 2002. *Ann Emerg Med*. 2005;45:655–658.

Chapter 6

Medical Support of the Tactical Athlete

Brian L. Springer, Douglas M. Kleiner, and John M. Wightman

OBJECTIVES

After reading this section, the reader will be able to:

1. State the roles of the tactical medical provider (TMP) in advising operational commanders on team fitness and nutrition for peak performance.
2. Outline basic principles of physical training and be able to provide an exercise prescription for basic aerobic and strength maintenance for a tactical operator.
3. List the two basic types of fitness tests and identify components from each test that is useful assessing the tactical operator's physical readiness.
4. Identify common acute and overuse injuries seen in tactical operations and describe management in the field as well as appropriate follow-up and referral.

INTRODUCTION

The performance of tactical operations places tremendous physical demands on the human body. Medical personnel must themselves be in the best physical condition possible. They must also be prepared to support the health and fitness of team members during all phases of preparation for, execution of, and recovery from tactical missions. The dangers inherent in these operations demand no less than peak mental and physical performance at all times. Failure to do so will, at best, complicate mission completion and, at worst, may jeopardize the safety of team members and civilians.

Tactical operators and their supporting tactical medical providers (TMPs) may be required to run, walk, or crawl long distances; avoid or scale multiple obstacles; climb stairwells or steep surfaces; or breach heavy barricades. In most cases, these tasks will be performed while wearing a heavy duty load, which may include a helmet, body armor, communications and weapon systems, ammunition, task-specific equipment, and medical supplies. Despite these necessary encumbrances, operators may—at a moment's notice—be required to deliver precise aimed fire, engage in hand-to-hand physical confrontation with an adversary, or move a hostage or bystander who cannot do so under their own power. In the event that an officer is incapacitated, a teammate may be required to drag or carry him or her—complete with their duty load—to safety.

Sports medicine is a very generic term. There are several disciplines within sports medicine, such as athletic training, exercise physiology, strength and conditioning, exercise science, biomechanics, kinesiology, sports nutrition, injury rehabilitation, physiological effects of human performance, motor learning, motor control, fitness, and wellness.

The term *tactical athlete* has been described in several sports medicine publications. It originated as a spin-off of the athletic trainers' campaign to include nontraditional occupations within their scope of practice by calling them "athletes" (e.g., the "industrial athlete"). Special weapons and tactics (SWAT) operators are often the most physically fit and the most physically active officers of the law enforcement agency; therefore, they are considered the "athletes" of the agency. Thus, these individuals are likely to sustain the same types of injuries as traditional athletes. The definition of an athlete is a person who is trained or skilled in exercises, sports, or games requiring physical strength, agility, or stamina. The tactical operator is unquestionably an athlete who requires these attributes for the successful completion of duties. To ensure mission safety and success, the TMP requires the knowledge and skills needed to maintain health and peak performance among team members and the ability to rapidly diagnose and treat athletic injury. These enable the TMP to advise the tactical commander on the fitness of human resources for the assigned duties and tasks expected of them.

PHYSICAL PERFORMANCE

Fitness

Regular exercise not only benefits the team member during the performance of duties, but provides for a healthier lifestyle. By promoting physical activity among all personnel, the TMP promotes wellness within the team, which leads to better performance of many tasks. There is also strong evidence that participation in regular exercise prevents work absenteeism through reduction of musculoskeletal complaints and sick days requested (1,2).

Some advantages of regular exercise are listed in Box 6.1 (3). A myriad of information on exercise benefits is available through the National Institutes of Health (*www.nlm.nih.gov/medlineplus/exerciseandphysicalfitness.html*). Another useful resource for the TMP is the Gatorade Sport Science Institute Web site (*www.gssiweb.com*), which is an excellent source of information on training, nutrition, and hydration. The American College of Sports Medicine (ACSM) Web site (*www.acsm.org*) contains links to consensus statements on the medical care of athletes.

BOX 6.1. Advantages of Regular Exercise.

Strengthening the cardiovascular and respiratory systems:
Regular exercise improves lipid profile, decreases the risk of coronary artery disease and hypertension, and enhances lung capacity.

Strengthening muscle and bone:
Weight-bearing exercise maintains muscle strength and bone density, which may prevent osteoporosis and falls associated with aging.

Weight management:
Exercise burns off excess calories, which would otherwise be deposited as fat and potentially lead to the development of obesity.

Prevention of diabetes:
By burning off blood glucose and helping maintain a proper weight, regular exercise can prevent the development of type-2 diabetes mellitus, which is linked to a myriad of health problems including heart and kidney diseases.

Stress management:
Regular exercise activates serotonin and norepinephrine in the brain helping to relieve stress and stave off depression. Endorphin release during exercise also helps alleviate mental stress.

Reduced cancer risk:
Regular exercise has been linked to reduced rates of prostate, breast, and colon cancers.

Improved sleep:
Regular exercise ensures proper sleep hygiene essential for maximal mental focus while on duty.

Exercise is defined as an activity by activated muscles that generate force. This includes all physical activities in tactical operations (e.g., running, crawling, climbing, pulling, physical manipulation of a weapon). Any exercise can be quantified by the physical characteristics of muscular action (4):

- *Force*: the product of an object's mass and the acceleration imparted to it
- *Work*: the product of force exerted on an object and the distance it moves (no time limit)
- *Power*: the amount of displacement (work) over time
- *Torque*: the degree to which force rotates an object around a fulcrum
- *Strength*: the maximal force that a muscle can generate at a specified velocity

General Strength and Endurance Training

The tactical officer may require any given combination of strength and endurance over a highly variable period of time. Exercise training as preparation for operations must encompass the development of muscular strength as well as cardiorespiratory endurance. The ultimate goal is the development and maintenance of a high degree of physical fitness. The ACSM's position stand, *The Recommended Quantity and Quality of Exercise for Developing and Maintaining Cardiorespiratory and Muscular Fitness, and Flexibility in Healthy Adults*, gives a detailed overview of the primary components of physical fitness (5).

- *Cardiorespiratory fitness*: the ability of the cardiovascular and respiratory systems to perform at aerobic (i.e., oxygen-consuming) capacity
- *Body composition*: the relative amounts of muscle, bone, and fat in the body, which is affected by the balance between cardiorespiratory and strength training
- *Muscular strength*: a muscle's ability to generate maximal force
- *Muscular endurance*: a muscle's ability to generate repetitive force
- *Flexibility*: the ability to move a joint or joints through a full range of motion

To carry out his or her role as a health advisor to the team, the TMP should have a fundamental understanding of how the human body performs during a physical challenge. The motor unit is the simplest functional component of muscle activity, consisting of the activating nerve—or motor neuron of the peripheral nervous system—and all of the muscle fibers that neuron innervates. Electrochemical impulses are transmitted from the central nervous system through the motor neuron to cause an all-or-nothing excitation at the motor endplate with contraction of those fibers.

Muscle fiber types can grossly be divided into type-1 (slow-twitch) fibers and type-2 (fast-twitch) fibers. Type-1 fibers rely predominantly on aerobic metabolism, which makes them resistant to fatigue, but they have a limited capability to produce high forces rapidly. Type-2 fibers rely primarily on anaerobic metabolism. They can generate high forces rapidly, but fatigue quickly. The type and intensity of activity determines the preferential recruitment of fibers (6). The degree of muscle force is dependent on the frequency of activation of the motor unit and the number of individual motor units that are recruited. Contraction of the fibers generates force that may be used to develop movement or resist movement against an external source (7).

Muscles involved in physical activity are arranged through a complex system of levers, wherein the various joints act as a fulcrum. Muscles are grouped into combinations of agonists and antagonists, with primary movement initiated by contraction of the agonist, and joint stabilization and braking of the limb controlled by contraction of the antagonist. Agonist/antagonist muscles will switch roles depending on the specific motion of the joint. Muscles are connected to bone either through direct attachment of muscle fibers or through fibrous connective tissue known as tendon. Ligaments are fibrous tissues that attach bone to bone and provide stability at the joint. Through highly coordinated contraction and relaxation of specific muscles and muscle groups, the human body is able to generate a variety of coordinated movement.

- *Concentric muscle action*: occurs when motor unit activation generates sufficient force to overcome resistive force resulting in muscle shortening where the opposite ends of the muscle are drawn toward one another

- *Eccentric muscle action*: occurs when resistive force exceeds the tension generated in the motor unit resulting in muscle lengthening

- *Isometric muscle action*: occurs when muscle force equals resistive force and there is no net change in muscle length

Strength is most often developed through resistance training, generating force against resistance provided by free weights, machines, or one's own body weight. This results in muscle hypertrophy (i.e., enlargement in muscle fiber mass, but not number). This occurs disproportionately among type-2 fibers. Aerobic conditioning is attained through endurance exercises such as running, biking, or swimming. Aerobic conditioning results in increased maximal oxygen uptake in the trained musculature, which allows the athlete to perform at a given intensity with greater ease. Additionally, both resistance and endurance training result in neural, endocrine, and vascular changes that facilitate performance of exercise.

The *exercise prescription* is a means of developing a basic exercise regimen aimed at achieving and maintaining an adequate level of general fitness. Exercise prescription is not designed to directly affect the ability to perform operational tasks, but rather serves as an indirect means to develop the physical abilities to enable the performance of tactical operations. The FITT mnemonic may be used for exercise prescription: frequency, intensity, type, and time. Recommendations for the performance of cardiorespiratory and strength training may be found in Table 6.1. These recommendations are tailored toward the concerns and needs of the tactical athlete.

TABLE 6.1. FITT Recommendations for Exercise Prescription (29).

	Cardiorespiratory Training	Strength Training
Frequency	Most individuals should engage in moderate-to-vigorous activity most days of the week.	Resistance training should be performed 2–3 times per week. It may be accomplished before, during, or after cardiovascular training.
Intensity	Intensity should be dictated by individual fitness goals, but a general goal is to maintain a heart rate in the range 70%–85% of the difference between 220 beats per minute minus age (in years).	For muscular strength training, at least one set of 8–12 repetitions for each major muscle group (minimum of 8 to separate exercises) should be performed with the goal of full fatigue by the last repetition.
Type	Type should be influenced by operational requirements. Most will consist of running. Bicycle-mounted law-enforcement officers should emphasize cycling. Rescue personnel may need to add climbing and swimming. Cross-training may be necessary for many (e.g., Marines), but can also alleviate the boredom of a routine. Injuries may require a different a temporary modification of exercise type to maintain cardiovascular fitness until returned to full duty.	Resistance training may be performed using free weights, weight machines, flexible-tubing apparatus, or a host of other manufactured equipment. However, gravity and body weight can serve the same purpose, and may have the advantage of direct correlation to task-specific training (e.g., pull-ups for raising one's body weight onto a roof). Adding duty load to some of these exercises will increase the resistance and add a sense of realism.
Time	Activity does not need to be consecutive, and may be divided throughout the day. Approximately 30–60 minutes of physical activity should be accumulated on most days of the week.	Increased number of sets for each major muscle group is not required. As the workout becomes more advanced, the individual may divide these workouts throughout the week (e.g., 1 day of chest and shoulders, 1 day of back and arms, and 1 day of hips and legs).

Stretching and maintenance of flexibility are poorly understood regarding their contribution to the prevention of injury. Certainly, recent evidence has shown that acute stretching prior to exercise can actually reduce performance (8). Controlled stretching of trained muscles should be accomplished several times weekly to ensure adequate muscular control through a useful range of motion. Extreme flexibility, although an aesthetic necessity in certain sports, is not a required attribute for the tactical athlete.

Task-Specific Training

Sports conditioning can be thought of as a pyramid. At the base is general athletic fitness, which makes up the bulk of training. Above this lies sport-specific athletic fitness, such as the ability to jump, sprint, and pull up one's body weight. At the peak are task-specific skills. In the case of tactical operations, these might include sprinting in full gear, handling a ram, or running a mile in full gear then being able to take an aimed shot (9).

Optimal general training for the tactical officer would be a combination of strength and endurance training, especially given that an operator may have to serve multiple roles in a given operation. An example would be comparing a breacher to a defensive lineman in football. Both perform tasks that are comparatively static, but require strength and proper leverage. A professional football team will usually have the option of specialty training a select group of individuals to fill the lineman role. A law enforcement SWAT team or infantry fire team may or may not have adequate personnel to do the same, and the hazards of the tactical environment may create a situation where a different, less specifically trained individual must fill that breacher role. Therefore, all team personnel must meet minimum strength and endurance requirements to provide depth as well as breadth to the group's ability to accomplish tasks necessary for mission accomplishment.

Training should concentrate on tasks the team members will perform. Specificity holds that training is most effective when exercises are similar to the activity in which improvement is sought. Although general fitness training should consist of whole-body exercise routines, supplementary exercises similar to the activity should be implemented to provide a training advantage (7). Some controversy remains, however, as to the use of weighted objects when performing tasks. Performing movements against resistance is useful for building strength, but will not necessarily improve performance of that specific movement when unburdened.

The most effective means to design a SWAT-specific or similar program is to individualize training regimens to the most common functions of the team. Reviewing previous missions can provide a valuable resource for training plans. For example, a team covering a relatively rural jurisdiction may find that missions require members to traverse long stretches of unimproved land. This may be done at a run, a controlled pace consistent with a patrol, or at a crawl when maximum concealment is required. Urban teams may find that they are more frequently climbing through windows, up stairs, and onto rooftops. These maneuvers should be practiced frequently while in full duty load.

Fitness Testing Standards

Some controversy exists as to ideal testing standards for tactical officers. However, many agree that operational fitness standards must meet several criteria to be considered reflective of job-related tasks. The content of the test must reproduce critical fitness-related functions of the specific job, be able to predict who can and cannot perform those functions, be based on scientific validity as evidenced by standards of care put forth by ACSM, and be nondiscriminatory with respect to age, sex, race, or physical handicap (10–12).

The two basic schools of thought revolve around the fitness test battery, as represented by the Cooper Institute for Aerobic Research's (CIAR) Law Enforcement Physical Fitness Test and job-task simulation, as represented by Operational Tactics' (OpTac) Operational Fitness Requirements for SWAT officers. The CIAR test examines the physical fitness components that are underlying factors for performance of specific tasks, whereas the OpTac examination has the officers perform the actual tasks most likely to occur during operations. Both tests (Tables 6.2 and 6.3) are designed to be administered in a specific order, and all team members are expected to pass all aspects of testing, regardless of age, sex, height, or weight.

Neither type of test provides a clear advantage. Although the fitness battery may have stronger scientific validity, it is still only predictive of overall operational performance. Job-task simulations may better represent specific abilities but fail to encompass a broader definition of fitness critical for the ever-changing tactical environment. The use of both standards to evaluate the abilities of tactical operators is recommended.

Regardless of assessment type, each individual should be tested for adherence to accepted standards on a routine and predetermined basis. A fitness battery should be administered at least annually and preferably semiannually or quarterly to ensure the operator is adequately physically fit. A task-specific battery should be administered at least semiannually, but preferably quarterly during each season, because clothing and tactical gear may vary with environmental conditions. Operators who fail any portion of their fitness test should be given at least 4 weeks to train and prepare before being required to retake and pass the entire test. A second failure should mandate referral up the chain of command and consideration of light-duty status until a decision on fitness for full duty is made.

▶ **TABLE 6.2.** Cooper Institute for Aerobics Research Physical Fitness Test for Public Safety.*

Test Component	Rationale
Vertical jump	Tests anaerobic power and explosive leg power; highly predictive of ability for sprinting and dodging, jumping and vaulting
1-minute sit-up	Tests core body muscular endurance; predictive of ability for lifting and carrying, dragging/pulling/pushing, crawling, short (<2 minutes) and prolonged (>2 minutes) use of force
300 meter run	Tests anaerobic power; highly predictive of ability for sprinting and dodging
Maximum push-up or bench press	Push-up tests upper body muscular endurance, predictive of ability for lifting/carrying, dragging/pulling/pushing, crawling, and use of force. Bench press test muscular strength, highly predictive of same
1.5 mile run	Tests aerobic capacity; highly predictive of ability for sustained pursuit, prolonged (>2 minutes) use of force

*Scoring based on absolute standards (single cutpoints) determined in law enforcement validation studies as fitness standard that must be attained by everyone regardless of age, gender, or handicap. Cooper Institute for Aerobics Research has validated minimal fitness requirements for multiple federal, state, and municipal agencies.

Nutrition and Hydration

Nutrients serve three basic functions in the human body: energy production, tissue growth and repair, and regulation of physiological processes. The greatest concerns to the tactical athlete during operations will be energy production as well as regulation of performance and temperature homeostasis through fluid consumption. Fuel use is ultimately determined by the intensity and duration of the exercise performed. Energy from exercising muscle comes from three main sources: the phosphagen system, the nonoxidative system, and the oxidative system. The end result of all three is the generation of adenosine triphosphate (ATP), which when broken down, provides the energy required for muscle contraction.

Metabolic Fuels

The phosphagen system converts ATP to adenosine diphosphate (ADP) releasing energy in the process. ADP is converted back to ATP by creatine phosphatase. This system is anaerobic (i.e., requires no oxygen), provides all-out muscle contraction for approximately 5 seconds, and is limited by presence of the substrate creatine.

The nonoxidative system is also anaerobic, generating ATP from the breakdown of readily available sugars (through a process called glycolysis) or of the body's carbohydrate stores (through a process called glycogenolysis), thereby providing additional anaerobic energy for high-intensity activity up to 2 minutes. A by-product of nonoxidative metabolism is the generation of lactic acid, which

▶ **TABLE 6.3.** Operational Tactics Operational Fitness Requirements for SWAT Officers.*

Test Component	Rationale
1-mile run in 12 minutes or less	Represents reasonable distance officer could be expected to run on a tactical operation
60-yard run carrying one-person ram or 45-lb dumbbell, wearing gas mask, in 15 seconds or less	Reasonable task in order to breach a door or deliver ram to assigned breacher
30-yard low-crawl wearing gas mask, within 60 seconds	Practical distance to crawl into a perimeter position or intelligence-gathering position
Climb 6-ft fence unassisted within 10 seconds	Reasonable task required to prevent undue delay on-scene
5 vertical raises (pull-ups)	Demonstrates officer's ability to pull themselves onto ledges, balconies, and rooftops on multiple occasions during operations
5 vertical pushes (dips)	Demonstrates officer's ability to push themselves onto barriers, small fences, ledges, decks, and balconies on multiple occasions during operations
Climb eight flights of stairs (four floors) carrying 1-person ram or 45-lb dumbbell, within 30 seconds	Elevators may not be available/practical; reasonable task in order to breach a door or deliver ram to assigned breacher
Move heaviest team member 20 yards within 40 seconds	Demonstrate ability to perform officer rescue on all team members while in full-gear

*Test performed in order shown. Officers must wear full SWAT gear including tactical footwear. One-mile run performed carrying assigned unloaded shoulder-fired weapon system.

is thought to be a component of fatigue either through a direct effect on the muscle or through pH-mediated central nervous system effects (13).

The oxidative system is aerobic (i.e., requires oxygen) and is the main source of ATP at rest and during prolonged, low-intensity, endurance activity. The primary fuel sources are carbohydrates and fat. Oxygen consumption is tightly correlated with exercise intensity, and so the maximal ability of the body to extract and use oxygen during exercise is often used as a measure of endurance ability. This may be identified by the scientific term *VO$_2$max* in published literature.

As a general rule, exercise at or greater than 70% of maximal effort is fueled predominantly by glucose and glycogen, whereas lower levels are fueled by glycogen and fat. The longer the duration of the exercise, the greater the use of fat, accounting for 60% to 70% of energy for moderate activity lasting 4 to 6 hours. Muscle glycogen stores are usually depleted after 90 minutes of moderate-to-high intensity exercise, but a high level of training enhances the body's ability to preferentially burn fat, known as the glycogen-sparing effect.

For optimal performance, the majority of the athlete's diet should be carbohydrate-based (14,15). The athlete undergoing regular training sessions requires approximately 55 cal/kg/day. Carbohydrates should provide 60% to 70% of the total caloric intake or 6 to 10 g of carbohydrates per kilogram each day. Current fad diets that limit carbohydrate intake have no role for the tactical operator, and such diets may limit athletic and mission performance (16). Small carbohydrate feedings of about 30 to 60 g/hour during exercise lasting longer than 1 hour may improve performance. A beverage containing no more than 5% to 8% of carbohydrates is ideal. Greater amounts may impede gastric emptying. After exercise completion, consumption of carbohydrate (1.5 g/kg within 30 minutes, followed by an additional 1.5 g/kg within 2 hours) aids in repletion of glycogen stores.

Protein is essential for strength training, because its constituent amino acids provide substrate for synthesis of contractile muscle proteins. In endurance training, protein promotes increased concentrations of oxygen-carrying hemoglobin and myoglobin, as well as oxidative enzymes in the energy-generating mitochondria of individual cells. Protein intake of 1.2 to 1.4 g/kg/day will meet the needs of most athletes, although heavy strength-training athletes may need up to 1.7 g/kg/day. In most cases, the increased caloric demands of training result in an adequately increased intake of protein.

Fat should account for no more than 30% of total calories. A well-rounded diet consisting of adequate amounts of fruits and vegetables will meet the needs of vitamins and minerals. Vitamin supplements are rarely needed, except in cases of dietary restriction.

Nutritional supplements have become a multibillion dollar industry. Under the 1994 Dietary Supplements Health and Education Act, it is the burden of the Food and Drug Administration to prove that a product labeled as a supplement is harmful rather than the product demonstrate safety and efficacy prior to marketing. Studies backing claims of performance enhancement are usually poorly designed, lack adequate controls, and derive erroneous conclusions (17). As a general rule, the tactical officer should not believe any nutritional claims on dietary supplements or by those trying to sell a product or promote a diet (16).

Fluid and Electrolyte Balance

Hydration is critical for both the prevention of heat illness and ensuring maximal performance during operations. At rest, the average adult requires 2 of 3 L of water daily. Adults exercising in high heat may lose up to 2 L/hour. Body armor or chemical-biological-radiological personal protective equipment adds a tremendous heat burden that accelerates fluid loss. Sweat losses as little as 2% of body weight may significantly impair performance. Thirst is a poor indicator of hydration status, and many athletes replace only 30% to 50% of their fluid losses during exercise. Therefore, it is beneficial to regulate hydration by drinking according to schedule rather than thirst. During sweating, water losses are greater than electrolyte losses, but this is not a significant issue in most cases. The loss of 1 g of sodium through a 2lb sweat loss can be replaced by a balanced diet. However, during endurance exercise of 4 hours or longer, clinically important or life-threatening hyponatremia may result from excessive water intake, sodium loss, or both.

Previously published guidelines for hydration usually fail to consider the variability in the type, duration, and intensity of activity, environmental concerns, and differences in the individual athlete. The ACSM has recently revised their decade-old guidelines to address these concerns (18). They recommend the following:

■ Prehydrate with slow consumption of beverages (~5 to 7 mL/kg) beginning 4 hours prior to activity until dilute urine is produced.
■ Replacement of fluid during activity is guided by type, duration, and intensity of activity as well as environmental concerns; end goal is the maintenance of dilute urine output and prevention of >2% body weight reduction from baseline.
■ Recovery consumption of 1.5 L fluid for each kilogram of body weight lost during activity.

Water remains an appropriate beverage for fluid replacement in activities lasting less than 1 hour and for prolonged recovery when combined with consumption of normal meals. However, sport drinks containing electrolytes and carbohydrates are ideal for prehydration, maintenance, and rapid recovery. They are highly palatable, aid in preservation of glycogen stores, and help prevent dilutional hyponatremia.

The role of the TMP in providing appropriate nutrition and hydration recommendations cannot be overemphasized. An athletics-based nutritional balance with an emphasis on quality carbohydrates is required to provide the tactical operator with adequate energy stores during high-intensity operations. Operators often will forgo adequate fluid intake (to avoid the need to urinate during operations), yet even mild dehydration markedly affects performance. The TMP should ensure that enough fluids are being consumed during operations and should recommend a sports beverage be used in operations lasting longer than 1 hour.

THE CARE AND REHABILITATION OF INJURIES

Epidemiology of Injuries

Musculoskeletal athletic injuries are likely to be encountered by the TMP during both training and operations. The Casualty Care Research Center's database, although limited somewhat by low numbers, examined injury patterns based on operation type (19). They found that musculoskeletal trauma was a common cause of injury in 21% of high-risk warrant services, 29% of barricade and hostage-rescue situations, and 45% of civil disobedience-control operations.

A 2007 research paper was presented at the ACSM by the author of this chapter (DMK) entitled, "The Epidemiology of Injuries and Illnesses in SWAT Officers: The Tactical aAthlete." The purpose of this project was to produce descriptive data regarding the epidemiology of injuries and illnesses to tactical team members. The study design was a 12-month, prospective, observational design with a cohort of three SWAT teams in north Florida. However, the data set grew beyond the defined cohort due to multijurisdictional and mutual-aid agreements. These additional law enforcement officers present on the scene were not full-time members of the tactical teams studied and included support personnel or affiliates with other agencies. Descriptive statistics were used to describe the population and data. A total of 952 law enforcement officers (644 tactical officers) were observed from 17 different law enforcement agencies, during 47 missions (high-risk warrant service or call-outs involving barricaded suspects) and training, totaling 164.75 hours of mission activity. Injury surveillance data were collected with Injury Tracker (Montreal, Canada) ITPalm software, a commercially available athletic injury tracking software program. The medical profiles of every member of that agency's SWAT team was downloaded onto a Palm Personal Digital Assistant (PDA)

(Sunnyvale, CA), and any evaluations, treatments, procedures, or changes in the officer's condition were recorded on the PDA by the tactical medic/ certified athletic trainer (ATC) following each mission or training session. The results showed no "tactical" injuries (gunshot wounds, blast injuries, or knife wounds) were sustained during this observation period. A total of 13 injuries were sustained during the study period (0.078 injuries per hour). The injuries sustained by law enforcement officers during this period were musculoskeletal, small lacerations (not requiring suturing), or heat related illnesses, all of which occurred during training and were evaluated and treated by a CAT. The types of injuries sustained in training by these "tactical athletes" were remarkably similar to any other athletic practice or training setting involving physical activity. These unique descriptive data regarding the epidemiology of injuries and illnesses to SWAT team members illustrates the need for, and cost savings as a result of, medical support provided by medical personnel with knowledge and training in sports medicine.

Athletic injury can be divided into acute and subacute/chronic. Acute injuries include sprains of muscle or tendon, strains of ligaments, and contusions of both soft issue and bone. Subacute and chronic injuries are more related to overuse and include tendinosis and repetitive-stress injuries. Tactical operators who sustain any of these injuries require careful evaluation and treatment to ensure they remain capable of carrying out their assigned duties. Enabling them to make a full and uneventful recovery is another important goal of timely and accurate identification and management of potentially disabling injuries.

Orthopedic Assessment

Because many injuries to the tactical athlete are orthopaedic in nature, the orthopaedic evaluation is critical. Many physicians utilize the HOPS method of assessment, which stands for history, observation, palpation, and special tests. Medic level TEMS providers might use a more generic pneumonic for assessment, such as signs and symptoms, allergies, medications, post history, last meal, events (SAMPLE), or even deformities, contusions, abrasions, punctures-burns, tenderness, lacerations, swelling (DCAP-BTLS), pulse, motor, sensation (PMS), and maybe even "the 6 Ps" (pain, pallor, paralysis, paresthesia, pressure, pulses).

We believe that a thorough assessment is the key to a good evaluation. We like the following seven steps:

1. History
2. Observation/inspection
3. Bony palpation
4. Soft palpation
5. Range of motion
6. Neuro (dermatomes/myotomes/reflexes)

7. Special tests (dependent on knowledge base/skills of TMP performing assessment)

History is always the first and most important step in the process. With orthopedic injuries, a good historian can describe "classic" signs, such as crepitus in the knee after sitting for prolonged periods. A good history should include the mechanism of injury such as falling on an outstretched arm, signs and symptoms, and range of motion limitations.

Acute Injury

Shoulder

The shoulder is the most mobile joint in the human body, which places it at risk for traumatic injury. Stability of the shoulder is provided by the joint capsule, cartilaginous labrum, glenohumeral ligaments, and the muscles of the rotator cuff. Stability of the shoulder girdle is essential to the tactical officer; impairment of the shoulder will affect ability to climb, crawl, breach, operate a weapon system, and engage in open-hand combat.

Injury to the shoulder often occurs when external force is applied to the shoulder, either directly or indirectly. An example of direct force is an officer who attempts to breach a minor barricade with the point of the shoulder, injuring the acromioclavicular joint (ACJ). Indirect injury may occur when an officer attempts to tackle a subject with an outstretched arm, where the arm acts as a lever and forces the humeral head anterior. Traction on the brachial plexus may result in a temporary "dead arm" or the shoulder may dislocate completely.

Examination of the shoulder begins with observation, looking for obvious asymmetry or deformity. Feel for distal pulses, and check sensation along the extremity. Carefully palpate the shoulder girdle and ACJ for tenderness. Have the officer move the shoulder through a full range of motion, and then assess shoulder strength against resistance. Extreme limitations of motion should raise suspicion for acute fracture or anterior dislocation, and the joint should be immobilized pending radiographic analysis. TMPs comfortable with on-field reduction of anterior dislocation may attempt the procedure, but the officer should be immobilized following. Swelling and tenderness over the ACJ may indicate a fracture or separation. ACJ separations can be quite painful, and the officer should be placed in a sling for comfort and referred for radiographic evaluation. Fractures and first-time or recurrent dislocations should be referred to an orthopedic surgeon.

Recovery from acute shoulder injury is highly variable. Fractures within the shoulder girdle and complete dislocations often require prolonged immobilization and can take 6 to 8 weeks to heal. Rehabilitation from sprains, strains, and subluxation should be treated with initial sling immobilization for comfort, followed by early mobilization. After full range of motion has returned, a gradual strength training program using light weight or elastic bands is appropriate. During the recovery phase, the officer may perform light duties, but should not be placed back into active training until the following criteria are met:

- Full range of motion
- Strength within at least 75% of normal as compared to the opposite arm
- Subjective feeling of "confidence" in shoulder (i.e., the operator feels the affected joint is close to or completely back to normal)

Skill-specific rehabilitation may then be employed. Allow the officer to return to training, with progression of activities such as running, climbing, shooting, and grappling. Ensure the officer is capable of performing all assigned duties (both a fitness battery and job-task simulation testing are appropriate at this time).

Hand and Wrist

Hand and wrist injuries may occur secondary to falls, collisions with individuals or obstacles, and impact from thrown or launched objects and projectiles. Loss of function of the wrist, hand, or fingers may dramatically compromise the operator's abilities and extreme caution should be used in evaluation of these injuries. The TMP should maintain a low threshold for early specialist referral.

The scaphoid is the most frequently fractured carpal bone, most often due to falling on an outstretched hand (20). Due to its distal to proximal blood supply, scaphoid fractures are at high risk for nonunion. This injury should be suspected following a fall or contusion when tenderness is elicited in the anatomic snuffbox. Nondisplaced fractures may not be radiographically present for up to 2 weeks. Immobilize the wrist in a SPICA splint and ensure early follow-up. When fracture is suspected in spite of normal films, MRI or bone scan may be used to detect injury (21).

Tear of the ulnar collateral ligament of the thumb is referred to as Gamekeeper's thumb or Skier's thumb. Injury occurs due to fall on an outstretched hand with the thumb abducted or when the thumb is forcibly abducted, which may occur when grappling.

Examination reveals point tenderness on the ulnar aspect of the metacarpal phalangeal joint. Marked laxity of the joint, especially in comparison to the unaffected hand, may indicate a complete rupture, which mandates early referral to a hand specialist for surgical repair.

Common injuries to the distal interphalangeal (DIP) include mallet finger and jersey finger. Mallet finger occurs following impact to the tip of an extended finger with sudden forceful flexion of the joint that disrupts the extensor tendon. The operator will be unable to actively extend their DIP. Radiographs should be obtained to see if there is an associated avulsion fracture of the distal phalanx. Markedly displaced fractures or fractures involving >25% of the articular surface may require surgery. Otherwise, the DIP will need to remain splinted in flexion for a minimum of 6 weeks.

Jersey finger occurs from hyperextension of the DIP while actively flexing. Disruption of the flexor digitorum profundus results in an inability to actively flex the DIP joint. This may occur when an operator, in an attempt to tackle or throw an individual, gets their finger caught in that individual's clothing. Radiographs should be taken to look for avulsion fractures or other injury. Most cases of jersey finger will require operative repair, and early referral to an orthopedic surgeon is warranted.

Knee

The knee joint contains four bones: femur, tibia, fibula, and patella. The joint is stabilized against varus and valgus force by the medial and lateral collateral ligaments. Anterior translation of the tibia relative to the femur is checked by the anterior cruciate ligament (ACL); conversely, the posterior cruciate ligament (PCL) prevents posterior tibial translation. The medial and lateral menisci serve as cartilaginous bumpers within the joint, while providing stability during extremes of flexion, extension, and rotation.

Knee injuries occur secondary to twisting movements (with or without contact) and high-energy impact. A detailed history of the injury will assist in generating a differential diagnosis (22). Sudden changes in direction with the foot planted may cause sprain or rupture of the collateral ligaments or ACL, as well as meniscal tears. Abrupt hyperextension, especially when landing from height, may cause ACL rupture. Fall onto a flexed knee may cause sprain or rupture of the PCL.

Ask the position of the knee (flexed or extended) and the foot (free or planted) at the time of injury. Inquire as to the development of an effusion following the injury, and if the officer has subjective complaints of the knee "giving way" or otherwise feeling unstable. Inspect the knee looking obvious bruising or presence of a joint effusion. Check active range of motion, and palpate carefully for areas of soft tissue or bony tenderness.

If suspicion for a fracture is high, radiographs should be obtained at this time prior to further examination. Otherwise, stability of the knee should be checked relative to varus, valgus, anterior, and posterior stress. The Ottawa Knee Rules are a validated clinical decision rule that can be applied in the field (23). Obtain a radiograph in traumatic knee injury when any of the following is present:

- Age older than 55 years
- Inability to bear weight for four steps
- Tenderness over the head of the fibula or over the patella
- Inability to flex the knee to 90 degrees

Any officer with evidence of instability or effusion should be referred to a sports medicine specialist for further evaluation.

The greatest danger knee injuries pose to the tactical officer is instability and the risk of the knee "giving out" during operations. Even following the return of full strength and range of motion, traumatic forces on the knee may cause buckling with the officer going down and unable to continue operations. The use of a brace can provide adequate stability in cases of collateral or PCL injury; meniscal injury and ACL tear most often necessitate surgical repair prior to return to full duty.

Ankle

Ankle injuries are common in active adults. Ankle sprains account for 25% of all sports-related injuries (24). The ankle is composed of two joints; the talotibial joint is formed by the tibia, fibula, and talus; it allows for plantarflexion and dorsiflexion of the foot. The subtalar joint is formed by the talus and the calcaneus; it allows for inversion and eversion of the ankle. The ankle is stabilized by a complex of ligaments laterally and medially, as well as by a fibrous syndesmosis that secures the distal tibia and fibula.

Injury most often occurs by forced inversion of the foot, resulting in damage to the lateral ligaments. This may occur when ambulatory on an uneven surface or when landing from a jump. Forced eversion may stress the medial ligaments and, when combined with rotation of the foot, may injure the syndesmosis. Concurrent fracture is commonly seen at the distal tibia or fibula or at the base of the fifth metatarsal. The Ottawa foot/ankle rules are an effective means of screening who needs radiographic analysis and can be used by the TMP in the field (25). The officer should be sent for films, if any of the following are present:

- Inability to walk for steps at time of injury or time of evaluation
- Tenderness over the posterior lateral or medial malleolus
- Tenderness over the base of the fifth metatarsal
- Tenderness over the tarsal navicular

The goal of initial treatment is the reduction of pain and swelling. Application of ice and elevation of the extremity may provide analgesia and reduce soft tissue swelling. Crutches may be required initially, but weight bearing should be encouraged as early as possible. Range of motion should re-established early, and after the officer is ambulatory, strength training with elastic bands is appropriate. Athletic tape or a lace-up brace may be required during rehabilitation to maintain stability in the sprained ankle. After the officer has full strength and range of motion, functional training can commence. Ligaments are slow to heal, so bracing during activity should continue for several months, pending reevaluation.

It should be emphasized that should the officer sustain an ankle sprain during operations, and if that officer's role can not be readily filled, the tactical boot should remain on and tightly laced to provide compression and stability. Following operations, the boot may be removed, ice applied, and the officer examined in detail.

Subacute and Chronic Injuries

When the body's ability to heal is exceeded by repetitive stress, overuse injury occurs. In the subacute setting, an officer who pushes himself during a particularly strenuous operation may overstress a muscle-tendon unit or bone, with resultant weakness and soreness the following day. Most subacute injuries will resolve with several days of rest. Of greater concern is overuse injury that develops over weeks to months. This may be secondary to development of significant connective tissue pathology or of a stress fracture.

Tendinosis

The term *tendonitis*, which implies inflammatory change to the muscle–tendon unit has largely been discarded and replaced by the terms *tendinosis* or *tendinopathy*. Early overuse may encompass an inflammatory response, but chronic soft tissue injuries show histopathologic changes of tissue degeneration and cell death (26). Common sites of tendinopathy are in the rotator cuff muscles of the shoulder, the flexor and extensor muscle wads of the elbow, the patellar tendon of the knee, and the Achilles tendon of the ankle. Early intervention should consist of limitation of inciting activity, range of motion, and light resistance training. A nonsteroidal anti-inflammatory drug (NSAID) or acetaminophen is an appropriate analgesic. Assess the officer's ability to perform functional tasks prior to the return to duty. Treatment of these entities can be challenging, and the TMP should have a low threshold for referral to a specialist.

Stress Fractures

Stress fractures occur when microinjury to bone exceeds rate of repair. They most often develop over the course of weeks in parts of the body where bones are directly stressed by impact or are indirectly stressed by attached muscle. Common locations include the tarsal navicular, metatarsals, mid-to-distal tibia, femoral neck, sacrum, sternum, and proximal humerus (27). Common inciting activities include running (distance and speed) and weight training. There is usually a history of a recent increase in either activity duration or intensity. Early in the disease

process, the officer may complain of night pain following activity; as the injury progresses, pain will gradually impedes athletic activity as well as daily activities, such as walking. Physical findings usually reveal localized tenderness over the fracture site.

Radiographic abnormalities are not apparent until several weeks into the disease process, and may show only subtle signs such as elevation of the periosteum. Eventually, sclerosis of the bone becomes radiographically apparent, and a definite fracture line may appear. The TMP should have a low threshold for referring suspected stress fractures for radiographs. When clinical suspicion remains elevated, a bone scan or magnetic resonance imaging (MRI) can confirm the diagnosis prior to any radiographic change (28). In most cases, the officer needs to be withheld from high impact activities until the pain free; this is followed by a gradual progression of activities over several weeks to allow for skeletal adaptation. Exceptions, such as tarsal navicular or proximal fifth metatarsal stress fractures, are associated with high rates of nonunion and may require prolonged immobilization. Any suspected stress fracture should be managed by a specialist.

SPORTS MEDICINE PROFESSIONALS

An ATC is the most well-rounded, nonphysician sports medicine provider. The governing body for athletic trainers (the preferred term, as opposed to *trainers*, which can mean almost anything), is the National Athletic Trainers' Association (NATA). ATC are specialists in the care, prevention, and rehabilitation of athletic injuries. They have a variety of skills, most of which are "borrowed" from other disciplines (e.g., physical therapy, emergency medicine, massage therapy). The ATC credential requires a bachelor's degree.

Many physical therapists also have some sports training, although they are primarily trained in the rehabilitation of sports injuries and not necessarily in the management of acute injuries, such as trauma. There is a certificate of additional qualifications (certified clinical specialist) as a sports physical therapist, available from the American Physical Therapy Association.

Doctors of Chiropractic also have Diplomates of the American Chiropractic Board of Sports Physicians (DACBSP).

Doctors of medicine include allopathic physicians (MD) and osteopathic physicians (DOs). The physician's training in sports medicine is highly variable, depending on specialty. As a general rule, DOs have greater exposure to musculoskeletal care during medical school, but may or may not have continued exposure during specialized residency training. Subspecialization in primary care sports medicine is available through the American Board of Medical Specialties following completion of an approved fellowship. Orthopedic surgeons may specialize in surgical sports medicine following fellowship training.

SPORTS FITNESS PROFESSIONALS

In the "fitness" and "exercise" aspect of sports medicine, several private as well as nonprofit professional organizations certify individuals as fitness experts. Many of these are not credible. Those that are credible often have various layers of certifications ranging from the most basic to very well-respected credentials within the sports medicine community.

On the basic level, there are many well-known organizations that certify individuals as "personal trainers" or "fitness instructors." Many of these have been in existence for a long period of time and include entities, such as the American Council on Exercise, National Academy of Sports Medicine, and the Aerobic and Fitness Association of America, along with dozens more.

In addition to "personal trainers," many other lower-level and similar certifications exist, such as "aerobics instructor," "stretch trainer," and "group fitness leader." Most of these require only a basic certification examination and some can be obtained online.

The National Strength and Conditioning Association (NSCA) is one of the more scientifically respected organizations. NSCA offers several certifications to include the NSCA Certified Personal Trainer and the more prestigious Strength and Conditioning Specialist (CSCS). The CSCS credential requires a bachelor's degree.

The ACSM is arguably the most scientifically based and well-respected fitness organization in the country. ACSM offers a more medically based track and a fitness track for certification. The fitness track includes the ACSM Certified Personal Trainerand the ACSM Health/Fitness Instructor certifications.

Both the ACSM and the NSCA offer fellowship status to the most highly educated and advanced members of their organizations. A doctoral degree is required to be a fellow of the ACSM.

TAKE-HOME POINTS

1. TMPs must be able to advise operational commanders and other decision-makers on issues related to preventive medicine, overall health and nutrition, general physical fitness, and hydration schedules surrounding a variety of activities.
2. Components of physical training can be grossly divided into strength and aerobic fitness; the tactical environment demands that operators train both components to maintain operational readiness.

3. Neither the fitness test battery nor the job-task simulation should be considered alone as an ideal method of assessing operational readiness; a combination of both testing methods should be administered.
4. The TMP's role of in treatment of sports injuries should be immediate stabilization in the field, early mobilization and return to job-specific tasks, and prompt referral to higher care for any complicated injury.

SUMMARY

SWAT training and operations results in injury patterns similar to those seen in athletics. This is no surprise given the high degree of physicality required to carry out a tactical mission. TMPs will frequently be called on to evaluate and treat musculoskeletal injuries. Injury may occur during fitness training, mission training, or operations; regardless, proper diagnosis and treatment are essential in restoring the operator to duty as quickly as possible. By giving sound nutritional, hydration, and training guidance, the TMP helps to ensure team members achieve and maintain their highest levels of performance. Last, the TMP can help draft guidelines that will serve to assess operators' levels of fitness, and test their ability to perform mission-specific tasks.

REFERENCES

1. Van Amelsvoort LG, Spigt MG, Swaen GM, et al. Leisure time physical activity and sickness absenteeism: a prospective study. *Occup Med [Lond]*. 2006;56(3):210–212.
2. Hildebrandt VH, Bongers PM, Dul J, et al. The relationship between leisure time, physical activities and musculoskeletal symptoms and disability in worker populations. *Int Arch Occup Environ Health*. 2000;73:507–518.
3. Mayo Clinic Staff. *Exercise: 7 benefits of regular physical activity*. 26 July 2005. http://www.mayoclinc.com/health/exercise/HQ01676. Published 18 April, 2007.
4. Knuttgen HG. What is exercise? A primer for practitioners. *Physician Sports Med*. 2003;31:31–42.
5. Pollock ML, Gaesser GA, Butcher JD, et al. ACSM position stand on the recommended quantity and quality of exercise for developing and maintaining cardiorespiratory and muscular fitness, and flexibility in adults. *Med Sci Sports Exerc*. 1998;30:975–991.
6. Arnold P, Gentry M. Strength training: what the team physician needs to know. *Curr Sports Med Rep*. 2005;4:305–308.
7. Harman E. The biomechanics of resistance exercise. In: Baechle TR, Earle RW, eds. *Essentials of Strength and Conditioning*. Champaign, Illinois: National Strength and Conditioning Association; 2000: 25–56.
8. McNeal JR, Sands WA. Stretching for Performance Enhancement. *Curr Sports Med Rep*. 2006;5:141–146.
9. Herring SA, et al. The team physician and the conditioning of athletes for sports: a consensus statement 2007. http://www.aafp.org/online/en/home/clinical/publichealth/sportsmed/conditioning.html. Published 18 April 2007.
10. The Cooper Institute. Common questions asked about fitness for public safety. http://www.cooperinst.org/education/law_enforcement/law.cfm. Published 18 April 2007.
11. Brzycki M, Meyers SA. *SWAT Fitness*. Hagerstown, Maryland: Operational Tactics; 2003.

12. Brooks ME. Law enforcement physical fitness standards and Title VII. *FBI Law Enforcement Bulletin*. 2001;5:26–32.

13. Cairns SP. Lactic acid and exercise performance: culprit or friend? *Sports Med*. 2006;36:279–291.

14. Manore M. Exercise and the Institute Of Medicine Recommendations for Nutrition. *Curr Sports Med Rep*. 2005;4:193–198.

15. Manore M, Barr S, Butterfield G. American Dietetic Association: position of the American Dietetic Association, Dieticians of Canada, and the American College of Sports Medicine. Nutrition and athletic performance. *J Am Diet Assoc*. 2000;100:1543–1556.

16. Butler FK, Deuster PA. The ten commandments of nutrition: 2005. *J Spec Op Med*. 2005;5:34–42.

17. Pearce PZ. Sports supplements: a modern case of caveat emptor. *Curr Sports Med Rep*. 2005;4:171–178.

18. Sawka MN, Burke LM, Eichner ER, et al. American College of Sports Medicine position stand. Exercise and fluid replacement. *Med Sci Sports Exerc*. 2007;39:377–390.

19. Medical aspects of specific operations. In: Vayer JS, et al. *Protecting the Homeland: Emergency Medical Tactical Provider Program Student Manual*. US Immigration and Customs Enforcement, Federal Protective Service, Special Operations Division, Protective Medicine Branch; 2005:171–188.

20. Geissler WB. Carpal Fractures in Athletes. *Clin Sports Med*. 2001;20:167–188.

21. Brooks S, et al. The management of scaphoid fractures. *J Sci Med Sport*. 2005;8:181–189.

22. Solomon DH, Simel DL, Bates DW, et al. The rational clinical examination: does this patient have a torn meniscus or ligament of the knee? Value of the physical exam. *JAMA*. 2001;286:1610–1620.

23. Emparanza JI, Aginaga JR, et al. Validation of the Ottawa knee rules. *Ann Emerg Med*. 2001;38:364–368.

24. Mack RP. Ankle injuries in athletes. *Clin Sports Med*. 1982;1:71–84.

25. Steill IG, Greenberg GH, McKnight RD, et al. Decision rules for the use of radiography in acute ankle injuries: refinement and prospective validation. *JAMA*. 1993;269:1127–1132.

26. Maffulli N, Testa V, Capasso G, et al. Similar histopathological picture in males with achilles and patellar tendinopathy. *Med Sci Sports Exerc*. 2004;36:1470–1475.

27. Stanitski CL, McMaster JH, Scranton PE. On the nature of stress fractures. *Am J Sports Med*. 1978;6:391–396.

28. Gaeta M, Minutoli F, Scribano E, et al. CT and MR imaging findings in athletes with early tibial stress injuries: comparison with bone scintigraphy findings and emphasis on cortical abnormalities. *Radiology*. 2005; 235:553–561.

29. Armstrong LE, Brubaker PH, Whaley MH, et al, eds. *ACSM's Guidelines for Exercise Testing and Prescription Sixth Edition*. Maryland: American College of Sports Medicine; 2000.

Chapter 7

Medical Support to Military Operations on Urban Terrain

Frank L. Christopher

OBJECTIVES (Fig 7.1)

After reading this section, the reader will be able to:

1. Describe the unique challenges presented by MOUT operations.
2. Discuss strategies to mitigate those challenges.

HISTORICAL PERSPECTIVE

The population of the world is constantly evolving. Since the close of World War II (WWII), the percentage of the Earth's population that lives in urban areas has almost doubled from 28% in 1945 to 49% today. The trend of migration continues; by 2025, an estimated 58% will live in cities. Today, 1.5 billion people live in 887 different cities with a population of over 1 million each (1).

A continual rise in the number and concentration of urban areas, together with a stretching of infrastructure, limited resources, and unsteady economic bases has led, and will continue to lead, to a parallel increase in the number of armed conflicts occurring within densely populated areas (2). Although limited urban operations were conducted in WWII, Korea, and Vietnam, more recent events, most notably the invasions of Grenada and Panama, the 1993 actions in Mogadishu, and the latest actions in support of the global war on terrorism, have revolved largely around cities. In the United States, the vast majority of firearm homicides occur in urban areas, a statistic with significant tactical law enforcement implications (3).

Available literature on medical support to military operations in urban terrain (MOUT) is scant; a good overview was authored in 1999 by Colonel (later Major General) Lester Martinez-Lopez as an appendix to the Arroyo Center's working group report on urban operations (4). The landmark article by Butler, et al. in *Military Medicine* in 2000 (5–7) utilizes the Battle of Mogadishu as a framework for discussion of many specific aspects of providing care in an asymmetric urban environment and is a must-read for anyone planning to provide medical support to combat or SWAT operations in built-up areas. The Cen-

ter for Army Lessons Learned has an extensive online library of publications covering all aspects of MOUT operations available to Department of Defense personnel at *https://call2.army.mil/focus/urban-ops.index.asp*.

MOUT CHALLENGES

The Joint Staff's Handbook for Joint Urban Operations describes the typical urban environment as "a concentration of structures, facilities, and population and is the economic, political, and cultural focus of the surrounding area" (8). The individuals charged with constructing the medical support template for any urban operation must take each of these considerations into account while developing the tactical plan.

Training and Rehearsal

The key to success in providing medical support to MOUT operations is to ensure that everyone on the target is trained, rehearsed, and ready to react to any casualty producing situation. This may represent a significant shift in current training philosophies; classically, "shooters" shoot and medics treat the wounded. However, in close quarters battle, lives and success depend upon each individual becoming cross-trained. The 75th Ranger Regiment, based on lessons learned from urban operations in Somalia, maintain the training philosophy that for team success on the MOUT battlefield each ranger needs to be proficient in four areas: physical fitness, marksmanship, battle drills, and medical proficiency (9). Using the ranger paradigm, which has subsequently been adopted by multiple army

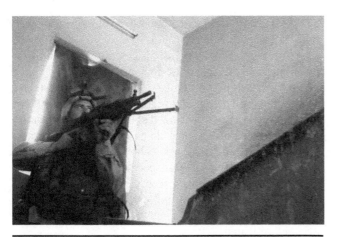

FIGURE 7.1. MOUT operations present unique challenges. (Courtesy of the 82D Airborne Division Public Affairs Office.)

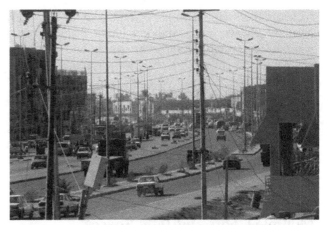

FIGURE 7.2. Traffic patterns, weather forecast, and security concerns must all also be evaluated and considered when determining primary and alternate evacuation routes. (Courtesy of the 82D Airborne Division Public Affairs Office.)

and marine light units, every soldier entering the objective is trained to provide basic lifesaving care, usually by completion of the Tactical Combat Casualty Care curriculum (10), which emphasizes three tenets: care under fire, tactical field care, and combat casualty evacuation care and is designed to prevent preventable death on the battlefield. This model is discussed elsewhere in this text. Additionally, every squad or section has at least one EMT-basic; every platoon includes at least one school-trained field medical professional.

Integrating casualty "play" into every training scenario and exercise well before starting actual combat operations will dramatically improve reaction, intervention, and survival. The utilization of "notional" casualties or casualty cards is insufficient to provide realistic training; specific individuals should be prompted to become "wounded" and the remainder of the team must then react, treat, evacuate, and be critiqued. Personnel should also rehearse what to do when the far-forward medic is the casualty. Alternatively, moulaged patients or computerized human patient simulators can be utilized as real-time training tools for first responders and medical personnel alike. Immediate treatment and evacuation of casualties off of the immediate objective without decrementing the fighting force must become a battle drill for all units conducting MOUT training exercises.

Treatment Capability and Location

Selecting a site as an initial casualty collection, triage, and evacuation point presents a significant challenge in the asymmetric MOUT environment. Ideally, this position will be free from the known enemy; be within casualty-carrying distance of the objective; be able to be secured; not be in the vicinity of friendly predesignated indirect fire targets; facilitate communication; provide cover, concealment, and weather protection; support lighting, suc-

tion, monitoring, or other specific treatment requirements; have at least two secure ground ingress and egress routes; and have the capability to safely accommodate a rotary-wing evacuation platform. Finding such an ideal site in the urban environment is frequently impossible and selecting the best location will require significant interaction with the intelligence, terrain analysis, and tactical leadership.

Medical and tactical leaders must jointly decide what medical capabilities and level of care will be brought into the fight. For smaller, "in-and-out" missions, a basic aid station may suffice; for larger operations, such as a cordon and search, resuscitative surgical and holding capability may be forecasted. Evacuation may be significantly limited; air evacuation is often impossible given obstacles and enemy threat, and ground evacuation may similarly be restrained, as was evidenced by the events of the Battle of Mogadishu. For this reason, planners must consider the possibility of providing an extended holding capacity. Traffic patterns, weather forecast, and security concerns must all also be evaluated and considered when determining primary and alternate evacuation routes (Fig. 7.2).

Types of projected injuries must also be considered; the casualties most often seen in MOUT operations are blast and overpressure, small arms, shrapnel, and burns. Hard walls, ceilings, and floors tend to "funnel" energy and projectiles, and wounds are often more severe than those inflicted by similar methods in an open environment.

Limited Individual Load

Military or paramilitary personnel conducting MOUT operations are significantly limited in what they can physically carry compared to their wheeled, armored, or even foot colleagues. One simply cannot maneuver a heavy rucksack, leg bags, "butt-pack," and body armor easily around hallways, doors, and up multiple flights of stairs without compromising surprise, stealth, and degrading combat effectiveness due to fatigue. Leadership at all levels will have to prioritize what items, including self- and buddy-aid items, are carried with each operator; likewise, accompanying medical personnel need to adjust their individual load to meet the anticipated casualty requirements of each mission set, while still maintaining personal safety and capacity to defend themselves and their patients.

Multiple Floors and Tight Spaces

Most civilian EMS personnel and military medics and corpsmen receive limited training in extracting wounded and injured personnel from small, enclosed spaces. However, MOUT operations may take place in the upper floors of multistoried buildings, requiring additional manpower to carry the casualty down multiple flights of stairs. Mechanical rooms, closets, bathrooms, and other small rooms can all hide casualties and can present a challenge for med-

ical personnel to treat and evacuate the casualty especially if the door opens into the room.

Before any MOUT operation is conducted, both first-responder and medical personnel must have knowledge of egress routes, how to remove doors and other obstacles, and should have the physical capacity and procedures emplaced to carry casualties long distances up or down stairs, to reach a safe point to provide more definitive treatment or evacuation. Such scenarios should be built into both routine training and mission-specific rehearsals to ensure that primary and secondary secure egress routes are available and understood and that any loss of combat power, such as soldiers needed to carry casualties out, is appropriately mitigated.

Doors and windows, after being breached, can easily become obstacles precluding effective treatment and evacuation (Fig. 7.3).

Communication

Critical to the success of any MOUT operation is for elements on the objective to be able to effectively

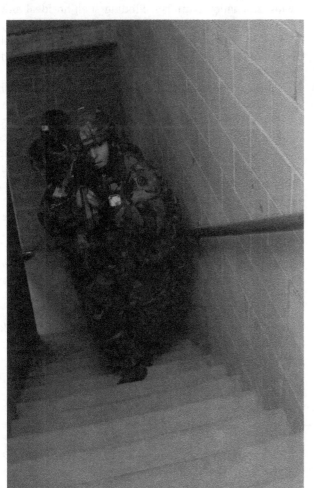

A

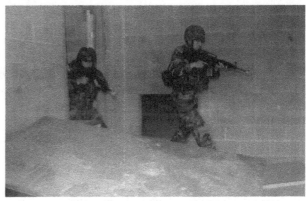

B

FIGURE 7.3. Before any MOUT operation is conducted, both first-responder and medical personnel must have knowledge of egress routes, how to remove doors and other obstacles, and should have the physical capacity and procedures in place to carry casualties long distances up or down stairs to reach a safe point to provide more definitive treatment or evacuation. (Courtesy of the 82D Airborne Division Public Affairs Office.)

communicate with each other, with supporting elements, and with a higher synchronizing headquarters. Effective communication prevents fratricide, enhances leaders' situational awareness, and allows for direct coordination of efforts at all levels. It is vitally critical for the supporting medical element(s) to be able to hear, understand, and act on the information they receive from the objective. This includes having the redundant capacity to communicate using prearranged and rehearsed hand signals, visual cues, or chemical lights to indicate the presence, location, nationality, and triage and/or evacuation category of any wounded or injured personnel.

Extrication

Soldiers and paramilitary personnel, when burdened with equipment, weapons, and ammunition, are generally heavy. If wounded, they may not be able to self-evacuate or assist those tasked to evacuate them in any way. If debris or other obstacles, stairways, and windows are to be utilized to evacuate wounded, an entire 10-man squad can become combat-ineffective if only two of their members become incapacitated. It then becomes critical for the tactical commander to have a system in place to provide additional personnel to enter the objective and withdraw the wounded. The commander must weigh the risks of generating additional casualties versus the benefits of not decrementing combat power on the objective; it is advisable to have a predetermined "trigger" for executing this option.

Casualty Marking and Triage

Although discussed extensively elsewhere in this text, one should consider the unique considerations of casualty marking and triage while in the close quarters or urban environment. Most notably, given the confined space and limited cover and concealment of operations conducted inside buildings, it may be most advisable to conduct initial triage at the first casualty collection point instead of at the point of injury. This should not, however, limit personnel from providing immediate live-saving treatment while on the objective or from delaying evacuation of the wounded from the close fight until the area is more secure. If conducted at night, use particular caution in utilizing visible sources (chemical lights) as casualty triage markers, because they may draw the attention of enemy snipers.

Existing Host-Nation Facilities

When conducting the medical intelligence preparation of the battlefield, planners should carefully consider the location, capability, security, and capacity of any medical facilities that exist within the local area of operations. Depending on the level of sophistication and infrastruc-

ture, these facilities may serve as a location to provide initial and stabilizing care to both friendly and enemy forces and may very well serve as the location for definitive care for any civilians that are injured or wounded as a result of the operation. Participating in a site survey and establishing personal relationships with host nation or city clinicians and administrators prior to the commencement of combat operations is highly advisable, if at all possible, although this must be weighed against the possibility of compromising operational security. In addition, any local emergency medical service (EMS) or other evacuation system may already be in place, and its personnel and equipment may be able to be leveraged (if permissive) or commandeered (if nonpermissive.) Many governmental organizations routinely monitor the medical capabilities and infrastructure of various countries; the Federal Research Division of the Library of Congress is one such comprehensive resource and is available at *http://lcweb2.loc.gov/frd/cs/cshome.html*.

Noncombatants/civilians on the Battlefield, Rules of Engagement and Entitlement, Translators, and Transfer of Care

When conducting MOUT operations in foreign countries, the operational planners, including the medical planners, must consider both the kinetic and nonkinetic effects of the operation on the civilian populace.

Civilian Casualties

In a large MOUT exercise conducted by the United States Marine Corps in 2002, between 17% and 40% of "non-friendly" casualties were civilian noncombatants. Civilian casualty rates were much higher in building-clearing operations than in "locate and attack" operations (9). Regardless of scenario, medical and tactical planners must incorporate a plan to locate, secure, triage, treat, and evacuate wounded noncombatants from the area. This must include detailed knowledge of the Rules of Engagement (ROE), rules of entitlement, or Status of Forces Agreements (SOFA), and also must include a detailed plan for transition of care from military or paramilitary forces to the local medical authorities, if those authorities have the capacity to provide an appropriate level of care.

Legal authorities must be involved and prepared to arrange financial reparations for medical and other claims which may be made against the military or paramilitary force. Information operations and public affairs offices must be well versed in the methodology of provision of medical care, so they can appropriately assist both in attaining the strategic and operational objectives and in keeping the civilian populace and media informed.

Translators with knowledge of basic anatomy and common medical questions are essential.

Supporting logisticians must also be prepared to receive deceased civilian casualties either from medical personnel or directly from the scene, and transfer or appropriately disposition human remains in accordance with the ROE or SOFA.

Diplomatic Issue–crossing Borders? Visas? VIPs?

If operating on foreign soil, leaders must plan contingency operations not only for fighting forces that become ill, injured, or wounded, but also for host-nation civilian noncombatants who are injured as a result of the conflict and cannot receive the appropriate standard of care in the host nation. Methodology to obtain passports, visas, and transportation, including critical care requirements, should be prearranged.

The unique requirements of senior leaders, not only of "friendly" military and paramilitary forces, but also of nonfriendly combatants and civilian leaders, must also be taken into account and planned for in the event that a requirement develops for them to be evacuated from the battle area.

Mass Casualty Producing Events

Medical personnel should plan for the worst possible scenario, when the number of casualties exceeds the capacity to provide care. During the prebattle analysis, leaders must develop a mass casualty plan. This plan must become a well-rehearsed battle drill synchronizing efforts to call forward additional medical personnel, equipment, evacuation vehicles, and a security element to handle the situation while the battle continues to unfold and medical personnel triage and treat. This plan must integrate tactical, logistic, and medical leaders (10).

CBRNE

Medical leaders must consider the possibility of encountering chemical, biological, radiological, nuclear, or high-explosive (CBRNE) armaments when conducting MOUT operations, especially if the target area is a suspected CBRNE manufacturing or storage facility. Specially trained and equipped personnel, equipment, and vehicles may be required to accompany the force to provide both care and decontamination capability; forces should be tailored to meet the specific mission requirements.

Resupply

It is inevitable that once casualties are treated, first responders and medical personnel at the casualty collection point

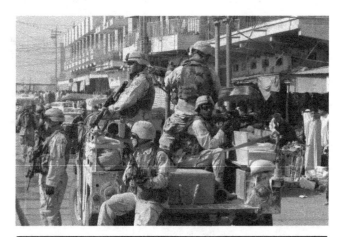

FIGURE 7.4. Medical evacuation (MEDEVAC) or casualty evacuation (CASEVAC) vehicles. (Courtesy of the 82D Airborne Division Public Affairs Office.)

will require resupply. An effective strategy for managing resupply requirements is to have predetermined, prestaged "speedballs" containing the medical equipment most likely to be required as the fight evolves and colocate that equipment with the other logistical items that are most likely to be needed as well, such as ammunition, water, and food. Given evacuation constraints and on-scene capabilities, this may include blood as well. Keeping vehicular and helicopter traffic to a minimum is a must in order to minimize additional risk.

Before starting the operation, the on-scene medical leader should determine what level constitutes a critical shortage of supply, and should establish a plan and radio codeword that automatically triggers a resupply operation, which may be as simple as kicking a box of supplies off of a vehicle, or as complex as the aerial delivery of palletized equipment. Secondly, medical evacuation (MEDEVAC) or casualty evacuation (CASEVAC) vehicles moving to and from the casualty collection point may be utilized as vehicles of opportunity to move additional (or unforcasted) requirements to the point of care (Fig. 7.4). These operations should be closely intertwined with resupply operations of other classes of supply and require significant prior planning with other logisticians, as well as the leaders of the security element that will accompany the mission.

Combatants Killed in Action

According to military doctrine, the remains of those combatants who are killed in action become the responsibility of the logisticians to evacuate and process. However, limited resources available on the objective and safety concerns during MOUT operations will likely preclude the insertion of any additional personnel who are not mission essential into the fighting force. Also, despite our best attempts, both friendly and unfriendly forces, as well as noncombatants, may perish after entering the medical care system. Regardless of circumstance, we must ensure that all remains are treated with the appropriate dignity and respect, and that the remains of enemy combatants and civilian noncombatants are treated in accordance with the generally accepted local custom. Prior planning for return of remains to civilian families or governmental authorities must be completed and rehearsals conducted. Although this usually falls outside of the medical "stovepipe," medical planners must be aware of the processes to deliver or to have remains evacuated from objective or off-objective treatment facilities. It usually is not advisable to transport wounded and killed combatants in the same vehicle or airframe; however, the tactical situation may preclude the use of multiple vehicles.

After Effects

Operations in the MOUT environment are often intense and violent. Medical leaders must ensure that military and paramilitary personnel who execute MOUT operations have the ability to ask for and receive medical, psychological, or spiritual care. Conduct of critical incident stress debriefings may also be considered.

TAKE HOME POINTS

1. MOUT operations present a variety of unique challenges that will change your usual approach to medical planning for combat operations.
2. Every person on the objective needs to be cross-trained and proficient in providing life-saving immediate medical care.
3. Integrate medical resupply into all resupply planning and operations.
4. No plan survives first contact!

SUMMARY

Planning for, and providing, medical support to MOUT operations poses a significant challenge to the medical, logistical, and tactical leadership. The best medicine, other than overwhelming fire superiority, is to train, practice, and inculcate the extrication, treatment, and evacuation of casualties at every training opportunity afforded the tactical unit. Ensuring cross-capability, integration of medical requirements into resupply operations, and development of mass casualty plans will save lives after the mission is begun. Developing a medical information operations plan with organic assets, embedded media, and the local press will also pay great dividends when the smoke clears.

REFERENCES

1. United Nations, Department of Economic and Social Affairs, Population Division. *Urban and Rural Areas 2003*. New York: United Nations; 2004.
2. Headquarters, Dept of the Army. *Urban Operations*. Washington: US Army; 2003. Field Manual 3-06.
3. Branas CC, Nance ML, Elliott MR, et al. Urban-rural shifts in intentional firearm death: different causes, same results. *Am J Public Health*. 2004;94:1750–1755.
4. Martinez-Lopez L. Medical support for urban operations. In: Glenn RW, Steeb R, eds. *The City's Many Faces: Proceedings of the RAND Arroyo-MCWL-J8 Urban Operations Conference*. Santa Monica: RAND Arroyo Center; 1999:305–331.
5. Butler F, Hagmann JH, Richards DT. Tactical management of urban warfare casualties in special operations. *Milit Med*. 2000;165:1–48.
6. Butler F, Hagmann J, Butler G. Tactical combat casualty care in special operations. *Milit Med*. 1996;161(suppl):3–16.
7. Hall MT, Kennedy MT. The urban area during support missions: case study–Mogadishu: applying the lessons learned, take 2. In: Glenn R, ed. *Capital Preservation: Preparing for Urban Operations in the Twenty-First Century–Proceedings of the RAND Arroyo-TRADOC-MCWL-OSD Urban Operations Conference, March 22–23, 2000*. Santa Monica: RAND Arroyo Center; 2001:546.
8. The Joint Staff. *Handbook for Joint Urban Operations*. Washington: The Joint Staff; 2000.
9. Marine Corps War-fighting Laboratory. *Millennium Dragon 02 Experiment After Action Review*. Quantico: Marine Corps Combat Development Command; 2002.
10. Volpe P. *"Medic! Medic!" A Personal Experience Monograph*. Carlisle Barracks: United States Army War College; 1996.

Hostage Survival

James L. Greenstone

OBJECTIVES

After reading this section, the reader will be able to:

1. Understand the guidelines for surviving a hostage situation.
2. Know what to do if taken hostage.
3. Recognize their responsibilities as they relate to the successful outcome of a hostage situation.
4. Facilitate "hostage survival."

HISTORICAL PERSPECTIVE

If you watch what is going on in the world, you know that hostage takings are not uncommon and that the reactions to these takings are varied. It is important to emphasize the need to know how to survive being taken hostage. This is especially true for personnel who will function in the tactical environment. This has been well recognized in the historic literature and reiterated in more recent publications (1,2).

It can be a tricky business that may be influenced by misconceptions and just plain bad ideas of what to do. Most professionals will tell you that their experience has made them good "negotiators," able to talk themselves in or out of almost anything. This author has witnessed this kind of thinking almost compromise a dangerous hostage situation where many lives were at stake. A negotiated release was jeopardized when the hostage refused to leave, preferring instead to remain as a captive because he thought that he could do a better job than the police negotiator, which is obviously the wrong thing to do. But, without training and forethought, any of us could fall victim to the same missteps.

As the chance of hostage and barricaded situations is possible in new places and under unique circumstances, knowing what to do, what is helpful and what is not assumes paramount importance. This is not a time for heroics or grandstanding. It is a time to know what to do and then to do it even under these very difficult circumstances. The trained professional in this situation may be the only trained person taken. That life and the lives of other hostages may well depend on this training paying off with large dividends for all concerned. If you are in the room, others will look to you for guidance. How you act is a matter of life and death.

Many say that they rely on "common sense" to get them through difficult situations. This author suggests that those who survive will do so, and do so much better, because of the "uncommon sense" that results from their training and their reliance on that training in difficult situations.

HOSTAGE SURVIVAL PHILOSOPHY

What to do if you are taken hostage? The action steps taken and concepts applied must be based upon proven approaches. Don't try to be a hero. Accept your situation, and be prepared to wait. This approach may help to calm others who are also taken.

It is important to follow instructions. Remember that the first 15 to 45 minutes are the most dangerous. Emotions are high on both sides. Minor errors become magnified in intensity and potential danger. Keep other captives calm. Reassure them that help is coming. This may help the situation and the authorities more than anything else you can do.

Do not speak unless spoken to, and then, only when necessary. This is not the time to assert your intellectual prowess or to tell the hostage taker that you are somehow special because you are a physician or the like. Try to rest and maintain your strength. This could be important later and in an extended standoff.

Do not make suggestions to the hostage taker. If the taker asks, answer. Otherwise remain quiet. Do not rely on the rules of the Geneva Conventions. They do not apply. In these cases, such reliance could get you hurt. Answer questions and do what you are told unless it is unconscionable for you to do so.

Do not try to escape unless you are absolutely sure that you will be successful. If you are going to try to escape, do it at the moment of capture. Your mental and physical abilities will be strongest at that time.

If you, or others, need medical attention or medication, inform your captors. This may help to develop human bonding between the hostage taker and the hostages. Let the hostage taker participate in the care of the ill or injured. Act as a guide or be of help to the hostage taker. It is harder to injure or kill someone to whom you are ministering.

Always be observant of the hostage taker and the surroundings. You may be released or escape, and your information may be helpful. Use your clinical observation skills to the maximum. The information you provide when released could prove invaluable.

Be prepared to answer the police/negotiator on the phone. Only give "yes" or "no" answers. If you have a chance to speak to authorities, listen to what they say to you and answer only what is asked. Remember, the bad guys will probably be listening to what you say. Try to remain calm while on the phone

Don't become argumentative. Avoid this to the greatest degree possible. Treat your captors like "royalty." Do nothing to threaten them. They want to believe that they are in charge. Let them.

Be patient. Remember and accept that highly trained personnel are attempting to secure your release. But, this may take a great deal of time. Time spent does not mean that there is not much going on outside your immediate awareness. There is much happening, and it is all designed to secure your release. Generally, it can be assumed that in a hostage situation, the longer the time spent, the greater the likelihood that no one will be hurt, and that the situation will be resolved successfully for all concerned. Remember this, although you may still find it very difficult to wait.

During a rescue attempt, lie low. When the police come in, make no sudden moves. This is not the time to assert who you are or to show your credentials. Wait until the rescue is over to explain medical needs. Remember, because you are a hostage, you will be regarded as such by the police. When rescued, expect to be handcuffed and searched. This will be done as a matter of policy. Let it happen.

TAKE HOME POINTS

1. Be prepared to wait.
2. Remember that well-trained personnel are working to secure your release.
3. Remain calm and keep faith with those with you.

SUMMARY

Almost anyone can survive a noncrisis situation, because we do it every day. For crisis situations, such as hostage takings, procedures are necessary to insure positive outcomes for all concerned. Further, the established procedures must be followed during these crisis situations. It is for just these situations that they are formulated. With this said, do not stop your thought processes. Pay attention to what is going on around you. Listen for clues that may hasten your release. Notice your captors and be able to identify them later as needed. Stay alive and well. Take care of yourself and others. In the final analysis, nothing is more important.

REFERENCES

1. Bolz F. *Hostage Cop*. New York: Rawson, Wade Publishers; 1979.
2. Greenstone JL. *The Elements of Police Hostage and Crisis Negotiations: Critical Incidents and How to Respond to Them*. New York: The Haworth Press; 2005.

Chapter 9

The Basics of Survival

John D. Schwartz and Paul J. Vecchio

OBJECTIVES

After reading this section, the reader will be able to:

1. Know the key elements of basic wilderness survival.
2. Be able to pack a basic survival kit that is appropriate for your mission needs.
3. Understand the differences between wilderness survival and survival in a tactical or "SERE" environment.

INTRODUCTION

When laypersons think of survival, they always think of man versus nature, making improvised shelters, finding water, making fires, and foraging for food. Although all of these things are part of survival, it really starts with your mind. Thinking ahead and anticipating the unexpected. Without using your mind and controlling your instincts, a person has no chance at survival.

Survival starts with the preparation for a trip, activity, or mission. Just as a medical practitioner goes through a medical threat assessment prior to deploying to a new operational area, the practitioner should also do a survival threat assessment to assess basic survival requirements for the area. This assessment should consider the possible environments that may be encountered in traveling to or from a location as well as the destination. Assessing the critical elements of survival for these environments can help the practitioner choose which equipment to add to or remove from their basic survival kit.

Most military and many civilian survival courses teach key words like SURVIVAL or STOP to help remember the key elements for survival. In most cases, this is counterproductive, because it focuses the learner on rote memorization rather than learning the important rationale for each key element. When a person understands the rationale for each element of survival, they will be better able to adapt and improvise as the situation demands. Most of survival is learning how to adapt to new conditions and improvise to meet the changing demands.

The Key Elements to Survival

The key elements to survival in their order of importance are: (i) your mind, (ii) first aid, (iii) shelter, (iv) fire, (v) signaling, (vi) water, and (vii) food. In almost all cases, the order of importance will stay the same. In some cases in the desert, fire might switch with water in order of importance, but fire is still high up on the list because deserts get very cold at night.

Your Mind

The first and most important element of survival is getting control of your thought process. This is very easy to say, but in reality is difficult to do. Our natural instincts use fear and panic to initiate a fight or flight response. This is how our ancestors were able to survive encounters with large predators. Today, our fight or flight responses are still very active and many of the drills in military and law enforcement training are intended to redirect and focus these natural instinctive responses. When someone refers to battle-hardened troops, they are referring to their ability to redirect and focus their natural instincts into a coordinated tactical response.

Most incidences that lead to a survival situation also challenge our ability to overcome our initial fear or panic. As a person becomes disoriented or lost, fear and panic slowly begin to take over. This is usually a slow creeping panic. At some point, increased apprehension causes people to start to rush. In most cases, they begin to search for clearings or higher ground. They think, "If only I can see where I am, I will not be lost." It is during this rushing state that experienced hunters and hikers will put down their packs or leave their guns propped against trees with the intention of returning once they get their bearings. The result is that without a good reference point (this is what they are looking for) they quickly lose track of where they left their equipment and the situation becomes much worse.

How does one control these feelings of fear and panic? The British SAS recommends sitting down and making a cup of tea. This is a great response. Sitting down will stop one's haste, which could lead to loss of equipment, injury, or further anxiety. Making tea forces one to break the chain of thought, which will continue to escalate toward panic. Once this chain of thought is broken and one's mind can be redirected, the person can later return to the original situation with a controlled and rational thought process. They can size up the situation, observe the environment, and assess their memories of how they came to be in the present situation. Sometimes a person can mentally backtrack and rethink how they got into the situation. The key is to slow down, think, and control fear and panic. Then assess the situation, form a plan, and start to think like a survivor rather than a victim.

First Aid

After having the proper mind set, first aid is the second most important element for survival. Situations like accidents and trauma can also challenge one's ability to think clearly. Shock or traumatic situations can induce a trance-like state. Victims have difficulty shaking off their initial shock in order to deal with the situation. Even minor injuries can reduce an individual's ability to function in an appropriate manner. This is where leaders and medical personnel seem to survive better than most people. The recognition of responsibility for others pulls them through more quickly. Medical providers are in many ways the quickest to recover, because of the role they play within the team. Personal health and the health of the team are critical for proper decision making. Because this is a book on tactical medicine, it is assumed the reader has a good understanding of first aid and, therefore, it will not be further discussed.

Shelter

The next key element to survival is shelter. Shelter is critical in almost every situation and environment. In a study of search and recovery (SAR) fatalities, 75% of the victims died within the first 48 hours due to exposure. In cold and wet environments, victims can quickly die from hypothermia without adequate shelter. In desert environments, shelter is essential to protect from the heat during the day and cold during the night. Proper shelter radically reduces water loss in these environments. In tropical environments, shelter is necessary to protect from rain and insects.

Clothing

Shelter starts with clothing. In almost all survival situations, never discard clothing. Try to keep your clothing clean and dry in cold environments. Layer your clothing to produce insulating air spaces. To prevent sweating and overheating, remove layers before climbing or performing strenuous activities. Protect your head and neck, because these are high heat loss areas.

In hot and dry environments, cover up with loose, light-colored clothing to prevent sunburn and minimize thermal absorption. Protect your head with a brimmed hat and your neck with a bandana. Wet your hat and bandana with saltwater, urine, or waste water to take advantage of evaporative cooling. In tropical environments, you should try to carry two sets of clothing. One set is for the daytime; it will be constantly wet and will protect you from thorns and biting insects. Keep the second set of clothing dry for sleeping at night and for protection from nocturnal insects.

Feet

In cold environments, it is always good to have plenty of room to move toes and to allow extra room for socks. Remember: air spaces are what create insulation. Insulated boots can also be very effective in hot dry climates. Temperature on the ground can exceed 65°C (149°F), so insulation in boots can actually reduce the amount of heat absorbed into the body. Boots in tropical environments need to be drainable. Also, pants should tuck into boots to prevent insects and leeches from crawling up your legs.

Eyes

In almost all environments, with the exception of tropical environment, sunglasses or another type of eye protection is needed to prevent eye fatigue and snow blindness. Improvised eye protection can be made by cutting horizontal slits through dark plastic jug material, bark, webbing, or any other appropriate material (see Fig. 9.1).

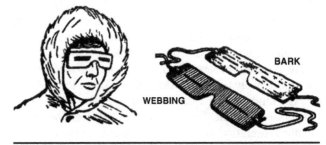

FIGURE 9.1. Improvised sunglasses. (Courtesy of US Army Survival Manual: FM 21–76 Department of Defense, June 1992.)

Choosing a Site for Shelter

The location where a person chooses to construct a shelter will go a long way toward helping them survive adverse conditions. A shelter location should help minimize the effects of cold, wind, rain, sun, insects, and hostile observation. Do not build shelters in exposed windy areas high up on a mountain. Locate shelters to take advantage of the sun in cold climates and the shade in hot dry climates. In a nontactical situation, it is best to place your shelter in a location where rescuers will look for you. If possible, locate near recovery sites. Never place your shelter under dead wood or "widow makers" (dead standing trees). It is always good if you can locate your shelter near a source of drinking water but not too close to stagnant water where insects are more likely to become a problem. Never locate your shelter under a solitary tree that could attract lightening or in a dry river bed that might be prone to flash floods. Avoid locations that are noisy, such as near fast flowing rivers or water falls, because the noise they produce may mask hearing rescuers or hearing pursuers in evasion situations. Also, assess the possibility of other hazards, such as lighting or an avalanche, in choosing a shelter location. Look for your shelter location early so you have time to set up, because once it becomes dark your options are severely limited.

In tactical situations, place your shelter in a location that can provide concealment from hostile observation from both the ground and air. Locate your shelter to provide several camouflaged observation points and escape routes. Minimize the disturbance to the area surrounding your shelter location. The site should be difficult to approach without being clearly seen. Make sure the shelter is small with a low silhouette and is irregularly shaped, because the human eye will pick up on any kind of pattern.

Making an Improvised Shelter

The most common mistake people make in constructing their shelter is making it too large. Smaller shelters are more efficient to build and are more effective at conserving body heat in colder climates. A shelter needs to protect you from rain, wind, snow, or sun. A practical shelter should be easy to build and only large enough to comfortably lie down in. Most survival books show elaborate shelters designed for weeks or months of service. In most cases, the energy expended in their construction is far too high and a small efficient shelter will provide better protection. In a tactical situation, several small irregularly placed shelters are more likely to go unnoticed than a single large shelter.

The kind of shelter one constructs is dependent on the materials available. Shelters can be made from almost all natural vegetation, turf, rocks, and snow, as well as a whole variety of man made materials, such as tarps or plastic sheeting. Natural shelters, such as caves, rocky crevices,

fallen trees, or large trees with low-hanging limbs, can provided the framework for simple efficient shelters. Caution should be exercised in evaluating caves and crevices as shelters. In some areas, they may be inhabited by snakes, scorpions, or other stinging insects. Because many caves and rock formations are formed by water, assess the impact of rain on their suitability.

Uprooted logs can make good natural shelters. Piling long sticks over the rooted section of a tree can make the base layer of an effective shelter. Another method is to dig out a small depression parallel to the fallen log and fill the depression with dry leaves or pine needles. Next, lay sticks and vegetation over the top of the log covering the depression. A person is then protected from both above and below. If snow is available, use it to cover the roof vegetation to provide an insulation layer to the shelter. Pulling material into the entrance can further reduce heat loss. Pine trees with low hanging limps can make very good natural shelters. Crawl in under the lower limbs and cut and tie these lower limbs ends higher up in the tree branches. This forms a hollow close to the tree trunk. Rain and snow are naturally funneled away from the center of the tree by the limbs. Vegetation can be piled in the space created next to the tree trunk to form a nest for sleeping. In snowy areas, more snow can be piled on the outer limbs to increase the weather resistance of the central part of the shelter. These kinds of shelters are also effective in tactical situations, because there is little change in the external appearance of the tree (Fig. 9.2).

Debris shelters are simple to build and provide weather resistant sleeping areas. Fasten two short poles together and then attach a third long ridgepole to form a V-shaped cave that is long enough and wide enough to accommodate a sleeping area. Continue to pile sticks and vegetation onto the shelter to create a weather resistant barrier. If a tarp or plastic sheeting is available, place this over the first layer

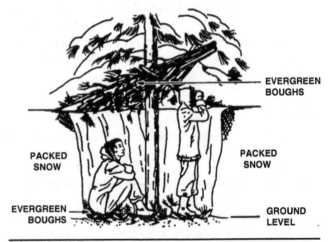

FIGURE 9.2. Pine tree snow shelter. (Courtesy of US Army Survival Manual: FM 21–76 Department of Defense, June 1992.)

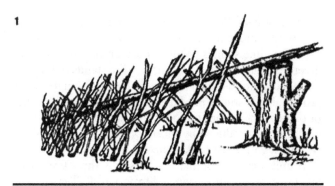

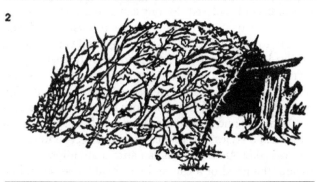

FIGURE 9.3. Debris shelter. (Courtesy of US Army Survival Manual: FM 21–76 Department of Defense, June 1992.)

and cover it with more sticks and vegetation to hold it in place. Fill the shelter with leaves or grass to create a nest to hold body heat (Fig. 9.3).

Snow is the most abundant insulating material to make shelters. Snow caves can protect survivors from wind and can hold heat for long periods of time. Caution should always be exercised when using an open flame inside any enclosed shelter. Carbon monoxide poisoning kills winter campers every year. Adequate ventilation should always be provided for any flame based heat source.

When the snow forms a crust, in some cases, a snow trench will work to create a shelter. Snow is dug out to create a trench. Pine boughs or blocks of cut snow are placed over the top of the trench to create a roof. Extra snow can then be piled on top to create an insulation barrier. Blocking off the entrance will seal the snow trench from wind and hold the survivors body heat inside.

Shelters in hot, dry climates need to offer protection from the sun in order to reduce water loss. The ground surface in these areas is extremely hot, so the shelter floor should be raised or dug down into the ground to avoid this excessive heat. If there is extra roof material available, layering the roof with an air space between the layers can significantly reduce the temperature within the shelter. Particularly important in desert survival is assessing the amount of effort which will be spent in making a shelter. Water loss is greatly increased with exertion, so simple, easily built shelters need to be considered when water supplies are limited.

Shelters in tropical, wet environments need to protect occupants from rain and insects. Shelters in the jungles need to be constructed above the ground to reduce dampness and the number of insects and snakes that inhabit the area. A water-resistant roof is also necessary to stay semidry.

Fire

The next most important factor affecting survival is fire. Fire provides warmth, light, and will lift your morale as night approaches and the temperature begins to fall. It will also provide a heat source to signal with, dry clothing, purify water, cook food, and keep biting insects at bay. Even in the desert, fire is very important as a nighttime signal and heat source, as nighttime temperatures drop greatly due to thermal radiation radiating back into a clear sky.

The location for a fire should be protected from wind and close enough to provide warmth to your shelter. You should clear the area of vegetation to prevent the fire from spreading. Watch for overhanging trees or deadwood. Keep fires small to keep them under control and to maximize the use of the available fuel supply. Never leave a fire that might jump to nearby vegetation.

Most plant material can be used as fuel with the exception of several poisonous species of wood or vine that can transmit poisonous resin through their smoke. Several examples are: poison wood, poison oak, and poison ivy. Many kinds of animal droppings make excellent fuel. In some areas of the world, local inhabitants burn "cow chips" exclusively for heating and cooking. Peat, when dry, will burn slowly and can be difficult to put out once started. Sometimes coal and charcoal can be found and will produce a very controllable fire. A mixture of oil and gasoline, when placed in a partially filled can of sand, will make an acceptable lamp or cooking stove. In some situations, animal fats can be used to make lamps or small stoves. In heavy snow or swamp conditions, a fire may be built on top of several green logs or on a raised platform to prevent the fire from extinguishing itself in the wet or snowy environment. Many kinds of rubber, plastic, and synthetic cloth will burn and produce thick black smoke that can be used as an effective signal in the desert or in snowy conditions.

Lighting Fires

Matches or lighters are by far the easiest way to make a fire. Keep matches in a waterproof container so that they will function when needed. Water and wind resistant matches are available and will withstand the outdoor environment longer than other common matches, but they are not waterproof as their label says. Small butane lighters will last a long time and are amazingly durable. Even after the butane from these lighters has been used, the spark produced by the flint can still be used to start fires. A commercially available magnesium rod and flint striker is one of the absolute best backup fire starters available. This device is durable, totally waterproof, and can be used for many fires. One of these should be included in every survival kit.

Other fire making devices all have significant drawbacks. Large lenses can effectively make fires when the sun is shining brightly. At other times, when fire may be most needed, a lens will be ineffectual. Shorting the poles of a car or airplane battery to make a spark can create fires. If fine steel wool has been included as tinder in your survival kit, you can use it to short circuit flashlight batteries and it will almost instantly start burning. Steel wool is an extremely effective tinder for most fire making and can be kept in a film canister or small baggy to prevent it from rusting. Spraying it with an oil protectant will help keep it from rusting and will make it burn even better. Signaling hand flares can also be used to make a good fire, but at the loss of one signaling device. In some cases, you may need fire to stay alive and the fire can then be used as a signal. The tradeoff has to be assessed carefully.

The many primitive friction methods of making fire are extremely difficult for "nonexperts." Without previous experience with these methods, their usefulness to make fire is limited and will not be discussed in any detail.

Signaling

Signaling is more important than water and food in most survival situations. In the majority of search and recovery missions (SAR), the victim is found within the first 48 hours. This is assuming someone knows to look for them. Preplanning will assure that someone will look for you. Protocols for checking in and out before and after a mission or activity should be established. When someone fails to make contact after a planned mission, a SAR sequence should automatically be triggered.

Today cell phones work in many areas of the world and satellite phone coverage is global. People can communicate from the high Himalayas to Antarctica. Satellite phones and global positioning systems (GPS) allow searchers to home in on exact locations. In some cases, weather may impede recovery, but it is just a matter of time before rescue reaches the location. Personal location beacons (PLBs) and emergency location transponders (ELTs) can bring rescues within range of more conventional signaling devices. In tactical situations, leave PLBs and ELTs off so as not to draw in hostile activity. Keep transmissions short and never transmit from your shelter location to prevent range-finding devices from homing in on your hideout. Follow all prearranged operational plans for recovery.

A mirror is a very effective daytime signaling device. Signaling mirrors can be seen from far beyond visual range. Pyrotechnic signals can be used effectively both day and night. Always follow the directions for each kind of device used. Smoke from flares and from ground fires make good day time signals. White smoke produced by placing green vegetation on top of a flaming fire stands out well on dark backgrounds, such as a green forest or jungle undergrowth. Black smoke produced by burning plastic, rubber, or oil products stands out best against snow and sand. Orange smoke produced by most commercial smoke flares will work with most backgrounds.

A universal sign of distress is usually three fires or orange squares set in a triangle formation. Reflective blankets or brightly colored clothing can be placed in a pattern to signify distress and assist in rescue. It is particularly important to set out a series of visual objects if you are holed up inside a shelter or are unable to assist further in your own rescue due to injury or illness. Sound can be an extremely effective signal when rescuers are close. Shouting is not particularly effective, because the human voice does not carry far and it uses a great deal of energy. Using a whistle in a series of three blasts is an effective universal distress code. Anything that can attract attention, such as raising the hood of a car, and convey distress should be used to bring rescuers to your location.

Water

Although water is essential to survival, most people can survive without it for at least 2 days even in hot climates. In cool, moist climates, people can live 10 to 12 days without water. Thirst or dehydration will cause weakness, fatigue, dizziness, headache, fever, and concentrated urine. Symptoms of dehydration include: loss of appetite, slow pace, apathy, impatience, anger, slurred speech, mental confusion, and hallucinations.

Most people require 2 to 3 quarts of water per day simply for bodily functions. This water requirement is greatly increased by heat exposure, exertion, cold exposure, high altitudes, burns, and illness. When water is available, drink it to maintain proper bodily function. When water is limited, try to reduce water loss by avoiding exertion, especially during the heat of the day. Try to stay above or below the hot surface of the ground. Avoid sunburn at all cost. If you do not have water, do not eat. Most foods will require more water for digestion than you gain from their consumption. However, there are some foods containing a large amount of liquid, which are exceptions to this rule. To limit water loss from your breath, try to breathe through your nose and limit talking. Avoid taking any diuretics, such as alcohol, and do not smoke.

To save existing water supplies, always collect water when the opportunity presents itself. Collect morning dew in a cloth and wring the water into a container. If it rains, you should always collect water. If you do not have containers, dig a hole and line it with plastic sheeting. After you have collected water in the hole, the extra plastic sheeting can be folded back over the top of the hole to prevent the water from evaporating.

Where to Look for Water

If any lakes, rivers, or streams are available, there should be no problem getting water. If water is not obviously available, then you must search for your water. Water can be found in valleys, ravines, and rock crevices. A seep or rock pool can sometimes be found containing water. Water will usually be found in areas where there is growing vegetation. When a dry river bed is on bedrock, water can sometimes be found under the gravel on the outside bend of the river. Again, vegetation will usually be the key for homing in on the source of water. If animals inhabit an area, they usually require water. Follow animal tracks to their source of water. When two trails intersect, most trails will intersect in a V pattern. The V in the pattern will most likely point in the direction of the water.

Some plants can provide drinkable water. Water vines found in some tropical areas of the world will provide palatable water. Always avoid any vine that has white milky sap. To obtain water from these vines cut the vine high up and then down low and water will start flowing out at the bottom. Catch the water in a container and taste for suitability. The water should be clear and have a slightly sweet woody flavor with no bitter taste. Young coconuts are also a good source of water. Ripe coconuts have a fair amount of liquid but can act as a laxative if too much is ingested. Water can also be found on desert islands by digging down to a thin freshwater lens. When rain falls on an island, it seeps through the ground and floats on the heavier saltwater. This lens stays for a long period of time and is the main source of water for many plants on the island. Slowly digging to the lens can provide (usually poorly tasting) fresh water. Mixing charcoal from your fire into the water can improve the taste.

Getting liquid from barrel cacti can be difficult. The outer husk of the cactus is very tough and armed with sharp spines. Once opened, the center of the cacti should be mashed and then squeezed through a cloth to extract the liquid. Place the mash in a cloth and form a ball. Keep twisting the ball of mashed cacti to extract as much of the liquid as possible. It usually has a rather bitter flavor. In some cases, it may be better to place the moist cacti flesh in a vegetation bag as described later.

When sources of water cannot be found, other methods of obtaining water might complement your existing supply. Water transpiration bags are one of the more effective means. A water transpiration bag consists of a clear plastic bag that is placed around a large leafy branch. The leaves will transpire water vapor into the bag. The vapor will then condense on the bags' inner surface and drip to the lower corner of the bag. The water can be extracted through a tube or the corner containing the water can be

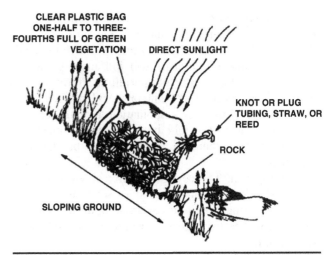

FIGURE 9.4. Vegetation bag on slope. (Courtesy of US Army Survival Manual: FM 21–76 Department of Defense, June 1992.)

raised, which causes the water to flow to a precut extraction hole. A vegetation bag is similar to the transpiration bag except the vegetation (such as cacti flesh) is placed in the bag and the bag is placed on a slight incline, so water vapor will condense on the inner surface of the bag and run to the lower corner (Fig. 9.4). These two methods are more efficient than a hand made solar still. Solar stills require significant digging and, in most cases, will cause you to lose more water in their construction than you will get from their water production (Fig. 9.5). A vegetation bag works in a similar fashion, yet requires minimal effort for construction. Commercial solar stills for sea survival work much more effectively and require little effort to deploy from the shore or a life raft.

Water from stills, vegetation bags, transpiration bags, cacti, and water vines require no treatment prior to drinking. All other sources require treatment to rid them of pathogenic organisms. Diarrhea or illness in a

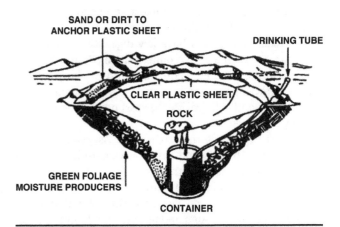

FIGURE 9.5. Below-ground solar still. (Courtesy of US Army Survival Manual: FM 21–76 Department of Defense, June 1992.)

water-limited environment can be a death sentence. Boiling water for a period of time is a proven method for dealing with most pathogens. The use of commercially available iodine or chlorine will kill most pathogens but has little effect on cryptosporidium. Filtration with hiking filters (rated to 0.2 microns) will remove everything except viruses. A combination of filtration and chemical treatment would be ideal, but in most survival situations, chemical treatment will be the most expedient.

It is important to recognize that in a survival situation no one should drink urine, blood, or sea water. Thirst is an overpowering condition but drinking urine, blood, or sea water will destroy a person's will to survive and hasten their death.

Snow and ice are an ideal source of water. However, avoid eating snow or ice if the energy necessary to melt it could induce a reduction of body core temperature. This may cause an individual to slip into hypothermia.

Food

Food, interestingly, is the least important element of survival. People have survived for as long as a month without food. Food is important for long-term survival, but not for the short term. Most survival books devote the largest sections to food procurement, yet it is the least likely factor to kill you in a survival situation. Hunger is debilitating for the first 3 to 5 days; after that, the body adapts and starts to break down its own fats and proteins to produce energy. Obviously, if this were to continue for a long period, the body would soon run out of energy, the kidneys would fail, and the person would die. In the short term, the body produces energy and the individual can continue to function, but at a reduced efficiency. Attention should be focused on attending to food needs once other factors required for survival are dealt with.

When finding food, the survivor needs to assess the value of the food energy versus the energy required to obtain it. Plants would seem like a good choice, because they are simple to obtain. This turns out to be wrong, because most wild plants have low digestibility and those that can be eaten safely require a detailed knowledge of species in the area. Few potential survivors have that in-depth knowledge. Animals provide a much higher nutritional value and will provide the most nourishment for the energy expended.

Almost everything that creeps, crawls, swims, or flies can be eaten. Insects and insect larvae are high in both protein and fat, and dig hunting requires low expenditures of energy. Looking for grubs around, under, and in rotten logs is an easy way to provide nourishment with minimal energy expenditure. Ants and termites are found in many areas of the world and can be easily caught. Desiccating insects in a can over a fire and then grinding them into a

paste or making them into a stew will make eating them more palatable.

Fishing hooks are useful for catching a variety of fish and can also be used to catch frogs and birds. Hand spears can be used to spear crabs, lobsters, and small sting rays in sandy shallows. There are a whole variety of mollusks, which can be collected in rocky shallows and tide pools.

A good stick can be used to kill frogs, snakes, and lizards. Sling shots can kill birds and larger lizards from a distance.

If a survivor had a rifle, he or she might be able to hunt a variety of mammals and birds. However, if no gun is available, catching mammals with snares is extremely difficult. Books are full of snare designs, yet trappers who are well practiced have about a 1:15 success ratio. This means that most people have little to no chance of success. If your survival kit were to have the metal parts of a commercial rat trap, you could set it up on a log and increase your odds to about a 1:3 success ratio. Rat traps can be used for small rodents as well as birds.

Clubs can potentially be used on several mammal species, but always be aware of the adults. Chop fishing with a machete at night can be very effective for catching a variety of fish. Also, some survival kits contain gill nets or fish poisons that can catch or kill fish.

The Contents of the Survival Kit

The survival threat assessment discussed at the beginning of this chapter will provide the key to the items needed in your survival kit. Certain parts of your survival gear should be carried on your person at all times. You should always carry your knife, compass, and matches with you. Other items may be carried with the survival gear in your pack or in your vehicle.

Your basic survival kit should contain several shelter making items. Clear plastic garbage bags or sheeting can be used for rain gear, improvised shelter, transportation bags, water containment sacks, and as an improvised sleeping bag. Your kit should also contain a length of cord for lashing shelter materials together. A reflective blanket and a sleeping bag can also be included in expanded survival kits. The basic survival pack should also have several fire making materials, such as a lighter and a magnesium/flint fire starter. These will be your backup for the matches you are carrying. Some form of tinder should be included in a waterproof container, such as the steel wool, discussed in this chapter. Expanded kits can include stoves and small lanterns as well. For signaling purposes, the survival kit should include a signaling mirror and a whistle at the absolute minimum. Other gear can be added based on the conditions of the mission. Personal location beacons and satellite phones can enhance rescue dramatically. Water purification tablets and a condom for water storage should be included in the basic kit. Extra water supplies or water filters may be most effective in some situations and can be included in the expanded kit. Fish hooks and line and the metal parts of a rat trap should be included in most survival kits for food procurement. A survival rife, sling shot rubber bands, or spear points might also be appropriate for some locations.

So, even as you plan for the survival conditions and pack your survival kit, remember the most important piece of survival gear is your head. Plan ahead, think, improvise, and learn to adapt to the conditions and you will be a survivor and not a victim of circumstances.

Principles of Survival, Resistance, Evasion, and Escape

As was discussed earlier in this chapter, survival situations can be extraordinarily challenging when it is simply man versus the harsh elements of extreme weather and climate, rough terrain, and other natural factors common to austere settings. When enemy forces, potentially unfriendly locals, and tactical considerations are added to the equation, then the challenges for survival can become overwhelming. This section will discuss the principles of survival, evasion, resistance, and escape (SERE) and will provide some tips for staying alive when the individual wants to avoid being found by the wrong people and move safely to a rescue location.

Survival

Survival in the context of SERE adds an entirely new dimension and level of challenge to an already difficult task. The term *nonpermissive environment* is often used to describe either a tactical setting or other hostile condition where overt procedures draw unwanted attention and security is paramount to survival. The basic prioritization of key elements to survival still hold true, but under nonpermissive conditions, security must be added to every facet of survival to ensure success. The following is a slightly modified list of the key elements to survival that were discussed earlier in this chapter. The priorities of survival from a SERE perspective are as follows: (i) your mind, (ii) security, (iii) first aid, (iv) shelter, (iv) fire, (vi) water, and (vii) food.

Notice that, once again, the mind is your most valuable asset, followed by the added element of security. As stated earlier, trying to survive in a nonpermissive environment is an overwhelming challenge and keeping the mind sharp and maintaining a constant situational awareness is crucial to success. Military personnel are very well equipped mentally through discipline and specialized training for overcoming the unique challenges associated with a survival situation, especially those that received formal SERE training prior to entering a hostile environment.

Evasion

It is essential to practice excellent camouflage and concealment techniques when trying to survive unnoticed in the wild. Any actions taken for survival should be accomplished with the least amount of observable movement as possible. Personal camouflage should be used to break the pattern of all lines of the human silhouette and make every attempt to blend in with the surrounding environment. Ideally, camouflage-patterned clothing should be worn and exposed skin should be covered by using commercially available camouflage kits commonly used by hunters and military personnel. If these items are not available, then the evader will need to improvise by using mud, grass stains, and soot from charcoal to break patterns on exposed skin, clothing, and equipment when operating in the field. Clothing that stands out against the terrain needs to be camouflaged with dirt and vegetation and anything reflective, such as glasses and watches, should be removed from sight or covered with something to keep it concealed. Strips of clothing and other materials can be used to break the pattern of equipment and if weapons were not already spray painted with some type of camouflage pattern before entering the operational area, then adding some strips of material to the weapon is fine as long as it does not interfere with the weapon's operation. Special consideration should to be addressed for optics, such as rifle scopes and binoculars, because their reflectivity can reveal your location. During the premission planning phase, it is advisable to pack a small amount of nylon stocking that can be stretched over the lenses of these types of optical systems. The nylon will greatly reduce the reflectivity and will still allow the operator to use the system effectively. When using vegetation as part of your camouflage system, remember to select the type of plant life that is prevalent in the area you are located. Do not pick one area clean, but rather take a few plants from a more spread out area. Be cautious that whatever impact you make on the vegetation will clue trackers to your presence and intentions. Also, be aware that vegetation used for camouflage will fade over time, so replace this frequently and change as needed when moving in different surroundings.

The evader needs to reduce making any sounds that reveals his or her presence while performing survival tasks and always practice good noise discipline techniques when moving. Natural sounds, such as the wind and rain, can help mask the sound of human footfall. Wrapping shoes with clothing can also help muffle the noises produced by movement. Any loose items or pieces of equipment that rattle during movement should be taped or wrapped so that they do not produce a sound when shaken. Talking between evaders should be avoided at all costs and the use of hand and arm signals should be used as a principle means of communication. Even low level talking can be detected from far away if conditions are just right and the evader's location will become compromised. Electronic devices, such as watch alarms, cell phones, and other noise-producing items, must be deactivated or put on the silent mode to avoid unwanted attention.

Light discipline is another essential practice that must be employed when hiding from the enemy. Any device that produces light in the visible and infrared spectrum is considered a high-risk item that can alert others to your presence. Most modern military and law enforcement organizations are equipped with night vision optical equipment with infrared light sources. Remember that the amplified light coming from the eye pieces of these devices can be seen from far away when viewed from the side, so make every effort to cover the light that "leaks" to the side with some type of masking material. Hostile forces that possess a night vision capability can also see infrared light sources that most night vision devices and targeting devices emit, so these are also risky to use and can compromise your position. Be wary that, if observed, an accidental discharge of a light source can draw just as much attention as an accidental discharge of your weapon.

Natural night vision is by far the safest means for the evader to use when operating in low illumination conditions. Natural night vision will improve over time for the evader as the pupils dilate and the evader gets accustomed to the dark. There will only be rare instances when a light source is necessary, such as reading a map at night or performing some other task that requires reading under low light. Whenever possible, use night vision devices and an infrared source in an area that affords maximum cover and try to be as low to the ground as possible. If all that is available is a standard flashlight, then covering the lens with a red filter (if available) or cover the lens completely with duct tape or other material and make a very small pin-sized hole in the covering. This will allow a small yet sufficient amount of light to escape. After this filter is constructed for the flashlight, then the evader should cover himself completely with a blanket, tarp, jacket, or other covering item so that no light escapes for others to see. Infrared light can penetrate some types of materials, so assess the threat and take the appropriate precautions.

The evader must seriously assess the risk versus benefit for making a fire. If a fire is absolutely necessary for survival due to extreme cold conditions, then great care must be taken to reduce the light signature and dissipate the smoke as much as possible. Build the fire near a tree which will help dissipate the smoke to a certain degree. It is usually more difficult to observe smoke during inclement weather, so this should also be taken into consideration. Thoroughly shield the fire from view by digging a pit 10 to 12 inches deep with a 6- to 12-inch opening at the top and keeping the flames below ground level. Dig a tunnel for air circulation approximately 10 inches away from the main fire pit about the same depth with a 6- to 8-inch opening. Choose an area for your fire pit with 360-degree screening,

if at all possible. Using a fire during dawn, dusk, and when the indigenous populous typically cooks, is also a good technique to reduce your signature. More sophisticated opponents that are looking for evaders may have thermal imaging devices and, therefore, building a fire would be a very high risk. Consider the situation and assess the threat before taking any actions that may reveal your location.

If a fire is out of the question, then remember that a shelter will help you conserve warmth and will assist in concealment. In the nonpermissive environment, the shelter needs to look like the immediate surroundings as much as possible, be constructed so it has a low silhouette, be small in size and of irregular shape, and be in a very secluded location that no one would normally walk.

In the natural world, predators are drawn to the motion that is made by their prey. When trying to hide from a human threat, movement will also be noticed by those that are hunting you. To mask your presence, always use terrain and natural cover to your advantage. Never travel on the top of a ridge or any terrain that you run the risk of silhouetting against. Do not disturb vegetation above the level of the knee and do not grab branches, vines, and shrubs to move them out of the way, it is better to use a small stick to gently push vegetation away as you move. Avoid scuffing bark on trees and logs and breaking branches, use shadows to your advantage, and walk as much as possible on hard surfaces so that you do not leave footprints. It is better to move in an irregular route to reduce the chances of being tracked and make frequent and irregularly spaced stops at points of concealment to survey the route and security situation ahead. If coming to a stop for a period of time, plan to make two right angle turns in the same direction and a third right angle turn in the opposite direction at locations that are conducive for not leaving signs of a turn or making any tracks. The idea is to slightly travel back toward the direction you came from and off of the main route. Find a hide site that allows you to overwatch the route you have traveled. If you are being tracked, the trackers will miss the signs of the turns and travel past you as you slip away to their flanks. If dogs are being used, this technique will probably not be successful. When dealing with dogs, the focus should be on defeating the dog handlers. This is accomplished by choosing a difficult route that will fatigue those in pursuit of you and select a route through areas that are impassable to humans that are walking upright. As discussed earlier, it is usually best to move at night, in bad weather, and when there is wind. Roads, trails, and other linear manmade objects present great risk to the evader. Only cross these danger areas after thoroughly assessing the threat from a concealed position. When crossing, use a bend in the road, shadows, and other aspects that afford the most security. Minimize your exposure to the road as much as possible. If the surface of the road or trail will cause you to leave foot prints, then take a piece of vegetation to scatter your tracks and cross the road while sidestepping with your foot parallel to the direction of the road.

Successful evasion relies heavily upon the navigation abilities of the individual and navigation is considered by some as both an art and a science. Entire books have been written on the subject and this chapter will only cover some of the essential concepts.

Handheld GPS devices are wonderful tools for navigating just about anywhere on the globe from the urban environment to the remote wilderness. This is a viable option as long as the batteries remain fresh and the terrain and foliage do not mask the signal from the constellation of satellites above. This being said, in addition to the GPS you pack in your bag, always include a backup method of navigation. The two essential items that should be taken into the operational area are a map and compass.

The map should be weatherproofed by either laminating or placing in a ziplock bag. The map should be "sterile" with no markings whatsoever. This security measure must be stressed to all members of the evasion team so that if the map falls into the wrong hands, it will not provide an opposition force with any useful intelligence. Some operators chose to write on the plastic laminate of the map with an erasable marker that can be wiped clean in a hurry. A more secure but difficult technique to master is to memorize key locations on the map while conducting premission planning and training before entering the operational area.

When preparing the map during the premission planning phase, cut and fold the portions of the map that are needed for the mission, but be sure to include marginal information needed to determine scale, distances, reference lines for the coordinate system, contour intervals (determines elevation for topographic maps), and the declination diagram (the angular distance between "true" north and "magnetic" north, which varies around the world). In addition to being waterproofed, the map should be placed in some type of map case that is tied onto the evader by a lanyard or other securing method.

A useful tool used in conjunction with a map is a protractor. This is slightly different than the common protractors used in geometry classes. Mapping protractors are very commonly used by the military services, but several civilian versions are available in the commercial market. This transparent navigational aid has printed information on one side and is placed on the map sheet with a graduated scale on the perimeter that indicates 360 degrees of angular measurement. The central area of the protractor usually has a crosshair that can be placed on any spot on the map and if the true north of the protractor is oriented in line with the true north vertical lines of the map, then the evader can determine directions from position to other locations of interest. Again, it important to note that in many parts of the world, true north differs from magnetic north and a careful inspection of the map's declination dia-

gram is required to avoid errors in conversion from "true" to "magnetic" directions (azimuths) from the map to the compass. Based on the type of protractor, several models have internal graduated scales for measuring distance for different scale maps and can assist in plotting locations using different coordinate systems.

Several types of compasses are commercially available and have multiple features that are very useful in the field. Some compasses have a built-in setting screw that allows the user to preset the declination angle as discussed earlier. Many compasses have luminous markings that allow use at night. Most of the better compasses are liquid filled, which helps dampen the oscillations of the north seeking needle that occur while moving. Almost all compassed possess a rotating bezel ring marked with a 360-degree scale so that a particular azimuth can be set and the evader can follow a specific direction while sighting in a distant point or when walking. Just like the map, the compass should be secured to the user to prevent accidental loss during movement, typically with a lanyard.

Determining distance on the ground is another skill that is highly useful to navigation. There are several different techniques. One simple method is to determine your "pace-count" in a premission setting by walking a measured distance (100 meters, for example) and counting how many times your left foot hits the ground. If this is done enough times, then the individual will know on the average how many steps are taken for a given length and through keeping track of these cumulative intervals, the evader will be able to determine distance traveled in the field. Of course the pace count will vary based on terrain, weight carried, day versus night, if running, if fatigued, in snow, etc. Accurate pace and distance determination can be established through repetitive training before the mission.

Navigation techniques vary greatly. In general, there are two types of land navigation: dead reckoning and terrain association. In dead reckoning, the evader follows a strict compass heading while keeping an accurate measure of distance through a pace count. This type of navigation works well in a flat environment that is devoid of recognizable terrain, but is impractical for densely vegetated or mountainous terrain. Terrain association uses the map and identification of terrain features (hill tops, saddles, ridges, valleys, spurs, draws, etc.) to determine location and find routes that are conducive to travel. Many find that the best way to navigate is to use a combination of the two techniques. A careful map reconnaissance should always be performed prior to actual movement and special note of stream crossings, roads, and difficult terrain should be considered in selecting the route during the planning phase. With the proper training and a good map, compass, and protractor, the evader can plot points on the map, determine azimuths that need to be followed on the compass through a simple conversion process, measure distance, and stay on course to a rescue location.

As with all military and law enforcement operations, a mission is more likely to succeed with implementing a well thought out plan. The more detailed the operation, the greater the necessity for an in-depth planning process and conduct of rehearsals for critical actions. When friendly forces enter into the operational area to execute the plan, it is not uncommon for unforeseen conditions to affect the original concept of the operation. In some cases, the degree of change is so dramatic and the threat is assessed as so high, that either part of or the entire mission must be aborted and the friendly forces find themselves in a situation where the primary method of extraction is no longer possible as originally conceived. The evaders must adapt to the new situation and seek recovery at another location using a set of preplanned procedures. This preplanned set of procedures is known as an evasion plan of action. This critically important annex to the overall operations plan will need to be developed before the operators enter the area where the mission is to be conducted.

Each organization has its own techniques, tactics, and procedures for developing and executing the evasion action plan. This is an extremely sensitive plan that needs to be prepared in isolation of other teams that may be operating in the area and only disseminated to those with a need to know to prevent accidental compromise if other teams are captured by enemy forces. It should be written so that it may be easily remembered by the evasion personnel concerned and with enough detail to give commanders and search and rescue assets the information that they will need in order to predict what the team on the ground is thinking when moving to predesignated rescue points within predefined boundaries. The predetermined rescue locations should be arranged in a corridor along a general compass heading toward friendly territory or other designated area. The plan should include phase lines along the general direction of travel and based on estimated movement time, specific locations need to be designated as safe sites and rescue sites. Within the evasion corridor, the team should always conduct surveillance of a potential rescue site to determine if it is safe to occupy and call for extraction.

The evasion action plan should include enough information to completely cover all means of radio and other technical communication methods, from encrypted voice to transponder beacons. Based on the threat, some enemy forces may have the means to triangulate the evader's location through radio direction finding techniques and, therefore, the evaders must assess the risk of making transmissions back to search and rescue assets. Other sections of the plan need to address all manner of coordinating instructions, alternate signaling methods, brevity codes, safe signals, duress signals, verification of evading personnel's identity, threat areas, resupply plans, potential friendly support assets in the area, to name but a few considerations.

Resistance and Escape

Many readers of this textbook have seen fictional and historically accurate films depicting the courageous efforts of heroes resisting their captors while being detained and ultimately succeeded against all odds in a daring escape back to friendly territory. An even greater number of books have been written on the subject by experts that have survived the horrors of being a prisoner of war and were able to tell their tale. There are several examples of resistance techniques and escape methods that may be derived from these films and books, but probably the best way to prepare for a detention situation is to attend training specifically dedicated to the subject of resistance and escape.

This open source text cannot delve into the details of this topic due to the law enforcement sensitive and classified nature of this topic. Several organizations have their unique standard operating procedures for what to do in a detained scenario and how to resist and escape from hostile forces. The leadership in each organization, whether it is military or law enforcement based, should require their cleared personnel to attend formal training in a high level risk SERE school, especially if these personnel are regularly exposed to operations where the threat of enemy capture is deemed high.

What can be said in this text is that the detained individual must refocus all efforts on the primary element of survival: your mind. This is the greatest (and may be the only) tool available to the resistor and potential escapee that is placed in a detained situation. The U.S. military has a code of conduct for those that find themselves in a prisoner of war status that is worthy of mention in this chapter. This code of conduct is divided into six articles and provides a common basis for how the military detainee should act while being held as a prisoner. This code provides the framework for the internal mental strength required to overcome the challenges of a detention setting. Although this may not directly equate to all detention scenarios that law enforcement personnel may find themselves in, there are commonalities in the theme of the military code of conduct from a mental focus perspective.

Article I: I am an American, fighting in the armed forces, which guard my country and our way of life. I am prepared to give my life in their defense.

Article II: I will never surrender of my own free will. If in command, I will never surrender the members of my command while they still have the means to resist.

Article III: If I am captured, I will continue to resist by all means available. I will make every effort to escape and aid others to escape. I will accept neither parole nor special favors from the enemy.

Article IV: If I become a prisoner of war, I will keep faith with my fellow prisoners. I will give no information nor take part in any action, which might be harmful to my comrades. If I am senior, I will take command. If not, I will obey the lawful orders of those appointed over me and will back them up in every way.

Article V: When questioned, should I become a prisoner of war, I am required to give name, rank, service number, and date of birth. I will evade answering further questions to the utmost of my ability. I will make no oral or written statements disloyal to my country and its allies or harmful to their cause.

Article VI: I will never forget that I am an American, responsible for my actions, and dedicated to the principles, which made my country free. I will trust in my God and in the United States of America.

If the opportunity presents to escape from a detained scenario, then the individual must make the call based on all available information. During escape efforts, failure is often met with dire consequences, but by the same token, detention without escape can have an equally grim outcome. All factors must be taken into consideration and the individual must decide what course of action to take. Once committed to escaping, the principles of survival and evasion must be strictly adhered to as discussed earlier in the chapter. The mental focus needs be centered on security and ultimately the recovery effort.

Surviving in the nonpermissive environment and adhering to the principles of SERE requires much more planning and advanced training above and beyond what is needed to stay alive in normal survival scenarios. Make training a priority during the premission phases and practice all the skills necessary for survival situations and detention scenarios whenever possible. Incorporate the various aspects of SERE into exercises and rehearsals so the first time the operators are faced with these unique conditions, it will not be during a real-world mission. Using the mind and keeping security as the highest priorities will give you the best chances of accomplishing your mission and getting through the challenges of surviving the natural and manmade threats that you will encounter in the operational area.

TAKE HOME POINTS

1. Your mind is the most important element that will influence your survival in both a wilderness or SERE survival situation.
2. Proper planning and anticipation of survival scenarios is essential in mission planning.
3. Formal SERE training can improve your chances of survival.
4. Food is lowest initial priority in survival situations.

CONCLUSION

No one intends on being in a survival situation; however, this is not an uncommon scenario. Individuals who are providing medical support for tactical operations are at an increased risk of this eventuality and should consider survival within their mission planning. Formal SERE training should be considered for the TEMS provider, especially for those involved in overseas operations.

Medical Concepts

Section Editor: PHILLIP L. COULE

Chapter 10

Penetrating and Explosive Injury Patterns

Ian S. Wedmore, John G. McManus, Jr., and Timothy A. Coakley

OBJECTIVES

After reading this section, the reader will be able to:

1. Discuss common physics of wounding from different penetrating
2. Describe wounding patterns from explosive and ballistic injuries.
3. Understand treatment and evacuation priorities for explosive and ballistic injuries.

INTRODUCTION

In the 21st century, it is an unfortunate fact that individuals on an expedition could become victims of penetrating or explosive trauma caused by accidents from hunting occurring nearby, becoming inadvertently shot while being caught up in political turmoil, or involved in an explosive event that is not uncommon in many parts of the world. The medical provider treating penetrating and explosive trauma in the austere environment is faced with multiple challenges to include: lack of medical supplies, prolonged evacuation time and distance, and lack of sophisticated care that is the standard for trauma care in the urban environment. This chapter will discuss the evaluation and treatment for penetrating and explosive injuries in the tactical environment.

Physics and Epidemiology

Ballistics

The available energy for a missile to inflict upon the body is dependent on the equation $E = 1/2MV^2$, where M is the mass of the bullet (larger bullets impart more energy), and V is the velocity of the bullet as it hits the tissue. Thus, in most cases, the potential damage is greatest with a high-velocity round, such as that seen with a modern assault rifles and high-velocity hunting weapons.

For missile injuries, there are two areas of projectile-tissue interaction. The first is a permanent cavity, which is a localized area of necrotic tissue and clot, proportional to the size of the projectile as it passes through. The second is a temporary cavity (cavitation) caused by the displacement of tissue away from the passage of the projectile. This results in an area of contusion and concussion some distance from the actual path of the bullet. The amount of damage done to tissue depends on the amount of energy transferred to the tissue as well as the elastic properties of the tissue itself. Elastic tissues, such as skeletal muscle, blood vessels, and skin, may be displaced significantly due to cavitation but then rebound with minimal permanent injury. Inelastic tissue, such as bone, brain or liver, handles cavitation poorly and tends to fracture resulting in significant damage. There is also a shock (sonic) wave that also passes through tissue and does not cause any appreciable clinical effect (1,2).

Despite the fact that the energy can be imparted to a tissue is potentially most dependent on V^2 the commonly held belief that high-velocity rounds always cause increased tissue damage is incorrect. Velocity is one factor in wounding. An increase in velocity does not de facto increase the amount of tissue damage. High-velocity rounds, if they do not impact bone or relatively inelastic tissues, such as brain or solid organs (liver), shatter or yaw in the tissue they may pass through the body, imparting little destructive energy (3). For example, the amount of tissue damage in the first 12 cm of a M-16A1 bullet wound has relatively little soft tissue disruption, similar to that of a 0.22 caliber long rifle bullet, which has less than half the velocity (4). Although the human thigh is approximately 12 cm wide in the average individual, it can be seen that a high-velocity round may pass through the body before it imparts any significant energy outside of the bullet path.

It has been suggested that high-velocity bullets will yaw in the tissue, increasing damage. Projectiles yaw in flight, which can create irregular wounds; however, unless a projectile hits an intermediate target, the amount of yaw in flight is insignificant. Yaw, in tissue, is in fact also seldom a consideration, as the bullets will not yaw until it penetrates deeply into the body. The AK-47 bullet, for example, yaws, but not until it has penetrated 25 cm into tissue (thus, in most cases, the bullet has already passed through the body before it has reached a depth sufficient to yaw) (5). The AK-74 assault rifle round, however, does yaw relatively early (about 7 cm of penetration), which may cause increased tissue damage.

Fragmentation of a bullet will also lead to increased tissue damage. The bullet fragments deviate out of the original bullet path in a multitude of directions and velocities causing damage to all the tissue they pass through. Although full metal jacket military rounds, in accordance with the Hauge agreement of 1899, are designed to remain intact in the body and many will, in fact, fragment after a certain distance in tissue. For example, the M-193 bullet of the M-16A1 rifle reliably fragments after traversing about 12 cm of soft tissue (6). Thus, again the bullet may have passed through the body before it fragments or if it enters tissue >12 cm in depth, it may cause significant damage due to multiple fragments formed. Military rounds and assault rifles are designed to wound (although often

severely) rather than kill, because wounded individuals require greater resources to evacuate and care for than those killed outright (7).

It has been often stated that exit wounds are always greater than entrance wounds. This has been shown to be frequently not the case and has no bearing on care, which is always in response to the wound regardless of whether it is an entrance or exit wound (8).

Explosive

An explosion is caused by the rapid chemical conversion of a liquid or solid material into a gas with a resultant kinetic energy release. Low-kinetic explosives (gunpowder) release energy slowly by a process called deflagration. In contrast, high-kinetic explosive detonation involves the almost instantaneous transformation of the physical space occupied by the original solid or liquid material into gases, filling the same volume within a few microseconds, and is, therefore, under extremely high pressure (Fig. 10.1). The highly pressurized gasses expand rapidly and compress the surrounding environment, generating a pressure pulse, which is propagated as a blast wave. This blast wave is called overpressure or blast wind. As a blast wave passes through the body, it causes damage by several different mechanisms. Patients injured from explosions usually suffer from a combination of blast, blunt, penetrating, and burn trauma (Table 10.1).

Propagation of overpressure waves down range is dependent on the environment. There are several related phenomena of a blast waves that can cause considerably more damage to the victim. Coupling occurs when one blast wave converges with another or multiple waves. The waves are additive in their destructive nature to the tissue. Reflected waves occur when the explosive force reflects off of a structures or surfaces. Both of these types of waves usually occur together in closed spaces such as buses, buildings, or streets between buildings. The cumulative force exerted on the body from reflected and coupled wave's increases the risk of primary blast injuries. The caregiver has to have a high clinic index of suspicion when evaluating these patients exposed to such situations.

Tympanic membrane (TM) rupture is a good marker for significant exposure to blast waves. The average kinetics necessary to incur such an injury can also cause occult or delayed primary blast injuries. When a ruptured,

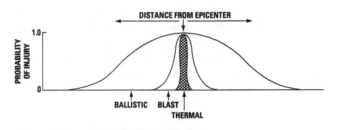

FIGURE 10.1. Explosive injury forces.

▶ **TABLE 10.1. Categories of Explosive Injuries.**

Category	Mechanism	Injury Type
Primary	A form of barotrauma, unique to explosions, which causes damage to air-filled organs.	■ Blast lung ■ TM rupture and middle ear damage ■ Abdominal hemorrhage and perforation ■ Globe (eye) rupture ■ Concussion
Secondary	Penetrating trauma caused by the acceleration of shrapnel and other debris by the blast.	■ Penetrating ballistic (fragmentation) ■ Blunt injuries ■ Eye penetration
Tertiary	Casualty becomes a missile and is propelled through the air, with typical patterns of blunt trauma.	■ Fracture and traumatic amputation ■ Blunt chest and abdominal trauma ■ Impalement ■ Closed and open brain injury
Quaternary	All other explosion-related injuries, illnesses, or diseases that are not due to primary, secondary, or tertiary mechanisms.	■ Burns (flash, partial, and full thickness) ■ Crush injuries ■ Exacerbation of underlying conditions (i.e., Asthma, COPD, angina) ■ Inhalation injury

TM, tympanic membrane; COPD, chronic obstructive pulmonary disease.

TM is seen in a patient exposed to explosive forces, a thorough evaluation needs to be performed even in the absence of significant injuries. Delayed presentations of occult bowel wall, pulmonary, and neurological injuries are common. Observation and repeated assessment needs to be performed for approximately 24 hours as most occult injuries will be recognized during this time.

Weapon Types

Low-velocity weapons: (<2,000 feet/sec and typically <1,100 feet/sec) do not as a general rule cause significant cavitation and have less propensity to cause significant soft tissue damage. Almost all civilian handguns are prime examples; these cause the majority of urban penetrating injuries.

High-velocity weapons: (>2,000 feet/sec) have the potential to cause significant soft tissue damage due to cavitation and include the M-16, M-4 carbine, AK-47, and AK-74 assault rifles. High-velocity civilian hunting rifles have a propensity to cause the most significant tissue damage. They fire large bullets at high velocity and the bullets are not metal jacketed, so they fragment quickly and yaw quickly. These bullets are designed specifically to impart massive tissue damage early (9). Unjacketed bullets in fact can cause a wound cavity up to 40 times the size of a jacketed bullet (10).

Explosive Devices

Because of the current increased terrorist threat and occurrence in many countries, multiple different explosive devices can be purposefully or accidentally encountered by adventure seekers even outside of previous "war" zones. Most accidental explosive injuries occur from handling or encountering mines, improvised explosive devices (IEDs), unexploded ordnance (UXO), such as grenades, and ammunition. In Afghanistan alone, the death and injury rate was 150 to 300 per month from accidental UXO encounters even before the current war.

An IED is often difficult to detect because it is made up of common items and can consist of almost any type of material and initiator. It is a "homemade" device that causes injury or death by using explosives alone or in combination with toxic chemicals, biological toxins, or radiological material. IEDs can utilize commercial or military grade explosives, homemade explosives, or military ordnance and can be found in varying sizes, functioning methods, containers, and delivery methods.

Commonly Encountered Assault Weapons

The AK-47 rifle is probably the most common weapon seen throughout the world. When firing the standard full metal jacketed bullet, there is a 25 cm path of relatively minimal tissue disruption before the projectile begins to yaw. This is why relatively minimal tissue disruption may be seen with some wounds. The AK-74 rifle utilizes a smaller 5.45-mm round compared to the AK-47. As previously mentioned, the AK-74 round tends to yaw early at 7 cm; therefore, it is more likely to cause increased tissue damage.

The M-16A1 and M-4 carbine fire a 55-grain full metal jacketed bullet (M-193) at approximately 950 m/sec. The full metal jacketed bullet penetrates about 12 cm before it yaws to about 90 degrees, flattens, and then breaks at the

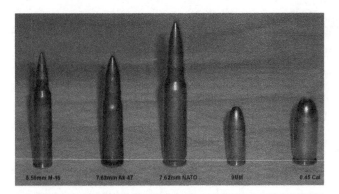

FIGURE 10.2. Standard full metal jacket military rounds found commonly throughout the world.

cannalure (a groove placed around the midsection of the bullet) (4) (Fig. 10.2).

There are many types of bullets now being used in weapons, such as incendiary rounds, designed to set fire to whatever they hit. Hollow point or "dum dum" bullets are designed to flatten when they hit tissue and, thus, increase tissue damage earlier upon striking the target and not penetrate objects. Armor piercing rounds designed to penetrate the light armor of vehicles. Clinically, this myriad of rounds will cause lesser or greater tissue damage, and there is nothing relevant for wound care based solely on what type of round was fired (11).

In summation, the most important determinant of tissue damage is the amount of energy transferred to the tissue rather than whether the wound is caused by a high- or low-velocity injury. A high-velocity weapon may pass through the body imparting little energy to the tissues and, thus, result in a wound similar to a low-energy transfer wound. The depth to which a bullet penetrates can affect the severity of the injury; wounds that penetrate to great depth without exiting the body will yaw and fragment imparting significant damage to the tissues. Bullet fragments that hit bone can result in significant tissue damage as well as the creation of secondary missiles and trauma. Each wound must be approached individually. Those that cause massive tissue injury require more extensive debridement regardless of being caused by high- or low-velocity projectiles.

Shotgun Wounds

Shotguns at close range are among the most destructive of all weapons as they disperse all of their energy into the affected tissue within a short distance. Shotgun wounds sustained at short ranges (<3 m) can be particularly devastating with massive tissue destruction, and the shotgun wadding also penetrates the wound leading to soft tissue contamination and bacterial proliferation (12). In contrast, however, shotguns wounds sustained at a distance may cause minimal injury (13). Short-range shotgun

wounds will usually require extensive debridement and wound care best carried out in an operating room (14,15). Field care will be as for all wounds: control of bleeding and, if possible, removal of necrotic tissue and copious irrigation of the wound.

Management of Soft Tissue Wounds

Military wounds and therefore also penetrating wounds sustained in the austere environment are all considered to be contaminated wounds. Treatment should, therefore, proceed based on this assumption.

Non–life-threatening Wounds

Non–life-threatening wounds will typically involve an extremity. These will most often be penetrating wounds, which penetrate through the tissue and exit the body, or grazing wounds, which do not penetrate deeply into body. Several standard principles apply to the treatment of all penetrating wounds. These principles include: (i) adequate wound excision; (ii) adequate wound drainage; (iii) immobilization until the soft tissues are healed; (iv) antibiotic therapy; and (v) secondary closure or coverage (16). All wounds will require these principles to be applied to some extent.

The wound should be debrided minimally of any obviously dead tissue at the entrance and exit. Conservative debridement of only obviously necrotic tissue is preferred to overexuberant debridement of tissue that may be potentially salvageable (17). The excision of necrotic tissue should remove enough skin from the entrance and exit wounds to allow for adequate wound drainage.

The wound must then be adequately irrigated. This requires the wound to be irrigated with a pressure of at least 7 PSI pressure at the wound surface (18,19). Pressure of 7 PSI can be generated by using a 30- to 60-cc syringe with an 18-gauge needle or catheter on it. The quantity of fluid utilized is enough to make the wound appear "clean," although as general rule use at least 250 cc per wound at minimum. Larger volumes are better than smaller, and there really is no such thing as "too much wound irrigation."

Although sterile saline or water is the hospital standard for wound irrigation, tap water has been show to be just as effective without any increased risk of wound infection (20–23). In the austere environment, neither sterile saline, sterile water, nor tap water is usually available. Therefore, any potable water source may be utilized. If water is drinkable, it will be effective. Hydrogen peroxide, bleach solutions, antibiotic solutions, and iodine solutions are no more effective than water for wound cleansing and may actually be deleterious as many of these solutions are tissue toxic.

The wound after irrigation is loosely packed with gauze to allow for free drainage. After the wound is dressed, it can be left covered until definitive care is reached (up to 72 hours). The dressing need only be removed, evaluated or changed if there is increased drainage, pain, or fever develops. The injured extremity should be splinted to prevent further soft tissue damage. Penetrating extremity wounds should be treated with antibiotics as soon as possible. This will be covered later under the antibiotic section of this chapter.

Penetrating wounds from projectiles should never be closed primarily. This will lead to an increased risk of infection (24,25). These wounds if required can be closed secondarily 3 to 6 days after the initial injury. This delay allows the bodies host defenses to reduce the wound bacterial counts back down to zero at which time closure can be carried out with a minimal effect on cosmetic outcome. The exception to this would be areas with significant vascularity where primary closure is associated with a minimal infection risk. This includes the face and scalp. These areas may be closed primarily after wound irrigation.

Individuals with penetrating wounds of the extremities are not required to be NPO during their evacuation. They can be given oral liquids for rehydration, can take oral medications, and if evacuation will be prolonged, they can eat normally.

Debridement Considerations

In the past, it been considered dogma that all high-velocity projectile tracts must be fully excised and explored, due to the effects of the temporary cavitation. Previous literature has suggested that cavitation caused significant injury requiring extensive debridement, up to 30 to 40 times the diameter of the round (26). This has turned out to be untrue. The larger cavitation diameter occurs rarely and is probably based on high-velocity hunting rounds. As previously discussed, temporary cavitation may not occur in many high-velocity wounds due to their passing through tissue before obtaining the depth at which cavitation occurs. Elastic soft tissue (skeletal muscle, blood vessels, and nerves) generally heals uneventfully and does not require excision, provided the blood supply remains intact. Temporary cavity effects are analogous to blunt trauma. Animal studies have shown that extensive debridement is not required in most high-velocity wounds (27,28). These most recent studies on high-velocity wounds found the administration of antibiotics rather than extensive debridement to be the most important factor in decreasing the wound infection rate.

Bullet Removal

Despite what most Hollywood movies would suggest, the removal of a bullet from a gunshot wound is not required in most cases. Bullets are, in fact, not "sterilized" by firing

(29). The majority of the contamination from a penetrating missile comes from the skin surface and any clothing or surface debris carried into the wound by the projectile. These contaminants are "sucked" into the wound by the vacuum effect of the temporary cavitation as it collapses on itself (30). The contamination is treated by conservative debridement and irrigation. Lead or copper poisoning does not occur from bullets unless they penetrate and reside in a synovial or cerebral spinal fluid filled space. Bullet removal, therefore, is only required in cases of penetration and lodgment in the synovial spaces of the body or cerebral spinal fluid filled neural structures. Bullets in soft tissue are quickly covered by avascular fibrous scar tissue, which prevents uptake of the metal (31).

Fragmentary Wounds

Shrapnel or fragment wounds are now the most common cause of civilian injuries in third world conflicts (32). Unfortunately, this also means that individuals venturing into austere regions for expeditions are more likely to be injured by fragments rather than bullets. Shrapnel and fragment wounds are managed according to the degree of tissue damaged, although, in general, small fragments are similar to low-energy transfer projectiles, such as handgun wounds. Large fragments may cause wounds similar to high- or low-velocity projectiles. Hand grenade fragments usually tend to cause limited soft tissue injury because the fragments do not penetrate deeply. They also do not typically result in comminuted fractures (33). They can often be treated by conservative debridement of obviously dead tissue, irrigation of the wound, and dressing (34,35). Similar to bullets, fragments in soft tissue do not require removal, and doing so may lead to excessive morbidity from the probing and incisions used to retrieve the fragments (36). In general, if the fragments are superficial and easily removed without complication, this can be done. If they are deeper and require substantial removal effort, they should be left in place unless infection develops at the site or criteria as discussed under bullet removal above occur. The International Committee of the Red Cross, based on experience gained in multiple austere theaters, recommends that soft tissue fragment wounds of <1 cm in size that do not have an associated hematoma or vital structure involvement should be managed conservatively (37). This practice was successfully used by a deployed British Field Hospital during the recent Iraq conflict (38). Large fragment wounds are treated with debridement and excision as required based on the wound.

Fractures

Fractures from penetrating missiles and explosives are splinted and stabilized as are fractures from any traumatic cause. However, fractures from high-velocity wounds tend to have a greater comminution rate (39) and, thus, are less likely to be well stabilized without surgical intervention. Fractures from low-velocity, low-energy gunshots tend to behave similarly to closed fractures and have a low incidence of infection (16). Antibiotic prophylaxis is recommended for all fractures associated with high-velocity wounds (40). In the urban setting, antibiotics may not be required for low-energy transfer wounds, although they are recommended for use in contaminated wounds with associated fractures. As all austere penetrating wounds are considered "contaminated," all penetrating wounds in these environments with or without fractures should receive prophylactic antibiotics.

Pelvic fractures will typically be stable fractures. If unstable, however, stabilization should be undertaken as soon as possible to minimize pelvic bleeding (41). In the austere environment, this is best carried out by use of some type of pelvic binder. The most easily performed method is to "sheet" the pelvis: a sheet is folded to the width of the pelvis, placed under it, and tied across the anterior pelvis. This is a very effective method of temporary stabilization (42).

Special Treatment Considerations

Hemorrhage Control

In the austere environment bleeding must be controlled as quickly as possible. The standard teaching of direct pressure and then the use of pressure points has for years been the standard. This remains the mainstay for mild to moderate bleeding in the austere environment. For severe bleeding with long transport to care times, this approach will not always work effectively. Particularly in the case of penetrating trauma and the often high associated incidence of significant venous or arterial bleeding, this approach may not be appropriate. In the combat setting, tourniquets have returned to the forefront of care for the control of major bleeding; they have the same utility for austere use.

The use of tourniquets does remain unquestionably controversial, and tourniquets have little utility in the urban setting with rapid transport times to definitive care. Conversely, in the hands of knowledgeable medical providers, tourniquets can prevent morbidity and save the life of a wounded individual in the austere setting. Modern tourniquets are light, fast, and effective, and with proper use, lead to rapid control of bleeding and the saving of lives with no increase in morbidity. In the Vietnam War, 10% of those who died of penetrating wounds died from compressible hemorrhage; that is, bleeding that could have been controlled with the use of the tourniquet (43).

In the combat setting, the tourniquet is utilized in two ways: (i) for immediate control of bleeding for a casualty while still under enemy fire (where direct pressure may not be able to be effectively applied initially) and (ii) for control

of bleeding when direct pressure and pressure points are not effective. Another advantage of modern tourniquets is that they can be applied and control bleeding quicker than direct pressure and use of pressure points, thus preventing blood loss until adequate dressings can be applied to control the bleeding and the tourniquet then removed. This is particularly important if there is only one person available to render aid and bleeding control. The placement of the tourniquet allows the provider to treat more severe injuries initially and then address the bleeding when more immediate life threats are controlled. Even if there are no other life threats, rapidly placing a tourniquet allows the provider to utilize both hands to place an effective pressure dressing. It is unlikely but not impossible that you would be under fire on an expedition; however, these other reasons for the use of tourniquets provide their greatest utility for austere use.

Why are tourniquets not used routinely? Tourniquets have lost favor for civilian use due to the morbidity associated with prolonged or inappropriate use. Recent military studies have found that tourniquets both save lives and have little associated morbidity even if placed for inappropriate reasons provided they were removed within several hours (44,45). The tourniquets now used by the military are quick and effective. The use of ad hoc tourniquets are much less likely to be effective and are much more likely to lead to severe morbidity through there use. The tourniquets of choice by the U.S. Army are the CAT tourniquet and the SOFFT tourniquet. In a comparative study of commercially available tourniquets, the combat application tourniquet (CAT) was found to be the best combination of compactness, lightweight, and least painful in addition to effectively stopping arterial blood flow as measured by Doppler (46).

A tourniquet can be applied and left in place for up to 2 hours with minimal morbidity to the effected extremity (this is the maximum duration tourniquets are left in place during orthopedic surgery without morbidity). A 2006 study on tourniquet use in orthopaedic surgery (tourniquet duration <2 hours) found the risk of complications to be 1 in 2,442 uses and permanent injury risk to be 1 in 31,742 uses (47). Tourniquets left on for 6 or more hours require the limb to be amputated distal to the tourniquet. Between 2 and 6 hours morbidity is unclear and depends on a multitude of factors, but the longer a tourniquet is left in place the higher the likelihood of limb loss.

A tourniquet is properly applied by applying it 1 to 2 inches proximal to the bleeding (Fig. 10.3). After a tourniquet is in place and bleeding is controlled, the wound may have further dressings, a pressure bandage, and or advanced hemostatic dressings applied. The tourniquet can then be loosened to see if bleeding is controlled. If it is, the tourniquet should be left in place, but not tightened during evacuation. If bleeding restarts, the tourniquet can be retightened to control the bleeding.

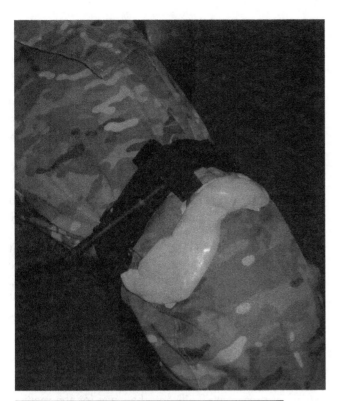

FIGURE 10.3. CAT tourniquet applied to leg "wound."

Advanced Hemostatic Agents

Recent advances in hemorrhage control include the development and fielding of modern hemostatic agents. The two most commonly utilized are zeolite granules (QuikClot) and Chitosan dressing (Hemcon bandage or Chitoflex bandage). Both have been shown in animal models to control severe venous and arterial hemorrhage (48,49). Both have seen significant use in the Afghanistan and Iraqi conflicts. A new form of modified Chitosan powder (Celox) is now commercially available as well. Chitosan (Hemcon) has been shown in an observational case series to be effective in controlling the bleeding of many penetrating wounds without significant side effects (50). These dressings are most appropriate and effective when utilized where tourniquets cannot be utilized (e.g., neck, axilla, or groin). They can also be applied after a tourniquet has been placed to control the bleeding. If effective in their placement (bleeding controlled), the tourniquet can be removed. All three agents are FDA approved for external use.

In the event of a penetrating groin or axillary wound with severe bleeding that cannot be controlled with a tourniquet, the best option available at this time would be the application of an advanced dressing and direct pressure. The author's first choice would be to stuff Chitoflex or pieces of Hemcon dressing into the wound and then place a pressure dressing. Pressure would then be manually maintained as best as possible and hypotensive resuscitation utilized to limit bleeding and allow clotting to occur in the wound. However, if a patient has massive bleeding from wounds that cannot be controlled by standard pressure dressings or tourniquets, use of any of these products is indicated to stabilize the patient. Application of either QuikClot or Celox has been shown to be effective when used in such wounds (Fig. 10.4).

Antibiotics

The use of prophylactic antibiotics in penetrating wounds in the literature is based on the type of wound (high vs. low velocity) and contamination. The literature universally supports the use of prophylactic antibiotics in high-velocity wounds (51–53). Shotguns are treated like high-velocity wounds due to the massive tissue destruction they inflict.

The use of prophylactic antibiotics in low-velocity wounds is much less clear. In low-velocity wounds in the urban setting, provided there was little wound contamination, good wound care and irrigation was undertaken and there was no advantage found to the use of prophylactic antibiotics (54–56). In the literature on low-velocity wounds, however, antibiotics are recommended for wounds with any contamination. Penetrating wounds in the austere environment are de facto considered contaminated and should be treated with prophylactic antibiotics. This is also true for fractures caused by penetrating wounds. In the past, for minimally contaminated wounds, a cephalosporin has been the recommended first-line prophylaxis. If the wound is heavily contaminated, penicillin was recommended to be added to prevent clostridial infection. If a heavily contaminated wound also involves a

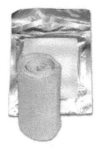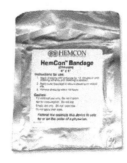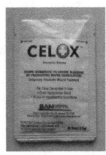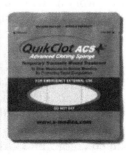

FIGURE 10.4. Commercially available hemostatic dressings.

fracture, then gentamicin should be added. These recommendations were all based on the ideal: IV antibiotic use in a hospital setting. In ideal circumstances, IV antibiotics would be given immediately after wounding. This, however, is impractical for the austere setting, because IV antibiotics require significant supplies and effort to administer. Fortunately, there are very effective oral antibiotics with excellent oral bioavailability, which can be given at the time of wounding with near equivalent efficacy to IV antibiotics.

The limited side effect profile (57) and ability to use in penicillin and sulfa allergic individuals as well as the once daily dosing recommends the fourth generation fluoroquinolones as the oral agent of choice for penetrating wounds in the austere environment (58). The fluoroquinolones, gatifloxacin or levofloxacin, are nearly 99% orally bioavailable and cover the bacteria typically involved in penetrating wounds. Of these two agents, gatifloxacin has the best coverage of Gram positive, Gram negative, and anaerobic bacteria to include clostridium (59). They can be given by mouth shortly after wounding to those with extremity wounds to decrease the risk of wound infections. If levofloxacin is utilized, then better coverage of anaerobes will have to be added. Clindamycin or metronidazole can be utilized (60). These antibiotics are also effective for penetrating torso injuries.

Penetrating abdominal and pelvis wounds will require IV or IM antibiotics as the individual cannot be given oral medications. A second generation cephalosporin with anaerobic coverage has previously been recommended for single-agent coverage of penetrating abdominal wounds (61). A 2000 meta-analysis of antibiotic use in penetrating abdominal trauma recommends the following antibiotics or combinations: cefoxitin, gentamicin with clindamycin, tobramycin with clindamycin, cefotetan, cefamandole, aztreonam, and gentamicin alone (62). Regardless of which antibiotic regimen is chosen, if an IV is not available, then giving IM antibiotics reasonable option.

Hypothermia Prevention and Patient Packaging

Penetrating trauma patients who become hypothermic have a poor prognosis. Hypothermic patients become coagulopathic, which greatly hinders hemostasis (63). This will worsen and complicate any hypovolemic shock that would otherwise occur. It was recognized in World War I that patients with penetrating injuries must be kept warm to decrease mortality. In the austere setting, this requires packaging the patients in multiple layers of insulation for transport. The patient can be laid on a "space blanket" and then wrapped in blankets and sleeping bags in several layers dependent on available materials. The use of chemical heat packs in between layers has been found to be effective in preventing heat loss (64).

TAKE HOME POINTS

1. High-velocity round wounds do not require aggressive or extensive debridement based solely on their velocity. Treat the wound not the weapon velocity.
2. Small (<1 cm) fragment wounds without associated hematoma or vital structure involvement can be managed conservatively with minimal debridement and irrigation. The fragments do not need to be removed.
3. Tourniquet use can be life saving in penetrating trauma. The goal of tourniquet use in penetrating trauma in the austere setting is to place it quickly to save loss of blood and then to remove the tourniquet as soon as possible once bleeding is otherwise controlled.
4. All penetrating wounds in the austere environment are considered contaminated and, therefore, should be given prophylactic antibiotics at the time of wounding. Fourth generation fluoroquinolones make an excellent oral antibiotic choice for extremity and torso wounds.

SUMMARY

Penetrating and explosive injuries in the austere environment present a significant challenge for the medical provider. Basic ATLS principles must be modified to adapt to the prolonged evacuation times to definitive medical care as well as the limited availability of medical supplies. The basics, however, remain unchanged with airway control, restoration of effective breathing, and hemorrhage control being the highest priorities. After the secondary survey is complete, wound care can be undertaken with minimal debridement, copious irrigation, and early administration of antibiotics to decrease morbidity and mortality.

REFERENCES

1. Harvey EN, Korr IM, Oster G, et al. Secondary damage in wounding due to the pressure changes accompany the passage of high-velocity missiles. *Surgery*. 1946;21:218–239.
2. Fackler ML. Wound ballistics: a review of common misconceptions. *JAMA*. 1988;259:2730–2736.
3. Santucci RA, Chang Y-J. Ballistics for physicians: myths about wound ballistics and gunshot injuries. *J Urol*. 2004;171:1408–1414.
4. *NATO War Surgery Handbook*. 3rd ed. Washington: Government Printing Office; 2004.
5. Barach E, Tomlanovich M, Nowak R. Ballistics: a pathophysiologic examination of the wounding mechanisms of firearms: part I. *J Trauma*. 1986;26:225.
6. Fackler ML. Wounding patterns of military rifle bullets. *Int Defense Rev*. 1989;1:59.
7. Ordog GJ, Wasserberger J, Balasubramanium S. Wound ballistics: theory and practice. *Ann Emerg Med*. 1984;13:1113.
8. Hollerman JJ, Fackler ML. Gunshot wounds: radiology and wound ballistics. *Emer Radiol*. 1995;2:171–192.
9. Barach E, Tomlanovich M, Nowak R. Ballistics: a pathophysiologic examination of the wounding mechanisms of firearms: part I. *J Trauma*. 1986;26:225.
10. DeMuth WE Jr. Bullet velocity and design as determinants of wounding capability: an experimental study. *J Trauma*. 1966;6:222.

11. Silvia AJ. Mechanism of injury in gunshot wounds: myths and reality [Confronting Forensic Issues]. *Crit Care Nurs Q*. 1999;22:69–74.
12. Ordog GJ, Wasserberger J, Balasubramanium S. Shotgun wound ballistics. *J Trauma*. 1988;28:624–631.
13. Ordog GJ, Wasserberger J, Balasubramanium S, et al. Civilian gunshot wounds: Outpatient management. *J Trauma*. 1994;36:106–111.
14. DeMuth WE. The mechanism of shotgun wounds. *J Trauma*. 1971;11:219–229.
15. Sherman RT, Parrish RA. The management of shotgun injuries: a review of 152 cases. *J Trauma*. 1963;3:76–86.
16. Bartlett CS. Clinical update: gunshot wound ballistics. *Clin Orthop Rel Res*. 408:28–57.
17. Fackler ML. Ballistic injury. *Ann Emerg Med*. 1986;15:1451–1455.
18. Rodeheaver GT, Pettry D, Thacker JG, et al. Wound cleansing by high pressure irrigation. *Surg Gyn Obst*. 1975;141:357–362.
19. Pronchik D, Barber C, Rittenhouse S. Low- versus high-pressure irrigation techniques in Staphylococcus aureus-inoculated wounds. *Am J Emerg Med*. 1999;17:121–124.
20. Valente JH, Forti RJ, Freundlich LF, et al. Wound irrigation in children: saline solution or tap water? *Annal Emerg Med*. 2003;41:609-616.
21. Bansal BC, Wiebe RA, Perkins SD, et al. Tap water for irrigation of lacerations. *Am J Emerg Med*. 2002;20:469–472.
22. Griffiths RD, Fernandez RS, Ussia CA. Is tap water a safe alternative to normal saline for wound irrigation in the community setting? *J Wound Care*. 2001;10:407–411.
23. Moscati R, Mayrose J, Fincher L, et al. Comparison of normal saline with tap water for wound irrigation. *Am J Emerg Med*. 1998;16:379–381.
24. Bowyer GW, Ryan JM, Kaufmann CR, et al. General principles of wound management. In: Ryan JM, Rich NM, Dale RF, et al., eds. *Ballistic Trauma*. London: Edward Arnold; 1997.
25. Coupland RM, Howell PR. An experience of war surgery and wounds presenting after 3 days on the border of Afghanistan. *Injury*. 1988;19:259–262.
26. Rybeck B. Missile wounding and hemodynamic effects of energy absorption. *Acta Chir Scand*. 1974;450 (suppl):1.
27. Fackler ML, Breteau JP, Courbil LJ, et al. Open wound drainage versus wound excision in treating the modern assault rifle wound. *Surgery*. 1989;105:576.
28. Mellor SG, Cooper GJ, Bowyer GW. Efficacy of delayed administration of benzylpenicillin in the control of infection in penetrating soft tissue injuries in war. *J Trauma*. 1996;40:S128.
29. Adams DB. Wound ballistics: a review. *Mil Med*. 1982;147:831.
30. Thoresby FP, Darlow HM. The mechanism of primary infection of bullet wounds. *Br J Surg*. 1967;54:359–361.
31. Berlin R, Gelin LE, Janzon B, et al. Local effects of assault rifle bullets in live tissues. *Acta Chir Scand*. 1976;459 (suppl):1–84.
32. Coupland RM, Samnegaard HO. Effect of type and transfer of conventional weapons on civilian injuries: retrospective analysis of prospective data from Red Cross hospitals. *BMJ*. 1999;319:410–412.
33. Coupland R. Hand grenade injuries among civilians. *JAMA*. 1993;270:624.
34. Gray R. War Wounds: Basic Surgical Management. Geneva: International Committee of the Red Cross; 1994.
35. Bowyer GW. Management of small fragment wounds in modern warfare: a return to Hunterian principles. *Ann R Coll Surg Engl*. 1997;79:175–182.
36. Bowyer GW. Management of small fragment wounds: experience from the Afghan border. *J Trauma*. 1996;40:170–172.
37. Coupland RM, Korver A. Injuries from antipersonnel mines: the experience of the International Committee of the Red Cross. *BMJ*. 1991;303:1509–1512.
38. Hinsley DE, Rosell PAE, Rowlands TK, et al. Penetrating missile injuries during asymmetric warfare in the 2003 Gulf conflict. *Brit J Surg*. 2005;92:637–642.
39. Robens W, Kusswetter W. Fracture typing to human bone by assault missile trauma. *Acta Chir Scand*. 1982;508 (suppl):223–227.
40. Dahlgren B, Almskog BA, Berlin R, et al. Local effects of antibacterial therapy (benzyl-penicillin) on missile wound infection rate and tissue devitalization when debridement is delayed for twelve hours. *Acta Chir Scand*. 1982;508 (suppl):271–279.
41. Zura RD, Bosse MJ. Current treatment of gunshot wounds to the hip and pelvis. *Clin Orthop Related Res*. 408:110–114.
42. Routt ML Jr, Falicov A, Woodhouse E, et al. Circumferential pelvic antishock sheeting: a temporary resuscitation aid. *J Orthopaed Trauma*. 2006;20 (suppl 1):S3–S6.
43. Maughon JS. An inquiry into the nature of wounds resulting in killed in action in Vietnam. *Mil Med*. 1970;135:8–13.
44. Mabry RL, Holcomb JB, Baker A, et al. US Army Rangers in Somalia: An analysis of combat casualties on an urban battlefield. *J Trauma*. 2000;49:515–529.
45. Lakstein D, Blumenfeld A, Sokolov T, et al. Tourniquets for hemorrhage control in the battlefield–a four year accumulated experience. *J Trauma*. In press.
46. Walters T. Testing of battlefield tourniquets. US Army Institute of Surgical Research. Paper presented at: Advanced Technology Applications for Combat Casualty Care 2004 (ATACCC) Conference; Aug 16–18 2004; St. Petersburg, FL.
47. Odinsson A, Finsen V. Tourniquet use and its complications in Norway. *J Bone Joint Surg*. 2006;88:1090–1092.
48. Sondeen JL, Pusateri AE, Coppes VD, et al. Comparison of 10 different hemostatic dressings in an aortic injury. *J Trauma*. 2003;54:280–285.
49. Acheson EM, Kheirabadi BS, Deguzman R, et al. Comparison of hemorrhage control agents applied to lethal extremity arterial hemorrhages in swine. *J Trauma*. 2005;59:865–875.
50. Wedmore IS, McManus JG, Pusateri A, et al. A special report on the chitosan-based hemostatic dressing: experience in current combat operations. *J Trauma*. 2006;60:655–658.
51. Howland WS, Ritchey SJ. Gunshot fractures in civilian practice. *J Bone Joint Surg*. 1971;53A:47–55.
52. Patzakis MJ, Harvey JP, Ivler D. The role of antibiotics in the management of open fractures. *J Bone Joint Surg*. 1974;56A:532–541.
53. Bowyer GW, Rossiter ND. Management of gunshot wounds of the limbs. *J Bone Joint Surg*. 1997;79B:1031–1036.
54. Simpson BM, Wilson RH, Grant RE. Antibiotic therapy in gunshot wound injuries. *Clin Orthop*. 2003;408:82–85.
55. Marcus NA, Blair WF, Shuck JM, et al. Low velocity gunshot wounds to the extremities. *J Trauma*. 1980;12:1061–1064.
56. Dickey RL, Barnes BC, Kearns RJ, et al. Efficacy of antibiotics in low-velocity gunshot fractures. *J Orthop Trauma*. 1989;3:6–10.
57. Walker RC. The fluoroquinolones. *Mayo Clin Proc*. 1999;74:1030–1037.
58. Mather R, Karenchak LM, Romanowski EG, et al. Fourth generation fluoroquinolones: new weapons in the arsenal of ophthalmic antibiotics. *Am J Ophthalmol*. 2002;133:463–466.
59. Ackerman G, Schaumann R, Pless B, et al. Comparative activity of moxifloxacin in vitro against obligately anaerobic bacteria. *Eur J Clin Microbiol Infect Dis*. 2000;19:228–232.
60. Brooks GF, Butel JS, Morse SA. Infections caused by anaerobic bacteria. Jawetz, Melnick, Aderberg's Medical Microbiology 23E. New York: Lange Medical Books/McGraw Hill; 2001:268–269.
61. Osmon DR. Antimicrobial prophylaxis in adults. *Mayo Clinic Proc*. 2000;75:98–109.
62. Luchette FA, Borzotta AP, Croce MA, et al. Practice management guidelines for prophylactic antibiotic use in penetrating abdominal trauma: the EAST practice management guidelines work group. *J Trauma*. 2000;48:508–518.
63. Holcomb JB, Pusateri A, Harris RA, et al. Dry fibrin sealant dressings reduce blood loss, resuscitation volume, and improve survival in hypothermic coagulopathic swine with Grade V liver injuries. *J Trauma*. 1999;47:233–242.
64. Hamilton RS, Paton BC. The diagnosis and treatment of hypothermia by mountain rescue teams: a survey(abs). *Wild Enviro Med*. 1996;7:28–37.

Operational Medicine Environmental Considerations

Bret T. Ackerman and Ian S. Wedmore

OBJECTIVES

After reading this section, the reader will be able to:

1. Describe the operational medical impact related to altitude effects and illness.
2. List presenting signs and symptoms and describe the initial treatment for cold environment injuries resulting from frostbite, trench foot, and hypothermia.
3. Discuss the pathophysiology, presentation and treatment of heat related illnesses from mild heat related illness to the life-threatening emergency of heat stroke.

HISTORICAL PERSPECTIVE

The environment and its effects on the body during tactical operations has always been a medical concern. Frostbite, for example, has accounted for over 1 million American casualties in World War I, World War II, and the Korean Conflict. The German army on the Eastern front performed over 15,000 amputations in 1942 solely for frostbite (1). The global war against terrorism has increased the requirement for providers to be knowledgeable in this area. Operations in Afghanistan occur at elevations well over 12,000 feet and potentially higher. The battle at Roberts Ridge occurred at 10,240 feet and most of operation Anaconda took place at elevations above 11,000 feet. Bagram Airfield itself is at a 5,000-foot elevation. This location provides challenges in altitude as well as cold. Operations in Iraq result in heat stress for many months of the year, as do operations for much of the year in Afghanistan, the Philippines, and Africa. Tactical operations in the continental United States (CONUS) can result in extremes of heat, cold, and altitude that can place the tactical provider at risk for an environmental injury or illness.

Altitude Effects and Illness

As altitude increases, barometric pressure and temperatures decrease. The decrease in barometric pressure results in a drop in the partial pressure of oxygen, and, therefore, hypoxia occurs in persons breathing ambient air at altitude. The relative concentration of oxygen remains the same 21% as that at sea level, but the relative drop in overall pressure of the ambient environment results in a decrease in partial pressure of oxygen at the alveolar level that results in a decrease in diffusion of oxygen across the alveolar arterial interface, and hypoxemia can ensue from this drop in pressure to cause oxygen diffusion. For example, at sea level barometric pressure is 760 mm Hg, and oxygen is 21% of the composition of air. At 12,000 feet (3,658 meters), the barometric pressure is only 483 mm Hg, resulting in a 40% drop in available oxygen per breath. Complicating the decrease in oxygen pressure to diffuse oxygen into the blood is an increased propensity to develop pulmonary edema secondary to a variety of factors that are not completely understood but are in part due to the relative drop in ambient pressure and changes in vascular tone in response to hypoxia and altitude changes. Similar changes in the brain can result in cerebral edema. Operators exposed to the low pressures and hypoxia of altitude will certainly suffer from a decrement in physical ability as well as the possibility of developing mild to severely debilitating or life-threatening illness.

Incidence of Altitude illness

The effects of altitude may be noticed at elevations as low as 1,500 meters (5,000 feet); the level at which the body begins to manifest a physiologic response to altitude. Symptoms of illness related to altitude, however, are rarely seen below 2,000 meters (7,000 feet) (2). The incidence of altitude illness increases with higher elevations but is also dependent on the rate of ascent. Experience provides a guide as to what percentage of personnel can be expected to be affected by altitude illness and the reduction it will have on personnel efficacy.

- 20% to 25% of visitors to between 7,000 to 9,000 feet developed altitude illnesses (3).
- 67% of climbers of Mt. Rainier who ascend to 14,400 feet in 36 hours develop altitude illness (4).
- Indian soldiers flown rapidly to over 10,000 feet had a high incidence of acute mountain sickness (AMS) and a 2% to 15% incidence of high altitude pulmonary edema (HAPE) with an associated high mortality (5).

The incidence of altitude illness is also affected by individual susceptibility, level of exertion, and age. The only good predictor of the likelihood of developing altitude illness is a prior history of altitude exposure and previous altitude illness. If a person had a previous incidence of altitude related illness and the altitude and ascent rates do not change, then one is likely to become just as ill or do just as well as previously.

Pathophysiology of Altitude Adaptation

Pulmonary Response

The initial response of the body to exposure to altitude is to increase the respiratory rate in an attempt to normalize PaO_2, resulting in a reduction of CO_2. This is first noted at approximately 1,500 meters of elevation (6). This rapidly results in a respiratory alkalosis that is compensated by an excretion of bicarbonate through the kidneys to attempt normalization of the pH. At the summit of Mt. Everest (29,000 feet), resting respiratory rates of 50 to 60 have been recorded.

Cardiovascular Response

The resting heart rate increases with altitude until the body is acclimatized, at which point it returns to normal. The maximum heart rate decreases with altitude. At very extreme altitudes, the two approach each other impacting the maximum work effort of the individual. Changes that occur in the vascular are poorly understood. The most important changes that occur are that of the pulmonary vasculature and cerebral blood flow. The hypoxia that results from the drop in ambient pressure results in pulmonary vasoconstriction, and an idiopathic inflammatory response in the pulmonary capillary bed. This inflammatory response results in leaky capillaries and resulting pulmonary edema. A similar inflammatory response may occur in the cerebral vasculature resulting in cerebral edema.

Hematopoietic Response

There is an increase in relative concentration of red blood cells (RBC) at altitude, initially due to hemoconcentration from the bicarbonate induced diuresis from the kidneys. When a person is exposed to high altitudes, there is also an increased production of erythropoietin, which leads to a true increase in RBC mass about 5 to 7 days after altitude exposure.

Immunologic Response

Cellular immunity is compromised at altitude and all individuals are to some extent immunocompromised because of this. Any pre-existing infection will tend to be somewhat refractory to treatment while at altitude.

Renal Response

Due to the respiratory alkalosis created from hyperventilation, a diuresis is normal on arrival at altitude as the kidneys excrete bicarbonate. Most people will exhibit polyuria at altitude, which is an indication of proper adaptation.

Ocular Effects

Altitude exposure negatively effects color vision, most predominantly in the blue-yellow range (7). Individuals who have undergone radial keratotomy (RK) should not go to elevation as the ocular hypoxia causes a distortion the RK scar. PRK does not appear to have this same issue (8).

At extreme elevations over 17,000 feet high, altitude retinopathy is common. On funduscopic exam, numerous ruptured blood vessels can be seen. Fortunately, there is typically no effect on the vision and the retinopathy usually resolves after return to sea level.

Prevention of Altitude Illness

Prevention of altitude illness is preferred to treatment. Those with altitude illness will be impaired to carry out operational missions. Staged acclimatization is the most effective technique of preventing altitude illness. When an altitude of 2,500 meters is reached, the altitude where an individual sleeps should be increased no more than 600 meters a night. Intermittent daytime altitude exposure is also effective in acclimatizing personnel to altitude.

Pharmacologic Prophylaxis

Acetazolamide

Acetazolamide is the most extensively studied of pharmacologic prophylactic agents for prevention of altitude illness. It inhibits carbonic anhydrase, which results in bicarbonate excretion by the kidneys and decreased production of cerebrospinal fluid. It is 75% effective in preventing altitude illness in individuals who rapidly ascend between 4,000 and 4,500 meters (9,10). Acetazolamide's method of action enhances the bodies' acclimatization to altitude by assisting in the excretion of bicarbonate.

The prophylactic dose is 125 to 250 mg PO twice a day starting 24 hours prior to ascent and continuing for 48 hours after altitude arrival. This is a lower dose than previously mentioned in the literature, but it is effective. The lower dose is designed to reduce the side effects while maintaining effective prophylaxis. The side effects of acetazolamide include polyuria, peripheral paraesthesias, nausea, and myopia (due to its effect of reducing intraocular pressure). It is also a sulfa-based drug and, as such, should not be utilized by those with a sulfa allergy. Reactions to acetazolamide have been reported in persons with no prior allergy and who are not allergic to sulfa drugs and, therefore, a test dose should be considered before travel (11).

Dexamethasone

Dexamethasone is also useful for the prevention of altitude illness and is as effective initially as acetazolamide (12,13). It does not facilitate acclimatization as acetazolamide does and has the significant side effects common to all steroids such as withdrawal rebound, emotional liability, immune suppression and others. It may be used by individuals with sulfa allergies. Discontinuation of dexamethasone while at altitude often results in the rapid return of altitude illness symptoms. There are anecdotal reports of death due to sudden discontinuation (14).

The combination of dexamethasone and acetazolamide appears to be the best prophylaxis for unacclimatized individuals who must ascend quickly to high altitudes and function well on arrival for a short duration mission, such as a rescue or raid (15). This combination has been shown to be effective in reducing illness in individuals going from 12,000 to 17,000 feet in 2 hours, a movement profile that would likely mimic military or tactical operations. In this operation, acetazolamide 500 mg sustained release every day as well as 4 mg Dexamethasone every 12 hours was utilized and no subject on the combination reached symptom threshold for AMS (16). The standard dexamethasone dose for prophylaxis is 4 mg PO every 6 hours, although 4 mg PO twice a day may be effective (17).

Gingko Biloba

The literature on gingko biloba is mixed in its efficacy in preventing AMS with results ranging from 100% effective to no better than placebo (18,19). Because standardization of gingko extracts in nutraceuticals is nonexistent, it makes interpretation of these studies difficult. Expert opinion suggests that if the gingko formulation is good then prophylaxis may be attained. The present recommendation for dosing is 120 mg PO twice a day. The side effect profile of gingko is minimal, leading to its recommended use. There are case reports of gingko effecting platelet function and potentially causing bleeding, but this increased bleeding risk has not been substantiated in actual bleeding studies in patients on gingko.

Medications that have been shown to be ineffective:

- Magnesium
- Naproxen
- Phenytoin
- Nifedipine (for AMS) (20)
- Antacids
- Montelukast

Acute Mountain Sickness

AMS the most common form of altitude illness. The symptoms begin shortly after arrival at high altitude, typically 3 to 24 hours after ascent. Symptoms reach peak severity in 24 to 72 hours and usually subside over the course of 3 to 7 days, but the duration is variable. Up to 40% of people who develop AMS will have symptoms at 7 days and up to 13% after 1 month.

AMS is the initial part of the spectrum of altitude illness and they are both likely extensions of the same underlying pathophysiology. After developing AMS, further ascent without an acclimation period usually exacerbates symptoms and can result in HAPE and high altitude cerebral edema (HACE).

Symptoms:

- Headache
- Dizziness
- Dry cough
- Nausea
- Emesis
- Malaise
- Anorexia

The differential diagnosis includes: flu, dehydration, exhaustion, hangover, viral syndrome, arterial gas embolism, and carbon monoxide poisoning.

Those with AMS should not advance their sleeping elevation nor ascend higher until the symptoms abate (typically 24 to 48 hours); however, it is not necessary to descend if symptoms are not severe.

Treatment medications include all those previously described for prophylaxis, but at potentially higher doses.

- Acetazolamide 125 to 500 mg PO BID
- Dexamethasone 4 to 8 mg followed by 4 mg q6h
- Low-flow oxygen
- Symptomatic treatment with prochlorperazine (also increase HVR)
- APAP or nonsteroidal anti-inflammatory drugs for symptomatic treatment of the headache

- Hyperbaric therapy: compression in a portable fabric hyperbaric chamber (such as a Gamow bag) can be effective in rapidly improving AMS symptoms.

HACE

HACE is brain edema caused by altitude exposure due to vasogenic changes in response to low barometric pressure and hypoxia. This vasogenic edema affects mostly the white matter of the brain. Although most individuals who ascend to high altitudes are likely to develop some minimal degree of cerebral edema, most of it is subclinical and with mild or nonexistent symptoms. As the edema increases, it becomes more symptomatic and potentially fatal. HACE can occur as low as 2,430 meters (8,000 feet), but the vast majority of cases occur above 3,600 meters (12,000 feet). Untreated HACE can worsen over 1 to 3 days or may become fulminate and result in death in <12 hours.

Fatal HACE is seen most often in people who have severe AMS symptoms and continue to ascend.

HACE represents the end stage of cerebral AMS. Symptoms include:

- Severe headache
- Emesis
- Altered mental status
- Ataxia: this is the pathognomonic sign of HACE; anyone with truncal ataxia at high altitudes has HACE until proven otherwise.

HACE treatment:

- Anyone suspected of or suffering from HACE must descend or be evacuated immediately.
- Mortality without descent is significant.
- Dexamethasone 8 mg followed by 4 mg q6h by any route available: IV, IM, PO
- Oxygen 2 to 4 L/min
- Hyperbaric therapy (Gamow bag or equivalent), if descent is not possible.
- If reascent must occur, wait at least 72 hours after symptom resolution at a lower elevation.

HAPE

HAPE, untreated, has an extremely high mortality. The pathophysiology is due to a breakdown in the vascular alveolar barrier and "leaky lungs," markedly elevated pulmonary artery pressures, and regional over-perfusion of the lungs. It is a noncardiogenic pulmonary edema; therefore, vascular fluid overload is not the issue and treatments typically utilized for cardiogenic pulmonary edema (such as nitrates and loop diuretics) will not be efficacious.

HAPE occurs in more than 10% of the people ascending above 3,700 meters; the onset is typically 2 to 4 days after rapid ascent to altitudes >2,438 meters (11,500 feet). Because it is normal for one to desaturate somewhat with sleeping, the onset or sudden worsening of HAPE at night is common.

HAPE Early Symptoms:

- Nonproductive cough
- Increasing nocturnal cough
- Rales can occasionally be noted on exam, but this is NOT pathoneumonic for HAPE
- Dyspnea on exertion greater than others at that altitude
- Fatigue, often manifested by falling behind others in activities
- Weakness with decreased tolerance for physical activity and increased time for recovery after physical exertion
- A fit individual who is suddenly always falling behind at altitude should be suspected of developing HAPE.
- Resting tachycardia and tachypnea greater than induced by altitude alone
- **Dyspnea at rest: this symptom indicates HAPE is imminen.**
- Once symptoms appear, HAPE can progress very rapidly (<12 hours) to coma and death.
- Nail beds and lips may be more cyanotic than other climbing members.

HAPE progressive symptoms:

- The cough produces frothy and sometimes pink or bloodstained sputum.
- Rales become more numerous and widespread.
- Wheezing may develop.
- Lung sounds progress to being audible (without stethoscope), especially when the individual is supine.
- Orthopnea may occur (<20%).
- Progressive hypoxemia causes dyspnea and cyanosis.
- Marked hypoxia by oximetry
- Mental status deteriorates with progressive confusion and sometimes vivid hallucinations (due to hypoxemia).
- Obtundation, coma, and death occur without treatment.
- Subfebrile/low-grade febrile temperature <38°C (100.5°F)

Dyspnea *at rest* and cough should be considered to be the onset of HAPE.

DELAY IN TREATMENT OF PROGRESSIVE HAPE USUALLY RESULTS IN DEATH!

HAPE Treatment:

- Depends on severity.

- Descent is mandatory; descent of even a few hundred meters (300 to 1,000 meters) is helpful and even curative in mild cases and lifesaving in severe cases.
- Mortality in severe cases can approach 50% if descent can not be accomplished rapidly.
- O_2 by mask or cannula.2 to 6 L/min (mild) or 4 to 6 L/min by mask (moderate and severe). DO NOT DELAY DESCENT.
- Hyperbaric therapy in a portable fabric hyperbaric chamber may be lifesaving: this should be utilized if descent cannot occur.
- Nifedipine 10 mg TID sublingually or 20 mg PO. A second 10 mg sublingual dose can be administered in 15 to 20 minutes, if no improvement in symptoms is apparent (followed by 30 mg TID).
- Nifedipine should not be used in lieu of descent; supplemental oxygen or treatment in a hyperbaric bag is appropriately used in conjunction with each of the other therapies.
- Dexamethasone my improve HAPE by stabilizing or decreasing the vascular endothelium leakage and as such can be utilized as well. Use HACE treatment doses.
- In all cases, move to lower elevation; if resolved, wait at least 72 hours before attempted return to previous elevation.
- Salmeterol has been shown to be effective for HAPE treatment; albuterol should also be effective due to the same mechanism (21).
- Other drugs that reduce pulmonary artery pressure, such as sildenafil, phentolamine, and hydralazine, have also been shown to be effective in reducing HAPE, although they have not been as well studied as nifedipine.

Prophylaxis

In individuals known to be very susceptible to HAPE who *must* ascend to an elevation where they have developed HAPE in the past, prophylaxis can be utilized.

Nifedipine has been shown to be effective prophylaxis of HAPE in susceptible individuals (22). Salmeterol or albuterol may also have some prophylactic benefit.

High Altitude Pharyngitis and Bronchitis

This is a common condition occurring typically after 2 to 3 weeks at altitude; it is not a true illness, but rather an inflammatory response to the environment from breathing cold dry air. It may represent the most common altitude-related condition seen at altitude (23). It is not life threatening and requires only symptomatic treatment. Its greatest significance is in being able to differentiate it from the onset of HAPE. Some key discriminators are the time-frame: this develops after a longer time at altitude; HAPE develops 2 to 4 days after the arrival at a new altitude.

Most important, the patient will *not* have dyspnea at rest. If there remains any doubt, treat as if HAPE is the diagnosis. Symptomatic treatment includes lozenges and the wearing of a scarf over the mouth.

Tactical Considerations

Proper acclimatization with graded ascents of intermittent altitude stays prior to combat operations is the ideal method of altitude acclimatization. Three weeks of intermittent altitude exposure (4 hours a day for 5 days a week) can reduce the incidence of altitude illness. This approach can be utilized by having personnel do training missions at altitude prior to an actual prolonged combat mission at altitude. For example, in Afghanistan, newly arrived unacclimatized troops would benefit from a few weeks of air assault training onto the surrounding high peaks, returning to Bagram in between. Acclimatization gained by time spent at a high altitude will last at least 8 days after the return to sea level.

Acetazolamide is effective in reducing AMS symptoms, but it also reduces exercise/work ability (24). This effect has been well shown when acetazolamide is taken at low elevations. It is unclear if this reduction in work ability is overcome by the decrease in AMS and increased acclimatization. Although, in at least one study, the workload was not reduced when acetazolamide was utilized at altitude.

For short duration missions to high elevations with unacclimatized troops, the best pharmacologic prophylaxis is dexamethasone and acetazolamide in combination. If troops are to utilize dexamethasone, a few trial doses at low elevation are warranted to determine those who develop significant psychological side effects from its use.

Cold Environment Injuries

Cold environments have inflicted its own unique constellation of injuries on participants in tactical operations both directly and in combination with separate medical illness or traumatic injuries. Complications of cold environments have had marked impacts on the military expeditions, notably Hannibal during his crossing of the Alps in 218 B.C. the American army garrisoned at Valley Forge in the winter of 1777 to 1778, World Wars I and II, Korea, and the Falkland War (25). One of the more recent examples are the deaths of several army ranger students who died of complications of accidental hypothermia in 1995 due to immersion in water during cold temperatures (26).

Frostbite and Trench Foot

This section will discuss frostbite and trench foot. Both of these conditions have a long history of negatively affecting military operations and have the potential to impact tactical operations in extended operations. Frostbite can extend from superficial to deep with associated significant tissue damage.

Frostnip

Frostnip is not true frostbite as freezing is limited to skin surface only, no tissue is actually damaged. This occurs when there is freezing of water on the skin. The skin appears red or minimally swollen and resolves quickly with warming. The significance of frostnip is that it signals the imminent likelihood of frostbite developing.

Frostbite

Frostbite by definition requires there to be frozen tissue and actual tissue damage. The depth of tissue involvement cannot be initially determined while the limb is frozen. This does not, however, alter the initial therapy.

Symptoms and clinical appearance:

- The skin initially becomes numb.
- The affected limb appears mottled, bluish, or yellowish.
- The limb feels waxy or frozen.
- The skin feels stiff or woody.

Treatment and Transport Decisions

The decision as to where to initiate treatment of frostbite will depend on the evacuation time or availability of evacuation. The ideal is rapid evacuation to a facility that can perform rapid rewarming *and* ensure no recooling of the injured extremity. The outcome of a frozen extremity is *not* directly related to overall time frozen, but more importantly to method of rewarming and any subsequent refreezing.

If evacuation requires walking on frozen feet, then *no attempt* at rewarming should be initiated and patient should ambulate on the frozen extremities. The goal is to prevent any refreezing of an extremity once it has thawed out. Thawing the tissue and having it refreeze will cause substantial damage and is far worse than a longer period of being frozen.

If evacuation is available and of short duration (a few hours only), the patient's extremity should be splinted and padded with dry dressings and protected from heat sources that would slowly rewarm the extremity. The extremity should also be protected from mechanical damage if at all possible.

> THE GREATEST DAMAGE TO TISSUE AND POOREST OUTCOME IS CAUSED BY FREEZING, THAWING, AND REFREEZING. THIS SHOULD BE AVOIDED AT ALL COSTS.

Frostbite Treatment

The best outcome for frostbite has been found to be that of rapid rewarming (27). This is done by immersing the extremity in gentling circulating water at 40°C to 42°C (104°F to 108°F, which is similar to a very warm hot tub). Temperatures above and below this range produce a worse outcome. The extremity is rewarmed until pliable and erythematous at the most distal areas (28).

Once rewarming has been completed, edema will appear within a few hours and vesicles within the next 6 to 24 hours. The appearance and location of this edema and vesicles will allow one to estimate to some extent the severity of injury.

> RAPID REWARMING IS THE TREATMENT OF CHOICE.

Frostbite Grading

Frostbite grading utilizes a system similar to the old system of grading thermal burns. The location and type of edema and vesicles that appears when rewarming is completed determines the grading.

- First degree: erythema/edema at distal involved sites, no vesicles
- Second degree: clear fluid filled vesicles, extend to distal areas
- Third degree: deeper vesicles, purple/hemorrhagic
- Forth degree: involvement of deeper structures, may be difficult to determine initially
- A more clinically useful grading typically divides injuries into superficial (first and second degree) or deep (third and forth degree).

Treatment of Vesicles

Treatment of superficial frostbite vesicles is often debated. The reasoning to debride vesicles is based on analysis of the vesicular fluid, which has been shown to contain thromboxane and prostaglandins (25). Theoretically, these substances if they remain in contact with the injured tissue will cause continued tissue ischemia and injury. This is the basis for the recommendations of some that the vesicles should be debrided or at least have aspiration the contents of the vesicle. The application of topical aloe vera is often recommended as it is a thromboxane inhibitor.

The argument against the debridement of vesicles is that the vesicle maintains a barrier to infection. This is particularly true of deep, hemorrhagic vesicles where there is a significant breakdown in the endothelial barrier. Most experts recommend that deep frostbite vesicles (which are hemorrhagic) be left intact. Aspiration can be considered.

The preponderance of literature evidence and expert recommendation is to:

- Debride clear or milky vesicles and apply topical aloe vera.
- Utilize IV or PO NSAIDs simultaneously: ibuprofen is an effective thromboxane inhibitor.
- Do not debride hemorrhagic vesicles.

General Treatment Considerations

These are consensus recommendations from the treatment protocols and literature up to the present time.

- Ibuprofen or ketorolac are given as systemic thromboxane/prostaglandin inhibitors.
- Tetanus immunization should be given if not up to date.
- Antibiotic prophylaxis with antistreptococcal agents is recommended by some treatment protocols for 48 to 72 hours.
- Presently this means penicillin G 500,000 units every 6 hours. This is continued for 72 hours as it is a prophylactic treatment.
- Should cellulitis develop, it is treated as normal and the penicillin is stopped.
- Dry loose dressings should be applied.
- Cigarette smoking/nicotine use is contraindicated during treatment due to its effect on the micro-vasculature.
- Daily hydrotherapy is recommended, but is outside the scope of this text.
- Pain control with NSAIDS and narcotics will need to be utilized.
- Large doses of narcotics may be required.
- There is *no* role for surgical intervention/debridement of necrotic or potentially necrotic tissue in the initial stages of frostbite treatment.
- The cold injury will self-demarcate over the course of several weeks through "dry gangrene."
- Frostbite cases will require prolonged hospital care (9 days on average); therefore, all but the most trivial should be evacuated to more definitive care as soon as possible.

Trench Foot (Immersion Foot)

A familiar condition to military physicians of prior wars this condition is now fortunately infrequently seen. It occurs from wearing wet boots and socks for a prolonged period, typically several days or longer. As opposed to frostbite, trench foot occurs most commonly in nonfreezing temperatures of 0°C to 12°C, but it can also occur at higher temperatures from prolonged water emersion. When this condition develops at warm temperatures from prolonged water exposure, it is known as *warm water immersion syndrome*. A lack of exercise or leg and foot movement and the associated venous stasis of immobilization in the

nonfreezing cold are felt to be part of the etiology of this condition. Tight, wet boots are also a major etiological factor in trench foot.

Trench Foot Symptoms and Signs

- A sensation of feet being "cold and numb" or "walking on wool"
- Itching, numbness, or paresthesias of the feet
- On exam, the foot may appear swollen with the skin mildly blue, red, or black.

Trench Foot Treatment

Trench foot treatment differs from frostbite in that rapid rewarming is NOT the preferred treatment. The extremity should be dried and allowed to slowly rewarm. The extremity should not be massaged and any mechanical trauma is to be avoided. Further cold and moisture exposure is of course to be avoided. Vesicles may develop in trench foot and are not to be debrided; however, any necrotic or infected tissue is to be removed. Further care is supportive with standard wound care and treatment of infection if it develops.

The pain of trench foot may be debilitating and last weeks to months; pain control should be provided as required with NSAIDs and narcotics. Those with trench foot require evacuation as it often leads to weeks to months of pain and disability. Adjunctive medications may be required to treat the neuropathic pain often seen in trench foot (29).

Rapid rewarming is NOT the treatment of choice in trench foot.

The treatment of warm water immersion foot is to dry the affected feet and allow them to remain dry at least overnight Warm water immersion foot can be prevented by allowing an individual's feet to dry overnight or by the application of silicone grease to the soles of the foot every 24 hours (30).

Hypothermia

"No one is dead until they are warm and dead (31)."

Hypothermia can develop in any military or tactical situation, and the emergency medical providers supporting these operations should recognize the environmental and medical etiologies capable of inducing this potentially fatal yet preventable illness, the signs and symptoms of the stages of hypothermia, and the prehospital and hospital treatment options.

Hypothermia is defined as a core body temperature of <95°F (<35°C) (31,32). Between 1979 and 1998, it was the reported cause of death of 13,970 persons in the United States (33). Primary or accidental hypothermia occurs when normal heat conservation mechanisms cannot overcome the low environmental temperature (34). Secondary hypothermia occurs when heat conservation mechanisms are altered by underlying illness or injury (35) and is a complication of systemic disorders including trauma, cancer, sepsis, endocrine disorders, such as hypothyroidism, hypothalamic dysfunction, and hypoglycemia, ethanol or other drug ingestion, or iatrogenic (administration of cool intravenous [IV] fluids) (33). Hypothermia can affect persons who are exposed to a cold environment due to injury or unexpected cold weather, especially if the affected person is wet (36). Although wilderness exposure is the classic cause, most cases of hypothermia occurs in urban settings (36).

Temperature Regulation

Heat exchange flows from areas of higher temperatures to lower temperatures. The body dissipates heat to the environment by five mechanisms: radiation, conduction, convection, evaporation, and respiration. Radiative heat loss is the transfer of thermal heat through air or space directly from the body to the environment (37). It occurs primarily from the head and exposed surfaces of the body to the environment; and accounts for >50% of heat loss (35). Conduction is the transfer of heat from two surfaces via direct contact with each other. This is the mechanism in hypothermia resulting from immersion in cool or cold water or prolonged wearing of wet clothing in cool temperatures. Conduction normally accounts for 2% to 3% of heat loss, but may increase to 25% in cold water (38). Convective heat loss occurs when the movement of the liquid or gas over a surface facilitates the heat exchange. It is the principle behind the concept of wind chill; the faster the wind blows across a surface, the more rapidly heat is carried away from the body (35). Evaporation cools the body surface through insensible moisture loss and sweating, and respiration transfers heat as it warms and moistens inspired air and evaporates in expired air (39).

Adaptive responses to counter heat loss or generate heat production are controlled in the hypothalamus and include peripheral vasoconstriction, skeletal muscle stimulation resulting in shivering, increased metabolic rate via thyroid and adrenal gland output, and behavior modifications, such as putting on more clothing or coming indoors (3). The very young, the elderly, and persons with altered mental status are at highest risk for developing hypothermia, as they are unable to mount the appropriate physiological and behavioral responses to the cold. Infants and children have larger surface areas-to-body mass ratios, whereas the elderly have less subcutaneous fat and skeletal muscle. Both result in faster cooling and lesser capability of generating heat. The elderly also have a higher incidence of chronic illnesses, which can impair thermogenic and heat conservation mechanisms.

Zones of Hypothermia

Mild hypothermia is defined as a core temperature between 35°C to 32.2°C (95°F to 90°F). Moderate hypothermia is defined as a core temperature between 32.2°C to 28°C (90°F to 82.4°F), and severe hypothermia is a core temperature of <28°C (82.4°F) (40). Most clinical thermometers do not measure below 34.5°C (94.1°F), and oral or axillary temperature measurements are usually not accurate with hypothermic patients, depending on the degree of vasoconstriction and impairment of the heat generating mechanisms affected. A rectal or esophageal temperature probe capable of measuring hypothermic temperatures is the most accurate (38). The esophageal probe should be placed to a depth of 24 cm. Rectal temperatures and most typically utilized, but care must be taken that the thermometer is not placed into cold or frozen stool.

Mild Hypothermia

Persons with mild hypothermia may appear pale and cool due to peripheral vasoconstriction, are usually able mount a shivering response, and have tachycardia and tachypnea. They can show varying states of altered mental status from decreased response time and difficulties with fine motor control to ataxia, confusion, and disorientation. The patient will also have cold diuresis induced by the increased renal perfusion from increased cardiac output (7).

Moderate Hypothermia

Patients with moderate hypothermia have lost the ability to shiver, stuporous, and have a slowing of their respirations, heart rate, and reflexes. Their blood pressure lowers; their pupils become dilated, and atrial dysrhythmias can occur. On electrocardiogram (ECG), the characteristic Osbourne J-wave may be seen at the junction of the QRS complex and ST segment (41).

Severe Hypothermia

Patients with severe hypothermia may appear apneic, comatose, have nonreactive pupils, and be areflexic. Their pulses may not be palpable, and they are prone to ventricular dysrhythmias and asystole. Life-saving procedures should not be withheld based on clinical presentation as intact neurological recovery may be possible after hypothermic arrest. Such patients should not be considered dead until they are warmed to near normal core temperature (42).

Pre-hospital Treatment

First-responder and prehospital medical personnel should make every attempt to prevent further heat loss in the hypothermic patient while handling him or her as gently as possible. The hypothermic myocardium is irritable due to the combination of hypovolemia, tissue hypoxia, acid–base fluxes, autonomic dysfunctions, coronary artery vasoconstriction, and increased blood viscosity (43). Injuries should be treated according to standard Basic Life Support (BLS) guidelines, and patients should be transported to a medical center as soon as possible.

Pre-hospital Treatment I

- Gently remove the patient's clothing, if wet.
- The patient should be kept dry.
- The patient should remain horizontal and be handled gently to avoid inducing arrhythmias.
- Do not massage, because this can prevent the patient's shivering response.
- IV fluids, warmed to 40°C to 42°C
- Do not use lactated ringers; D5NS is the fluid of choice. The cold liver cannot metabolize lactate. Wrap the patient in multiple layers of insulation, such as sleeping bags or layered coverings, to prevent further heat loss.
- Intubation and ventilation may be performed; do not withhold out of fear of inducing arrhythmias.

Pre-hospital Treatment II

Limit active rewarming to body's center/core only.

- The use of heated (40°C to 45°C), humidified air/O_2 is the method of choice.
- Norwegian personal heater pack (charcoal heater), warming tube can be placed into insulation wrap
- Forced air (Bair Hugger) with rigid frame
- Hot water bottles in groin/axilla (44)

Modifications of BLS and ACLS for Hypothermia

The 2005 American Heart Association (AHA) Guidelines for cardiopulmonary resuscitation (CPR) and emergency cardiovascular care (45) base therapy recommendations on the presence or absence of a perfusing rhythm. Patients with a perfusing rhythm will require passive external rewarming, active external rewarming, and active internal rewarming for mild, moderate, and severe hypothermia respectively. Severe hypothermic patients should also be considered candidates for extracorporeal membrane oxygenation. Hypothermic patients in cardiac arrest will require CPR with modifications to the BLS and advanced cardiac life support (ACLS) care and active internal rewarming.

Severely hypothermic patients may be bradycardic and bradypneic, but still perfusing. Rescue personnel want to insure they do not precipitate ventricular fibrillation by the mechanics of performing CPR on the irritable myocardium. If the hypothermic patients pulse is difficult to detect, the BLS provider should assess breathing followed by pulse for 60 to 90 seconds to confirm respiratory arrest, cardiac arrest, or bradycardia severe enough to require CPR

CPR

- Auscultate and palpate for at least 1 to 2 full minutes before determining the patient to be pulseless.
- Initiate CPR on a pulseless patient only if no cardiac monitor is available.
- If cardiac monitor shows any electrical complexes, DO NOT initiate CPR.
- CPR is appropriate, if the patient is in V-fib or asystole.
- CPR is contraindicated if patient has any signs of life, has obvious lethal injuries, or is frozen solid.
- CPR should be undertaken even if it can only be intermittent during transport.

If the initial rhythm in a hypothermic patient is ventricular fibrillation or pulseless ventricular tachycardia, the 2005 AHA Guidelines recommend the administration of one shock followed by resumption of CPR. If the patient does not respond to the defibrillation, further shocks should be deferred, CPR continued, and rewarming processes continued until the core temperature is raised to at least 30°C, because successful conversion to sinus rhythm is difficult at temperatures below 30°C (86°F) (45). The severely hypothermic myocardium is also unresponsive to cardiovascular drugs and pacemaker stimulation. For this reason, and to prevent the accumulation of toxic levels of these drugs due to decreased metabolism that accompanies hypothermia, the 2005 AHA guidelines recommend withholding IV drugs until the core body temperature is >30°C (86°F). If the core body temperature is >30°C, ACLS medications can be administered, but at increased intervals between doses.

Passive External Rewarming

Passive external rewarming is the treatment of choice for most patients with mild hypothermia (41). The patient is removed from the cold environment and insulating material placed around him or her. Patients must have an intact thermoregulatory system. It should be performed initially on all hypothermic patients and may be the only required treatment for otherwise healthy patients with mild hypothermia (38).

Active External Rewarming

Active rewarming is the direct transfer of exogenous heat to a patient. Active external rewarming techniques apply heat directly to the patient's skin. Techniques include radiant heat sources, such as heat lamps or a warming fire, immersion of the hypothermic patient in warm, 40°C (104°F) water, heating blankets, and forced air warming systems, such as the Bair-Hugger by Augustine Medical, Eden Prairie, MN (34). Warming fires and immersion are impractical in the medical treatment facilities, but can be options in the field if there is a prolonged delay in evacuation and the tactical situation permits. There are disadvantages to external rewarming. It may be ineffective in patients with poor peripheral perfusion. Peripheral dilation can lead to venous pooling, exacerbating the relative hypovolemia of most hypothermic patients and resulting in hypotension. Lactic acid washout from the periphery may result in worsening of the patient's acidotic state; this is termed rewarming lactic acidosis (34). Core temperature afterdrop is the continued decline in a hypothermic patient's temperature after removal from the cold. This is due to the temperature gradient that exists between the colder periphery and the warmer core. The cooling of blood that perfuses the colder extremities continues to cool the body core until this temperature difference is eliminated. In addition to continued drop in core temperature, a decline in mean arterial pressure can also occur (46). Some recommend that if external rewarming is used, the heat source should be applied to only the thorax, leaving the periphery vasoconstricted (42).

Arteriovenous Anastomoses Warming (AVA)

AVA warming can be an effective method of external rewarming without increased risk of after-drop. To utilize the technique, immerse hand, forearms, feet, and calves in water heated to 44°C to 45° C. This opens AVAs in the digits causing increased flow of warmed venous blood to the heart and body core in preference to the periphery thus the decreased afterdrop risk (47).

Active Core Rewarming

Active core, or central, rewarming supplies heat to the body's core first; rewarming proceeds from the core outward. Humidified air and oxygen, either via mask or endotracheal tube, heated to ≤45°C (115°F) will provide an excellent source for alveolar heat exchange without causing thermal burns to the patient's airway (43). IV fluids should be warmed to a maximum of 40°C (104°F) (38). Gastric lavage and bladder irrigation with warmed fluids are two other techniques, but there is a risk of fluid and electrolyte fluxes if not managed carefully (41). Peritoneal lavage with heated crystalloid at 40°C (104°F) at 10 to 20 mL/kg of body weight is suitable for severe hypothermic patients (48,49). Closed pleural lavage is an active core rewarming method that when performed with sterile saline at 40°C to 42°C, infused anteriorly, and continuously drained from the posterior midaxillary tube, approximated the heat transfer with peritoneal lavage (13). Extracorporeal rewarming is the most efficient means of rewarming. Cardiopulmonary bypass using the femoral vessels is the most common technique used, but continuous arteriovenous rewarming techniques and venovenous bypass techniques are also available (50,51). Hemodialysis and mediastinal lavage with warm fluid via open thoracotomy have also been used successfully. Gastric lavage has been utilized in the past, but is no longer recommended.

Disposition

Otherwise healthy patients with mild hypothermia that have been rewarmed easily in the emergency department may safely be discharged to a warm environment. Patients with higher degrees of hypothermia should almost always be admitted for continued monitoring, treatment, and workup of underlying medical disorders, if indicated. Most hypothermic patients do not require transfer to a tertiary care center; however, patients with severe hypothermia are best managed in facilities capable of performing cardiopulmonary bypass.

HEAT ILLNESS

Heat stress has affected human operations throughout history. Examples appear in the Old Testament, Homer's *Iliad*, Alexander the Great's campaign against King Darius of Persia, and the Crusades, as well as modern cases from the American Revolutionary to the Vietnam Wars. Multiple terms have been coined including the terms *sunstroke*, used during the American Civil War, *heatstroke*, used during the Spanish-American War, and *tropical fatigue*, used during World War II. Hot and humid environments, potential lack of acclimatization time, and the operational clothing and protective equipment worn all combine to put the assaulter and support personnel at increased risk of heat illness.

Heat illness is a spectrum ranging from mild heat edema to the life-threatening emergency heat stroke (52). Medical personnel who support such operations must be prepared to treat the entire spectrum of heat injuries in military or law enforcement personnel, victims and suspects, and bystanders, as well as take an active role in recommending the command enforce procedures that help prevent or decrease the effects of heat stress during such operations.

Environmental Considerations

Hot environments are not required for heat illnesses to occur; all forms of heat injury can occur in cool or cold temperatures if heat dissipation is prevented as in persons conducting exertional activities while wearing too heavy or too many layers of clothing. Anticholinergic medications, such as the antidiarrheals, antipsychotics, and antinausea medications, interfere with heat dissipating mechanisms. Sympathomimetics, such as over-the-counter decongestants, or illicit drugs, such as amphetamines and cocaine, can increase heat production.

Pathophysiology of Heat Illness

The mechanisms of heat dissipation are covered in the section on hypothermia. Failure to dissipate heat results in heat stress and overload. Heat stress damages organisms by three mechanisms: proteins denature and intracellular processes are interrupted resulting in cell death, multiple inflammatory mediators are released, and injury to the vascular endothelium results in increased vascular permeability, activation of the coagulation cascade, and disseminated intravascular coagulopathy (53). If untreated, severe heat injury will result in multiple organ failure.

Heat Acclimatization

Acclimatization or acclimation is the process of physiologic adaptation to repeated heat stress, usually requiring ten to sixty days to occur (54). Cardiovascular conditioning results in increased skin blood flow to dissipate heat without reducing oxygen delivery to the major organs. Activation of the renal-angiotensin-aldosterone system results in increased retention of sodium, which allows for expansion of plasma volume, and increased volume of sweat secreted. This factor is paramount to stress to commanders and troops as heat acclimatization results in an *increased* water requirement. The increase in glomerular filtration rate improves the kidney's ability to resist exertional rhabdomyolysis (55).

Heat Edema

Heat edema is swelling of the hands and feet due to cutaneous vasodilatation and pooling of interstitial fluid in dependent extremities (52). It is self-limited, usually resolving with elevation of the extremities.

Heat Syncope

Heat syncope is fainting due to peripheral vasodilatation usually combined with dehydration; it is seen most frequently in poorly acclimatized persons (56). It is self-limited, resolving with supine positioning. Oral rehydration usually is sufficient for volume replacement. The most important consideration is differentiating heat syncope from altered level of consciousness due to heat stroke. In heat syncope, the core temperature of the patient will not be elevated.

Heat Cramps

Heat cramps are painful muscle spasms usually occurring after several hours of exertion usually combined with heavy sweating and ingestion of large volumes of water (57). Usually related to salt deficiency, they are usually benign and respond with ingestion electrolyte-containing solutions (52).

Heat Cramps Treatment

- Mild cases can be treated with oral 0.1% to 0.2% salt solutions. Salt tablets should not used.
- Most "sports drinks" (diluted 1:1 with water) are effective for mild cases.
- IV NS or LR provides rapid relief in more severe cases.

Heat Exhaustion

Heat exhaustion is a clinical syndrome characterized by volume depletion that occurs as a result of heat stress (58). Although the previous forms of heat illness are not as severe, heat exhaustion, if not properly treated, can progress to the potentially fatal heat stroke. Heat exhaustion is classified as water depletion and salt depletion heat exhaustion. Water depletion heat exhaustion occurs in persons, classically military personnel, athletes, or laborers, who are working in hot environments with inadequate fluid replacement. Invalid patients with poor access to water in non–air conditioned or poorly ventilated rooms are also at risk for water depletion heat exhaustion. Salt depletion heat exhaustion occurs over a longer time period, and is due to a combination of heavy sweating coupled with volume replacement with hypotonic solutions. Most heat exhaustion patients present with combined water and salt depletion (2).

Patients with heat exhaustion usually present with vague and nonspecific symptoms including weakness, fatigue, headache, nausea, vomiting, and orthostatic lightheadedness. Their core temperature may be normal to elevated but is usually <40°C. They can be tachycardic, unless they are on medications that blunt this response, such as β-adrenergic blockers, and they may have signs of orthostatic hypotension. Most will be sweating and have some clinical sign of at least mild dehydration.

Field treatment of heat exhaustion patients includes removing them from the hot environment to a cool, shaded place, allowing them to rest, and removing excess clothing, and rehydrating them with an oral electrolyte-containing solution. If their dehydration is marked, or if there is any concern of electrolyte abnormalities, IV normal saline should be administered until they are hemodynamically stable. All heat exhaustion patients should be evaluated in an emergency department for fluid and electrolyte assessment and continued treatment. Free water deficits should be replaced slowly so as not to decrease the serum osmolality too quickly and iatrogenically precipitate cerebral edema. Further discussion on laboratory evaluation will be discussed in the section on heat stroke as the laboratory testing is similar.

Young, otherwise healthy patients with no significant laboratory abnormalities and who respond quickly to treatments do not require hospitalization. Patients with require cautious fluid and electrolyte replacement, elderly, or patients with comorbid conditions that put them at high risk for immediate recurrence should be managed as inpatients. If there is any question as to whether the patient has heat exhaustion or heat stroke, treat him or her for heat stroke.

Heat Exhaustion versus Heat Stroke

The distinction between heat exhaustion and heat stroke is difficult. It is generally accepted that heat illness is a spectrum of disease with an unclear distinction and progression between its entities. Individuals who do not respond dramatically to rest and fluid-electrolyte repletion should be observed for 24 hours with laboratory surveillance for the delayed complications of heat stroke. Encephalopathy, coagulopathy, or persistent elevations of body temperature suggest probable severe heat stroke. Because renal and hepatic complications of heat stroke can be delayed 48 to 72 hours, any evidence of renal or hepatic injury during the initial 24 hours of observation should lead to the presumptive diagnosis of heat stroke.

Heat Stroke

Heat stroke is defined clinically as a core body temperature >40°C and central nervous system (CNS) dysfunction resulting in delirium, convulsions, or coma. It represents a true medical emergency. From a pathophysiology basis, an alternative definition has been proposed: a form of hyperthermia associated with a systemic inflammatory response, leading to a syndrome of multiorgan dysfunction in which encephalopathy predominates (59). Common to either definition are both elevated temperature and severe CNS dysfunction. There are two forms of heat stroke: classic or nonexertional heat stroke and exertional heat stroke.

Classic or nonexertional heat stroke occurs in the very young, elderly, or debilitated who are exposed to elevated temperatures for a prolonged period of time, usually at rest, and who lack the ability to dissipate heat as can healthy older children and adults (55). Examples include children left unattended in vehicles and home-bound individuals in poorly ventilated rooms during heat waves. Exertional heat stroke occurs when a patient produces more metabolic heat than can be dissipated into the environment resulting in heat retention and elevated core body temperature (60). Examples include athletes, laborers, military and tactical personnel training, working, or operating in hot environments or in cold environments with too much clothing and equipment.

The signs and symptoms of heat stroke are very similar to heat exhaustion, and as stated earlier, heat exhaustion, even if aggressively treated, can proceed to heat stroke. Skin manifestations can vary. Patients with nonexertional heat stroke may have dry skin, whereas patients with exertional heat stroke usually are sweating profusely. Emphasis here is that first responders through all levels of medical providers should not use the presence or absence of sweating as diagnostic criteria for heat stroke. Nausea, vomiting, and diarrhea can occur. Patients with both heat exhaustion and heat stroke usually present with tachypnea. Unless on beta adrenergic agonists, most patients will be tachycardic, and heat stroke patients frequently can be hypotensive (56). As stated previously, treat heat exhaustion as heat stroke if there is any sign or suspicion of severe CNS dysfunction.

After initial treatment in the field, all patients with suspected heat stroke should be further evaluated in an emergency department. Laboratory abnormalities and complications associated with heat stroke include leukocytosis, elevated transaminases, and elevated creatinine phosphokinase. Coagulation studies should be drawn, and serum electrolytes checked. Sodium can be normal, high in severe free water deficits or low if aggressive rehydration with hypotonic fluids has been given. Serum potassium can be low, normal, or high. Lactic acidosis is frequently present and hypocalcaemia and hypoglycemia are not uncommon. Rhabdomyolysis, acute renal failure, and disseminated intravascular coagulopathy are complications that can result from heat stroke (52).

Field Treatment

Attention to the ABCs are always paramount, but specific to heat injury. The key to the treatment of heat stroke is rapid cooling (55) as morbidity and mortality is directly related to the duration and intensity of the elevated temperature (61). At the first suspicion of significant heat illness, first-responders should remove the patient from a hot environment to a cool, shaded area. All clothing and equipment should be removed. Multiple, acceptable methods are available to cool the hyperthermic patient; the one chosen depends on availability of materials and monitoring requirements of the patient.

Ice water or cold water immersion is an effective method of rapidly lowering core body temperature, with cold water immersion being more tolerable to patients than immersion in ice water (61). Disadvantages for immersion include: cold or ice water may induce shivering in the patient, resulting in continued heat production by the patient; ice water is very uncomfortable for the patient to lie in as well as the medical staff to work with; sanitary issues with the bath water occurs if the vomiting or diarrhea happens; and electronic monitoring is difficult with the patient immersed in water (61).

More frequently, after the patient is stripped of all clothing and equipment, cool water is sprayed over the patient's skin along with fanning. This combines conduction, evaporation, and convection methods to dissipate the heat. Ice or cool packs can be applied to the patient's axillae, neck, and groin to dissipate heat from the venous plexus that are in these anatomic areas. If the patient is aeromedically evacuated, flying with the doors open allows airflow through the cabin facilitating dissipation by convention. However, this can only be done if doing so would not put the aircraft, air crew, or patient in further danger.

If available, IV access should be obtained and 1 to 2 liters of fluid over 1 hour should be administered, because most patients, especially victims of exertional heat stroke, have some level of dehydration. Administration of further amounts should proceed more slowly as determined by the patient's level of hydration (62). The administration of larger amounts of IV fluids will not assist in temperature reduction and may precipitate pulmonary edema. Cooling measures can precipitate a shivering response in the patient, which can cause increased heat production. Gentle massaging of the patient can ameliorate some of the shivering. Pharmacological adjuncts will be mentioned in the next section.

Heat Stroke

- Prodromal symptoms include: dizziness (lightheadedness), weakness, nausea, confusion, disorientation, drowsiness, irrational behavior, syncope, seizures, or coma.
- Collapse is a universal feature of heatstroke.
- An individual who collapses after exercise in a warm environment with a core temperature of ≥40.5°C has heatstroke.
- Casualties who are **unconscious** and have a core temperature of ≥39°C have heatstroke.
- Core temperature is often lower upon arrival at a treatment area.
- Seizures occur frequently (>50% of cases) with heatstroke.

Lack of sweating is not a criterion for heatstroke.

The goal of heat stroke treatment is lowering the core temperature to 38.5°C to 39°C as rapidly as possible.

Hospital Treatment

On arrival to the hospital, the patient should have his or her ABCs reassessed, core temperature, rectal or esophageal, monitored continuously, or at a minimum every 5 to 10 minutes, and active cooling measures continued until his or her core body temperature is between 38.5°C and 39°C (52). Further active cooling can result in hypothermia; and even after active cooling measures have ceased, continuous close monitoring of core body temperature is important to detect any return of hypothermia and the need to reinstitute active cooling measures.

In the emergency department, cooling with spray mist and fanning is a common method as this does not interfere with the electrical monitoring equipment, however if the patient's core temperature remains dangerously elevated and is not responding to this, immersion in cold or ice water may be required. Other methods of cooling include wrapping the patient in cooling blankets, sheets soaked with cold or iced water, or a commercially available body cooling unit (63). Ice water and gastric or peritoneal lavages are not recommended, because they may cause water intoxication (59). Shivering and seizures are treated with benzodiazepines typically diazepam 5 to 10 mg IV.

IV fluids are maintained with infusions adjusted based on the patient's hydration status and free-water deficit. A urinary catheter may be placed to monitor the patient's urinary output. Most patients' mental status and blood pressure will improve with cooling; however, all patients with heat stroke should be admitted as inpatients after stabilization in the emergency department for closer monitoring. Patient's who fail to improve clinically or who have significant lab abnormalities or persistent CNS deficits should be admitted to an intensive care setting.

Outcome

Today, most patients should have good outcomes; the mortality rate should be <10%, if treated appropriately and quickly (52). Before 1950, heat stroke had a mortality rate of 40% to 75% (61). Long-term effects are rare, if they are treated correctly. In a case-controlled study of 21 young patients with heat stroke, none had any abnormal findings of physiological sequelae or heat tolerance at 6 months (64).

PREVENTION

Heat illness is a preventable illness, especially when due to exertion. With proper acclimatization, work–rest cycles, and fluid intake guidelines, most cases of heat illness should not occur. The U.S. Army Center for Health Promotion and Preventive Medicine in collaboration with the U.S. Army Research Institute of Environmental Medicine has developed heat injury prevention material and heat rest cycle recommendations, such as FM 21-10/MCRP 4-11.1D for use at U.S. Army installations (65). However, military and law enforcement personnel may find themselves in tactical situations that do not allow for the application of the exact recommendations set forth by the work–rest guidelines. Physical conditioning along with acclimatization, when acclimatization is possible, and proper fluid and food intake will mitigate them from becoming a heat casualty and jeopardizing the success of the mission. Commanders and supervisors should ensure that their personnel are taking every reasonable action possible to mitigate the effects of the heat on their personnel.

PREVENTION GUIDANCE: HEAT INJURY PREVENTION

Heat injury is easier to prevent than to treat and occurs most commonly in unacclimatized individuals during the first few weeks in a hot environment (66).

- Acclimatization to heat requires at least 7 to 10 days.
- Approximately 1 hour of progressively more difficult exercise, which is sufficient to induce moderate sweating each day, will maximize acclimatization. This can be accomplished by predeployment training in artificially warm environments, such as exercising in a sauna.
- Because heat acclimatization leads to the earlier onset of sweating and more dilute sweat, it may lead to increased water requirements.

> Water restriction/discipline leads to increased heat injury and is contraindicated.
>
> Acclimatization does not reduce, and may actually increase, water requirements.

- Individuals will on average not feel thirsty until dehydrated by1.5 L (1% to 2%) dehydrated.
- The gastrointestinal tract can adequately absorb only 1 to 1.5 L/hour. Consumption of greater volumes can lead to gi disturbance and possible hyponatremia.
- Daily rehydration should not exceed 12 L/day of water as this can lead to hyponatremia. This level of intake may not adequately replace water losses which can reach 15 L/day per individual.
- Salt depletion is rare and only tends to occur in individuals who are not heat acclimatized and do not consume normal meals.

> Salt supplements not routinely required and are only recommended in rare instances were adequate food with its normal sodium content is not eaten.

TAKE HOME POINTS

Altitude Effects and Illness

- HACE is seen most often in people who have severe AMS symptoms and yet continue to ascend.
- Dyspnea at rest indicates that HAPE is imminent. The presence of cough with dyspnea at rest heralds the onset of HAPE. Delay in recognition of HAPE and delaying treatment of progressive HAPE usually results in death and can occur in <12 hours from onset of symptoms.

Cold Environment Injuries

- The greatest damage and poorest outcome from frostbite is caused by the freezing, thawing, and then allowing refreezing to reoccur.
- The best outcome for frostbite is through the treatment of choice, which is rapid rewarming.
- Trench foot (immersion foot) is not treated the same as frostbite and rapid rewarming is not the treatment of choice for trench foot. Treatment of trench foot involves the extremity being dried and allowed to slowly rewarm the affected area.

Heat Illness

- The goal of heat stroke is lowering the core temperature to 38.5°C to 39°C as rapidly as possible.
- A lack of sweating is not a criterion for heatstroke.
- Water restriction/discipline leads to increased heat injury and is contraindicated.
- Acclimatization does not reduce, and may actually increase, water requirements.
- Salt supplements are not routinely required and are only recommended in rare instances were adequate food with its normal sodium content is not eaten.

SUMMARY

Tactical operations have been successfully executed in hot environments from ancient times to the current operations in southwest Asia. Key to success of these operations is to insure that tactical personnel are physically fit to accomplish these arduous missions in these horrific environments. When possible, acclimatization should occur and tactical personnel and their leaders should apply work-rest cycles as the tactical situation allows. Supply of and regular appropriate ingestion of water, electrolyte-containing fluids, and foods will keep the soldier or law-enforcement person from becoming a heat casualty. Regardless of how fit the individual is, he or she may still succumb to heat illness, as will enemy soldiers or law enforcement suspects, hostages, civilians on a battlefield, or bystanders near a law enforcement operation. Medical personnel should anticipate treating these heat casualties during an operation, instructing individuals to identify the early symptoms of heat illness in themselves and in their partners, and to initiate appropriate first-responder treatment when required. Tactical medical personnel should know how to aggressively treat heat injuries properly, and they should work with the operations personnel planning and conducting these operations to enact policies and procedures that will decrease the likelihood of heat injuries without compromising the safety of the soldier or law enforcement officers or the tactical success of the mission. Heat injuries are preventable, and when they occur, they are recoverable if the appropriate actions are taken quickly.

REFERENCES

1. Reamy BV. Frostbite: review and current concepts. *J Fam Prac*. 1998;11:34–40.
2. Szul A, ed. *Altitude Illness in NATO War Surgery Handbook*. 3rd ed. Washington: Government Printing Office; 2004.
3. Honigman B, Theis MK, Koziol-McLain J, et al. Acute mountain sickness in a general tourist population at moderate altitudes. *Ann Intern Med*. 1993;118:587.
4. Larson EB, Roach RC, Schoene RB, et al. Acute mountain sickness and acetazolamide: clinical efficacy and effect on ventilation. *JAMA*. 1982;288:328.
5. Singh I, Roy SB. High altitude pulmonary edema: clinical, hemodynamic, and pathologic studies. In: Hegnauer A, ed. *Biomedical Problems of High Terrestrial Elevations*. Springfield, Va: Federal Scientific and Technical Information Service; 1962;108–120.
6. Morris A. Clinical Pulmonary Function Tests: A Manual of Uniform Lab Procedures. Salt Lake City: Intermountain Thoracic Society; 1984.
7. Karakucuk S, Oner AO, Goktas S, et al. Color vision changes in young subjects acutely exposed to 3,000 m altitude. *Aviat Space Environ Med*. 2004;75:364–366.
8. Mader TH, Blanton CL, Gilbert BN, et al. Refractive changes during 72-hour exposure to high altitude after refractive surgery. *Opthalmology* 1996;103:1188–1195.
9. Forwand SA, Landowne M, Follansbee JN, et al. Effect of acetazolamide on acute mountain sickness. *N Engl J Med*. 1968;279:839.
10. Greene MK, Kerr AM, McIntosh IB, et al. Acetazolamide in the prevention of acute mountain sickness: a double blind controlled crossover study. *Br Med J*. 1981;283:811.
11. Tzanakis N, Metzidaki G, Thermos K, et al. Anaphylactic shock after a single oral intake of acetazolamide. *Br J Ophthalmol*. 1998;82:584.
12. Ellsworth AJ, Meyer EF, Larson EB. Acetazolamide and dexamethasone use versus placebo to prevent acute mountain sickness on Mount Rainier. *West J Med*. 1991;154:289.
13. Levine BD, Yoshimura K, Kobayashi T, et al. Dexamethasone in the treatment of acute mountain sickness. *N Engl J Med*. 1989;321:1707.
14. Rock PB, Johnson TS, Cymerman A, et al. Effect of dexamethasone on symptoms of acute mountain sickness at Pikes Peak, Colorado (4,300 m). *Aviat Space Environ Med*. 1987;58:668–672.
15. Schoene RB. Dexamethasone: by safe means, by fair means. *High Altitude Med Biol.* 2005;6:273–275.
16. Zbernhard WN, Schalick LM, Delaney PA, et al. Acetazolamide plus low–dose Dexamethasone is better than acetazolamide alone to ameliorate symptoms of acute mountain sickness. *Aviat Space Environ Med*. 1998;69:883–886.
17. Rock PB, Johnson TS, Larsen RF, et al. Dexamethasone as prophylaxis for acute mountain sickness. Effect of dose level. *Chest*. 1989;95:568–573.
18. Chow T, Browne V, Heileson HL, et al. Ginkgo biloba and acetazolamide prophylaxis for acute mountain sickness: a randomized, placebo-controlled trial. *Arch Internal Med*. 2005;165:296–301.
19. Roncin JP, Schwartz F, D'Arbigny P. EGb 761 in control of acute mountain sickness and vascular reactivity to cold exposure. *Aviation Space Environ Med*. 1996;67:445–452.
20. Hohenhaus E, Niroomand F, Goerre S, et al. Nifedipine does not prevent acute mountain sickness. *Am J Respir Crit Care Med*. 1994;150930;857–860.
21. Sartori C, Allemann Y, Duplain H, et al. Salmeterol for the prevention of high-altitude pulmonary edema. *N Engl J Med*. 2002;346:1631–1636.
22. Oelz O, Maggiorini M, Ritter M, et al. Prevention and treatment of high altitude pulmonary edema by a calcium channel blocker. *Int J Sports Med*. 1992;13 (suppl 1):S65–S68.
23. Basnyat B, Litch J. Medical problems of porters and trekkers in the Nepal Himalaya. *J Wild Environ Med*. 1997;8:78–817.
24. Garske LA, Brown MG, Morrison SC. Acetazolamide reduces exercise capacity and increases leg fatigue under hypoxic conditions. *J Applied Physiol*. 2003;94:991–996.
25. Paton BC. Cold, casualties, and conquests: the effects of cold on warfare. In: Pandolf KB, Burr RE, eds. *Textbooks of Military Medicine: Medical Aspects of Harsh Environments*. Vol 1. Washington: TMM Publications; 2001:313–349.
26. Milton Palmer. Arlington National Cemetery Website. http://www.arlingtoncemetery.net/mpalmer.htm. Published 23 August, 2006.
27. Entin MA, Baxter H. The influence of raped re-warming on frostbite in experimental animals. *Plast Reconstr Surg*. 1952;9:511–515.
28. McCauley RL, Hing DN, Robson MC, et al. Frostbite injuries: a rational approach based on the pathophysiology. *J Trauma*. 1983;23:143–147.
29. Szul A, ed. Frostbite. In: *NATO War Surgery Handbook*. 3rd ed. Washington: Government Printing Office; 2004.
30. Douglas JS Jr, Eby CS. Silicone for immersion foot prophylaxis: where and how much to use. *Milit Med*. 1972;137:386–387.
31. Auerbach PS. Some people are dead when they're cold and dead [editorial]. *JAMA*. 1990;264:1856.
32. Bessen HA. Hypothermia. In: Tintinalli JE, Kelen GD, Stapczynksi JS, eds. *Emergency Medicine: A Comprehensive Study Guide*. New York: McGraw Hill, 2004:1179–1183.
33. Danzl DF. Accidental Hypothermia. In: Auerbach PE, ed. *Wilderness Medicine*. 4th ed. Philadelphia: Mosby; 2001.
34. McCullough L, Arora S. Diagnosis and treatment of hypothermia. *Am Fam Physician*. 2004;70:2325–2332.
35. Hixon EG. Cold injury. In: DeLee JC, Drez D Jr, eds. *Orthopaedic Sports Medicine: Principles and Practice*. Philadelphia: WB Saunders; 1994:385–396.
36. Varon J, Sadovnikoff N, Sternback GL. Hypothermia: saving patients from the big chill. *Postgrad Med*. 1992;92:47–54, 59.
37. Sallis R, Chassay CM. Recognizing and treating common cold-induced injury in outdoor sports. *Med Sci Sports Exerc*. 1999;31:1367–1373.
38. Crawshaw LI, Rausch RN, Wallace, HL. Thermoregulation. In: Auerbach PE, ed. *Wilderness Medicine*. 4th ed. Philadelphia: Mosby; 2001:112–128.
39. Danzl DF. Accidental hypothermia. In: Marx JA, Hockberger RS, Walls RM, eds. *Rosen's Emergency Medicine: Concepts and Clinical Practice*. 6th ed. Philadelphia: Mosby; 2006:138.

40. Danzl, DF, Evan LL. Treatment of accidental hypothermis. In: Pandolf KB, Burr RE, eds. *Textbooks of Military Medicine: Medical Aspects of Harsh Environments*. Vol 1. Washington: TMM Publications; 2002:491–529.

41. Danzl DF, Pozos RS. Current concepts–accidental hypothermia. *N Engl J Med*. 1994;331:1756–1760.

42. Vassallo SU, Delaney KA, Hoffman RS, et al. A prospective evaluation of the electrocardiographic manifestations of hypothermia. *Acad Emerg Med*. 1999;6:1121.

43. ECC Committee, Subcommittees and Task Forces of the American Heart Association. 2005 American Heart Association guidelines for cardiopulmonary resuscitation and emergency cardiovascular care. Part 10.4 Hypothermia. *Circulation*. 2005;112:IV-136–IV-138.

44. Danzl DF, Pozos RS, Hamlet MP. Accidental hypothermia. In: Auerbach PE, ed. *Management of Wilderness and Environmental Emergencies*. 3rd ed. St Louis: Mosby; 1995:51–103.

45. Hamilton RS, Paton BC. The diagnosis and treatment of hypothermia by mountain rescue teams: a survey. *Wilderness Environ Med*. 1996;7:37.

46. Southwick FS, Dalglish PH Jr. Recovery after prolonged asystolic cardiac arrest in profound hypothermia: a case report and literature review. *JAMA*. 1980;243:1250–1253.

47. Hamlet MP. Nonfreezing cold injuries. In: Auerbach PE, ed. *Wilderness Medicine*. 4th ed. Philadelphia: Mosby; 2001:129–134.

48. Vanggaard L, Eyolfson D, Xu X, et al. Immersion of distal arms and legs in warm water (AVA rewarming) effectively rewarms mildly hypothermic humans. *Aviat Space Environ Med*. 1999;70:1081–1088.

49. Moss JF, Haklin M, Southwick HW, et al. A model for the treatment of accidental severe hypothermia. *J Trauma*. 198;26:68–74.

50. Otto RJ, Metzler MH. Rewarming from experimental hypothermia: comparison of heated aerosol inhalation, peritoneal lavage, and pleural lavage. *Crit Care Med*. 1988;16:869–875.

51. Gentilello LM, Codean RA, Offner PJ, et al. Continuous arteriovenous rewarming: rapid reversal of hypothermia in critically ill patients. *J Trauma*. 1992;32:316–327.

52. Goldman RF. Introduction to heat-related problems in military operations. In: Pandolf KB, Burr RE, eds. *Textbooks of Military Medicine: Medical Aspects of Harsh Environments*. Vol 1. Washington: TMM Publications; 2002:3–42.

53. Sanders AK, Boggess BR, Koenig SJ, et al. Medicolegal issues in sports medicine. *Clin Orthopaed Related Res*. 2005;433:38–49.

54. Lugo-Amador NM, Rothenhaus T, Moyer P. Heat-related illness. *Emerg Med Clin N Am*. 2004;22:315–327.

55. Schmidt EW, Nichols CG. Heat- and sun–related illnesses. In: Harwood-Nuss AL, ed. The Clinical Practice of Emergency Medicine. 3rd ed. Philadelphia: Lippincott Williams & Wilkins; 2001:1667–1670.

56. Knochel JP. Catastrophic medical events with exhaustive exercise: "white collar rhabdomyolysis." *Kidney Int*. 1990;38:709–719.

57. Grogan H, Hopkins PM. Heat stroke: implications for critical care and anaesthesia. *Bri J Anaesth* 2002;88:700–777.

58. Gaffin SL, Moran DS. Pathophysiology of heat-related illness. In: Auerbach PS, ed. *Wilderness Medicine*. 4th ed. Philadelphia: Mosby; 2001:240–281.

59. Vicario S. Heat Illness. In: Marx J, Hockberger RS, Walls RM, eds. *Rosen's Emergency Medicine: Concepts and Clinical Practice*. 6th ed. Philadelphia: Mosby; 2006:2254–2267.

60. Bauchama A, Knochel JP. Medical progress: heat stroke. *N Engl J Med*. 2002;346:1978–1988.

61. Roberts WO. Exertional heat stroke during a cool weather marathon: a case study. *Med Sci Sprts Exerc*. 2006;38:1197–1203.

62. Moran DS, Gaffin SL. Clinical management of heat-related illnesses. In: Auerbach PS, ed. *Wilderness Medicine*. 4th ed. Philadelphia: Mosby; 2001:290–316.

63. Epstein Y, Sohar E, Shapiro Y. Exertional heat stroke: a preventable condition. *Isr J Med Sci*. 1995;31:454.

64. Weiner JS, Khogali M. A physiological body-cooling unit for treatment of heat stroke. *Lancet*. 1980;1:507–509.

65. Royburt M, Epstein Y, Solomon Z, et al. Long-term psychological and physiological effects of heat stroke. *Physiol Behav*. 1993;54:265–267.

66. The US Army Center for Health Promotion and Preventive Medicine Heat Injury Prevention website. http://chppm-www.apgea.army.mil/heat/#_GTAAFS. Published 31 August, 2006.

Chapter 12

Medical Preplanning Considerations for Tactical Emergency Medicine Operations

Kermit D. Huebner and John G. McManus, Jr.

OBJECTIVES

After reading this section, the reader will be able to:

1. Describe the importance of medical considerations in preplanning phase of the tactical mission.
2. Describe some of the most important medical aspects that can affect mission outcome.
3. List tactical considerations that effect treatment, evacuation and logistical medical support.

INTRODUCTION

Providing tactical emergency medicine care can be a dangerous endeavor. Unlike most traditional emergency medical service (EMS) systems, tactical emergency medical service (TEMS) units must be prepared to provide care under fire in austere environments. Planning for medical support to tactical operations is vital to ensure appropriate medical support is provided in the right place at the right time without interrupting or interfering with tactical procedures. Although preplanning is vital, there are two competing truths that must be reconciled. First, "proper prior planning prevents poor performance" and second, "best laid plans always fall apart when bullets start flying." Although personnel must be able to adapt to the tactical situation, it is imperative that medical plans are incorporated seamlessly into the tactical plan and possible courses of actions on the objective should be reviewed and rehearsed prior to the event. This chapter will discuss planning considerations for tactical medical plans and effects of on-scene treatment and evacuation, logistics, and command and control.

PLANNING CONSIDERATIONS

Defining the Mission

In order to formulate an appropriate medical plan, planners must understand the proposed tactical plan. Medical planners must be intimately familiar with the tactical unit, its capabilities, as well as tactics, techniques, and procedures (TTP) that will influence courses of action on the objective. Knowledge of these components and an understanding of the tactical commander's philosophy will allow the medical planner to anticipate the medical support needs and develop a medical threat assessment. The military uses a well-defined process for deliberate planning: the military decision-making process (MDMP). This process consists of eight steps: (i) receipt of mission, (ii) mission analysis, (iii) course of action development, (iv) course of action analysis, (v) course of action comparison, (vi) course of action approval, and (vii) orders production (1). Medical planning should occur parallel to tactical planning. Remember, "good medicine" can sometimes be "bad tactics" and "bad tactics" can lead to mission failure.

The initial step is to develop the medical mission from the tactical mission. Key questions that need to be addressed include:

What medical support is required?
Where is the medical support needed?
When is the medical support needed?
What are the types of casualties anticipated and what is the likely casualty flow?

These questions can be better addressed after evaluating the following mission variables.

Enemy Capabilities

Number of Personnel

How many suspects are expected to be on-site? How many bystanders are anticipated to be on-site or in the immediate area? These numbers have a direct impact on the casualty estimate.

Weapons

What types of weapons systems is the enemy likely to employ? Although the goal of treatment is to treat the wound, not the weapon, consideration of the weapons types may allow the medical planner to better estimate the types of wounds that may be seen. During tactical assaults, the anticipated wounds would be expected to result from bullets; however, consideration must be paid to ballistic, blast, and thermal effects that may result from explosives. Gunshot wounds are the most common injuries sustained by suspects, followed by contusions and abrasions (2). On the conventional battlefield, multiple small fragment wounds of the extremities are the most common injury patterns seen (3). Tactical teams must also be aware of the potential for secondary devices.

Likely Enemy Courses of Action

What tactical intelligence is known about the suspects? Information that may influence medical actions includes the anticipated level of aggression of the suspects and suspected courses of action once the assault begins. As the situation unfolds, the zones of care on the objective may change and medical assets may need to be repositioned to provide timely medical care and evacuation.

Potential for CBRNE Agents

Is it possible that the targets have access to chemical, biological, radiological, nuclear, or high explosive materials? Each of these poses a unique set of challenges in the tactical environment. Chemical agents may consist of traditional chemical warfare agents, such as the mustard agents, pulmonary agents, nerve agents, incapacitating agents, and riot-control agents, as well as toxic industrial chemicals and materials. Biological agents of concern include: bacteria (such as *Bacillus anthracis* spores, *Francisella tularemia*, and *Yersinia pestis*), viruses (such as orthopox viruses, equine encephalitis, and viral hemorrhagic fevers), and toxins (such as botulinum toxin, ricin, and staphylococcal enterotoxin B). Ionizing radiation threats include alpha radiation, beta radiation, neutron radiation, and gamma rays. Tactical situations that may result in exposure to chemical, biological, radiological, nuclear and explosive (CBRNE) agents need additional preplanning to

include pre-exposure and postexposure prophylaxis, depending on the agent, as well as personal protective equipment (PPE) and decontamination requirements. Guidelines for medical management of chemical, biological, and radiological agents (4–6) are available and recommendations for prehospital PPE and decontamination have been published (7).

Environment

Topography

The environment and terrain layout can have significant effects on types of casualties to anticipate. Urban terrain consists of a mix of manmade and natural obstacles that may affect both tactical and medical courses of action. The limitations on routes of access, visibility, and the three-dimensional battle space are likely to result in close, violent contact. Data from urban combat in Somalia from July 1998 to March of 1999 revealed 125 casualties. Fifty-five percent of injuries resulted from bullet wounds and 31% from fragment wounds. Additional injuries included blunt trauma (12%) and burns (2%) (8).

Evacuation routes may be limited which can prolong extrication and increase the need for on-site medical care (9). Tactical operations in remote locations, especially with helicopter or airborne insertions, may also increase the need for on-site medical care or sheltering in place (10). Terrain may also be a predictor of the types of noncombat injuries that may be seen, for example, an increase in ankle sprains.

Climate

Climate may play an important role in preparing for noncombat injuries. Estimation of weather conditions is important for use of preventive measures to decrease the likelihood of cold weather and hot weather injuries. Guidance on proper hydration and work–rest cycles can decrease environmental casualties. Climate is also a factor for consideration of the types of evacuation platforms to use and may adversely affect functions and storage life of certain medical equipment and supplies.

Weather conditions may impact the ability to evacuate casualties. Although primary evacuation from the tactical site will be via ground transportation, in remote areas, aeromedical evacuation may be required to transport casualties to the nearest trauma center. Turbulence, limited visibility, and altitude restrictions may all adversely effect aeromedical evacuation (11).

Flora and Fauna

A detailed evaluation of the medical threat from poisonous plants and venomous animals should be conducted.

Preventive measures and avoidance instructions can be put forth to protect the tactical team. The presence of venomous animals may also affect medical logistics, including specific medical countermeasures, such as antitoxins.

Medical Treatment Capabilities

An estimate of the medical treatment capabilities that are needed on-site can be obtained by evaluation of the factors listed previously. Additionally, mitigating factors should be taken into account. The use of body armor in combat operations in Iraq and Afghanistan has resulted in increased survival rates and has led to a change in injury patterns sustained in combat. Experience has shown that the largest proportion of penetrating wounds of personnel wearing body armor are of the upper and lower extremities and of the head and neck (12,13).

Medical planners must balance the requirements of medical care on the objective versus the medical capabilities of the unit. Medical capabilities will vary from unit to unit, depending on the composition of the TEMS team and medical equipment available. The medical support package should be tailored to the tactical mission and may need expanded evacuation capabilities in certain situations. It is important to know what additional medical assets in the community may be leveraged, such as standard EMS for transport and aeromedical evacuation assets. Next, echelon medical support should be identified to include integration into the local trauma system.

Evacuation

TTPs for medical evacuation should be established for tactical team members within the hot zone. Casualty collection points (CCP) should be identified as rally points for those requiring medical attention. CCPs should be preplanned and coordinated with the tactical assault.

Primary and alternate routes of evacuation should be delineated in the medical plan, including evacuation routes from the CCPs to the safe zone and transportation from the safe zone to hospital facilities. Two key features of evacuation planning include time and distance. During the planning phase, each proposed evacuation route should be evaluated for the distance from patient pick up to the next level of care.

Medical evacuation vehicles available will vary between TEMS units. Medical evacuation (MEDEVAC) vehicles are dedicated medical vehicles that allow the provision of medical care while en route. Casualty evacuation (CASEVAC) consists of using nonmedical evacuation vehicles to transport casualties to medical care. CASEVAC vehicles may include vehicles organic to the tactical unit or vehicles of opportunity. In remote areas, aeromedical evacuation from the safe zone to the next level of medical care may provide more expedited transport to definitive care; however, use of aeromedical evacuation assets require additional planning to assign designated landing zones, may be limited by weather conditions, and may have difficulty landing in areas with electrical/telephone lines or other wires.

Command, Control, and Communication

Medical control should be incorporated into the tactical command post to direct medical assets and track casualties as the operation unfolds. TTPs should be developed within the unit for requesting evacuation assets and medical care. As the operation precedes, the delineation of the hot zone, warm zone, and safe zone may change requiring movement of medical assets in support of tactical maneuvers. Movement of medical personnel on the objective should be synchronized with the tactical plan.

Logistics

Units' standard operating procedures should include a basic load of medical supplies to be carried by TEMS personnel. Modifications to the basic load may be necessary depending on the type of mission, casualty estimates, and expected duration of the operation. Resupply procedures should be identified and included in the medical plan. During extended operations or those that experience a larger number of casualties, the use of preconfigured push-packages may be beneficial. Some examples of push-packages include IV kits, burn kits, and airway kits. Medical personnel can then request the specific push-packages to get the medical equipment needed on-site.

Issuing the Plan

After the plan is finalized, it should be included as an annex to the tactical plan and distributed to team members. The detailed instructions in the operations plan may be converted to a single-page table that highlights key points by phase of operation and includes command and control for the operation, landing zones, evacuation routes, casualty collection points, ambulance exchange points, decontamination points, communication frequencies, phase lines, and all medical treatment facilities and air evacuation triggers from the point of injury to the aircraft launch point (14).

The tactical rehearsal is a vital tool to disseminate the plan, ensure integration with the tactical plan, and highlight issues regarding medical support on the objective (15). This step-by-step walk through of all phases of the operation allows each component of the tactical plan to be viewed in an overlaying fashion. Efficient rehearsals will reinforce training, increase proficiency, reveal weakness and problems with the plan, synchronize actions of subordinate units, and improve team member's understanding of the concept of operations, and anticipated contingencies (16).

TAKE HOME POINTS

1. Medical planners must be intimately familiar with the tactical unit, its capabilities, as well as TTP that will influence courses of action on the objective.
2. "Good medicine" can sometimes be "bad tactics" and "bad tactics" can lead to mission failure.
3. An estimate of the medical treatment capabilities that are needed on-site can be obtained by evaluation of the environment, enemy capabilities, medical capabilities, and evacuation plan and routes, as well as logistical assets.
4. The medical portion of the tactical operational plan must be incorporated to form a seamless, cohesive plan that addresses each anticipated contingency. All team members should be thoroughly familiar with this plan.

SUMMARY

Medical planning for tactical operations can be difficult given the many variables that need to be addressed. Extensive planning is required to provide appropriate medical care in the right place at the right time to save live, limb, and eyesight. Moreover, the medical plan must be incorporated into the tactical operational plan to form a seamless, cohesive plan that addresses each anticipated contingency. These plans should be detailed, but flexible to adapt to the tactical situation. Critical considerations in development of the medical plan include enemy capabilities, the environment of the operation, casualty estimates, anticipated medical resources needed, evacuation platforms and routes available, tactical command and control, and logistics. After the plan is completed, it should be disseminated to team members as an annex to the tactical plan or as a medical support matrix. Rehearsal of operational plans and creation of standard tactics, techniques, and procedures will ensure members understand the medical plan.

REFERENCES

1. Department of the Army. *Staff Organization and Operations*. Washington: US Government Printing Office; Department of the Army: 1997. Field Manual 101-5.
2. Metzger JC, Marcozzi DE. *Tactical EMS*. In: Ciottone GR, ed. *Disaster Medicine*. Philadelphia: Mosby; 2006:297–301.
3. Burris DG, FitzHarris JB, Holcomb JB, et al. Weapons effects and parachute injuries. In: *Emergency War Surgery*. 3rd ed. Washington, DC: Borden Institute; 2004:1.1–1.15.
4. USAMRICD. *Medical Management of Chemical Casualties Handbook*. 3rd ed. McLean, Virginia: International Medical Publishing, Inc; 2002.
5. USAMRIID. *Medical Management of Biological Casualties Handbook*. 6th ed. Fort Detrick: 2005.
6. AFRRI. *Medical Management of Radiological Casualties Handbook*. McLean, Virginia: International Medical Publishing, Inc.
7. Stopford BM, Jevitt L, Ledgerwood M, et al. *Development of Models for Emergency Preparedness: Personal Protective Equipment, Decontamination, Isolation/Quarantine, and Laboratory Capacity*. Rockville, Maryland: Agency for Healthcare Research and Quality; 2005.
8. Mabry RL, Holcomb JB, Baker AM, et al. United States Army Rangers in Somalia: an analysis of combat casualties on an urban battlefield. *J Trauma*. 2000;49:515–529.
9. Department of the Army. *Military Operations on Urbanized Terrain*. Washington: US Government Printing Office; Field Manual 90-10, 1979.
10. Malish R, Devine JG. Delayed drop zone evacuation: execution of the medical plan for an airborne operation into Northern Iraq. *Milit Med*. 2006:171:224–227.
11. Shimanski C. *Helicopter Evacuation of the Injured Patient*. Wilderness Medical Society website. http://www.wms.org/pubs/heli_1.html.
12. Patel TH, Wenner KA, Price SA, et al. A US Army Forward Surgical Team's experience in Operation Iraqi Freedom. *J Trauma*. 2004;57:201–207.
13. Kosashvili Y, Hiss J, Davidovic N, et al. Influence of personal armor on distribution of entry wounds: lessons learned from urban-setting warfare fatalities. *J Trauma*. 2005;58:1236–1240.
14. Clay JD. The Medical Platoon Leader and Parallel Planning. Army Logistician. NOV–DEC 2004.
15. Sobczak SD. Combat Health Support Planning. *Army Logistician*. http://www.almc.army.mil/ALOG/issues/julaug96/ms953.htm. Accessed September 26, 2007.
16. Dept of the Army. *Medical Platoon Leaders Handbook: Tactics, Techniques, and Procedures*. Washington: US Government Printing Office; 2001. Field Manual 4-02.4.

Chapter 13

Triage

Julio R. Lairet and John G. McManus, Jr.

OBJECTIVES

After reading this section, the reader will be able to:

1. Describe the history of triage.
2. Discuss the importance of using certain physiologic criteria to determine triage categories.
3. Provide several examples of current triage systems.
4. Discuss triage principles that are unique to the tactical environment.

HISTORICAL BACKGROUND

Triage as we know it today has evolved from our many experiences throughout the years. Its origin is from the French word *trier*, which means to sort. During the Napoleonic era, Larrey was the first to establish a system in which soldiers requiring immediate care were attended to initially regardless of rank (1). He was also the first to initiate care of casualties while they were still on the battlefield prior to evacuating them to field hospitals (1).

World War I brought an important advancement in how casualties were managed. For the first time, patients were triaged at central casualty collection points after which they would be moved to receiving facilities. During World War II, a tiered approach to triage was implemented; casualties were treated in the field by medics after which they were directed to higher echelons of care. The implementation of this philosophy was responsible for saving more lives than any other advancement to date (1).

During the last two decades, the question of how we perform triage has re-emerged and taken its place on center stage. This new interest in triage has introduced many new systems designed to sort through patients in an attempt to identify which casualties need medical attention first.

TRIAGE PHILOSOPHY

Triage is defined as a process for sorting injured people into groups based on their need for or likely benefit from immediate medical treatment. It is an ongoing, "dynamic" method by which management of casualties is prioritized for treatment and evacuation. This is by definition a resource-constrained environment. The performance of accurate triage provides tactical emergency medical support (TEMS) with the best opportunity to do the greatest good for the greatest number of casualties. Triage of casualties merely establishes order of treatment, not which treatment is provided. However, during triage, TEMS providers should concentrate on performing necessary lifesaving interventions (LSIs), which could result in a new triage category of that patient. The provider must move quickly to the next patient and not spend large amounts of time with any one patient. LSIs during triage usually include:

- Opening the airway through positioning (no advanced airway devices should be used)
- Controlling major bleeding through the use of tourniquets or direct pressure provided by other patients or other devices
- Relieving a tension pneumothorax with needle decompression

In most situations, the number of victims during a tactical environment will not equal those of a mass casualty incident (MCI) or a disaster. Although resources may be limited, it is important to understand and be prepared to implement the principles of MCI and disaster triage if needed.

MCI triage is carried out across the United States on a regular basis by prehospital providers. During an MCI, the emergency care system becomes stressed, but is not overwhelmed. An MCI cannot be defined by an actual number of casualties, because the rate limiting step will be the capacity of the system and not the number of victims. In some systems, due to their limited resources, four victims could constitute an MCI, whereas in other systems it could take as many as 10 to 15 victims before the system became stressed. During an MCI, additional personnel can be quickly mobilized to support the operation and, therefore, maintain the appropriate number of resources for the number of casualties. The priority of MCI triage is to identify and care for the sickest casualties first.

During a disaster, the system becomes overwhelmed and the available personnel cannot support the number of victims. Because of the limited resources, a divergence occurs in the philosophy of triage. The priority is redirected from caring for the sickest victims to doing the most good for the greater number of patients. This is a difficult transition for most health care providers, because it is human nature to attempt to care for the sickest casualties. The initial objective of triage during a disaster is to identify the victims whose injuries can wait for care without risk (green or minimal) and establish which victims will most likely not survive even if care is rendered (black or expectant). After these two groups are identified, resources can be allocated to sort and care for the remaining casualties who will include those with serious (yellow or delayed) and critical (red or immediate) injuries.

When discussing triage, it is important to address two terms which are integral to performing triage: *undertriage* and *overtriage*. Undertriage refers to triage sensitivity in the identification of patients needing LSIs. The goal is to minimize the rate of undertriage, because a high rate will directly impact the mortality and morbidity of those casualties that are triaged to a lower category erroneously. Because it is impossible to achieve a 0% of undertriage, acceptable rates have been established as 5% or less (2).

Overtriage refers to the misclassification of a casualty into a higher category than they actually are. High rates of overtriage can also be problematic, because the system could be overwhelmed by casualties resulting in an increase in morbidity and mortality of critically injured patients (3). Rates of overtriage of up to 50% have been deemed acceptable in an effort to minimize the rates of undertriage (4).

TRIAGE SYSTEMS

Currently, there are several triage tools which are used in the prehospital setting to sort through casualties in MCIs and disasters. The most widely used system is simple triage and rapid treatment (START). This system was developed in 1983 by the Newport Beach Fire Department and Hoag Hospital in California; in 1994, the system was revised (5, 6). The goal of START triage is to identify injuries that could lead to death within 1 hour. This system focuses on respiratory status, perfusion, and the mental status of the casualty. It is important to understand the limitations of the START system as it was designed for conventional trauma and has recently been criticized as ineffective when used at the World Trade Center site on 9/11/01 (7).

In recent years, move, assess, sort, and send (MASS) triage has emerged as an alternative system for sorting casualties in the pre-hospital environment. This system was introduced by Drs. Coule and Schwartz as part of the National Disaster Life Support Programs (NDLS) (8). It utilizes a rapid grouping system based on the ability to walk and follow commands and assigning the standardized military triage categories based on clinician judgment as its foundation (immediate, delayed, minimal, expectant) (8). It is also a very user-friendly system, which will allow for rapid triage of multiple patients during a MCI or disaster with minimal training of law enforcement and first responders (Fig. 13.1).

The first phase of MASS triage is the "move" phase. All patients who are ambulatory are asked to relocate to a predetermined location where they will be classified as minimal until they are individually assessed (8). The remaining

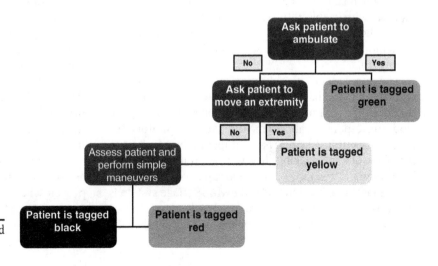

FIGURE 13.1. Move, assess, sort, and send (MASS) triage.

patients are asked to follow a simple command, such as moving an arm or a leg. To follow this command, the victims must have sufficient perfusion of the brain to remain conscious, they are initially classified as delayed (8). The remaining group of patients includes both the immediate and expectant group (8).

The second step of MASS triage is the "assess" phase; during this phase, the victims that are not moving are evaluated and immediate LSIs are administered (8). In addition to assessing those patients who are not moving, patients with obvious life-threatening hemorrhage or severe respiratory distress should also be assessed for LSIs. The assessment phase of MASS Triage involves the use of clinician judgment for determining the patients triage category. Simple maneuvers are performed, such as opening the airway and controlling a life-threatening hemorrhage. As additional providers are available to perform triage, they begin assessing the patients in the delayed and minimal initial groups. The order of priority for individual assessment is not moving, moving but nonambulatory, and finally the ambulatory group, as resources become available. After completion assess phase and all immediate life-threatening interventions are completed, the next phase of "sort" is carried out (8). Patients are then classified as immediate, delayed, minimal, or expectant (IDME) according to their injuries and moved to a casualty collection point for their triage category (8).

The "minimal" classification is assigned to the "walking wounded"; these are the patients who, under the move phase, were able to ambulate to a designated area. These patients will have minor injuries such as abrasions, contusions, and minor lacerations (8). Their vital signs will be stable, and although they require medical attention, it can be delayed for days if necessary without an adverse effect (8).

The "delayed" patients are those who are in need of definitive medical care, but should not decompensate rapidly if care is delayed initially (8). Examples of this group include: deep lacerations with bleeding controlled and good distal circulation, open fractures, abdominal injuries with stable vital signs, amputated fingers, patients who have developed anginal chest pain after a MCI, or hemodynamically stable head injuries with an intact airway (8).

The "immediate" classification is assigned to victims who need immediate medical attention due to obvious threat to life or limb (8). Patients under this group include: unresponsive, altered mental status, respiratory distress, uncontrolled hemorrhage, amputations proximal to the elbow or knee, sucking chest wounds, unilateral absent breath sounds, cyanotic patient, and rapid weak pulses (8).

The last classification under the MASS triage system is the "expectant" group. These are patients that have little or no chance for survival despite maximum therapy. Initially

resources should not be directed toward this group, because they will be needed to care for the other patients. As the event progresses and resources become available, comfort care should be given to these patients (8). One must remember that the sort phase is a dynamic phase in which patients will be retriaged as the event progresses (8). The last phase is "send." In this phase, victims are transported off the scene to the appropriate facilities (8).

Research evaluating the different triage systems has been limited. Currently, there have not been any prospective studies evaluating all the physiological criteria within the available triage systems. Individual physiological criteria used by different triage systems have been studied. In a study by Holcomb et al. (9), it was determined that a patient with a systolic blood pressure of <90 mm Hg and motor scores of <6 required a LSI 95% of the time. McManus et al. (10) studied the relationship between pulse character and trauma outcomes and determined that patients with a weak pulse were noted to have a mortality of 29% versus 3% for patients with a normal pulse character. Garner et al. (11) evaluated several triage systems retrospectively, including the severe injury and triage sieve, START, modified START, and CareFlight triage. In their study, they noted that the motor component of the GCS had a sensitivity of 72.6% and a specificity of 96.2% in predicting severe injury. Garner also noted that the sensitivity and specificity of the modified START triage system was 85% and 86% respectively.

TACTICAL TRIAGE

The tactical environment presents its own complex challenges not encountered in MCIs or disasters. Medical personnel may have to care for victims under fire. This creates a very hazardous condition in which priorities must be established. The goal is to move the patient out of the hot zone to an area where medical attention can be rendered safely.

On some teams, medical personnel may also have the additional duty of being a law enforcement agent. In this situation, establishing a safe perimeter during the breach must be their priority. It is indispensable that each team member carry out their primary assignment during the breach. Care for the victim will have to wait until the patient can be extracted to the warm or cold zone. After the victim is relocated to a safer environment, the patient can be assessed and initial LSIs carried out when indicated.

The tactical environment's uniqueness requires an algorithm specific for this field. Utilizing a standardized approach when triaging tactical casualties will aid medics in correct treatment and evacuation priority in the shortest amount of time. Utilizing simple, readily obtained indicators of the casualties physiologic state, assists in this process.

The triage process enables TEMS personnel to predict a patient's ability to survive or the need for a casualty to undergo an LSI, thus determining the urgency of treatment and the priority of the evacuation. Utilizing a standardized approach and readily obtained indicators of the patient's physiologic state, assists in this process. After a thorough review of all of the existing triage systems, there is insufficient evidence to support one system over the others. However, TEMS personnel should develop model guidelines for the initial triage of multiple patients with traumatic injuries at the scene of an incident.

One approach is the triage decision matrix depicted in Figure 13.2. Although this system is based on the evaluation of physiological criteria that are included in other triage systems, this decision matrix incorporates the unique aspects of the tactical environment and combat casualty care. The goal of this decision matrix is to identify the casualties that will need an LSI. As in other systems, the casualties will be sorted into minimal, delayed, immediate, and expectant categories.

Minimal (Green)

Casualties in this category are often referred as the "walking wounded." These casualties have minor injuries (e.g., small burns, lacerations, abrasions, and small fractures) and can usually care for themselves with self or buddy-aid. These casualties should still be utilized for mission requirements (e.g., scene security).

Delayed (Yellow)

This category includes those wounded who may need surgery, but whose general condition permits delay in surgical treatment without unduly endangering life or limb of the casualty. Sustaining treatment will be required (e.g., oral or IV fluids, splinting, administration of antibiotics, and pain control). Some examples of injuries in this category include casualties without evidence of shock, large soft tissue wounds, fractures of major bones, intra-abdominal or thoracic wounds, and burns that cover <30% of the total body surface area without airway involvement (TBSA).

Immediate (Red)

This category includes those casualties who require immediate LSIs and surgery. Injuries in this category consist of hemodynamically unstable casualties with respiratory obstruction, chest or abdominal injuries, massive external bleeding, and shock. These casualties may be unresponsive with weak radial pulses.

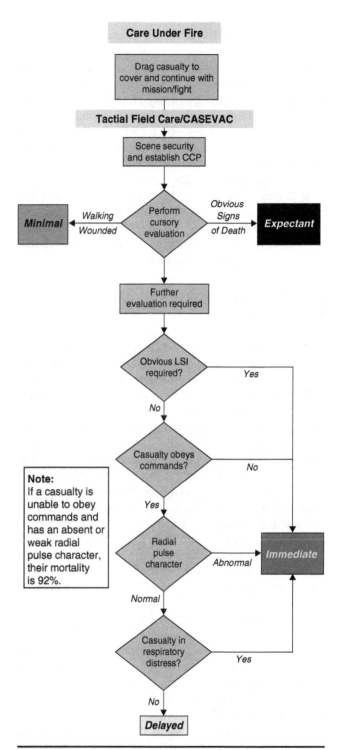

FIGURE 13.2. The US Army triage algorithm during tactical combat casualty care (From *PHTLS Prehospital Trauma Life Support: Military Version*. 6th ed. Philadelphia, PA: ElSevier; 2007, with permission.

Expectant (Black)

Casualties in this category have wounds that are so extensive that even if they were the sole casualty and had the benefit of optimal medical resource application, their survival would be highly unlikely. However, the expectant casualty should not be neglected. These casualties should receive comfort measures and pain medication, if possible. Some examples of expectant casualties are unresponsive patients with penetrating or blunt head wounds and casualties with absent radial pulses.

It is indispensable that the caregiver understand that triage is not a static activity. After the initial categorization of casualties, they should be retriaged on a continuous basis as their condition may change requiring that their triage category be upgraded.

DOCUMENTATION OF TRIAGE ACTIVITIES

Documentation of the patient's category and interventions is an essential phase in caring for casualties of disasters or MCIs. In many cases, this information is often the only data available for the emergency department personnel as they begin to care for the victims upon arrival to the hospital. Although there are many commercially produced triage tags available, they all have unique benefits and problems. To date, the perfect triage tag has not been created. Although it should be weatherproof, it should also be easy to write on. The triage tag should contain information such as patients identification, gender, the main injury or problem, interventions performed with times, the prehospital provider, emergency medical service (EMS) unit number and triage category. Another important aspect of the ideal triage tag is one that can be secured directly to the patient and not to the patient's clothing.

The importance of using triage tags during a disaster or an MCI can not be over emphasized. During the disasters which resulted from the attacks on the Pentagon and the World Trade Center, EMS systems encountered many challenges. During the rescue efforts at the Pentagon, triage tags were not implemented while in New York City EMS personnel ran out of tags during the third hour (11). As a result, it was difficult to establish what treatment the patients received during the prehospital phase of the rescue efforts. In addition, "EMS personnel were unable to provide accurate progress reports or retain information for legal documentation" (12).

When establishing a disaster plan, it is essential that communities agree on a single triage tag to be utilized. This will avoid confusion when different agencies respond to a disaster or MCI. After establishing which tag will be utilized, the next challenge involves rescuer education and familiarization with the triage tag. Some communities have overcome this challenge by implementing a plan called "triage Tuesday" (13). This plan implements the use of triage tags on all patients transported by EMS on Tuesdays.

CURRENT MILITARY DOCTRINE

Because the tactical environment provides limited equipment to aid the medic in triage decision making, optimal treatment and evacuation of casualties relies on easily utilized triage tools. The primary purpose of a triage tool is to ensure delivery of the right patient to the right medical asset at the right time. Currently, most multicasualty triage tools, as described previously, utilize the casualty's physiologic data to help determine priority. Physiologic data are used for triage, because they are readily obtainable at the site of injury and provide a snapshot of a casualty's stability. However, not all available physiologic data (i.e., respiratory rate, oxygen saturation) correlate with survival. Furthermore, not all physiologic data are useful or obtainable in a tactical situation. For example, the ability to accurately obtain a manual blood pressure or listen for a respiratory rate in a casualty is limited in most and impossible in some tactical environments.

As noted earlier, some physiologic predictors have a stronger association with the ability to predict patient mortality or the need for an LSI, particularly the motor component of the Glasgow Coma Scale (GCS) and the systolic blood pressure (9,15). These findings were similar to other studies that have attempted to correlate severity of injury and physiologic variables, particularly the casualty's level of consciousness. In addition, pulse character of the radial artery has been shown to correlate with the need for an LSI (10). A weak radial pulse suggests a casualty has a systolic blood pressure of approximately 80 mm Hg and a mortality of 29%. An absent radial pulse suggests a casualty has a systolic blood pressure of <50 mm and a mortality of 92%. Based on these studies, a triage decision matrix depicted in Figure 13.2 was developed.

When looking at this diagram, note the ability for a casualty to walk immediately places them into the "minimal" category. Remember, however, the assumption that triage is a continuous process and frequent reassessment is required. Casualties may move from one category to another. Triage occurs at every phase of tactical combat casualty care and a casualties situation may change based on this process. Therefore, if a casualty when initially triaged has an absent radial pulse and cannot obey commands, he has more than a 95% chance of requiring an LSI and should be placed in the immediate or even expectant category based on the tactical situation. However, in a trauma study by Holcomb et al., no patient died if their initial triage revealed a palpable radial pulse and the ability of the casualty to follow commands (9).

TRIAGE DURING THE THREE PHASES OF COMBAT CASUALTY CARE

Triage in the Care under Fire Phase:

1. Get the patients who are not clearly dead to cover.
2. Carry on with the fight. Return fire.

Triage in the Tactical Field Care Phase:

1. If the casualty can walk, he will do OK.
2. Perform an initial rapid assessment of the casualty for triage purposes. This is a quick initial check of the patient and should take no more than 1 minute per patient.
3. Talk to the casualty and check radial pulse. If the casualty is responsive and has a normal radial pulse character, he or she has more than a 95% chance of living.
   a. This casualty is in the minimal category.
4. If unresponsive and the casualty has a weak or normal radial pulse, the casualty has an increased chance of dying and may benefit from an immediate LSI.
   a. This casualty is in the immediate category.
5. If responsive, but the casualty has a weak or absent radial pulse, the casualty has an increased chance of dying and may benefit from an immediate LSI.
   a. This casualty is in the immediate category.
6. If unresponsive and the casualty has an absent radial pulse, the casualty has a 92% chance of dying.
   a. Casualties in this category are usually expectant.
7. If indicated, rapidly perform immediate LSIs. Move quickly.
8. Reverse treatment from ABC to CBA.
   a. The majority of casualties will have injuries that require hemorrhage control. It does no good to have a patient with a good airway but who has bled out.
9. Package them to move out of the area.

Triage in the CASEVAC Phase:

1. Retriage at each level. Categories and treatment requirements can and will change.
2. Use the increased diagnostic equipment available at this level to assist in triage.
3. Soft tissue injuries are common and may look bad, but do not kill unless they are associated with shock.
4. Bleeding from most extremity wounds should be controllable with a tourniquet or haemostatic dressing. CASEVAC delays should not increase mortality if bleeding is fully controlled.
5. Casualties who are in shock should be evacuated as soon as possible.
6. Casualties with penetrating wounds of the chest who have respiratory distress unrelieved by needle decompression of the chest should be evacuated as soon as possible.
7. Casualties with blunt or penetrating trauma of the face associated with airway difficulty should have an immediate airway established and be evacuated as soon as possible.
8. Casualties with blunt or penetrating wounds of the head where there is obvious massive brain damage and unconsciousness are unlikely to survive with or without emergent evacuation.
9. Casualties with blunt or penetrating wounds to the head where the skull has been penetrated, but the casualty is conscious should be evacuated emergently.
10. Casualties with penetrating wounds of the chest or abdomen who are not in shock at their 15-minute evaluation have a moderate risk of developing late shock from slowly bleeding internal injuries. They should be carefully monitored and evacuated as soon as feasible.

TAKE HOME POINTS

1. Triage does not mean treatment! Although LSIs are performed during initial triage, triage is used to prioritize treatment and evacuation priority!
2. Triage is a "dynamic" and ongoing process
3. Determine which triage system works best for you and your community.

SUMMARY

Triage during a tactical environment brings a unique set of challenges that must be overcome. Flexibility is crucial when approaching casualties during this environment, caregivers must be ready to adjust to the situation as it changes. Although there are some differences between normal prehospital triage and tactical triage, the goal is the same. We must identify which casualties require an LSI and get them to the right facility in a timely manner. In years to come, the field of triage will continue to change based on evidence medicine in an attempt to improve the outcome of victims. It is important to understand that while sorting patients is a difficult task, it is also an art that necessitates that rescuers are calm under stress and can react to evolving situations.

REFERENCES

1. Kennedy K, Aghababian R, Gans L, et al. Triage: techniques and applications in decision making. *Ann Emerg Med.* 1996;28:136–144.
2. Wesson DE, Scorpio R. Field triage: help or hindrance? *Can J Surg.* 1992;35:19–21.
3. Frykberg ER, Tepas JJ. Terrorist bombings: lessons learned from Belfast to Beirut. *Ann Surg.* 1988;208:569–576.
4. American College of Surgeons Committee on Trauma. Field categorization of trauma victims. *Bull Am Coll Surg.* 1986;71:17–21.
5. Super G. *START: A Triage Training Module.* Newport Beach, CA: Hoag Memorial Hospital Presbyterian; 1984.

6. Cone D, MacMillan D. Mass-casualty triage systems: a hint of science. *Academic Emergency Medicine*. 2005;12:739–741.

7. Asaeda G. The day that the START Triage System came to a STOP. *Academic Emergency Medicine*. 2002;9:255–256.

8. Coule P, Schwartz R, Swienton R. Advance disaster life support–provider manual. Chicago, IL: American Medical Association; 2003.

9. Holcomb J, Niles S, Miller CC, et al. Prehospital physiologic data and lifesaving interventions in trauma patients. *Milit Med*. 2005;170:7–13.

10. McManus J, Yershov A, Ludwig D, et al. Radial pulse character relationships to systolic blood pressure and trauma outcomes. *Prehosp Emerg Care*. 2005;9:423–428.

11. Garner A, Lee A, Harrison K, et al. Comparative analysis of multiple-casualty incident triage algorithms. *Ann Emerg Med*. 2001;38: 541–548.

12. Lessons Learned Information Sharing. Emergency medical services: triage tagging system http://www.LLIS.gov. Published July 12, 2005.

13. Vayer JS, Ten Eych RP, Cowen ML. New concepts in triage. *Ann Emerg Med*. 1986;15:927–930.

14. Meredith W, Rutledge R, Hansen AR, et al. Field triage of trauma patients based upon the ability to follow commands: a study in 29,573 injured patients. *J Trauma*. 1995;38:129–135.

Chapter 14

Tactical Combat Casualty Care

*Michael D. Shertz, Troy Johnson, Donald M. Crawford,
and John Rayfield*

OBJECTIVES

After reading this section, the reader will be able to:

1. Describe the differences between the military and civilian environment.
2. Identify the stages of care in the tactical and operational environment.
3. List the immediate medical interventions that can make the biggest difference in the tactical and operational environment.
4. Discuss current techniques in hemorrhage control, pain management, antibiotic therapy, and airway control.

INTRODUCTION

The advancements of modern medicine and technology create an enormous divergence between the civilian first world care and the care that is provided under the austere environment of operational and tactical medicine. One look at a the modern emergency department and the reliance on advanced monitoring and imagining technology makes the medical care practiced only a few years ago seemingly obsolete. In comparison, the austere operational and tactical environment has changed very little. Reliance solely on equipment that can be physically carried renders most modern conveniences untenable and unavailable. Looking at the casualty distribution during recent modern conflicts, several authors have discerned that seemingly simple interventions can make profound differences in survival. In this chapter, we will review some of these interventions and the applications during future operational scenarios.

HISTORICAL PERSPECTIVE

The link between medicine and the tactical environment has existed since antiquity. With the advent on intravenous fluids and early antibiotics during World War II, medical care on the battlefield has become more aggressive and invasive. Insights by physicians, such as Henry K. Beecher, started to question some of the earlier believed philosophies of the time and the push for active fluid resuscitation. Although noted in several publications, many of these concepts seemed to have been lost until Dr. Ron

Bellemy published his WDMED data from Vietnam in 1970 (1). Although this data identified life-saving interventions on the modern battlefield that may prevent unnecessary mortality, these concepts seemed to be eclipsed by a new and emerging advanced trauma life support (ATLS) system and certification that was coming of age. Thus, the civilian-based system worked very well in the modern established medical system of the continental United States but was not applicable to the battlefield or operational environment. This adherence to the ATLS guidelines continued even in the military environment until one day in 1996 outside FT. Bragg, North Carolina, at the Special Operations Medical Association Conference a former Navy Seal and a professor at the Uniformed Services University presented a lecture on a new concept, tactical combat casualty care (TCCC). The room was extremely skeptical about the seemingly outdated interventions Dr. Butler and Dr. Hagmann were presenting (2). These concepts were contrary to the established doctrine of ATLS. This debate continued for several years until animal data and practical operational experience provided data to validate TCCC principles. After two modern conflicts, TCCC is the currently being implemented for prehospital casualty care in the armed forces and is expanding to the civilian law enforcement community.

DIFFERENCES WITHIN THE PREHOSPITAL ENVIRONMENTS

It is important to note that there are significant differences in civilian and military (tactical) prehospital

▶ **TABLE 14.1.** Medical Support Differences in Civilian, Law Enforcement, and Military Operational Environments.

	Munitions	*Resources*	*Time on Scene*	*No. of Casualties*	*Scene Safety*
Civilian	Handgun, knife		Short	Small	Secure
Law Enforcement	Handgun, knife	Restricted	Medium	Medium	Potentially warm
Military	Rifle, fragmentation	Restricted	Long	Large	Potentially hostile

environments. The continuum moves from relatively safe civilian emergency medical services (EMS) through the more risky law enforcement EMS to the far forward and sometimes very high-risk military combat setting. Noting the differences within this continuum allows prehospital health care providers and tactical commanders to appreciate the different approaches that medical personnel take in these varied situations.

The first major difference seen is in the limitation of medical resources. The robust medical and trauma system enjoyed in the United States experiences extremely few occurrences were the medical system is overwhelmed. Couple this with the fact that many trauma related occurrences involve only a few of people and can be routed to different hospitals, the system is never truly stressed. However, the military environment and many austere operational law enforcement environments are all but denied this luxury. When things go wrong in these settings, multiple casualties and subsequent mass casualty situations can quickly arise. These situations often overwhelm the limited existing medical support structure. Thus, in a resource restricted environment of this nature, it is exceedingly important to know what interventions are going to make the greatest impact on the greatest number of casualties. In contrast, those interventions which will only serve to use up your precious resources must also be identified and avoided.

The second difference is in the type of casualties that are produced in the various environments. In the civilian trauma environment, blunt trauma represents the preponderance of casualties (i.e., motor vehicle accidents, falls) (3,4). In the military and operational environments, there is a significant increase in the number of penetrating traumatic injuries (gunshot, fragmentary, blast propellant wounds, etc.) (1,2,4–11). Blunt trauma and penetrating trauma patients are obviously treated differently, and the treatment for one patient will not always be warranted in another. Because of the increased complexity and number of combat casualties, additional training and knowledge of the TCCC guidelines are important for the operational and tactical medic.

The third difference manifests itself in the time that the casualty spends both in the field and during transport to the higher levels of care. Since the enacting of the National Highway Safety Act in 1966, the civilian evacuation times

are often measured in minutes due to high speed communication and response assets. This is not always the case in the operational or tactical environment. The influencing factors of nonsecure evacuation and extraction routes, prolonged evacuation times due to terrain, mission, or restricted resources (i.e., evacuation platforms) greatly impacts on the care and survival of casualties in these challenging environments. These special considerations must be factored into planning medical support for missions in the tactical or operational environment. Other factors when comparing the different environment are outlined in Table 14.1.

PREHOSPITAL CARE IN THE TACTICAL AND OPERATIONAL ENVIRONMENT

The committee on tactical combat casualty care (COTCCC) was founded in 2002 by the U.S. Special Operations Command with support from the Navy Bureau of Medicine and Surgery (BUMED). They are now the primary proponents for the military chapter in the prehospital trauma life support (PHTLS) course (12) and have defined the different operational settings in which medical care is provided in the tactical environment. Breaking up the operational setting into these categories allows medical personnel to concentrate their efforts on the most applicable interventions during that specific stage. The stages include care under fire, tactical field care, and combat casualty evacuation care (CASEVAC) (13).

1. *Care under fire* is just that, care rendered to a casualty while the casualty and the medical aid provider are under effective hostile fire. This is the "hot zone," where the risk of additional injury to the care provider and the casualty are extremely high. Medical equipment and opportunity to render care are extremely limited. The care under fire phase *is not* the time or place to be opening an aid bag and searching for a piece of equipment.
2. *Tactical field care* is the care that is delivered while in the field or operational setting while not under effective hostile fire. The ability of the medical provider to render care is still hampered by resources and the environmental conditions, but not by risk of hostile contact. This is the "warm and cold zones." This can also occur

at any point in time during training and missions where the medical provider is under these austere and challenging conditions. The medic must be aware that he could come under effective hostile fire once again and immediately transition into a care under fire phase. The difference between these two phases is crucial. Simply dragging a casualty 5 feet around the corner of a building could transition the medic from care under fire to tactical field care.

3. *Combat Casualty Evacuation Care* (CASEVAC) constitutes the care rendered to the casualty during evacuation. This can be via ground, aviation or watercraft. Although additional resources (equipment and personnel) may be prestaged in the evacuation platform, the environmental conditions that the care is provided under present their own special complexities (e.g., confined space, lack of access to patient's injuries, moving platforms). An additional note of clarification must be made in this stage in reference to the definition of terms. CASEVAC is defined in military field manuals as care rendered while on a tactical mission platform, whereas MEDEVAC is delineated as casualty evacuation on a dedicated medical platform (i.e., ambulance, medical aircraft) (13).

Civilian, nontactical, EMS providers participate in patient encounters that have the potential to utilize these three phases of care. The active participation of law enforcement officers makes "care under fire" an infrequent event; however, in 1999 during the Columbine shootings, EMS personnel were shot at by the perpetrators. With the exception of cases involving prolonged extrication, the tactical field care and CASEVAC stages are typically blurred as more and more EMS care is rendered en route to the definitive treatment facility

CARE WITHIN THE TCCC STAGES

Care Under Fire

The paramount concerns during this stage of care are transitioning to a safer environment and hemorrhage control. The first, transitioning to a safer environment, can be accomplished in many ways; suppressing the enemy's fire, physically moving the casualty and care provider from the hostile fire zone, or providing effective cover and concealment for the medical provider and casualty within the hostile fire zone. As the old saying states, "victory is the best medicine." Sometimes having the medical provider and casualty continue to participate in the suppression of the enemy is the most beneficial course in the long run. It is solely the decision of the tactical commander, and he makes that decision based on both the situation and knowing the limitations of providing effective medical care during this stage. Taking the medical care provider

away from his medical duties can have short-term benefits, but significant long-term disadvantages as well. The tactical commander must weigh all of these considerations in terms of the overall benefits for both the unit and the mission. Patient and care provider movement can be difficult under effective direct fire. The tactical commander's decision making process can be dominated by considerations of unnecessary or additional casualties for the time period that a specific casualty is exposed to direct fire. In addition, the commander must consider the impact of the loss of his potentially sole medical provider in these situations. If the casualty has any ability at self-movement to an area of cover or concealment, movement should be encouraged. Additional augmenting devices, such as rope or tubular nylon webbing, can also be thrown to the casualty to assist in his movement with minimal risk to the helping personnel. There are also many field carrying techniques, with one man and two man carries. A good description of these can be found in Chapter 8-5 of the *Army Field Manuel 8-10-6* or the *Prehospital Trauma Life Support (PHTLS) Manual* (12,14). Finally, providing cover or concealment for the casualty and care provider can be accomplished through the use of obscuring smoke munitions or providing ground vehicles with ballistic protection capabilities.

The focus of medical attention in this phase is to obtain hemorrhage control. A review of combat casualty data from Vietnam through today (1,2,7,10,15–18) clearly identifies that the vast majority of penetrating trauma occurs to the extremities. First identified by the WDMED database, the number one reversible cause of combat mortality is exsanguinating hemorrhage form extremity trauma (1). During this stage, hemorrhage control is ideally gained through the use of tourniquets. Although shunned for many years, tourniquets have now re-emerged as the standard of care in this environment due to their ease of use, rapid application, and complete stoppage of blood loss (2,19). Previous anesthesia literature on use of tourniquets during surgery has demonstrated that limited to no detrimental effects occurs with proper tourniquet placement for <2 hours (20).

Tourniquets can be rapidly applied in these unsafe, tactical environments with adequate hemorrhage control (19). There are many types of tourniquets currently on the market. The current tourniquet in use by the USSOCOM is the combat action tourniquet (CAT), and it is receiving very good reviews from current operators in the field (21). The benefit of using tourniquets like the CAT is that they exert significant direct pressure deep within tissue and can be rapidly applied with minimal training. Next to surgical control, it is the best way to gain rapid extremity hemorrhage control in almost all situations. Based on this view, both the American and Israel military, as well as the International Committee of the Red Cross (ICRC), have embraced tourniquets as an initial hemorrhage control option during a care under fire phase in order to achieve rapid control of bleeding (22). When applied as the first hemorrhage control option tactically, most can be converted to a less drastic hemorrhaged control option within 2 hours. However, when tourniquets are on for 6 hours or improperly applied, they may damage soft tissue and cause enough ischemic muscle to potentially necessitate amputation whether the tourniquet was really needed or not.

For injuries not amendable to tourniquet application, there are now several advanced technology bandages and hemorrhage control agents available on the market. A word of caution is warranted when using these advanced hemostatic bandages and hemorrhage control agents. In the care under fire stage, these can be difficult to apply and are only truly needed for injuries not amendable to tourniquet use. We will cover these agents in greater detail depth in the field care section.

The final note concerning the care under fire stage is the need for nonmedical provider's proficiency in the application of tourniquets. Many casualties may bleed out before a medical provider reaches them (23). Operators and nonmedical personnel must be proficient in conducting this task. The simple placement of a tourniquet will greatly increase the survivability of injured personnel on the battlefield.

Tactical Field Care

When out of the direct line of effective enemy fire, casualties need to be disarmed and stripped of all sensitive information. Weapons, ammunition, and other sensitive items, such as night vision goggles, should be retained by nonmedical personnel for turn in or reuse if the tactical situation demands. Alteration of the casualty's sensorium, due to either the effects of trauma, hemorrhage, or medication, can cause the casualty to confuse the intent of medical personnel and possibly use any retained weapons in a defensive mode. In addition, retained munitions subjected to improper handling may detonate harming health care providers or other friendly forces. During the disarming of the patient, the medic should survey for any additional sites of bleeding not initially identified in the care under fire stage. Previously unidentified wounds should be quickly addressed with either a tourniquet or a bandage/hemostatic agent where appropriate. Nonmedical personnel can hold direct pressure and provide elevation to sites not amenable to tourniquet placement. It is important to alleviate the skilled medical provider from this task in order that they may continue on with the patient's assessment or address other wounded personnel.

Airway, Breathing, and Circulation

The patency of an unconscious patient's airways should be assessed next. The jaw thrust or chin lift maneuver are easily executed. If the patient is breathing sponta-

neously and handling their own secretions, a nasopharyngeal airway should be inserted and the patient placed in the semiprone recovery position. This limits the risk of secretions, gastric products, or blood from being aspirated into the lungs (12). If the casualty does not have an open airway, is not handling his own secretions, or lacks a gag reflex, then a more definitive airway is warranted. In the tactical field care setting, an immediate cricothyroidotomy performed by trained personnel is now indicated for casualties with significant maxiofacial trauma, suspected airway thermal burns, or toxic exposure (12,24). For those patients lacking maxiofacial trauma, endotracheal intubation or supraglottic devices should be attempted per unit or regional protocol. Caution is warranted concerning this endeavor because once a casualty's airway is secured, a means of ventilating the patient must be provided and maintained. This requires, at a minimum, bag valve ventilation equipment and at least one dedicated person to continually bag/ventilate the patient until definitive care can be reached. In some scenarios (i.e., mass casualties), this may exceed the capability of local assets and should not be considered at the onset of medical operations. This is undoubtedly a difficult decision, but one that may ensure the greatest good is done for the greatest number of injured.

After the airway concerns are adequately addressed, evaluation of the patient's breathing begins. WDMED data of casualties suffered in Vietnam indicate that tension pneumothorax is the second leading cause of preventable combat mortality (1). Recent data indicate that this is less common today as a result of the improved level of ballistic protection now worn by combat troops (17). On the other hand, few law enforcement personnel have access to this level of body armor protection, and there still exists a significant number of penetrating chest injuries in this community. Subsequently, any patient with penetrating chest trauma and respiratory distress is assumed to have a tension pneumothorax. Previous studies have demonstrated that the usual signs and symptoms of tension pneumothorax are often difficult, if not impossible, to discern in the operational environment (25,26). Thus, the mechanism of injury, subjective symptoms, rapid respirations, and tachycardia should be ample evidence to warrant needle thoracostomy. Furthermore, evidence suggests that needle thoracostomy performed on patients without a tension pneumothorax accounts for minimal additional trauma, further reinforcing the benefits of early intervention (12). Medical personnel should be trained and equipped appropriately to perform this task in the field setting. Because of the well-developed pectoral muscles in our patient population, a 14-, 12- or 10-gauge needle, 2.5 or 3 inches in length, is necessary to ensure adequate penetration into the chest cavity is recommended (27,28).

Chest tube thoracostomy by nonphysicians is not advised in this setting and are potentially harmful due to the increased risk of infection and potential for additional tissue damage. Swine model studies show needle thoracostomy is effective for up to 4 hours in alleviating and preventing tension pneumothoraces (29). The significant additional risks of inserting chest tubes in contaminated, suboptimal environments are not warranted at this time. Continual monitoring of these patients ensures that the cannula remains patent and the patient stable. Open chest wounds should be covered with petroleum gauze at exhalation, and taped or dressed with a bandage. At no time should a dressing be place on a casualty without either continuous monitoring capability or needle thoracostomy.

Another common adjunct to pneumothorax management is the "Asherman Chest Seal." Despite utilization by several military forces worldwide, there is no published literature to show this device adds anything to the management of a pneumothorax. The best use for the device is as a protective hub around the Angiocath used for decompression. This necessitates cutting off the latex "flutter" valve to facilitate air movement both in and out of the catheter. Specifically, simple pneumothoraces by themselves usually do not cause death until they progress to tension. A tension pneumothorax by definition allows air in, but not out. If a Heimlich-type flutter valve is to be used after needle decompression to prevent additional airflow into the pleural space, special attention to the direction of the Heimlich-valve is crucial. Numerous case reports exist where these valves were placed backward or accidentally reversed. Reversal of the valve would allow airflow into the chest, but not out, which essentially creates a tension pneumothorax. Because simple open pneumothoraces are not by themselves a cause of death, it may be safer to leave the Angiocath open to the environment. As long as air flows both into and out of the Angiocath hub, tension pneumothorax usually can't occur on the decompressed pleural space.

After airway and breathing issues are adequately addressed, aid providers must re-evaluate the circulatory status. Tourniquets placed during the care under fire stage or during the initial disarming of the patient should be reassessed for their effectiveness in hemorrhage control. Dressings and hemostatic agents placed earlier require reevaluation and augmentation, if necessary. For the vast majority of wounds, a simple gauze dressing or pressure dressing will provide ample amount of hemorrhage control. Hemostatic agents should be reserved for wounds that are not amendable to pressure dressings, or for failure of initial dressing application, or to gain adequate control of bleeding. Of the agents currently on the market, HEMCON and QuikClot appear the most promising. HEMCON received approval for external use by the U.S. Food and Drug Administration (FDA) in November 2002. It is a proprietary formulation of poly-N-acetyl glucosamine, which fuses with the tissues to tamponade bleeding at the site of injury. Several studies show it's effectiveness in severe bleeding. Subsequently, it is the hemostatic agent of choice

for the U.S. Special Operations Command. QuikClot also received approval from the FDA for external use in 2002. It is the hemostatic agent of choice of the U.S. Marine Corps. QuikClot is a zeolite tetramer that absorbs water in the plasma through an exothermic reaction, concentrating clotting factors at the site of bleeding. It is also shown to be effective in severe bleeding, but can produce exothermic temperatures up to 90°C, producing burns, if not applied appropriately (30–33). It must be noted that there is controversy regarding the use of these dressings. When QuikClot, chitosan dressings, and fibrin sealant dressings were compared to the current U.S. Armed Forces bandage in an experimental swine model with 6 mm femoral artery punch lacerations (100% fatal if untreated), only the fibrin sealant dressing showed reduced bleeding and prevented exsanguinations. Neither the current military bandage, QuikClot, nor the chitosan dressing (HEMCON) prevented fatal exsanguinations in this model (34). Unfortunately, the fibrin sealant dressing is not currently commercially available and costs between $500 and $1,000 per dressing (35).

After the dressing is applied and hemorrhage control achieved, intravenous (IV) placement and fluid resuscitation can be addressed. This is yet another place where hospital treatment and field treatment diverge. Ideally, all patients would have IV access established, but in the resource-restricted field environment, only patients with a demonstrated need for fluid resuscitation, IV antibiotics or IV analgesia require IV lines. Wounded who can handle PO fluids should be encouraged to maintain good hydration and may not require an IV at this point. Casualties requiring IV fluid resuscitation need an 18-gauge angiocatheter placed in the most easily accessible vein. Eighteen-gauge angiocatheters are preferable because of their ease of insertion and relatively fast infusion times (1,36,37). If an IV cannot be obtained after several attempts, intraosseous infusion devices should be used (38). Several devices currently on the market utilize the sternum and tibia for intraosseous access sites. Tactical medical personnel familiarization and competency needs to be attained with at least one of these devices in order to gain vascular access when IV cannulation fails. Dislodgement of these all these devices is common; therefore, all access sites should be strongly secured in order to limit the chance of dislodgment during transport. We encourage the use of Velcro straps, suture, or other securing devices.

Intravenous Fluids and Access

Current recommendations on fluid resuscitation are guided by the bleeding status of the casualty. If a patient's bleeding is stopped, then controlled resuscitation with IV normal saline or oral fluids can occur. Casualties with uncontrolled hemorrhage (either internal or external) require a hypotensive resuscitation protocol (39,40). During hypotensive resuscitation, clinical evaluation is imperative. The systolic blood pressure only loosely correlates with adequate perfusion, therefore, it is only used as a definitive resuscitation guide in those patients whose clinical function cannot be assessed (i.e., head injury or altered mental status). In a head injured patient with altered mental status, a target systolic blood pressure of 90 mm Hg or greater needs to be maintained in order to ensure adequate cerebral blood flow (41–46). Correlation with cognitive function and/or urine output is often a better indication of adequate perfusion. A patient whose cognitive function deteriorates or becomes unconscious requires an immediate fluid challenge. The optimal type of fluid for resuscitation is still under debate. Lactated ringers has fallen out of favor due to both its small retained intravascular fluid volume (20% of infused volume after 1 hour) (47,48) and potential contribution to cell death (49,50). Normal saline is still commonly used, but it also suffers the shortfall of a small retained intravascular volume as well as a significant weight per liter of 2.2 lb. Recent literature indicates the optimal resuscitation fluid may be hypertonic saline (5% to 7.5%) due to its cerebral protective nature and small volume requirements (250 cc) (41–46). The problem is that hypertonic saline is not currently manufactured in bulk and is very difficult to obtain. Hetastarch solutions, including Hespan (6% hetastarch) and Hextend (6% hetastarch), which contain balanced electrolytes, a lactate buffer, and physiological levels of glucose, also meet the small fluid requirements. Administration of 500 cc of Hetastarch solution expands intravascular volume by 800 cc. The recommended Hetastarch solution administration is two 500 cc boluses (12). Mixed hypertonic-hetastarch solutions are currently undergoing review at the time of this publication and warrant close tracking for future use (51,52).

Following circulatory assessment, casualties need a thorough primary and focused secondary assessment. It is critical to identify any missed injuries at this time. Collecting a brief medical/surgical history, medications and allergies is necessary to avoid further injury and to guide treatment. A complete physical assessment (and reassessments) is important in the unconscious or altered patient, especially when evacuation times are prolonged.

Analgesia

The treatment of pain and suffering must never be forgotten or neglected in this environment. It is important to note that suffering includes both pain and anxiety. The perception of pain by the patient is exacerbated by poor communication regarding their medical care. Patients are particularly concerned with loss of life, loss of function, and changes in lifestyle when injured. It is imperative that medical providers address these concerns and provide appropriate analgesia to the injured.

Analgesia administration should proceed in a step wise fashion. A regimen using 1,000 mg of acetaminophen alone or in conjunction with 800 mg of ibuprofen is shown to be effective for mild pain (53). Moderate to severe pain analgesia indicates the use of opiates or ketamine. Oral, sublingual, or transbuccal analgesic preparations provide adequate analgesia in patients without IV access. A recent study using oral transbuccal fentanyl citrate (OTFC) during Operation Iraqi Freedom showed efficacy in controlling pain (54). Intranasal ketamine appears to have promise as well (53). Studies continue to evaluate the efficacy of these products in varied environments. Patients with IV access should receive opiates. The initial 5 mg IV dose of morphine sulfate can be repeated every 10 minutes until achievement of adequate pain relief or until respiratory depression occurs. Continual monitoring is required when giving opiate medication or ketamine because of potential respiratory compromise. Intramuscular or subcutaneous injections are suboptimal because of the delay in systemic absorption and significant adverse effects, such as hypotension, following resuscitation due to rapid absorption from the tissues once circulation is restored.

Antibiotics

Failure to administer antibiotic therapy to patients in the prehospital setting contributes to unnecessary morbidity and mortality. Patients tolerating oral fluids can take oral preparations of fluoroquinolones with good gastrointestinal absorption and broad spectrum coverage. The current recommendation from the TCCC committee is gatifloxacin (12). Gatifloxacin is no longer marketed, so moxifloxacin is the preferred alternative. It is a broad coverage antibiotic that is cost effective and temperature stable. IV antibiotics of choice include cefotetan, ertapenem, or a fluoroquinolone (55). These antibiotics are preferred for their broad-spectrum coverage and longer dosing times (12 to 24 hours).

Hypothermia

Hypothermia, acidosis, and coagulopathy are often referred to as the "lethal triad" in trauma patients. The association of hypothermic coagulopathy with high mortality has been well described. As many as 66% of trauma patients arrive in emergency departments manifesting hypothermia (temperature <36°C). Approximately 80 % of nonsurviving patients have had a body temperature <34°C. This level of hypothermia causes coagulation proteins to not work, thus exacerbating the bleeding problem. The effect of hypothermia on coagulation results from inhibition of enzyme activities and platelet function, as well as increased fibrinolysis.

Prevention of hypothermia (<34°C) should be emphasized in military and civilian tactical operations.

Hypothermia occurs regardless of the ambient temperature and occurs with equal frequency in cold and hot climates. Attention to hypothermia prevention will decrease the deleterious effects of heat loss and decrease deaths from uncontrolled hemorrhage. Prevention of hypothermia is much easier than treatment of hypothermia. Therefore, prevention of heat loss should start as soon as possible after wounding. This will be optimally accomplished in a layered fashion with rugged, durable products located close to the point of injury, especially during ground and air evacuation. Use of both external warming adjuncts as well as warmed fluids may aid in hypothermia prevention.

CASEVAC Care

CASEVAC affords the opportunity to bring additional equipment and personnel forward to assist in casualty care. Prior planning for deployable push packs and personnel packages significantly augments this stage of tactical casualty care. Adaptability is the key to success in this endeavor and prior coordination for the use of electronic monitoring devices, heating elements, infusion devices, and even blood products on the evacuation platform invites success in patient care. Identifying and mitigating the limitations in weight, room (cube), and function are imperative prior to executing the CASEVAC mission. Casualties may require ongoing care during CASEVAC and engaging in procedures on a platform for the first time while moving in both the horizontal and vertical plane can be enlightening as well as difficult. Despite the inherent challenges, the CASEVAC platform presents an opportunity to significantly increase the provided medical support to the casualty. Attention, while en route with the casualty, should be directed to continuing evaluation, monitoring, preventing hypothermia, establishing IVs, fluid resuscitation, and additional procedures as necessary (e.g., definitive airways, splinting). CASEVAC platforms allow for medical resupply to the medical personnel on the scene. Push packs (prepackaged medical resupply) have worked very well in both conventional and unconventional units. The contents of push packs can be standardized or vary greatly from mission to mission.

TAKE HOME POINTS

1. Medical providers in the tactical environment must understand principles of TCCC.
2. ATLS other courses taught for in-hospital medicine are often not feasible or applicable to the tactical medical environment.
3. Rapid control of hemorrhage and addressing airway and breathing problems can result in decreasing morbidity and mortality.

4. The three phases of TCCC are used to help providers understand the medical care that can be rendered during a tactical mission.

SUMMARY

The tactical environment presents both a difficult and sometimes exotic place to administer medical care. It is critical to understand the different stages of tactical medical care and to know the significant interventions for each stage in order to maximize patient care. Important concepts include hemorrhage control, relief of tension pneumothoraces, controlling pain, and early antibiotic administration.

REFERENCES

1. Wound Data and Munitions Effectiveness Team. *The WDMET Study.* Bethesda: Uniformed Services University of the Health Sciences; 1970.
2. Butler FK, Hagmann J, Butler EG. Tactical casualty care in special operations. *Milit Med.* 1996;161(suppl):3–16.
3. Engelhardt S, Hoyt D, Coimbra R, et al. The 15-year evolution of an urban trauma center: what does the future hold for the trauma surgeon? *J Trauma.* 2001;51:633–638.
4. Biffl WL, Harrington DT, Majercik SD, et al. The evolution of trauma care at a level I trauma center. *J Am Coll Surg.* 2005;200:922–929.
5. Bellamy RF. *Combat Trauma Overview. Textbook of Military Medicine: Anesthesia and Pre-Operative Care of the Combat Casualty.* Washington: Dept of the Army; 1994:1–42.
6. Reister FA. *Battle Casualties and Medical Statistics: US Army Experience in Korea.* Washington: Dept of the Army; 1973.
7. Mabry RL, Holcomb JB, Baker AM, et al. United States Army Rangers in Somalia: an analysis of combat casualties on an urban battlefield. *J Trauma.* 2000;49:515–528.
8. Chambers LW, Rhee P, Baker BC, et al. Initial experience of US Marine Corps forward resuscitative surgical system during Operation Iraqi Freedom. *Arch Surg.* 2005;140:26–32.
9. Stevens RA, Bohman HR, Baker BC, et al. The US Navy's forward resuscitative surgery system during Operation Iraqi Freedom. *Milit Med.* 2005;170:297–301.
10. Champion HR, Bellamy RF, Roberts CP, et al. A profile of combat injury. *J Trauma.* 2003;54(suppl):S13–19.
11. Bellamy RF. The causes of death in conventional land warfare: implications for combat casualty care research. *Milit Med.* 1984;149:55–62.
12. McSwain M, Frame S, Salomone J. *Prehospital Advanced Life Support.* 5th ed. St Louis: Mosby; 2003:387, 388.
13. US Army. *Army Field Manual 8-43.* Fort Bragg: US Army Special Operations Command; 2000.
14. US Army. *Army Field Manual 8-10-6.* Washington: HQ Dept of the Army; 2000 April 14. http://www.brooksidepress.org/Products/OperationalMedicine/DATA/operationalmed/Manuals/fm8_10_6/toc.pdf Accessed September 27, 2007.
15. Holcomb JB, Stansbury LG, Champion HR, et al. Understanding combat casualty care statistics. *J Trauma.* 2006;60:397–401.
16. Holcomb, JB. The 2004 Fitts lecture: current perspective on combat casualty care. *J Trauma Injury Infect Crit Care.* 2005;59:990–1002.
17. Gawande A. Casualties of war–military care for the wounded from Iraq and Afghanistan. *N Engl J Med.* 2004;351:2471–2475.
18. Fox CJ, Gillespie DL, O'Donnell SD, et al. Contemporary management of wartime vascular trauma. *J Vasc Surg.* 2005;41:638–644.
19. Lakstein D, Blumenfeld A, Sokolov T, et al. Tourniquets for hemorrhage control on the battlefield: a 4-year accumulated experience. *J Trauma.* 2003;54:S221–S225.
20. Barash PG, Cullen BF, Stoelting RK. *Clinical Anesthesia.* 5th ed. Philadelphia: Lippincott Williams & Wilkins; 2006:1123–1124.

21. Walters TJ, Wenke JC, Kauvar DS, et al. An observational study to determine the effectiveness of self-applied tourniquets in human volunteers. *J Prehosp Care*. 2005;9: 416–422.

22. Lakstein D, Blumnfeld A, Sokolv T, et al. Tourniquets for hemorrhage control on the battlefield: a four year accumulated experience. *J Trauma*. 2003;54(suppl):S221–S225.

23. Carey ME. Analysis of wounds incurred by U.S. Army Seventh Corps personnel treated in corps hospitals during Operation Desert Storm, February 20 to March 10, 1991. *J Trauma*. 1996;40:S165.

24. Salvino CK, Dries D, Gamelli R, et al. Emergency cricothyroidotomy in trauma victims. *J Trauma*. 1993;34:503.

25. Mines D. Needle Thoracostomy fails to detect a fatal tension pneumothorax. *Ann Emerg Med*. 1993;22:863.

26. Chen SC, Markmann JF, Kauder DR, et al. Hemopneumothorax missed by auscultation in penetrating chest injury. *J Trauma*. 1997;42:86–89.

27. Britten S, Palmer SH, Snow TM. Needle Thoracocentesis in tension pneumothorax: insufficient cannula length and potential failure. *Injury*. 1996;27:758.

28. Givens M. Needle thoracostomy: implications of computed tomography chest wall thickness. *Acad Emerg Med*. 2004;11: 211–213.

29. Holcomb JB, Pusateri AE, Kerr SM, et al. Initial efficacy and function of needle thoracocentesis versus tube thoracostomy in a swine model of traumatic tension pneumothorax. *J Trauma*. In press.

30. Pusateri AE, Delgado AV, Dick EJ Jr, et al. Application of a granular mineral-based hemostatic agent (QuikClot) to reduce blood loss after grade V liver injury in swine. *J Trauma*. 2004;57:555–562.

31. Wright JK, Kalns J, Wolf EA, et al. Thermal injury resulting from application of a granular mineral hemostatic agent. *J Trauma*. 2004;57:224–230.

32. Wright FL, Hua HT, Velmahos G, et al. Intracorporeal use of the hemostatic agent QuickClot in a coagulopathic patient with combined thoracoabdominal penetrating trauma. *J Trauma*. 2004;56:205–208.

33. Alam HB, Chen Z, Jaskille A, et al. Application of a zeolite hemostatic agent achieves 100% survival in a lethal model of complex groin injury in Swine. *J Trauma*. 2004;56:974–983.

34. Acheson EM, Kheirabadi BS, Deguzman R, et al. Comparison of hemorrhage control agents applied to lethal extremity arterial hemorrhages in swine. *J Trauma*. 2005;59:865–874.

35. Pusateri AE, Holcomb JB, Kheirabadi BS, et al. Making sense of the preclinical literature on advanced hemostatic products. *J Trauma*. 2006;60:674–682

36. Aeder MI, Crowe JP, Rhodes RS, et al. Technical limitations in the rapid infusion and intravenous fluid. *Ann Emerg Med*. 1985;14:307.

37. Hoelzer MF. Recent advances in intravenous therapy. *Emerg Med Clin North Am*. 1986;4:487.

38. Dubick MA, Holcomb JB. A review of intraosseous vascular access: current status and military application. *Milit Med*. 2000;165:552–558.

39. Mapstone J, Roberts I, Evans P. Fluid resuscitation strategies: a systematic review of animal trials. *J Trauma*. 2003;55:571–589.

40. Revell M, Porter K, Greaves I. Fluid resuscitation in prehospital trauma care: a consensus view. *Emerg Med J*. 2002;19:494–498.

41. Vincent JL, Berre J. Primer on medical management of severe brain injury. *Crit Care Med*. 2005;33:1392–1399.

42. Gruen P, Liu C. Current trends in the management of head injury. *Emerg Med Clin North Am*. 1998;16:63–83.

43. Chestnut RM. Guidelines for the management of severe head injury: what we know and what we think we know. *J Trauma*. 1997;42:S19.

44. The Brain Trauma Foundation. The American Association of Neurological Surgeons. The Joint Section on neurotrauma and critical care. Resuscitation of blood pressure and oxygenation. *J Neurotrauma*. 2000;17:471–478.

45. Pinto FCG, Capone-Neto A, Prist R, et al. Volume replacement with lactated ringer's or 3% hypertonic saline solution during combined experimental hemorrhagic shock and traumatic brain injury. *J Trauma*. 2006;60:758–764.

46. Prehospital hypertonic saline resuscitation of patients with hypotension and severe traumatic brain injury: a randomized controlled trial. *Surv Anesthesiol*. 2005;49:250–251.

47. Rainey TG, Read CA. The pharmacology of colloids and crystalloids. In: Baltimore CB, ed. *The Pharmacologic Approach to the Critically Ill Patient*. Baltimore: Williams & Wilkins; 1988:219–240.

48. Carey JS, Scharschmidt BF, Culliford AL, et al. Hemodynamic effectiveness of colloid and electrolyte solutions for replacement of simulated blood loss. *Surg Gynecol Obstet*. 1970;131:679.

49. Deb S, Martin B, Sun L, et al. Resuscitation with lactated Ringer's solution in rats with hemorrhagic shock induces immediate apoptosis. *J Trauma*. 1999;46:582–588.

50. Deb S, Sun L, Martin B, et al. Lactated Ringer's solution and hetastarch but not plasma resuscitation after hemorrhagic shock is associated with immediate lung apoptosis by the up-regulation of the Bax protein. *J Trauma*. 2000;49:47–53.

51. Kramer GC, Perron PR, Lindsey DC, et al. Small volume resuscitation with hypertonic saline dextran solution. *Surgery*. 1986;100:239.

52. Wade CE, Grady JJ, Kramer GC. Individual patient cohort analysis of the efficacy of hypertonic saline/dextran in patients with traumatic brain injury and hypotension. J Trauma. 1997;42:S61–S65.

53. Wedmore IS, Johnson TR, Czarnik J. Pain management in the wilderness and operational setting. *Emerg Med Clin North Am*. 2005;23: 585–601.

54. Kotwal RS, O'Connor KC, Johnson TR. A novel pain management strategy for combat casualty care. *Ann Emerg Med*. 2004;44:121–127.

55. Butler F, O'Connor KC. Antibiotics in tactical combat casualty care. *Milit Med*. 2003;168:911–914.

Chapter 15

Critical Casualty Evacuation from Tactical Settings

John M. Wightman, Mark E. Gibbons, Mark E. Gebhart, and James E. Brown

OBJECTIVES

After reading this section, the reader will be able to:

1. State the roles of the tactical medical provider in advising operational commanders on evacuation contingencies.
2. List at least four key differences in evacuation considerations between tactical and non-tactical settings.
3. Identify the two most crucial elements to consider when choosing between two or more evacuation options for critical casualties.
4. Outline the major elements of planning and coordinating evacuation assets before and during tactical missions.

INTRODUCTION

Medical personnel supporting tactical operations must plan for the rescue and evacuation of casualties to sources of care beyond the scope or capabilities of those at the scene. Crisis situations may develop during any phase of operations. These can affect bystanders, adversaries, or operators. Critically ill or injured casualties will almost always require supportive care or definitive management at a hospital or trauma center. Concise and flexible contingency planning affirms the role of the tactical medical provider (TMP) as the operational commander's medical advisor. TMPs plan, coordinate, and facilitate expeditious transportation of casualties from the scene to an appropriate emergency department (ED) or specialty referral center while maximizing the level of care during patient movement or transition of care. Preparation for foreseeable medical or nonmedical crises is essential for mission success.

Medical care during evacuation (MEDEVAC) can be conducted over the earth's surface, through its atmosphere, or some combination of these. Organized ground-evacuation systems have been employed since the Napoleonic Wars of the 19th century. Tactical casualty evacuation (CASEVAC) by rotorcraft was introduced during the Korean War, but MEDEVAC by air was really expanded and refined by both military and civilian organizations since the Vietnam War (1).

The development of civilian out-of-hospital medical response shares a direct relationship with the military. The early 1970s witnessed an explosion of educational programs as a large pool of veteran Vietnam medics transitioned to civilian emergency medical services (EMS) providers. Following a seminal white paper just before this period (2), legislatures across the nation recognized the possibilities for reducing mortality, and moved quickly to implement these and other programs to initiate a new era of out-of-hospital medical care in the United States.

In any health care system, each separate component is interrelated and relies upon the others. The out-of-hospital portion is vitally important. Actions taken by all providers in the evacuation chain influence subsequent care and ultimate outcome of critical casualties (3). Medical skills brought to the tactical arena will vary widely—from civilian EMS providers of basic life support (BLS) to highly trained and experienced tactical physician-paramedic teams.

Although the medical literature regarding tactical emergency medical support (TEMS) continues to grow, there is still precious little evidence regarding the efficacy of recommended techniques and procedures. Nonetheless, practitioners of TEMS—whether law enforcement, military, or other—prepare for and face a variety of difficult challenges. Many of these would tax even the most experienced out-of-hospital providers. On-scene management and tactical evacuation of seriously ill or injured casualties are on one extreme of this spectrum. The dedication, training, experience, planning, and on-the-spot judgment of a TMP may be the only hope for casualty survival, regardless of whether there is literature evidence to support any specific course of action (COA). Extrapolations from the military and nontactical literature may be made in some cases, but must be critically reviewed for applicability to any given system or situation.

TACTICAL VERSUS NONTACTICAL SETTINGS

From its very conception in the late 1980s, TEMS has focused on mitigating risk in a high-risk environment. This has been done by conducting preventive services for team members and augmenting personnel, planning for medical support of training and mission operations, providing medical advice to commanders and other decision-makers (i.e., being their "medical conscience"), and managing the sequelae of illnesses and injuries in a variety of settings. When faced with critical casualties, the expected stressors of out-of-hospital care are only compounded by direct threat of injury from adversaries, low-light or high-noise environments, restrictive personal protective equipment (PPE) (e.g., gloves, body armor, chemical-biological-radiological (CBR) masks and suits), inability to directly or immediately access casualties in some scenarios, and casualties potentially being friends or co-workers.

Operational security (OPSEC) is a risk-management tool used to deny adversaries information about a tactical unit's intentions and capabilities (4). Polices and procedures must exist to identify and protect critical information that could compromise mission accomplishment. In part, it was a breach of OPSEC during the raid on the Branch Davidian Compound near Waco, Texas on February, 28 1993 that contributed to 32 operator casualties (four fatal gunshot wounds, 20 nonfatal engagement wounds, eight nonfatal injuries) and seven adversary casualties (3 fatal and four nonfatal gunshot wounds). During the planning phase of Operation TROJAN HORSE, a dispatcher in the local EMS system informed a friend in the media that three ambulances had been placed on standby for Monday (1 March) by the Bureau of Alcohol, Tobacco, and Firearms. A paramedic also told a reporter at the scene of an unrelated accident that "something big" was going to happen on Monday (5).

During the planning, as well as execution and debriefing, of tactical operations, all personnel must ensure the commander's OPSEC guidance is not violated. TMPs must have a systematic process to obtain critical information,

identify and analyze potential threats, assess risks and vulnerabilities, and implement appropriate countermeasures for medical threats, while maintaining the necessary level of security. Should unintentional exposure of mission-critical information occur, unit and team commanders must be briefed without delay to determine any potential impact on the planned mission.

Establishing scene safety prior to rescue is common to both tactical and nontactical settings. Although some threats may be different, a higher level of risk may be acceptable during TEMS. Each tactical unit's commander allocates medical assets based on resource availability and perceived risk. Military units have different missions, methods, and resources than typical law enforcement units, though overlap in many principles, concepts, and techniques should be leveraged where possible.

EVACUATION SYSTEMS

When planning for the possible evacuation of critical casualties, TMPs must have solid understandings of the capabilities and limitations of a wide variety of transportation platforms ranging from improvised litters to mobile intensive care units (MICUs). Manual carries are discussed in Chapter 19. Preplanned surface evacuation vehicles are usually ground ambulances, but they could be watercraft in some scenarios. Preplanned air evacuation from tactical settings is most often accomplished by helicopter, but airplanes may be required for longer distances. Vehicles of convenience can be employed when absolutely necessary, but this usually represents a failure of premission contingency planning.

Box 15.1 provides some key questions related to evacuation platforms. Some missions may require specialized rescue, evacuation, or medical assets. Underground and underwater operations are an example. Breeching or cutting tools are others. Occasionally, potential patients may be known to require medications not typically carried by TMPs or civilian EMS.

▶ **BOX 15.1. Some Questions Related to Evacuation Platforms.**

Terrain and weather considerations

- Is the casualty being exposed to weather conditions until pick-up, such that it might be detrimental to outcome?
- Will a tactical or technical rescue be required before the casualty can be moved to an evacuation platform (e.g., extrication from a collapsed structure or mangled vehicle, high-angle movement from a building or off a mountain)?

- If considering a ground response with an off-road segment, can the specific vehicle get in and out without becoming immobilized? If not, could the casualty be moved to a site that is more accessible?
- If considering use of a rotocraft, is there a suitable HLZ that can rapidly be found by the flight crew? If the location could be found but no HLZ exists, does the aircraft have hoist equipment and a trained crew? If neither, could the casualty be moved to a site that is more accessible or would ground evacuation be more appropriate from time and level-of-care standpoints?
- Can the vehicle be used in the existing weather? If using an air asset, is the aircraft and flight crew instrument-rated? If using a watercraft, can the casualty be safely transferred to it in rough conditions? Even if using a ground vehicle, does the weather prevent an unsafe condition that would delay the response (e.g., flash flood, hurricane, tornado)?

Vehicle specifications

- How many casualties can be safely accommodated from space and en route-care standpoints?
- Is there more than one available, if the number of casualties exceeds the space available or a vehicle is unavailable for maintenance reasons?
- Will the vehicle require armor, intrinsic defensive weapon systems, or security escort into and out of the scene or along the transportation route?

Special equipment for locating pick-up or transfer sites

- Map and compass
  - Most surface vehicles will only have a map, but do they have a compass for off-road navigation? All air vehicles will have both.
  - Do the on-scene tactical personnel have a compatible map and a compass for either providing the responding crew an azimuth or navigating to a more suitable pick-up site?
- GPS
  - Does the responding vehicle have GPS capability, especially with a moving-map display?
  - Do on-scene tactical personnel have the capability of providing coordinates in the same system used by the vehicle crew?
- Visual aids
  - Does the responding vehicle need equipment such as a high-intensity spotlight, night-vision goggles (NVGs), or forward-looking infrared (FLIR)?
  - Do on-scene personnel need search lights or flashlights, chemical illumination sticks, signal flares, visual or infrared strobes, infrared-reflective panels or tapes, smoke grenades, fluorescent panels, or other marking equipment?

Crew specifications

- What will be the highest level of care required?
  - Is a BLS unit staffed by emergency medical technicians (EMTs) sufficient for field care while gaining a time advantage over the availability of more advanced care?
  - Is ALS provided by a paramedic, nurse, or physicians' assistant (PA) necessary for their additional skills to be applied during transportation?
  - Is a MICU with care provided by or under direct supervision of a physician required for survival of a critical casualty?
- Is security still a concern?
  - Can the responding crew know the site of operations or witness anything at the scene, or will the pick-up site have to be moved for security purposes?
  - Will the TMP or an operator have to accompany any casualties to prevent inadvertent release of sensitive information by a casualty with altered mental status or one who will be treated with mind-altering medications during the course of their care?
  - Will security elements be able to accompany suspects [or enemy prisoners of war (EPWs)] throughout all phases of evacuation?

Nonstandard medical equipment

- Will technical equipment for extrication or high-angle rescue be required?
  - Most ground and air ambulances will not have this equipment intrinsic to the responding vehicle, though some helicopters may have a hoist for vertical extraction.
  - Most organizations with the necessary specialized skills to retrieve casualties will have personnel with medical training to care for the injured during the technical-rescue phase of the evacuation.
- Will equipment such as a Kendrick Extrication Device (KED), Sked stretcher, Stoke's basket, or other specialized litter be necessary for casualty transportation?
- Will decontamination be required before loading in an ambulance?
- Could the evacuation vehicle bring needed equipment or supplies to the scene for early intervention before evacuation?
  - A transport ventilator may be better than a bag-valve device for longer distances or multiple casualties.
  - Starting blood products at the scene and en route might be more beneficial than waiting until hospital arrival.

- Some illnesses—or transportation delayed sufficiently for infections to be established—might require parenteral antibiotics or vasopressors for support.
- Some medications typically carried by TMPs could be rapidly exhausted in some scenarios, such as exposure to a chemical nerve agent, which might require more atropine than the 6 mg supplied in Mark-I antidote kits.
- Some patients might require a specific medicine that can be brought to the scene instead of immediately evacuating the casualty.

Medical communications between TMP and evacuation crew

- How are various vehicle types requested?
- Is there a dedicated and secure radio frequency for continued communication while the vehicle is en route and during transportation to a hospital?
- If the TMP accompanies the casualty to the hospital in an aircraft, is there an extra headset for communicating with the crew?

Ground Evacuation

Federal Standard KKK-1822-E defines types and standards for ambulances in the United States and Canada. The three current categories of ground vehicle are based on different chassis-cab styles: type-I, light-duty trucks; type-II, passenger/cargo vans; and type-III, medium-duty trucks. More recently, another version has been developed based on the chassis-cab of heavy-duty trucks. The civilian public-service sector uses the term *ambulance* to describe a unit staffed and equipped to operate at the BLS level. The term *medic* is used to define a unit staffed and equipped to provide advanced life support (ALS). A MICU is a ground-transport vehicle staffed and equipped to provide physician-directed critical care, either in person or through advanced-practice paramedics or critical care nurses. National minimum-equipment lists exist for each category. EMS and TEMS medical directors may add equipment and supplies to ambulance or medic units under their control.

A backboard, Stokes basket, or Sked may help modularize critical TEMS equipment if space permits. The Sked and similar rescue systems perform functions of basket-type stretchers, yet are lighter weight and can be stored in more compact forms. They have proven to be highly versatile for TEMS evacuation missions by ground or air. Many helicopter crews use them for hoisting operations too. Intrinsic patient straps on all these rescue devices can help secure several items on one man-portable platform. By compartmentalizing specialized equipment, the whole package can be delivered to the casualty or hoisted as a unit. By placing critical equipment together, confusion is avoided when team members not familiar with medical equipment must retrieve items for the TMP.

The United States and some other military organizations have their own built-in system to transport casualties from point-of-injury to initial medical care. Any reliance on civilian EMS organizations to support law enforcement tactical operations will be limited to whatever is available in the community or region. The primary advantages of ground-based vehicles are:

- more ready availability, largely due to the numerical ratio of ground over air assets;
- potential to preposition closer to operations;
- dispatch from a base to most incident scenes with minimal difficulty; and
- ability to drive directly to the casualty in many circumstances.

Some EMS systems may have the capacity to dispatch ground MICUs staffed with crews who also staff air ambulances on other shifts. This makes the only key consideration the time to stabilization or definitive care. Disadvantages of ground-based platforms include:

- dependence on various skills of responding crews, even within a training category: BLS, ALS, or MICU;
- inability to access rugged or vertical terrain, including some buildings; and
- potentially lengthy transport times to definitive care, especially when far away or in heavy city traffic.

Some of these problems can be mitigated when the ground vehicle is dedicated to the tactical unit and prepositioned near the outer perimeter.

Air Evacuation

One obvious advantage of air evacuation is speed. A less-commonly considered benefit is the advanced medical skills most crews bring to the scene or the point of transfer from ground to air. Disadvantages associated with air assets include:

- fewer available vehicles;
- inability to position near the location of the mission, due to noise compromising OPSEC;
- increased security required for forward staging;
- time to arrival if not prestaged; and
- need for support resources, including local ground units.

Contemporary military commands and civilian flight programs may operate fixed-wing, rotary-wing, or a combination of both aircraft types. This is dictated by the list of potential missions, conceivable operating environments, and budgetary constraints. Civilian hospital-based flight programs frequently have the single mission profile of MEDEVAC. Public-safety aircraft often support multiple missions such as law enforcement, search and rescue, and firefighting—with or without the capability to also perform MEDEVAC operations.

Civilian air ambulances come in a wide variety of aircraft but are most commonly staffed and equipped similar to MICUs. An exception, which is more common in tactical military settings, exists when a utility helicopter or cargo airplane is being employed as a MEDEVAC asset. As long as the crew has ALS capability, the civilian literature on helicopter transportation does not support any advantage of a nurse-nurse team over a nurse-paramedic combination (6,7). It remains inconclusive regarding any putative superiority of onboard physicians in the United States (8,9), although there seems to be demonstrable benefits in Australian (10) and German (11,12) systems.

Similar to their rotary-wing counterparts, civilian evacuation organizations normally convert fixed-wing aircraft then permanently dedicate them to an aeromedical evacuation (AE) mission. They are almost always staffed and equipped for critical care. The military more commonly modifies passenger or cargo aircraft for each AE mission as necessary. Within the continental United States, the Air Force's C-21A (military version of the Lear Jet 35A)—often in combination with the self-contained life support for trauma and transport (LSTAT) system—can be used for single patients, although space is just as limited as in a helicopter. When more than one patient requires transportation simultaneously, the C-130E/H/J is employed for shorter distances or the C-17A for longer distances. Expedient aircraft, such as tankers, can also be used. These military assets are staffed with an AE crew typically composed of two flight nurses and three AE technicians. The equipment they carry is for care of stable patients only. When seriously ill or injured casualties require evacuation, the AE crew is augmented by a critical care air transport team (CCATT) composed of one intensivist physician, one nurse experienced in critical care, and one cardiopulmonary technician (13,14). Their equipment package is designed to manage up to three ventilator-dependent patients, any of whom may be only initially stabilized and are at risk for later clinical deterioration during evacuation.

The primary advantage of fixed-wing AE is the ability to move critical casualties long distances without, or with minimal, refueling stops. Larger aircraft offer more room to continue casualty resuscitation and stabilization en route, as well as the ability to carry more than one patient at a time. The most significant disadvantage is the requirement for a runway, which may not be in close proximity to tactical operations or definitive-care facilities. Critical casualties must be moved by ground or air conveyance to the runway, transferred to the airplane, flown to a different location, and then transported again by ground or air from the destination airport to the hospital. Even in relatively mature combat theaters, military hospitals are rarely close enough to runways that some ground component is not required on each end of the evacuation. Lack of thorough planning and coordination for each phase only

places casualties at increased risk for death or permanent disability.

PLANNING FOR THE WORST

The best method of evacuation for any particular situation involving critical casualties depends on many parameters. The two most crucial elements to consider for planning and execution of these evacuations are time available for transport and treatment capabilities en route (15). Premission variables include:

- scene security
- natural and manmade hazards to transportation assets
- terrain and weather
- availability and maintenance status of transportation resources
- estimated response and transportation times
- capabilities of local and regional medical facilities

Intramission variables include:

- casualty status
- number of casualties
- persistent threats
- continuing mission requirements
- diversion status of destination facilities

These are certainly not all-inclusive lists. General phases of evacuation planning are listed in Box 15.2. These are discussed in more detail in the following paragraphs of this section.

> **BOX 15.2. Planning Considerations for Casualty Evacuation.**
>
> 1. Receive mission briefing from commander or designee.
>   - Freedom and constraints related to specified and implied tasks
>   - Degree of authority and independence for task completion
>   - Guidance on level of operational security during planning
> 2. List critical facts and assumptions on which planning and decisions will be made.
> 3. Identify and analyze potential medical threats.
>   - Illnesses
>   - Operational injuries
>   - Engagement injuries
>   - Environmental exposures
>   - Chemical, biological, or radiological (CBR)
>   - Effects of contamination
>   - Need for decontamination
>   - Effects of sustained operations (if applicable)
>   - Water and food

- Work–rest cycles
- Circadian rhythms
- Operator medications
4. Assess risks and vulnerabilities.
   - Medical histories of adversaries and bystanders largely unknown
   - Potential for illness, injury, or fatigue of critical personnel
     - Commander
     - Operators with unique skills
     - Tactical medical providers (TMPs)
   - Time available to plan may not allow complete assessment
     - Likely threats
     - Possible countermeasures
     - All evacuation options
   - Vulnerabilities of tactical environment
     - Inability to directly or immediately access casualties in some scenarios
     - Low-light or high-noise environments
     - Restrictive personal protective equipment (PPE)
   - Planned evacuation asset might not available when requested
     - Unable to contact
     - Vehicle on another call
     - Maintenance issues
     - Weather
   - Stress of casualties potentially being friends or coworkers
   - Negative press following media coverage
5. Locate medical capabilities and rescue/evacuation assets.
   - Tactical team
   - Community in area of operations (AO)
   - State or regional resources (e.g., heavy rescue, technical rescue)
6. Prepare possible COAs based on potential contingencies.
   - Present plans to commander
   - Receive commander's selection and additional inputs for modifications
   - Continue to refine plans until accepted by commander
7. Implement countermeasures.
   - Skills training
   - Equipment adjusting
   - Mission briefing
   - Execution rehearsing
   - Appropriate supervising
   - Continuous reassessing
8. Execute the plan.
9. Observe, supervise, re-evaluate, and adjust as necessary while operations progress.

Receive Mission

The unit commander or operations officer should brief their staff, outline intentions, and provide guidance before developing final mission plans. A senior TMP should be part of this staff with authority to offer candid input regarding medical implications of plans and foreseeable medical consequences of decisions. To do this, TMPs must have a working knowledge of ground and air medical resources available to support any operation. These include assessments of medical capabilities at the scene (intrinsic tactical element plus any preplanned augmentation), potential EMS responders, and several potential destination hospitals.

Dedicated EMS assets are tools. If used correctly, they can contribute to saving lives. If used improperly, they may jeopardize valuable personnel and compromise the likelihood of mission completion without casualties. In a civilian law enforcement setting, flashing ambulance lights or the inadvertent overflight of an adversarial target by a medical helicopter could increase a suspect's aggression or destroy any trust developed through prior negotiations. In wartime military settings, detection of the evacuation platform may lead to capture or destruction of the vehicle and personnel onboard. Crews must have solid understandings of designated routes and avoidance areas, which allow uncompromised approaches to designated ground entry control points (ECPs) and helicopter landing zones (HLZs).

List Facts and Assumptions

TMPs make evacuation triage decisions based on time, not distance, and this must be considered in premission planning and coordination. Although some increased time is inherent in greater distance, it is not the only factor involved. There is certainly a difference between helicopter straight-line flight time at 160 miles per hour and ground-vehicle road-dependent drive time at an average speed of 40 miles per hour; but this simplistic approach ignores a myriad of other factors.

Assuming that a scene has been secured, an ambulance standing by between the inner and outer perimeters might be able to drive a critical casualty to an appropriate ED in less time than a helicopter can fly from the same facility to the scene, conduct high and low reconnaissance of an unfamiliar HLZ, approach and land, receive the casualty (possibly by ground vehicle from the actual incident site), and return to the hospital. One study conducted in two California counties found a statistically faster total response time with a helicopter when more than 10 miles from a trauma center, if air and ground were requested simultaneously (16). However, the average difference was <5 minutes out of more than 40 minutes total time, and outcomes were not examined. When the distance resulted in ground transport times of 80 ± 5 minutes, total air times were 50 to 75 minutes. Therefore, about 20-minutes difference or about 20-miles distant might be good initial guidelines in similar civilian metropolitan settings.

When working away from dense urban areas where air transport expedites patient delivery, TMPs should consider setting up "hot pads" for rotorcraft to deliver resources or launch MEDEVACs. Staging areas for larger operations should be at offsite locations that allow secure parking for multiple ground and air vehicles, along with crew shelter and logistical support.

Unsecured scenes further complicate the time it takes to rescue casualties and move them to an evacuation platform outside the inner perimeter. A full-service medical center might be a block away, yet it could take hours to evacuate casualties to it.

A map of U.S. trauma centers is kept up to date by the American Trauma Society's Trauma Information Exchange Program Web site (17). Regional trauma centers, designated by state authority or verified by the American College of Surgeons as level-I or level-II, provide comprehensive trauma care (18), but other hospitals and medical centers may be more appropriate in certain circumstances. Not all critical casualties result from trauma, and stabilization of nonsurgical casualties may be possible in smaller EDs or equivalent military units.

Depending on the tactical situation, illumination, available field equipment, and the TMP's level of emergency medical skill; rapid medical or surgical interventions at an outlying ED may be beneficial for some problems. These might include:

- controlling proximal extremity hemorrhage
- managing difficult airways
- inserting chest tubes
- x-raying the chest for occult air or fluid
- administering blood products

Some facilities, particularly in the deployed wartime military setting, may even be capable of damage-control surgery for internal hemorrhage prior to transfer to a center more appropriate for definitive care.

With regard to rural settings and long transportation times, one small study in New York found mortality rates similar to national averages when trauma patients were first resuscitated at outlying facilities. Patients who died before transfer did so in median time of 42 minutes (19). A more recent study from the same state further determined that total out-of-hospital time was not an independent predictor of trauma mortality (20). These results must be interpreted cautiously, because the care provided at the initial hospitals were not sufficiently detailed to readily extrapolate to other settings.

Analyze Threats

Within the OPSEC constraints placed on TMPs by their commanders, intelligence is gathered and both medical and nonmedical issues are considered for every evacuation contingency prior to their emergent need. Generic threats of medical significance include:

- potential psychological impact of events
- environmental temperature and moisture extremes
- prolonged duration of operations
- access to potable water and safe food
- primitive or improvised electrical and heating sources
- chemical, radiological, or other hazardous materials
- person-to-person communicable illnesses
- vector-borne diseases
- human waste products or bodily remains
- contaminated needles and other sharp items
- ability to assess potential casualties in low-light or high-noise environments
- external threats that impact ingress and egress evacuation routes

There are likely a host of additional threats to the well-being of teammates and other individuals. Many may be specific to any particular mission type, geographical location, time of year, and other factors. Some may be identified by operators and some by TMPs, but all must be incorporated into plans and repeatedly reassessed during mission execution.

Assess Risks and Vulnerabilities

Risk is inherent in any tactical operation. The U.S. Army uses the mnemonic METT-TC to remind planners to assess risks related to *mission* objectives and tactics, *enemy* objectives and capabilities, friendly *troops* employable, *time* available, *terrain* and expected weather, and potential *civilian* interactions. Other organizations can apply similarly standard categories. Information regarding risks is obtained through individual and unit experiences plus intelligence gathering and directed reconnaissance. Each risk identified is assessed for its potential impact on operations. The unit commander makes the final decision as to how much risk is acceptable and what countermeasures will be implemented to mitigate it.

The prime vulnerability when relying on evacuation platforms extrinsic to the tactical unit is their potential incapacity to respond to the pickup location in the time required to make a difference in a critical casualty's outcome. For example, one published study revealed that up to a third of helicopter evacuation missions might be aborted after they are requested, with weather being the most common reason for inability to respond (21). Other causes of response failure, which might also affect ground vehicles, include:

- wind and weather extremes
- communication failure

- inability to locate the scene
- inaccessible terrain
- unsecured pickup locations

Depending on jurisdictional and many other systemic factors, an unplanned general request for EMS assistance could summon hordes of medical responders, thereby creating additional congestion on ingress and egress routes. Command personnel may have a difficult time communicating with these personnel once dispatched. Responding EMS providers may be inadvertently placed in harm's way. These and other factors may make an already chaotic scene unmanageable. A staging location away from the area of operation and an ECP may help temper the potentially negative impact of well-intended responders.

Locate Evacuation Assets

TMPs must plan on the appropriate level of care as well as the time it will take to move the care to the casualties or deliver the casualties to the care. This is accomplished by combining the medical assets intrinsic to the tactical unit and those external units or organizations that can be dedicated to the mission or called during contingencies. *When resources are constrained, a tiered approach— from tactical to nontactical providers or BLS to ALS—is one solution.*

BLS is usually able to prevent further injury, conduct rapid casualty assessments, control external hemorrhage, administer supplemental oxygen, employ bag-valve-mask ventilation, perform cardiac compressions, immobilize the spine, and splint fractures. ALS adds the capabilities to accomplish advanced airway interventions, infuse intravenous crystalloid fluids, monitor cardiac electrophysiology, and administer medication therapy. In many situations, however, sound BLS skills coupled with perceptive time-awareness may prove superior to ALS in the field. The rapid evacuation of critical casualties with appropriate care en route may allow BLS responders the opportunity to contribute to excellent outcomes despite less training and only basic equipment. One article from urban Los Angeles reported that trauma patients requiring artificial ventilation were five times more likely to survive with a bag-valve-mask technique than with ventilation following endotracheal intubation (22).

Responses can be "tiered" by progressively increasing capabilities from initial BLS to interval ALS to final hospital-based care. In the tactical setting, the decision to send high-value low-density medical assets into potentially hostile environments may also lead to plans to tier the response. The tiered approach is used frequently by both civilian and military response systems where and when there is not enough ALS capacity to serve the size of a given geographical area or volume of requests for field care. Military units often call different levels of care "echelons" as

casualties progress through the evacuation system from point of injury or illness to whatever level of care is necessary to definitively manage their problem. As each level in a tiered system transfers care to the next higher, the lower level can be put back into service to respond to or receive more casualties.

When determining possible evacuation platforms and the medical capabilities of their crews, the literature contains several studies indicating superiority of air over ground in select circumstances. A review of published civilian experiences from the mid-1980s to mid-1990s revealed collective survival benefits ranging from one to 12 additional lives saved per 100 patients transported (23). However, when trauma victims were retrieved directly from the field, no survival benefit was realized in Pennsylvania's trauma system over the same decade (24). On the other hand, Maryland's flight program documented a lower mortality for the most severely injured subset of trauma patients (25). These results differed from two other statewide studies that found helicopter evacuation had a significant impact for patients who were not at the extremes of trauma severity (i.e., moderately but not mildly or severely injured) (26,27). Blunt trauma (28,29), serious head injuries (30,31) and burns may be specific groups who might benefit more from air evacuation, though different system characteristics and research methodologies make any blanket conclusions difficult. *The best evacuation platform is the one that gets the casualty to the necessary facility in the right amount of time with an appropriate level of care en route.*

Finalize Plans

TMPs should prepare two or three potential COAs for the commander's consideration. These should be based on a thorough assessment of potential contingencies combined with meticulous planning to the extent that time and OPSEC allow. Each COA should be recommended for specific reasons. The commander may accept, modify, or reject any or all of these. The process is recursive until a final medical support plan, which includes evacuation methods, is complete.

Written extraction and transportation plans should be developed and briefed to all involved personnel. Standard operating procedures (SOPs) may be used in many circumstances, but often have to be modified or rewritten for extended operations or unusual settings. TEMS team leaders should brief command personnel on original plans, and provide periodic updates when they are modified or command is transferred. When OPSEC guidance does not limit premission communication with specific evacuation resources, training, briefings, and rehearsals will facilitate near-seamless transfer of medical care from one vehicle to another or one team of providers to another.

OPERATIONAL DECISION-MAKING

The unique aspects of tactical operations require that TMPs adapt to rapidly changing situations to ensure effective evacuation of critical casualties. Figure 15-1 provides a skeleton for the phases of casualty evacuation. The initial consideration in a tactical setting involves whether or not to attempt casualty rescue if there is a continuing threat to potential rescuers. Some evacuation decisions can be made using remote assessment. If a casualty is thought to be critical and the anticipated evacuation asset is not on scene, the request can be made before the casualty is actually retrieved. Of course, the staging area for the ground or air vehicle must be secured. After the casualty has been

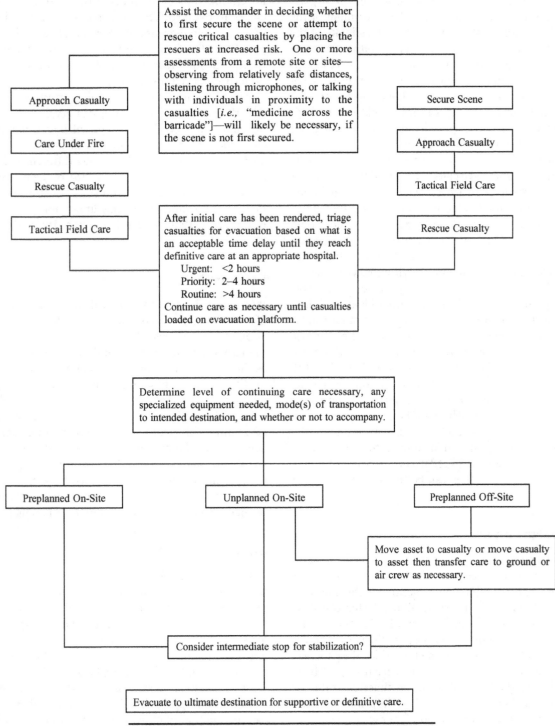

FIGURE 15.1. Tactical considerations for casualty evacuation.

rescued and tactical field care administered, a final decision on evacuation mode and en route patient management can be made.

Evacuation Triage

As outlined in Chapter 13, *triage for treatment* is categorized as immediate, delayed, minimal, expectant, and dead. Terms used during *triage for transport* are urgent, priority, routine, and convenience. An assessment of the casualty's physiological status leads to an estimate of the maximum delay until stabilization or definitive care need be provided. Urgent patients require these interventions within 2 hours from the time of assessment. Priority patients are expected to tolerate a delay of up to 4 hours. Routine and convenience categories should not apply to casualties who were ever considered critical at any point in time, even if stabilized in the field.

The assigned evacuation category does not necessarily parallel the current triage category for field treatment. For example, a casualty with a gunshot wound to the abdomen may not require immediate interventions in the field, if relatively stable hemodynamically. Such a casualty would properly be placed in the delayed treatment category, yet an urgent evacuation might be warranted for potential occult internal bleeding and developing peritonitis. When necessary, the TMP must emphasize the importance of transport to the appropriate level of care for either illness or injury to the transporting providers. Patients with moderate-to-severe injuries appear to have better chances of survival when managed at level-I trauma centers than those primarily treated at other types of hospitals (32). The TMP should make efficient use of transport resources, particularly in multicasualty incidents. Noncritical routine or convenience patients may be placed in spare spaces of vehicles transporting those more seriously ill or injured. Retaining less seriously ill or injured operators at the scene under the supervision of a TMP may be necessary for mission accomplishment; they can be transported at a later time.

Transportation Mode

When determining whether ground or air medical transport is more appropriate, the TMP must consider many factors before making a recommendation to the unit commander. Although air transport allows faster transport times; the delay to launch, fly to, and land at the scene—plus the logistics required to transport the patient to the waiting aircraft, brief the crew, and transload the patient—may negate the positive aspects of faster transport from the incident to the hospital. Turnover times can often be reduced, if the flight crew is staged on the primary ground conveyance then used for transport from scene to aircraft. The medical team can be briefed on patients' conditions

and assist with critical interventions during movement to a waiting aircraft at an HLZ or runway.

Depending on the capabilities of the tactical medical element, the evacuation team may possess more advanced or specialized skills to care for critical casualties. In an urban setting with helicopters dispatched from a centrally located trauma center, direct evacuation from the scene made little difference for victims of noncranial penetrating trauma, unless the skills of the flight crew were necessary in the field. This occurred <7% of the time, even when the initial ground EMS responders could only provide BLS (33). Similar results were found for two countywide but still metropolitan systems transporting mostly blunt-trauma victims (34,35).

The literature must be carefully scrutinized for urban, suburban, or rural study settings; interval stops at outlying hospitals; and severity and types of injury. Some reports concluded there was a reduction in mortality (19,25,27–29,36), whereas others found no difference (24,26,33–35,37) or even potential harm (38) by using air ambulances. The relatively low numbers of deaths in all studies make generalizable statements impossible, so TMPs must be familiar with the issues then weigh risks and benefits in each case.

Stay or Go

It is imperative that the medical capabilities at the scene of an ongoing tactical operation not collapse due to evacuation of a critical casualty. TMPs may wish to accompany the casualty to the ED to continue care en route or act as the medical advocate for the patient at the destination facility. However, bystanders, adversaries, and operators will continue to be at risk until threats are secured and the scene is cleared. The evacuation platform may have its own capabilities sufficient to continue patient management. If adequate for the casualties' problems, it may be best to simply transfer care and follow-up at the hospital later. If the casualties must be accompanied by some or all of the tactical medical element, alternative arrangements must be made to provide for support of any ongoing mission.

Intermediate Stops

Although a regional medical or trauma center may be the best destination for supportive or definitive care, one or more intermediate stops at less-capable hospitals may be necessary for logistical reasons too. For example, the most logistically time-efficient HLZ for air evacuation might be a helipad, parking lot, or field next to a closer but smaller hospital. An interval stop might also allow the TMP to return to ongoing operations after the casualty has been passed to an appropriate level of care, either a critical-care evacuation platform or the local hospital's ED. Recent changes in the Emergency Medical Treatment and

Active Labor Act (EMTALA) have made it possible for direct transfers from ground to air vehicles without any legal requirement for stabilization inside the ED between these evacuation legs (39). An additional consideration is that, if casualties are evacuated into an outlying hospital first and the TMP does not remain with them, further decisions about transfer to a higher level of care may be out of the hands of the TMP.

Necessary Delays

Only vitally needed procedures should delay transportation of critical casualties, who by definition require more resources than can be delivered in the out-of-hospital setting. Most civilian EMS protocols indicate that appropriate scene times for trauma patients should generally be <10 minutes. As opposed to those with serious injuries, some patients with critical illnesses may benefit from out-of-hospital interventions before evacuation.

Other problems can cause additional delays to total evacuation times. Casualties requiring extrication from mangled vehicles or collapsed structures may need critical care support during the processes of freeing them. Casualties who have been exposed to chemical, radiological, or toxicological agents will require decontamination prior to placement in a medical evacuation vehicle, so that off-gassing of vapors, close proximity to radioactive sources, or direct patient handling do not adversely affect the providers.

TAKE HOME POINTS

1. TMPs must be able to advise operational commanders and other decision-makers on issues related to preventive medicine, contingency planning, emergency care at the scene, and appropriate evacuation choices.
2. When evacuating critically ill or injured casualties from a tactical setting, consideration must be given to the compounding effects of the out-of-hospital environment, continuing tactical and medical threats, restriction of vision and dexterity by PPE, and the psychological effects of casualties potentially being friends or coworkers.
3. The two most crucial elements to consider in planning and execution of critical evacuations are the time available to complete all aspects of transport and the level of care and treatment capabilities en route to a hospital ED or specialty center.
4. Planning for the contingency of a sudden need to evacuate critical casualties—be they bystanders, adversaries, or operators—involves a thorough understanding of the types and capabilities of various platforms that could be possibly employed or requested in a given area of operations.

SUMMARY

In addition to acting as medical operators, who directly care for critical casualties in difficult out-of-hospital settings, TMPs must also be advisors to and the "medical conscience" of their unit commanders, who in turn are ultimately responsible for all outcomes of operations. In the event that critical casualties occur, the commander will look to TMPs to rapidly recommend realistic evacuation options. Subsequent recommendations will be based on assessments of the tactical situation, the casualties' conditions, and their likelihoods of survival. Decisions must be made in the high-stress environment of a tactical out-of-hospital setting, while simultaneously providing care to those casualties and continuing to support other aspects of ongoing operations. Meticulous planning, thorough coordination, sound judgment, and decisive action are the skills needed to fulfill this obligation.

APPENDIX FOR HELICOPTER OPERATIONS

Safety is the paramount concern when operating around aircraft, particularly when a helicopter is used for the rapid evacuation of critical casualties. All steps required to load patients onto a hoist or into a helicopter on the ground must be accomplished in a deliberate yet unhurried manner. *In every instance without fail, ground personnel must heed the direction of the flight crew, so as not to compromise the safe completion of evacuation operations.*

Requesting Evacuation

TMPs must identify the methods used to request air evacuation within each jurisdiction, and stay within these parameters. If not simply requested through the 9-1-1 system, helicopters are most often obtained through a regional dispatch center specific to the individual flight program. These centers are accustomed to asking for the information necessary for that program to accomplish its portion of a mission, thus making the most efficient use of limited time in a critical situation. Some of these flight programs may be able to also offer ground MICU evacuation.

The aircrew must first be able to locate the pickup site. The operational commander may not make this the responsibility of the TMP—who may be medically managing one or more critical casualties—at the time of request, but the TMP should have had significant input to determining potential HLZs during premission planning. Primary and secondary sites should have been identified. Detailed reconnaissance before mission execution may not have been possible, due to OPSEC concerns, as the best HLZs are often close to the target location. Ideally, an operator would have visually inspect all contingency landing and transfer sites during the planning phases of an operation and noted the global positioning system (GPS) coordinates. These could either be programmed into the navigation systems of preplanned evacuation platforms before missions or relayed to dispatchers when a request for evacuation is made.

Alternatively, the TMP could single out open areas that with relative certainty will accommodate any aircraft that could potentially be requested. Intelligence obtained from aerial photographs and corroborated with investigators is another premission technique useful in locating suitable HLZs. If street-level mapping is available, identifying locations near the area of operations that typically have adequate space to land multiple aircraft may be possible. Schools, shopping malls, large industrial areas, office complexes, and military installations may provide easily identifiable HLZs for responding aircraft. The use of computer-based navigation programs, GPS devices with moving-map displays, and open-source or classified satellite imagery have greatly enhanced the TMP's ability to remotely gather exact coordinates for HLZs during the planning phase. However, the TMP must confirm that the method of labeling coordinates (e.g., latitude & longitude, universal polar stereographic (UPS) map, military grid) is compatible with traditional navigation methods such as pilotage and dead reckoning.

Designating Landing Zones

Unless casualties will be hoisted to a hovering rotocraft, a HLZ must be designated for the aircraft to set down. The first considerations are space and visibility. A good rule of thumb for most medium-sized helicopters is an area 100 feet in diameter. When surrounding obstructions are not tall, and other hazards are minimal and easy to see, the pilot-in-command may accept 40 feet less, particularly if the narrowest area is perpendicular to the wind direction. Whenever possible, helicopters land and takeoff into the wind. At night, the space should be increased by at least 40 feet in all directions. Within the OPSEC guidelines established by the commander, visibility and illumination can be enhanced by vehicle emergency lights on roofs and headlights pointed toward the HLZ. Infrared devices may be necessary in some nighttime tactical situations. Lights should not be pointed at the aircraft, unless requested by the aircrew.

Additional considerations include security, slope, surface, and scatter—the 4 S's. Security considers both adversarial threats and crowd control, including the potential need to stop traffic if a road or highway landing is considered. Slope is important so that the aircraft can set firmly on the ground without its main rotor blades continuing to generate lift and consequent high-velocity downwash. Most helicopters used for MEDEVAC can only land with 10 degrees to 15 degrees of slope. The landing surface must also be able to support the weight of the aircraft, and be free of upward protrusions and downward holes. Long grass makes it difficult for the aircrew to determine touchdown risks. Scatter refers to possible dirt, dust, snow, smoke, or debris that can be sucked into the aircraft's rotor systems or blown into nearby personnel and equipment. The downward and outward wind created by a landing helicopter can easily exceed 100 miles per hour. Any lose debris will be accelerated into nearby buildings, vehicles, or people. It may also be pulled toward the aircraft causing damage or negatively impacting flight. Inadvertent "brown out" or "white out" from swirling dust or snow, respectively, may cause the pilot to lose visual reference to the ground during landing, creating a dangerous situation for both aircrew and ground personnel.

Assisting Aircraft Approach

There are many techniques for guiding a helicopter to and into a HLZ, but most should only be practiced by experienced individuals. Less-experienced ground personnel can help by identifying obstructions and other hazards around an HLZ (e.g., antennae, buildings, trees, poles, wires, fences). If the aircrew is having difficulty locating the HLZ, ground personnel can identify nearby landmarks or communicate an azimuth, which involves telling the aircrew what the compass heading from the HLZ to the aircraft is. Pilots can then calculate a back-azimuth to turn toward the HLZ. The individual in communication with the aircraft advises the crew when he or she can see the aircraft then further assists by helping them make any corrections necessary to locate the HLZ. It is often best to reference the aircrew to the desired location using simple directions such as "45° to your right" or "to your left of the tall smokestack." If the tactical commander permits, emergency lighting can be left on until the aircraft locates the HLZ. What remains illuminated during their approach and landing will be at the discretion of the pilot on the controls.

Loading Casualties

Once on the ground, the pilot will flatten the pitch of the main rotor blades. They still produce some wind, but will no longer force as much air down toward the ground and outward along the surface. On the other hand, the crew may not shut down engines, so rotors continue to turn. The tips of overhead and tail rotors move at many hundreds of feet per second. They can crush a person's skull or severe a body part in an instant. *Ground personnel should never approach a helicopter without being explicitly directed by a crewmember where, when, and how to do so.*

Typically, a nonpilot crewmember will disembark the aircraft to meet with security and medical personnel, receive a briefing, and give instructions for loading procedures. Although patients may be loaded through doors in the side of the aircraft or rear doors under the tail boom depending on aircraft type, certain safety precautions are common to most helicopters. All loose articles on the casualty, litter, and rescue personnel—especially headgear without chin straps—must be removed or secured. At least four personnel should carry the litter for safety in case one person stumbles or falls. This will also make lifting easier for all rescuers.

Hearing and full eye protection should be mandatory for all personnel approaching a helicopter with spinning rotors. Patients are moved to the aircraft head first, so blowing debris will be less likely to strike their eyes or enter their respiratory system. The initial track toward the aircraft will usually be within 45 degrees of its nose in full view of and in eye-contact with the pilot on the controls, and only after a crewmember has authorized it either verbally or by hand gestures. Normally, a crewmember will personally escort all ground personnel to and from the helicopter.

All personnel should keep their heads low during their advance, because gusts of wind can cause main rotor blades to flap down to <4 feet above the ground in some models. If there is a slope, the approach will always be from the downhill side, where there is more rotor clearance. No object should ever be carried vertically or above shoulder height. When next to the aircraft, rescuers may stand to help lift the patient into the cabin. *Nobody should ever be farther rearward than the most rearward edge of a side-loading door or a litter's length behind a rear-loading door.* The tail rotor spins so fast that it may be impossible to see, especially with illumination less than bright sunlight or if viewed edge-on when close to the aircraft.

Patient loading will be directed by the aircrew. Rescuer departure from the vicinity of the aircraft will usually be made by the same path as it was approached, keeping all heads low. Additional safety precautions include never smoking, running, or throwing objects within 200 feet of a helicopter.

Accompanying Patients

If a TMP must accompany a critical casualty, additional safety precautions must be observed. The aircrew will determine whether or not the TMP will require a vest tethered to a hardpoint in the aircraft interior or must be seat belted. Sometimes, seatbelts will only be required for take-off and landing. Often though, the TMP may be required to sit in the cockpit, because there may not be enough room in the casualty compartment. When the TMP possesses more medical expertise than the aircrew—which will usually only be the case when the TMP is a physician accompanying a nonphysician crew—only verbal advice can be provided in this situation. Military helicopters more often have a medical crew with less training than advanced-practice nurses and paramedics. There are usually two pi-

lots occupying the cockpit, but the casualty compartment is usually much bigger than in a civilian aircraft, so it is less likely that the TMP will be required to be stationed away from the casualty.

When critical care must be administered to a casualty during flight, crew members of civilian air ambulances will usually be the best to accomplish it for a number of reasons. First, they are the most familiar with the availability and location of their equipment and supplies, as well as the constraints placed on care by the configuration of the aircraft interior. Second, nonphysician crewmembers usually practice under protocols developed by a physician-level medical director; plus they can call their base hospital by radio for specific advice, if necessary. Third, if operating in a state or territory other than one in which the TMP is licensed, statutory regulations may limit what care the TMP can provide in that jurisdiction.

The main advantage of accompanying the casualty to the interval or final destination is to act as that person's advocate throughout the entire evacuation sequence and at the hospital to ensure the best possible care for that casualty and maintain OPSEC to the degree possible. The onset of illness or mechanism of injury can be more accurately communicated to the receiving physicians and surgeons. If the casualty is a teammate, the TMP should also know the individual's personal information and medical history, so it can be conveyed to hospital personnel in situations when the casualty cannot do it for himself or herself. Moreover, the TMP can keep the casualty's family and the team's chain of command informed of status, progress, and additional needs within the limits allowed by the federal Health Insurance Portability and Accountability Act (HIPAA) in civilian institutions in the United States.

REFERENCES

1. DeLorenzo RA. Military and civilian emergency aeromedical services: common goals and different approaches. *Aviat Space Environ Med.* 1997;68:56–60.
2. Committee on Trauma and Committee on Shock, Division of Medical Sciences, National Academy of Sciences, National Research Council. *Accidental Death and Disability: The Neglected Disease of Modern Society.* Washington: National Research Council; 1966.
3. Hoff WS, Schwab CW. Trauma system development in North America. *Clin Orthop Relat Res.* 2004;422:17–22.
4. Interagency OPSEC Support Staff. *Through the Eyes of the Adversary: Operations Security for Public Safety Agencies.* http://www.ioss.gov/contact_Us.html
5. Bentsen L. *Report of the Department of Treasury on the BATF Investigation of Vernon Wayne Howell.* http://www.carolmoore.net/waco/waco-treasury-report1.html. Accessed September 27, 2007.
6. Burney RE, Hubert D, Passini L, et al. Variation in air medical outcomes by crew composition: a two-year follow-up. *Ann Emerg Med.* 1995;25:187–192.
7. Wirtz MH, Cayten CG, Kohrs DA, et al. Paramedic versus nurse crews in the helicopter transport of trauma patients. *Air Med J.* 2002;21:17–21.
8. Baxt WG, Moody P. The impact of a physician as part of the aeromedical prehospital team in patients with blunt trauma. *JAMA.* 1987;257:3246–3250.

9. Hamman BL, Cué JI, Miller FB, et al. Helicopter transport of trauma victims: does a physician make a difference? *J Trauma*. 1991;31:490–494; discussion 494.

10. Bartolacci RA, Munford BJ, Lee A, McDougall PA. Air medical scene response to blunt trauma: effect on early survival. *Med J Austral*. 1998;169:612–616.

11. Schmidt U, Frame SB, Nerlich ML, et al. On-scene helicopter transport of patients with multiple injuries—comparison of a German and an American system. *J Trauma*. 1992;33:548–553; discussion 553–555.

12. Biewener A, Aschenbrenner U, Rammelt S, et al. Impact of helicopter transport and hospital level on mortality in polytrauma patients. *J Trauma*. 2004;56:94–98.

13. Grissom TE. Critical care air transport: patient flight physiology and organizational considerations. In: Hurd WW, Jernigan JG, eds. *Aeromedical Evacuation: Management of Acute and Stabilized Patients*. New York: Springer; 2002:111–135.

14. Grissom TE, Farmer JC. The provision of sophisticated critical care beyond the hospital: lessons from physiology and military experiences that apply to civil disaster medical response. *Crit Care Med*. 2005;33(suppl 1):S13–S21.

15. Polk JD, Fallon WF. Indications and considerations for emergent evacuation of the peacetime casualty. In: Hurd WW, Jernigan JG, eds. *Aeromedical Evacuation: Management of Acute and Stabilized Patients*. New York: Springer; 2002:13–26.

16. Diaz MA, Hendey GW, Bivins HG. When is a helicopter faster? A comparison of helicopter and ground ambulance transport times. *J Trauma*. 2005;58:148–153.

17. American Trauma Society. *Trauma information exchange program (TIEP)*. http://www.amtrauma.org/tiep/reports/publicreports.html. Published 15 April, 2006.

18. American Trauma Society. *American College of Surgeons Committee on Trauma Classification System of Trauma Center Care*. http://www.amtrauma.org/tiep/reports/ACSClassification.html. Published 15 April, 2006.

19. Veenema KR, Rodewald LE. Stabilization of rural multiple-trauma patients at level III emergency departments before transfer to a level I regional trauma center. *Ann Emerg Med*. 1995;25:175–181.

20. Lerner EB, Billitier AJ, Dorn JM, Wu Y-WB. Is total out-of-hospital time a significant predictor of trauma patient mortality? *Acad Emerg Med*. 2003;10:949–954.

21. Lawless J, Tallon JM, Petrie D. Aborted air medical missions: a 4-year quality review of a Canadian province-wide air medical program. *Air Med J*. 2005;24:79–82.

22. Eckstein M, Chan L, Schneir A, Palmer R. Effect of prehospital advanced life support on outcomes of major trauma patients. *J Trauma*. 2000;48:643–648.

23. Gearhart PA, Wuerz R, Localio AR. Cost-effectiveness analysis of helicopter EMS for trauma patients. *Ann Emerg Med*. 1997;30:500–506.

24. Brathwaite CEM, Rosko M, McDowell R, et al. A critical analysis of on-scene helicopter transport on survival in a statewide trauma system. *J Trauma*. 1998;45:140–144; discussion 144–146.

25. Kerr WA, Kerns TJ, Bissell RA. Differences in mortality rates among trauma patients transported by helicopter and ambulances in Maryland. *Prehosp Disas Med*. 1999;14:159–164.

26. Cunningham P, Rutledge R, Baker CC, Clancy TV. A comparison of the association of helicopter and ground ambulance transport with the outcome of injury in trauma patients transported from the scene. *J Trauma*. 1997;43:940–946.

27. Jacobs LM, Gabram SGA, Sztajnkrycer MD, et al. Helicopter air medical transport: ten-year outcomes for trauma patients in a New England program. *Conn Med*. 1999;63:677–682.

28. Baxt WG, Moody P, Cleveland HC, et al. Hospital-based rotocraft aeromedical emergency care services and trauma mortality: a multicenter study. *Ann Emerg Med*. 1985;14:859–864.

29. Thomas SH, Harrison TH, Buras WR, et al. Helicopter transport and blunt trauma mortality: a multicenter trial. *J Trauma*. 2002;52:136–145.

30. Di Bartolomeo S, Sanson G, Nardi G, et al. Effects of 2 patterns of prehospital care on the outcome of patients with severe head injury. *Arch Surg*. 2001;136:1293–1300.

31. Davis DP, Peay J, Serrano JA, et al. The impact of aeromedical response to patients with moderate to severe traumatic brain injury. *Ann Emerg Med*. 2005;46:115–122.

32. MacKenzie EJ, Rivara FP, Jurkovich GJ, et al. A national evaluation of the effect of trauma-center care on mortality. *N Engl J Med*. 2006;354:366–378.

33. Cocanour CS, Fischer RP, Ursic CM. Are scene flights for penetrating trauma justified? *J Trauma*. 1997;43:83–86; discussion 86–88.

34. Phillips RT, Conaway C, Mullarkey D, Owen JL. One year's trauma mortality experience at Brooke Army Medical Center: is aeromedical transportation of trauma patients necessary? *Milit Med*. 1999;164:361–365.

35. Shatney CH, Homan SJ, Sherck JP, Ho C-C. The utility of helicopter transport of trauma patients from the injury scene in an urban trauma system. *J Trauma*. 2002;53:817–822.

36. Boyd CR, Corse KM, Campbell RC. Emergency interhospital transport of the major trauma patient: air versus ground. *J Trauma*. 1989;29:789–793; discussion 789–790.

37. Arfken CL, Shapiro MJ, Bessey PQ, Littenberg B. Effectiveness of helicopter versus ground ambulance services for interfacility transport. *J Trauma*. 1998;45:785–790.

38. Falcone RE, Herron H, Werman H, Bonta M. Air medical transport of the injured patient: scene versus referring hospital. *Air Med J*. 1998;17:161–165.

39. 68 Federal Register §53221-53264 (2003).

Chapter 16

Medical Care of In-Custody Individuals

Robert F. Mulry, Alexander M. Silverstein, and William P. Fabbri

OBJECTIVES

After reading this section, the reader will be able to:

1. Describe the operational, legal, and ethical justifications for the provision of appropriate medical treatment to persons in legal custody.
2. Describe medical concerns associated with assumption of custody, transport of the prisoner, and transfer of custody at the medical or booking facility.
3. Describe methods and potential hazards associated with patient restraint.
4. Identify situational and individual factors associated with increased risk of sudden death while in custody.
5. Describe elements of the medical preplan for a tactical operation.

INTRODUCTION

The act of taking an individual into custody begins a relationship where the custodial officer assumes responsibility for the health and welfare of the individual taken into custody. This relationship should be viewed as a continuum, beginning with the act of taking the individual into custody and ending only when responsibility for the individual is assumed by another governmental agency or the individual is released.

Responsibility for the health and welfare of a prisoner may last only a brief period of time. It may simply entail ensuring that a prisoner is properly secured in a transporting patrol car with a seatbelt. However, it may also involve complex medical monitoring due to chronic medical conditions while the prisoner is transported over great distances. Considerations, such as fitness for confinement, the appropriateness of certain physical restraints, the potential for preexisting injury or illness, security of law enforcement personnel, medical preplanning, and documentation, should all be addressed.

The views expressed in this article are those of the authors and do not necessarily represent the views of the Federal Bureau of Investigation or of the United States Government.

This chapter will address the essential elements of medical support and medical preplanning as it relates to law enforcement agency responsibilities for individuals in custody. The period examined is from the point of initial interaction with tactical law enforcement until arrival at a medical treatment facility, or in the case of subjects without medical needs, at the initial arrest processing location. Medical support provided in military or correctional settings is beyond the scope of this discussion.

ASSUMPTION OF CUSTODY

Upon receiving an individual in custody, it is the individual law enforcement officer's responsibility to assure that provisions for United States standards of health care are available to the in-custody individual with appropriate consideration of security and tactical safety issues.

Appropriate medical treatment of subjects in custody is mandated for both operational and ethical reasons. Provision of medical care can positively impact the relationship between the prisoner and escort, potentially leading to beneficial intelligence or investigative outcomes. To do less risks potential complaints of withholding of medical care for punitive purposes. The withholding of adequate medical care may be viewed as excessive force, an unconstitutional act in violation of the Fourth Amendment right to be free of unreasonable seizure. Federal courts have held that "a pretrial detainee's constitutional right to medical care, whether in prison or other custody, flows from the procedural and substantive due process guarantees of the Fourteenth Amendment" (1). In a legal context, when a law enforcement officer takes custody of a prisoner, a duty to provide adequate health care may then arise. Failure to provide such health care may be viewed as a breach of that duty and expose the officer and his or her agency to civil liability.

If the escorting law enforcement officer is the arresting officer, a determination of the health status of the prisoner can rapidly be made based on the circumstances of the arrest and the physical appearance of the prisoner. If an application of force was necessary during the arrest, there may be a higher likelihood that the prisoner may have sustained injuries.

If tactical safety and security considerations permit, a trained prehospital medical provider, such as an emergency medical technician (EMT) or paramedic should be summoned to the scene of the arrest to determine the extent of the injuries or illness and whether medical treatment is required. If this is not possible, medical assistance should be accessed as soon as possible, meeting emergency medical service (EMS) personnel at a prearranged, secure location nearby. The presence of trained medical personnel, either as part of the tactical team or staged nearby, allows for rapid evaluation of in-custody individuals prior to transportation from the crisis site. The inclusion of a medical component in the operational plan reduces delay in access to EMS care and enhances the stability of the site during the critical period following tactical activity. The latter can significantly reduce the risk of additional injury to operators, subjects and bystanders following the arrest.

MEDICAL CONSIDERATIONS OF PRISONER TRANSPORT AND TRANSFER OF CUSTODY

Law enforcement officers responsible for the transportation or escort of prisoners should be aware of the potential for exposure to body fluids or respiratory-communicable diseases through contact with the prisoner. The use of personal protective equipment (PPE) including disposable nonlatex examination gloves and surgical masks in addition to standard tactical eye protection can greatly reduce infectious disease risk exposure of law enforcement officers. Expeditious transfer of sick or injured prisoners to trained medical personnel prior to transport will also reduce the risk to officers of body fluid contamination during transport.

In the event that the prisoner is received from another agency, a determination should be made as to the health status of the prisoner prior to accepting custody. If a preexisting medical condition exists and circumstances of the arrest permit, documentation should be obtained in advance regarding the diagnosis, the prisoner's condition, treatment received, medications required, and special considerations for transportation. In the case of a prisoner with a complicated medical condition or any condition that may require treatment during transport, a trained medical provider should be part of the prisoner escort team. When the prisoner is known or suspected significant medical history, a face-to-face report from the sending facility medical staff should be received prior to the transfer of custody. Where special security risks or considerations exist for the prisoner, it is beneficial to have a sworn officer as the medical provider. This allows the officer/medical provider to perform law enforcement functions while intervening medically when necessary. This also helps to ensure a high level of operational security during transit and minimizes the size of the escort team.

Tactical law enforcement teams at a destination jurisdiction may receive prisoners extradited from other jurisdictions, transporting them to the site of initial processing or confinement. The involvement of tactical teams in these transfers is sometimes required because of the high-risk nature of the subject involved or the need for enhanced security to ensure the safety of the prisoner. A medical annex to the operational plan for such missions is required, as in any tactical mission. As these subjects may be received following prolonged transport by ground or aircraft, pre-existing medical conditions may become problematic while en route. This eventuality should be reflected in the medical plan.

If the prisoner is received from a governmental agency of a country other than the United States, an independent medical practitioner should accompany the prisoner escort team receiving the subject. This medical provider should perform a thorough physical examination of the prisoner prior to custody being accepted. The physical diagnosis requirements of this examination usually require skills beyond conventional EMS training. A certified physician assistant (PA-C), registered nurse practitioner (RN-P) or physician with experience in prehospital or primary care medicine is appropriate for this task. This examination should be recorded in detail and should accompany the prisoner to the point of processing for confinement. Again, if a serious or complicated medical condition exists, a face-to-face report should be given by the escort team medical provider to the receiving facility medical staff.

RESTRAINT CONSIDERATIONS

The method and amount of restraint required for the prisoner may have a significant impact upon transport plans, including the number of escort personnel required, chosen mode of transportation and level of medical support needed.

From both medical and legal standpoints, the techniques used for prisoner restraint should be the minimum required to ensure the safety of the escort personnel as well as the compliance of the prisoner.

For the short distance movement of a prisoner, a common law enforcement transport technique is to place the handcuffed prisoner in a transport van or car. Handcuffs are usually applied with the prisoner's hands behind his or her back when used by police as the sole means of physical restraint to prevent the combined use of the joined arms and the handcuff device as a weapon. Single-use disposable plastic wrist restraints, commonly referred to as "flex-cuffs," frequently used in situations involving the arrest of multiple subjects, are used in a similar fashion.

If a car is used for transport, the prisoner is often placed in the back seat. If the vehicle is without a cage, an escorting officer is likely to be seated behind the driver. If the prisoner has a predetermined medical condition or an injury, a sworn officer who is also a medical provider may be used as one of the transporting officers.

This makes a medically trained officer available to immediately recognize and address medical issues that may arise, even in the course of a relatively short duration transport. Prisoner transport vans are used in the initial arrest phase in some jurisdictions, particularly when arrests of large numbers of subjects are anticipated. Because officers often do not accompany the subjects or have controlled access to the rear of the van during transport, these vehicles are often unsuitable for transport of subjects with confirmed or suspected medical concerns.

Subjects received from extraditions involving long distance transport may be received from the transporting officers in prisoner transport belts. Transport belts allow for the prisoner's hands to be located in the front, yet still remain secured close to the body. This method increases prisoner comfort and reduces wrist trauma due to friction, reduced circulation, and nerve impingement. This arrangement facilitates monitoring of distal neurovascular status of the hands and also facilitates prisoner self-toileting.

Prisoners classified as ambulatory in conventional medical operations without suspected injury of the limbs may often be transported safely by car using the standard restraint methods described. Any subject with injuries deemed by the treating EMS personnel to be at risk for exacerbation en route should be monitored by a medically trained officer regardless of the mode of transport. Due to the risk of a prisoner becoming noncompliant or assaultive, officer and health care provider safety is always paramount. The use of vehicle or aircraft safety belts, in addition to handcuffs or a transport belt, provides an added layer of restraint to protect the escorting officers

and protection of the prisoner from injury in the event of a vehicular accident.

If a prisoner's condition requires ambulance transportation, he or she must be restricted to the stretcher gurney. Soft restraints should be used on all extremities whenever a prisoner is transported by ambulance. Although this is unusual in general EMS practice, it should be remembered that the patient is in a custodial status and that both restraint and officer escort are required to prevent escape or self-injury. Close medical observation is required due to the potential for unexpected medical deterioration, choking hazards and attempted self-injury. Some officers and jurisdictions require a law enforcement suitable restraint, such as handcuffs, to supplement the soft restraints usually associated with stretchers. Care must be taken in this situation to ensure the ability to deliver care to the subject in the event of a medical emergency during transport and to monitor the distal neurovascular status of any extremity handcuffed to a stretcher.

A prearranged procedure for transfer of a stretcher-borne subject in custody should be in place with medical facilities listed in the medical operational plan.

A restrained prisoner may attempt to spit at or bite the escorting officers. The application of a surgical face mask to the prisoner will provide an additional layer of protection to the officers. The mask should be loose fitting, permitting the escorting medic to monitor respiratory effort. Escorting officers should conscientiously address the threat of exposure to communicable diseases from the prisoner's body fluids. All transporting officers should have medical examination gloves and eye and face protection immediately available on their person. In many cases, this personal protective equipment is best worn as a precaution any time that attendants and escorts occupy the close quarters of a vehicle with a prisoner.

With proper application and careful monitoring, appropriate physical restraints are usually sufficient to achieve safe transport of subjects from the arrest site to the initial arrest processing or medical treatment facility. Modification of restraint to the mutual satisfaction of both security precautions and medical care requirements is routinely achievable when transporting a nonambulatory person in custody.

A special note should be made regarding restrictive four-limb restraints used in some law enforcement settings. A recurring scenario in some reports of deaths of persons in custody describes the prisoner's hands being restrained behind the back, the prisoner then placed in a face down position, often in a restrictive posture, either on the floor of the passenger compartment of a car or through further restraint of the legs flexed dorsally behind the back in a "hog tie" fashion, also referred to as "hobble-restraint." Fatalities associated with this procedure have been postulated to result from so-called "positional asphyxia" due to interference with thoracic and abdominal excursion. While the physiologic basis for positional asphyxia as the terminal event in these cases has been questioned in some studies (2), this preterminal scenario nevertheless continues to be described frequently in the forensic medicine literature (3–5). In addition, the authors can individually attest to anecdotal experience involving restrained subjects, often with clinically obese habitus, exhibiting marked respiratory distress following restrictive supine restraint, relieved by positional change to a lateral decubitus position.

Factors implicated in sudden death following physical restraint include substance intoxication (5,6), altered sensorium of uncertain cause and/or chronic cardiopulmonary or other medical conditions (8,9). It has been postulated that metabolic acidosis plays a role in cases of "excited delirium," with continued struggling by the subject against the restraints, followed by subsequent sudden death. The contribution of these comorbid factors to presumed ventilatory insufficiency produced by the hobble restraint has not been addressed by (2,11) and is not amenable to human study. It is prudent for law enforcement and EMS personnel to mutually understand the potential hazards of prone restraint (12), particularly in the setting of altered mental status, suspected cardiopulmonary illness, obesity, or large habitus

Although at least one consensus study advises against the use of hobble-type restraint in conventional EMS (13) operations, some tactical law enforcement situations may continue to require at least temporary use of restrictive four limb restraint. Constant monitoring of the prisoner's condition (i.e., respiratory rate and effort) is required should this type of restraint be used with reduction of restraint as soon as is consistent with the safety of all present on scene. An early indication that the prisoner may be experiencing difficulty breathing is an increase in combativeness or agitation. This change may be easily overlooked (13) during a chaotic arrest situation, especially in the setting of the presence of multiple, possibly belligerent or noncompliant subjects.

As a general principle, the prisoner should be placed in a head up or lateral recumbent position whenever possible with a transition to the least restrictive restraint method consistent with control of the subject, regularly confirming that he or she can adequately breathe. Prisoners identified as requiring EMS transport should be four-point restrained as previously described, because hobble-type restraint is not consistent with the ability to rapidly administer care en route.

Although all arrest subjects warrant observation and assessment, some prisoners should be recognized as being at increased risk for medical complications. Factors, such as pre-existing medical conditions, obesity, suspected drug use, altered mental status, and the means utilized by officers to subdue the subject, such as carotid restraints (15) (i.e., "choke holds"), combined arm-leg restraint, the use of impact weapons (e.g., ASP batons, nightsticks, blackjacks), oleoresin capsicum ("O.C.," "pepper") spray, conducted energy weapons (Taser-type devices) (16), or other non-

lethal force application, identify a subpopulation of arrest subjects who warrant careful, close, and continuous assessment.

Preliminary studies confirm the potential for sudden deterioration in the condition of subjects who present with mental status changes or admitted drug use. Although comprehensive data are not yet available, one preliminary study (17) of 100 in-custody deaths found each of these factors present in over 50% of the cases. Of special concern to tactical officers and medics is the observation that more than half of these cases in this study involved collapse of the subject within the first hour after the arrest.

Persons in custody who exhibit violent behavior where limit-setting measures and physical restraints are ineffective raise issues of safety for law enforcement officers, health care providers, the prisoner, and the public. Prisoners who continue to struggle violently despite physical restraint without evidence of respiratory distress, especially where mental status is questioned, should be treated as a medically unstable emergency (18) warranting close observation, expedited evacuation to a medical facility, and consideration of applicable EMS chemical restraint protocols.

The extent of knowledge applicable to the use of sedation in the early phase of police custody is limited. Studies in the United States, United Kingdom, and Australia regarding the use of sedation for control of acute agitation are largely limited to nonemergency in-patient settings (19). There is no drug available offering complete safety from adverse side effects and, therefore, the risk and benefits of chemical restraint should be considered to prevent the prisoner from harming himself or others.

If chemical restraint is considered, a physician must be consulted prior to the administration of any medications for purpose of restraint. A pre-established protocol may be useful in facilitating this consultation. The jurisdictional EMS protocol for sedation of a patient with significant injuries or an acute severe illness is appropriate for the management of persons in custody meeting those injury or disease criteria. Existing protocols may also apply to persons requiring aeromedical evacuation, as this mode of transport is not consistent with a combative patient. This is not to suggest that patient treatment protocols be applied in arrest situations absent injury or illness solely for purposes of sedation of an alert, healthy person in custody. Thorough documentation must be completed regarding the necessity for this technique, including the behaviors necessitating sedation, mental status of the patient prior to sedation, name of the physician consulted, medication orders received, dosage and route of administration, and all medical monitoring regularly recorded.

Chemical restraint protocols may involve butyrophenone neuroleptic medications, such as haloperidol or droperidol, or benzodiazepines, such as lorazepam or midazolam. Intravenous administration offers a short dose-response interval which hastens control of the patient and facilitates close observation, but may not be practical given the combative nature of the patient. The degree of combativeness of the prisoner may require intramuscular dosing with attendant patient-variable delay of action (20) and need for prolonged observation.

Droperidol gained favor in the emergency department and EMS use, in part because of its relatively rapid action, even by the intramuscular route (21,22). The use of droperidol in the United States, Canada, (23) and the United Kingdom has been complicated by concerns regarding proarrhythmic prolongation of the QT interval, a side effect implicated in some fatalities (18,24). The scientific rationale for a 2001 U.S. Food and Drug Administration (FDA) warning applied to specifically to droperidol versus other butyrophenones and the relevance of these concerns in clinical practice is controversial (26,27). Manufacturer recommendations for obtaining a preadministration medical history and electrocardiogram (ECG) monitoring (28) are impractical in the context of a violent subject in the field, effectively removing droperidol specifically and butyrophenones in general (28) from use in the EMS.

The use of the so-called second generation or atypical anti-psychotic agents, such as risperidone and clozapine, for control of delirium or agitation has not been specifically studied or listed as an indicated use. The latter medication is not available for parenteral use. Cardiac side effects, such as tachycardia, are also described in the literature (28).

Short-acting benzodiazepines have not been implicated in cardiac conduction disturbances, although their use in an EMS population with a high incidence of alcohol intoxication warrants caution. One study suggests the possibility of increased respiratory depression potential with midazolam versus that of droperidol in a clinical study (22), whereas another survey of 71 prehospital sedation cases suggested an increase in critical care admissions, a presumed result of increased cardiorespiratory monitoring requirements for persons sedated with midazolam after droperidol use was discontinued (32). The shorter duration of action of midazolam warrants current consideration as a reasonable alternative to the butyrophenones in the EMS setting with appropriate attention to respiratory status throughout transport.

Persons under arrest are also at risk for self-destructive behavior. A study of deaths in custody in Victoria, Australia (33) totaled 96 deaths in custody, 45 of which occurred prior to entry into a correctional environment. Of this latter figure, 12 deaths (26%) were the result of suicidal actions, twice the number of deaths in the sample attributed to drug toxicity and four times the number deemed to result from natural causes such as cardiovascular events. A comprehensive review of the international literature undertaken to identify risk factors associated with self-injurious behavior in police custody (34) identified the first 3 hours in custody as a period of high risk of self-injurious behavior, presumably due to the degree of

stress and fear associated with the prospect of incarceration. In addition to an association between alcohol intoxication and self-injury, the study identified males 20 to 30 years of age with no previous arrest history at higher risk for impulsive self-destructive behavior. Less surprisingly, older males previously convicted of violent crimes or sex offenses were also identified to be at high risk to attempt self-harm in custody.

In the unfortunate event that a prisoner expires while in the custody of law enforcement officers, courts will evaluate the objective reasonableness of the officers' actions. Officers are protected by qualified immunity against civil suit when their conduct is objectively reasonable, even when that conduct infringes on a constitutional right. Officers who reasonably, but mistakenly, use excessive force are entitled to immunity under the law (35). Among the factors to be considered would be the amount of force used to affect the arrest and to maintain custody of the prisoner. No more force than is absolutely necessary to affect an arrest and safely maintain custody is permitted. However, the safety of law enforcement officers must first and foremost be considered when decisions on level of force are to be made. Prehospital health care provider awareness of potential risk factors and constant prehospital medical surveillance of at-risk prisoners will contribute to a finding of objective reasonableness in such cases.

THE TRANSPORTATION PLAN

There are several considerations to take into account when planning for the transportation of a prisoner, including the time and distance to be traveled, special security considerations, medical requirements, mode of transportation, and compliance of the prisoner.

The time and distance to be traveled may be inconsequential, such as moving across town, or may involve prolonged travel from a remote location by vehicle or aircraft. Long-distance transports require consideration of the number of escort personnel required to ensure continuous vigilance, nutritional requirements for the escort detail as well as the prisoner, and sleeping accommodations for the detail, drivers/aircrew, and prisoner. These considerations may also affect the type of vehicle or aircraft used. For example, the reduced duration of transport may justify the use of aircraft versus ground travel.

It is imperative that a thorough evaluation of support requirements regarding the duration of the transport and mode of transportation be made prior to the commencement of the transport to ensure that adequate security personnel, aircrew or drivers, waypoints, and logistics support are provided. This may also include finding safe layover locations that can provide adequate security, medical infrastructure, and logistics support.

Special security considerations include the preplanning of safe medical treatment facilities that can provide assistance en route, security of vehicles or aircraft if an emergency layover is required, and preclearance of personnel who may be called upon to assist along the route in the event of a medical emergency. The knowledge that a specific individual at a hospital is prepared to assist in the event of an emergency is invaluable in the context of a high security, highly sensitive prisoner movement. Emergency physicians and trauma surgeons associated with facilities supporting the home jurisdiction are a valuable resource in selection of contingency medical centers and staff along the planned route of travel.

All subjects should be searched for traditional or improvised weapons by the arresting officer prior to transport. It is appropriate for medical personnel to confirm that this has been accomplished prior to loading the subject for transport, requesting the escorting officer to repeat the search if any question arises. The medical provider must exercise extreme care in assuring that medical treatment items are kept out of the reach of the prisoner. Items such as needles, scalpels, splints, or other supplies that can be used as weapons (36) may be easily secreted by the prisoner and can inflict serious injury to law enforcement officers or medical personnel.

MEDICAL PREPLANNING

Medical preplanning for prisoner movements, whether long or short distance, should include the following:

1. Distance/duration of the movement.
2. Medical history/medical condition/medical requirements of the prisoner.
3. Level of medical training of the medical operator appropriate to support the mission.
4. Medical equipment and medical supplies required to support the mission.
5. Medical considerations for the escort team. This may include required immunizations, insect repellent and chemoprophylaxis for vector borne diseases such as malaria and availability of safe nutrition and water sources. Additionally, the possibility of the presence of a communicable disease, such as tuberculosis, in the prisoner should be considered and precautions taken. On prolonged transport, common travel-related illnesses amongst the escort team should be anticipated and planned for accordingly.
6. Within the context of security, medical preplanning should include emergency action plans in the event of a medical or traumatic emergency during the movement. If the movement entails local transport via automobile, the closest hospital and the closest trauma center should be identified prior to the commencement of the movement. In prolonged transport movements, preplanning should include global positioning system (GPS) identification of medical treatment facil-

ities in proximity to the ground route, airport, or heliport/landing zone. Before including a facility in the plan, the planner should determine the suitability of the facility. Information, such as the trauma center level designation or the presence and suitability of an emergency department, is imperative. Ideally, a trauma center will have a level I or II designation, and an emergency department will have a board certified emergency medicine physician continuously present. During international travel, the U.S. Department of Defense has facilities that offer multiple advantages, including security, diplomatic protection, superior airfield facilities, and enhanced standards of medical care.

FITNESS FOR CONFINEMENT

Every prisoner who has sustained an injury or is suffering from a medical illness must be afforded adequate medical care. Following the provision of indicated field care, a determination needs to be made by a physician or other qualified medical professional that the prisoner is fit for confinement in a detention facility. Again, the medical history and physical diagnosis skill required for this determination are consistent with the training of a PA-C, RN-P or physician level practitioner. Fitness for confinement should be documented by the medical professional, including time and dated history and physical data, documenting the subject's condition at the onset of and during transport as well as at the time of transfer of custody upon arrival at the detention facility.

Any injury or illness of the prisoner must be addressed and afforded U.S. standards of medical care appropriate to the injury or illness. Most detention facilities in the United States employ medical support staff but are not equipped or staffed to address the severely ill or injured. Experience has shown that these facilities will often refuse to accept a prisoner with an incompletely evaluated and treated injury or unstable medical condition. The medical operator must, during the preplanning phase, identify a facility where medical clearance will be obtained prior to confinement. If serious medical issues exist with the prisoner, a medical detention facility such as hospital prisoner ward, or provision of an around-the-clock security detail in a conventional hospital setting should be anticipated during the preplanning phase.

TAKE HOME POINTS

1. Rapid determination of the health status of a prisoner is indicated when the application of force is required to secure the subject, conducted by prehospital medical personnel, either as part of the tactical team or staged nearby.

2. Restraint methods typically used by police may require modification if injuries are suspected or ambulance transport is required. Restraint systems and personal protective equipment is required to ensure the safety of the prisoner, officer, and EMS crew while permitting delivery of emergency care as required en route.

3. Factors implicated in sudden death in custody include altered sensorium, "excited delirium," suspected substance intoxication, large habitus, and chronic medical conditions.

4. In cases of continued violence despite limit setting and conventional restraint, judicious use of an approved EMS chemical restraint protocol is preferable to supine, "hobble," or other forms of unconventional restraint.

5. Precautions against prisoner attempts at intentional self-harm are advised, particularly in the initial hours following arrest.

SUMMARY

Medical care of the person in custody may include medical screening following use of force, immediate care after an injury has occurred, care during EMS transport, precautionary observation during prolonged transport, and/or clearance for confinement at a destination facility. Proper preplanning and the use of appropriate medical personnel will greatly simplify medical care of the prisoner, improve the safety of the escorting officers, and ensure the protection of the Constitutional rights of the prisoner.

Typical restraint methods used in law enforcement may require modification in prisoners with injuries deemed by EMS personnel to be at risk for exacerbation en route, whether or not ambulance transport is required. The minimum degree of restraint consistent with the safety of the prisoner, officers and the public is indicated. Special caution is indicated in prisoners with altered sensorium, suspected substance intoxication, obese or large habitus, or suspected chronic medical conditions. Expedited evacuation under close observation to a medical facility and consideration of applicable EMS chemical restraint protocols is indicated in violent subjects who fail to respond to conventional limit setting and physical restraint. Unconventional forms of restraint, including four limb and supine restraint, should be avoided.

REFERENCES

1. *Wagner v. Bay City*, 227 F.3d 316, 324 (5th Cir 2000).
2. Chan TC, Vilke GM, Neuman T, et al. Restraint position and positional asphyxia. *Ann Emerg Med.* 1997;30:578–586.
3. Reay DT, Fligner DT, Stillwell AD, et al. Positional asphyxia during law enforcement transport. *Am J Forensic Med Pathol.* 1992;13:90–95.
4. Howard JD, Reay DT. Positional Asphyxia. *Ann Emerg Med.* 1998;32:116–117

5. O'Halloran RL, Lewman LV. Restraint asphyxiation in excited delirium. *Am J Forensic Med Pathol.* 1993;14:289–295.
6. Bell MD, Rao VJ, Wetli CV, et al. Positional asphyxia in adults. *Am J Forensic Med Pathol.* 1992;13:101–107.
7. O'Halloran RL, ibid.
8. Stratton SJ, Green K. Sudden death in individuals in hobble restraints during paramedic transport. *Ann Emerg Med.* 1995;25:710–712.
9. Reay DT, Howard JD. Restraint position and positional asphyxia (setter). *Am J Forensic Med Pathol.* 1999;20:300–301.
10. Chan TC, et al. op. cit.
11. Chan TC, Neuman T, Clausen J, et al. Weight force during prone restraint and respiratory function. *Am J Forensic Med Pathol.* 2004;25:185–189.
12. Laposata EA. Positional asphyxia during law enforcement transport [letter]. *Am J Forensic Med Pathol.* 1993;14:86–87.
13. Kupas DF, Wydro, GC. Patient restraint in emergency medical services systems. *Prehospital Emergency Care.* 2002;6:340–346.
14. Kupas DF, ibid.
15. Reay DT, Eisele, JW. Deaths from law enforcement neck holds. *Am J Forensic Med Pathol.* 1982;3:253–258.
16. Vilke G, Johnson W, Castillo EM, et al. Evaluation of in-custody deaths proximal to use of conductive energy devices. *Ann Emerg Med.* 2006;48:23-24
17. Ho JD, Reardon RF, Heegaard WG. Deaths in police custody: an 8-month surveillance study. *Ann Emerg Med.* 2005;46:94.
18. Brice JH, Pirrallo RG, Racht E, et al. Management of the violent patient. *Prehospital Emergency Care.* 2003;7:48–56.
19. Knott JC, Taylor DMcD, Castle, DJ. Randomized clinical trail comparing intravenous midazolam and droperidol for sedation of the acutely agitated patient in the emergency department. *Ann Emerg Med.* 2006;47:61–67.
20. Burdick W. A prospective, double-blind, randomized trial of midazolam versus haloperidol versus lorazepam in the chemical restraint of violent and severely agitated patients. *Ann Emerg Med.* 2005;45:93.
21. Thomas H, Schwartz E, Petrilli R, et al. Droperidol versus haloperidol for chemical restraint of agitated and combative patients. *Ann Emerg Med.* 1992;21:407–412.
22. Hick JL, Mahoney BD, Lappe M, et al. Prehospital sedation with Intramuscular droperidol: a one-year pilot. *Prehospital Emergency Care.* 2001;5:391–394.
23. Wooltorton E. Droperidol: cardiovascular toxicity and deaths. *Can Med Assoc J.* 2002;166:932.
24. U.S. Food and Drug Administration. FDA strengthens warnings of Droperidol. http://www.fda.gov/bbs/topics/ANSWERS/2001/ANS01123.html. Published October 18, 2006.
25. Brice JH, op. cit.
26. Shale JH, Shale CM, Mastin WD. A review of the safety and efficacy of droperidol for the rapid sedation of severely agitated and violent patients. *J Clin Psychiatry.* 2003;64:500–505.
27. Kao LW, Kirk MA, Evers SJ, et al. Droperidol QT prolongation and sudden death; what is the evidence? *Ann Emerge Med.* 2003;41:546–558.
28. American Association of Health System Pharmacist. AHFS Drug Information. American Association of Health System Pharmacists. American Hospital Formulary Service. Bethesda, Maryland. 2006:2356–2500.
29. AHFS Drug Information. ibid. pp. 2384–2389.
30. AHFS Drug Information. ibid. pp. 2356–2384.
31. Knott JC, et al. op. cit.
32. Martel M, Miner J, Fringer R, et al. Discontinuation of droperidol for the control of acutely agitated out-of-hospital patients. *Prehospital Emergency Care.* 2005;9:44–49.
33. Petschel K, Gall, JA. A profile of deaths in custody in Victoria, 1991–96. *J Clin Forensic Med.* 2000;7:82–87.
34. McCleave, NR, Latham, D. Self-injurious behavior in police custody. *J Clin Forensic Med.* 1998;5:13–26.
35. *Wagner*, at 321, citing *Gutierrez v. City of San Antonio*, 139 F.3d 441 (5th Cir. 1998).
36. Hayden JW, Laney C, Kellermann AL, et al. Medical devices made into weapons by prisoners: an unrecognized risk. *Ann Emer Med.* 1995;26:739–742.

Chapter 17

Operational Performance and Preventive Medicine

Scott E. Young and Guillermo J. Pierluisi

OBJECTIVES

After reading this section, the reader will be able to:

1. Discuss previous preventive measure strategies used in tactical operations.
2. List specific potential medical risks for tactical personnel.
3. Discuss health surveillance and maintenance.
4. Describe strategies used for mitigation of potential medical threats.

HISTORICAL PERSPECTIVE

The practice of tasking personnel to preventive medicine duties within the U.S. Armed Forces (or would be U.S. Armed Forces) dates back to the Revolutionary War (1). One of General George Washington's first general orders issued at Headquarters, Cambridge, Massachusetts, July, 4 1775, addressed to line officers whom he held responsible for the health of their men, reads:

> All officers are required and expected to pay diligent attention to keep their men neat and clean; to visit them often at their quarters, and inculcate upon them the necessity of cleanliness, as essential to their health and service....They are also to take care that necessarys (latrines) be provided in the camps and frequently filled up to prevent their being offensive and unhealthy.

History has also shown us that the implementation of preventive medicine interventions is needed in every field operation. Furthermore, it has shown us that any omission or delay in the implementation, laxity in the enforcement or lack of surveillance after implementation can be most deleterious to the field units. For example:

1. During World War II, 95% (November 1942 to August 1945) and 77% (November 1942 to August 1945) of the U.S. Army hospital admissions in the Pacific and European Theaters of Operations, respectively, were for disease and nonbattle injuries (DNBI) (2). During the winter of 1943 alone, frostbite caused more casualties among the port gunners on B-17 and B-24

bombers (due to exposure to cold air rushing by at more than 200 miles per hour as they opened the doors to fire their machine guns) than all other sources combined (3).
2. During Operation Desert Shield-Storm (1990–1991), despite our general success against DNBI, sporadic outbreaks of diseases and preventable injuries occurred when preventive medicine principles were ignored. A food outbreak affecting 648 individuals working on the flightline in Jeddah, Saudi Arabia, occurred on January 20, 1991 (4). The implicated food source was a locally catered meal served throughout the day. In Desert Shield preventable injuries were responsible for most deaths among U.S. soldiers (5). The 3rd Armored cavalry regiment outpatient sick call records reflects that noncombat orthopedic trauma and unintentional injuries accounted for the greatest number of lost duty days and evacuations from theater (6).
3. During the early phases of Operation Restore Hope in Somalia (1992–1993), epidemic mosquito borne malaria and dengue occurred in an infantry battalion, affecting nearly 10% of the troops. Command emphasis on personal protective measures was lacking (5).

The incidence of preventable illness during tactical operations is not acceptable, because the teams are usually small and can become completely ineffective with the loss of only a few of the teammates. Because of this, the medical personnel of tactical operation teams must be very aware of the types of injuries and preventable illnesses seen in this work environment.

Operational Performance and Preventative Medicine Philosophy

The tactical medic's job is to maximize mission success by providing appropriate medical care before, during, and after missions. The most important aspect of this job is to prevent injury and illness from occurring, not just treating injury as it occurs. Tactical operations are inherently dangerous, and minimizing the risk to operators not only keeps them safe and injury free, but also ensures the success of the mission. Most special operations units have operators with unique attributes and capabilities. The loss of one of these members (e.g., sniper) to a preventable injury, such as a corneal abrasion from a tree branch, can significantly impact the success of a mission.

Injury prevention starts with adequate medical planning. Predicting medical threats associated with specific situations and developing medical assets and transport systems to accommodate potential injuries will help to minimize morbidity and mortality in the hazardous tactical environment.

Preparing operators before deployment with appropriate physical conditioning, health surveillance and immunizations will also help to ensure mission success. By addressing these issues prior to deployment, the provider will minimize medical equipment needs and will be able to inform the mission commander of any significant health-related issues that may impact operator performance.

Physician level medical oversight is essential in establishing good preventative medicine in the tactical community. This ensures the best guidance to the tactical medical provider, and protects the medical team in the event of an untoward outcome. The licensed practitioner is ultimately responsible to the tactical commander for all preventative medicine measures applied by members of the tactical medical team.

Preventative medicine in the operational environment has a broad scope, covering topics from food handling to immunizations to injury prevention during incidents. By addressing these issues before, during, and after deployment, the tactical medic will help to ensure operator well being and mission success.

MECHANISMS OF PREVENTION

Surveying Potential Medical Risks

The tactical medical provider should take as much time as possible leading up to deployment to assess the potential medical threats that members of the tactical team may face based on the intelligence given for a particular situation. The amount of time tactical medical personnel have to complete this planning may be minutes to weeks, depending on the type of incident. When developing a written survey of possibly medical hazards, the medic should work closely with the mission commander to ensure that he/she is informed of potential risks/complicating factors associated with a given situation and can possibly make alterations in mission planning where needed. This information should be documented in a concise, legible format so that it can be easily distributed to team members as needed.

The following is a list of data to be included in the development of medical risk survey. For each category, the survey should identify all conceivable risks and propose solutions to prevent operator illness or injury in a brief and easily referenced manner (Fig. 17.1).

1. Incident specific risks: Opposition weapon systems, known or possible chemical/biological warfare agents, preplanned evacuation routes, weapon systems utilized by the tactical team, entry methods, and other specific threats and hazards that members of the tactical team may face based on the situation.

2. Environmental health threats: Extreme heat or cold, hydration needs, nutritional needs based on the intensity of operator activity, sanitation considerations, risks associated with local wildlife/plant life, and specific risks associated with unique terrain (i.e. mountainous, desert, waterborne, etc).

3. Disease concerns: Should include diseases not covered by standard vaccinations, potential food borne illness, body fluid precaution risk, and region specific disease concerns as dictated by local departments of health or the Center for Disease Control.

4. Climate/weather forecast: Climate can be predicted based on location and time of year. An extended forecast should be obtained, in the event of prolonged or sustained operations. These can also be updated actively during deployments.

5. Regional medical assets: If air/ground evacuation support for casualties is not part of the deploying unit, the tactical medic should be aware of local/regional medical assets available from the civilian community, or possibly the military. If the potential exists for the utilization of medical evacuation assets outside of the tactical team, consideration should be made to informing these services in advance of the operation. This release of intelligence is clearly dependent on the secrecy of the situation.

6. Medical facilities: In addition to planning for casualty evacuation, the tactical medical team should know locations and distances to the closest medical facilities, the closest trauma center, and the closest burn center. Locations for hyperbaric chambers should also be noted if dive operations are planned. The ability to communicate with such facilities including radio frequencies and telephone numbers should be obtained. An assessment of the capabilities to include trauma center designation, ED physician staffing capabilities,

<u>Mission</u>: High-risk warrant service

<u>Date/Time</u>: 15 May 2000, 0525

<u>Location</u>: 1120 Elm Street, Anywhere, TX, USA GPS 44.44 N 55.55 W

Mission Specific Risks:
1. Hostile threats: small arms fire, potential "booby" traps
2. Accidental injuries: Motor vehicle crashes; lacerations and abrasions; back injury from improper lifting

<u>Recommendations</u>: All personnel should wear full body armor with hearing and eye protection and have respiratory protective masks immediately available. Appropriate safety gear should be employed when riding in a motor vehicle, including lap and shoulder restraints; riding on running boards and tailgates should be avoided. The medical status of each member of the tactical team should be reviewed prior to deployment.

<u>Environmental Threats</u>:
1. Heat injury and dehydration: Body armor and clothing add significant insulation and can raise core body temperature.

<u>Recommendations</u>: Individuals should dress in layers to facilitate the removal of excess clothing when possible. Personnel should be given easy access to water and sports drink. Members should be encouraged to drink often with the goal of clear to pale yellow urine. A latrine should be easily accessible to team members.

<u>Disease concerns</u>:
1. Food borne disease: Improperly kept food can lead to significant gastrointestinal distress, with an incubation time of 2 to 12 hours.

<u>Recommendations</u>: Refrigerated foods should be kept at 45°F (7°C) and hot foods should be kept at 140°F (60°C) at all times. Personnel should wash hands with soap and water before eating.
2. Arthropod borne disease: Insects such as ticks and mosquitoes harbor significant diseases, including West Nile virus, Lyme's disease, and others.

<u>Recommendations</u>: Team members should utilize insect repellants with DEET at 20% to 35% on skin, keep sleeves rolled down, and treat uniforms with permethrin.
3. Blood borne pathogens: Members of the team can be exposed to diseases such as HIV and hepatitis B and C through the body fluids of all individuals involved in a mission.

<u>Recommendations</u>: All personnel should use contact precautions (at least latex or tactical gloves) when handling individuals, either hostile or civilian. Consider eye protection based on the situation, and all uniforms and equipment exposed to body fluids should be cleaned and decontaminated as appropriate.

<u>Climate/Weather</u>: The predicted high/low temperature for May 15 is 76°F/52°F. There is a 20% chance of rain in the morning. The predicted sunrise/sunset is 0642/1854.

<u>Regional Medical Assets</u>:

Anytown Fire/EMS Service	(111) 222-3333 (Business)
123 A street	(111) 222-3334 (Fax)
Anytown, TX 11223	911 (Emergency)

Comments: Operates 4 MICU units 24/7. HAZMAT, high angle rescue, and swift water teams available.

Anytown Medevac Services	(111) 222-1234 (Business)
123 A street	(111) 222-1235 (Fax)
Anytown, TX 11223	

Comments: One helicopter with a two-patient capability. Empty weight: 4,976 lb. Maximum gross weight: 7,056 lb. Cruise speed 120 knots. Endurance 2:30 hours, LZ 100' X 100', 10-minute response to mission location.

<u>Medical Facilities</u>:

Anytown Trauma/Burn Center	(111) 222-5555 (Business)
123 A street	(111) 222-5556 (Fax)
Anytown, TX 11223	

Comments: Level I trauma center with burn unit.

Anytown Community Hospital	(111) 222-6666 (Business)
123 A street	(111) 222-6667 (Fax)
Anytown, TX 11223	

Comments: Community hospital with 15-bed emergency department.

<u>Major Airfields</u>

Anytown Airport	(111) 222-7777 (Business)
123 A street	(111) 222-8887 (Fax)
Anytown, TX 11223	

Comments: Airfield Data: Two runways; Runway 1: Aircraft size max: 747 to 400

<u>Additional Contacts</u>:

Anytown Poison Control (111) 2-POISON
Anytown Animal Control (111) 2-ANIMAL

**Consider adding maps of local area if not familiar to tactical team members.

FIGURE 17.1. Sample Medical Risk Assessment

ancillary service availability (e.g., CT scan), presence of a helipad and its specifications, and which specialties are represented at the facility should be obtained in the planning phase.

7. Hazardous materials teams (HAZMAT): Contact information for local/regional/national HAZMAT services should be available regardless of whether or not this type of threat is anticipated.

Most of this information can be obtained via the internet and possibly a few phone calls. For the medical facilities and regional medical assets, face-to-face contact is the ideal option, as it helps them understand the mission and what to possibly expect in the event of casualties. This interaction is clearly limited by the level of operational security, which needs to be clearly established by the mission commander prior to any data collection. The ATF raid on the Branch Davidian compound in Waco, Texas, was compromised by an OPSEC breach for medical planning and extreme caution must be used when interacting with outside agencies and civilian EMS.

Because the time from the start of incident planning to actual deployment is extremely variable, it is important for the tactical unit to maintain records of previous risk surveys, which can be reused in the event of a return to the same location or environment. By developing a thorough risk assessment survey, the tactical medic can help prevent a great deal of unnecessary injuries as well as be better equipped to handle medical incidents as they occur.

Immunizations/Health Surveillance

Tactical operator health prior to deployment, as well as during missions, can have a significant impact on both morbidity and mortality in addition to mission success. The tactical medic, especially when integrated with a unit, will likely be more aware of "minor" issues, such as nagging ankle injuries or "colds," which could potentially impact operator performance. These health issues must be dealt with appropriately, possibly with commander involvement, to help prevent injury to the operator as well as others in the unit.

Dental health maintenance is another essential aspect of team health surveillance. The development of severe dental pain or infection during an operation could cause the loss of a key operator, and potentially jeopardize the mission. All members of the tactical team should undergo routine yearly dental evaluation, and more importantly, should address any issues that arise immediately to prevent the development of significant pain and/or infection. The tactical medical provider should also be familiar with basic dental emergencies and how to resolve minor problems in a field situation. These skills may prevent the unnecessary loss of a member of the tactical team, and thus help to ensure mission success.

> **TABLE 17.1.**

CDC Recommended Immunizations

Annual influenza
Hepatitis B
Measles/mumps/rubella (MMR)
Tetanus/diphtheria with a booster every ten years (every 5 years if injured)
Varicella
Annual tuberculosis exposure test
Consider smallpox vaccine
Consider anthrax vaccine

Health surveillance is particularly critical immediately postdeployment. Each member of the team should be briefly assessed for any minor/major injuries and other health issues that may have occurred during an operation. Tactical medical providers must address these issues as soon as possible to prevent the development of chronic medical problems that may lead to a loss of a member of the tactical team. The team leader should be made aware of any mission related health issues as they arise.

All members of the tactical team should receive the routine vaccinations recommended by the Center for Disease Control for health care workers (see Table 17.1). This includes influenza annually, hepatitis B, measles/mumps/rubella (MMR), tetanus/diphtheria with a booster every 10 years (every 5 years if injured), and varicella. A tuberculosis exposure test should be administered yearly for all members of the tactical team. Also, depending on the mission location and requirements, anthrax, and small pox vaccines should be considered. When deploying to specific regions, especially outside the United States, the most up-to-date recommendations for specific immunizations can be obtained at www.cdc.gov, or 1-800-232-4636/1-877-394-8747.

Nutrition/Food Handling/Sports Supplements

Transmission of all food borne illnesses is always preventable if foods are procured, stored, prepared, and served properly (7). Foods that require refrigeration should be kept below 45°F (7°C) at all times, except when required elsewhere for preparation and serving. Hot foods should be kept hot [140°F (60°C) or above]. Food handlers must be screened for current illnesses prior to be allowed to serve foods. Food handlers should wear gloves during food preparation and serving. Food handlers should also be provided adequate field hand washing facilities and supplies (e.g., soap, paper towels) so they can wash their hands prior to food preparation and serving. Hand washing is the most effective general method for the prevention of human-to-human transmission of diseases. In environments where soap and water are not readily available, alcohol-based waterless hand sanitizer can be effective for reducing disease transmission and illness. Catered foods should be inspected to assure adequate preparation prior to serving it to the tactical operations team. The pre-operation use of immunizations (e.g., hepatitis A) and antimicrobial agents to prevent food borne diseases should be considered when applicable.

Performance enhancing nutrition is an evolving science with new products becoming available on a frequent basis. From creatine to electrolyte enhanced hydration solutions, athletes of all kinds are using more of these products to maintain peak performance. Some of these supplements may be useful in the operational setting, whereas others are potentially harmful. Creatine is a supplement commonly used to provide increased muscle energy, size, and strength for short-term, intense physical activity (i.e., weight training), but has little evidence of value in sustained exercise (i.e., running, cycling). Its use is somewhat controversial, and several cases of exertional rhabdomyolysis have been attributed to creatine consumption associated with significant exertion (8,9). Creatine should be used with caution and possibly avoided completely if tactical operations are likely to require significant exertion for an extended period of time.

The use of electrolyte and carbohydrate containing hydration solutions (i.e., Gatorade, Powerade, etc.) can be very beneficial, especially when operating in a heated environment. A wide variety of sports bars and gels are also available, providing portable, easily digested nutrition. Although they are not intended to be used as meal replacements, these products can give members of the tactical team simple and complex carbohydrates while "on the go." It is important that members of the tactical team experiment with these products during high- and low-intensity training operations to help determine which flavors and brands are tolerated the best. Appropriate implementation of nutritional supplements can boost operator moral, help maintain efficiency during high-intensity operations, and assist in preventing heat-related illness.

Critical Incident Stress Management

Members of the tactical team are likely to be exposed to situations that produce an acute stress reaction. These situations include, but are not limited to, the injury or death of a team member, injury or death of a hostage, and visibly disturbing trauma. The stress of these situations may be magnified by the operator's fatigue, lack of sleep, and duration of exposure to the stressful environment. If this reaction is not addressed promptly, more severe conditions, such as posttraumatic stress disorder (PTSD), may develop. The short- and long-term signs and symptoms that present with stress related problems threaten the readiness of the tactical operations team.

The preventive intervention against this threat is the early identification of individuals with personal problems. This task is not an easy one to complete. Medical personnel who are fully integrated in their tactical team and know the team members will have a better chance to succeed in identifying those in need of support. The support should be in the form of assistance in ventilating their stress. Military as well as civilian studies have shown that recognizing and treating the symptoms of acute stress immediately can prevent them from crystallizing into clinical PTSD (10). Officers who develop an acute stress reaction should be treated close to the team (proximity), as soon as possible (immediacy), by providing them an explanation of their symptoms (e.g., temporary; a normal reaction to stress; will not prevent them from returning to duty (expectancy)] (11).

Work-Rest Cycles and Sleep/Wake Aids

Lack of sleep, stressful conditions and prolonged activity can lead to poor decision making, reduced performance, injury to members of the tactical team, and may even lead to mission failure. The implementation of appropriate work–rest cycles can maximize operator performance and enhance mission success. In general, each individual should be allowed more than 4 hours of uninterrupted sleep in a 24-hour period. Clearly this can't occur for all members of the team at the same time. The best time frame for this rest to occur is from midnight to 0600. The rest of the times, in descending order of preference are 1300 to 1800, 1800 to 2400, and 0600 to 1200. Another potential solution is rotating members of the team through each job as possible, while giving one or two members some time for a 1-hour "power nap." This can significantly enhance performance and improve moral. The sleeping/rest area for members of the tactical team should be in a safe, comfortable, and preferably quiet area. This will maximize the amount of quality rest each member gets.

The use of sleep/wake aids is an evolving science as new medications are frequently being released that have fewer side effects and varying durations of action. Their use is somewhat controversial, with much anecdotal success and failures. The best way to determine the appropriate use of sleep/wake aids for tactical operators is to utilize them in training. This will give the medical personnel, team leader, and team members a better idea on how each medication affects their cognitive and physical performance. Each individual is likely to have unique reactions to each agent. Some of the more commonly utilized medications and their recommended usage by the manufacturer are listed subsequently.

Sleep Aids (See also Chapter 18)

1. Zolpidem tartrate (Ambien): Doses are typically 5 to 10 mg PO. The half-life ($T\frac{1}{2}$) is 2.5 hours (12).

2. Zolpidem tartrate extended release (Ambien CR): Doses are typically 6.25 or 12.5 mg PO. The $T^1/_2$ of the medication is 2.8 hours, but the way the medication is delivered once taken by the user is over a greater period of time, and thus the drug "effects" will be sustained longer (13).
3. Zaleplon (Sonata): Doses are 5 and 10 mg PO. The $T^1/_2$ is 1 hour (14).
4. Eszopiclone (Lunesta): Doses are 1, 2 and 3 mg PO. $T^1/_2$ is 6 hours (15).

Wake Aids (Also see Chapter 18)

1. Modafinil (Provigil): Doses are 100 and 200 mg, with a maximum of 400 mg/day. The $T^1/_2$ may be as much as 15 hours, especially if multiple doses are taken (16). Modafinil is a relatively new drug, and potentially serious side effects may be unreported. The use of this medication in the operational setting is new and should be approached with some caution.
2. Dextroamphetamine (Dexedrine): Doses are 5 to 60 mg PO. The $T^1/_2$ is approximately 12 hours (17).

The timeframe of effects for each medication is somewhat predictable in the average healthy tactical operator. For the sleep aids, the individual will likely be able to return to duty after 3 to 4 $T^1/_2$ of the medication. Therefore, without using these medications in training or prior to deployment, the type/duration of effects on members of the tactical team cannot be safely predicted. If using sleep aids, it is also advisable to consider "checking" the individual's lethal and less-lethal weapons to prevent accidental discharge or inappropriate use while under the influence of medications. It is important to note that each medication can potentially be habit forming and should only be used for short (<1 week) periods of time. Multiple anecdotes exist of persons taking sleep medications in the field while underestimating their rapid onset, which placed themselves or others in danger. Therefore, explicit instructions regarding their rapid onset should be provided to persons taking such medications.

Preventing Injury During Deployment

Medical threats are inherent to the practice of tactical operations (18). The extensive use of dangerous equipment including firearms, explosives, breaching devices, high light and sound intensity producing distraction devices, rappelling equipment, and vehicles with exterior mounted equipment and weapons pose many threats to tactical operators. The wide variety of threats faced by the tactical team from opposing forces, including chemical and biological materials, nonfiring weapons (e.g., knifes, batons), physical force, improvised explosive devices (IEDs), blood, feces, saliva, and urine also threaten the well-being of the tactical operators. Motor vehicle crashes are always

a danger during tactical operations. Also, the use of bulky protective equipment, even though necessary, may present a threat to the tactical officers, because it increases the risk for heat related illnesses (19).

The best approach for minimizing and preventing injuries from these potential risks is education and enforcement of preventative measures. Many of these threats can not be completely avoided but their potential detrimental health effects can be minimized if members of the tactical team wear the proper protective clothing during operations (e.g., helmets, eye protection, hearing protection, masks, ballistic vests, uniforms made of fire retardant and liquid impermeable material, knee pads, elbow pads, gloves, and boots), refrain from wearing unnecessary clothing or jewelry, and follow all standard operating procedures and emergency motor vehicles operations guidelines. Protective gear should fit well, be appealing to the operator (i.e., most tactical team members will not wear eye protection if it is not visually appealing), and most importantly, should be well used by the team members in training prior to deployment.

Arthropod born illnesses can be a significant threat depending on the location and environment that operators are deployed to. Appropriate preventative medications should be distributed to members of the tactical team when endemic disease (e.g., malaria) is a potential threat. Prophylactic medication recommendations for specific regions can be obtained through the Centers for Disease Control, and at *www.cdc.gov*. Treating uniforms with permethrin 0.52% and having operators utilize some type of topical arthropod repellant can go a long way in preventing potentially life-threatening illness.

The tactical medic should perform a screening examination of all individuals detained by the tactical team during an operation. Screening for injuries can help to prevent an untoward outcome of the detainee while under custody, and evaluating for possible communicable diseases can help prevent the transmission of an illness to members of the tactical team. Any findings should be reported to the mission commander and appropriate treatment and/or isolation measures should be instituted as soon as possible.

A wide variety of combat hearing protection is available, each providing different levels of protection. The most ideal earplugs utilize three phalanges to filter out loud sounds while maintaining adequate hearing for lower intensity sounds. The least effective hearing protection is the standard foam earplugs, which are not acceptable for use in tactical operations. They do not provide sufficient protection and prevent the transmission of voice and quieter sounds (such as rifle bolts).

It is important that the tactical medical provider enforce the adherence to safety guidelines and use of protective gear to help minimize preventable injury to the tactical team (20). It is equally essential that all members of the tactical team utilize assigned safety equipment during training operations so that they are clear on the physical limitations associated with their gear.

TAKE HOME POINTS

The development of a medical threat survey prior to deployment is critical in preventing unnecessary injuries to tactical team members, and more importantly, can help ensure mission success.

- Maintaining immunizations and adequate surveillance of operator health between deployments will help to preserve the continuity of the tactical team.
- The use of work–rest cycles and careful application of sleep/wake aids can improve the physical and mental performance of members of the tactical team.
- Strict adherence to preventative safety measures, including appropriate physical conditioning and proper protective clothing will help to minimize nonhostile operator injury and prevent the loss of key specialties of the tactical team.
- Addressing critical incident stress with immediacy, proximity and expectancy will help to prevent long-term PTSD.

SUMMARY

Preventative medicine is the most important part of the tactical medic's job. Tactical operations are inherently dangerous, and tactical teams are typically small, relying on each individual to perform a specific function. By minimizing unnecessary injury and illness, the tactical medical provider can help maintain the operating efficiency of the tactical team, and most importantly, ensure mission success.

REFERENCES

1. Bayne-Jones S. *The Evolution of Preventive Medicine in the United States Army, 1607–1939*. Washington; Office of the Surgeon General, Dept of the Army; 1968.
2. Disease of Military Importance (SC 25-152). Fort Sam Houston: Academy of Health Sciences, US Army; 1975.
3. Heiskell L. Hypothermia and frostbite: considerations in cold weather special operations. *The Tactical Edge*. 1992;10:26–29.
4. DeMaio J, Bailey L, Hall K, et al. A major outbreak of foodborne gastroenteritis among Air Force personnel during Operation Desert Storm. *Milit Med*. 1993;158:161–164.
5. Withers BG, Erikcson RL, Petruccelli BP, et al. Preventing disease and non-battle injury in deployed units. *Milit Med*. 1994;159:39–43.
6. Wasserman GM, Martin BL, Hyams, KC, et al. A survey of outpatient visits in the United States Army forward unit during Operation Desert Shield. *Milit Med*. 1997;162:374–379.
7. Withers BG, Erikcson RL, Petruccelli BP, et al. Preventing disease and non-battle injury in deployed units. *Milit Med*. 1994;159:39–43.
8. Kuklo TR, Tis JE, Moores LK, et al. Fatal rhabdomyolysis with bilateral gluteal, thigh, and leg compartment syndrome after the Army Physical Fitness Test. A case report. *Am J Sports Med*. 2000;28:112–116.
9. Sandhu RS, Corno JJ, Scalea TS, et al. Renal failure and exercise-induced rhabdomyolysis in patients taking performance-enhancing compounds. *J Trauma*. 2002;53:761–763; discussion 763–764.
10. Armfield F. Preventing post-traumatic stress disorder resulting from military operations. *Milit Med*. 1994;159:739–745.
11. Military Leadership. *Field Manual 22-100*. Washington: Headquarters, Dept of the Army; 1990: 59.
12. Ambien. New York, NY: Sanofi-Synthelabo Inc; 2004.
13. Ambien CR. New York, NY: Sanofi-Synthelabo Inc; 2005.
14. Sonata. Philadelphia, PA: Wyeth Pharmaceuticals Inc; 2004.
15. Lunesta. Marlborough, MA: Sepracor Inc; 2005.
16. Provigil. West Chester, PA: Cephalon Inc; 2004.
17. Dexedrine. Research Triangle Park, NC: GlaxoSmithKline; 2006.
18. Carmona R, Rasumoff D. Medical aspects of the Force Continuum. *The Tactical Edge*. 1994;12:69–71.
19. Yeskey KS, Llewellyn CH, Vayer YS. Operational Medicine in Disasters. *Emerg Med Clin North Am*. 1996;14:429–438.
20. Pierluisi GJ. *Medical Support for Tactical Law Enforcement Operations: The Role of Injury and Illness Prevention* [master's thesis]. Pittsburg: University of Pittsburg School of Public Health; 1999.

Sustained and Continuous Operations

Bradley N. Younggren and Benjamin Harrison

OBJECTIVES

After reading this section, the reader will be able to:

1. Define continuous and sustained operations.
2. Explain what effects sustained operations can have on cognition, decision making, and fine motor skills.
3. Describe some of the pharmaceuticals that are available that can help with both sleep and alertness as is mission required.
4. List the other practical aspects of sustained operations that must be considered prior to execution of such a mission.

HISTORICAL PERSPECTIVE AND DEFINITION

If the human body requires approximately 8 hours of sleep per day for the average person, then one could assume that operations could be extended up to 16 continuous hours. This crude definition does not take into account other integral factors, such as level of activity and complexity of functioning required. Nevertheless, it does serve as a foundation from which we can define such operations, thereby classifying the existing research and identifying areas for further studies.

Researchers have started to recognize that there may be differences between short-term sustained operations (SUSOPS) and long-term sustained and continuous operations. It might be most effective to define short-term SUSOPS as any time of continuous operations for a period of time <1 week. Long-term SUSOPS can, therefore, be defined as any time >1 week in duration. It is important to point out that these are fairly arbitrary definitions that will continue to evolve as a larger body of literature develops to support these concepts. Currently, this helps explain some of the different physiologic effects we see in both instances.

THE EFFECT OF SUSOPS ON THE HUMAN BODY

There are numerous scenarios where tactical operators are required to perform for longer periods of time than would be considered the norm. The human body is known to respond to a number of stressors to include fatigue, sleep deprivation, and a negative energy balance (1). Studies have looked at these factors in a number of different research scenarios in both short-term and long-term SUSOPS. Interestingly, there appears to be some differences between the two types of operations. Most civilian tactical operations will be more short term in nature. As such, that information will most likely be more pertinent to the medical director of a special weapons and tactics (SWAT) or special response team (SRT).

There are some commonalities that apply to both scenarios that are worth reviewing. It is apparent that both acute and chronic exercise will cause core temperatures to be lower when exposed to cold because of a larger peripheral heat loss (2,3). The shivering response is also blunted in SUSOPS, which could potentially contribute to lower core body temperatures. Additionally, the increased heat gradient generated could lead to larger losses in core body temperatures (1).

Short-Term SUSOPS

Most of the research on SUSOPS has centered on the effect cold exposure has on the physiologic response mechanisms in the human body. Although providing excellent research, this preference has also highlighted the need for researchers to begin looking at the effects of long-term operations in hot, air environments.

Researchers have shown that repeated, intermittent exposures to cold water over a 10-hour period can blunt the shivering response (4). This is important because shivering is one of the body's mechanisms to generate heat and increase core body temperature. Additionally, Castellani et al. showed that in an 84-hour SUSOP with cold air exposure, there was a greater fall in core body temperature than compared to controls (5). This fall in core body temperature was hypothesized to be due to either a blunted shivering response or to a larger thermal gradient which resulted in greater losses in core body temperature. It is difficult to isolate one stressor as the cause of the blunted shivering response, but it is thought that fatigue plays a role in the recalibration of the response to cold (6–8).

Interestingly, in Castellani's study the vasoconstrictor response was not impaired as was anticipated. In fact, it appears to be enhanced, thereby exhibiting a pattern referred to as insulative acclimatization. This process transfer's heat to the subcutaneous muscles to support exercise, while decreasing the amount of heat lost to the environment (1).

Research has also shown that underfeeding can contribute to impaired thermoregulatory response to cold (9–11) even in the presence of normal plasma glucose. This change appears to be most prevalent in the presence of exercise. In SUSOPS, we need to anticipate whether individuals are going to be moving or sedentary during the mission, and plan accordingly. It is very important to point out that these effects were evident even in the presence of eating; individuals just weren't meeting their metabolic demand in the presence of exercise.

Long-term Sustained and Continuous Operations

Although these are more likely relevant in the military arena, it is still useful to review some of the changes that occur over longer periods of time. In general, there is an increased risk of hypothermia over time. This is from the combined effects of three factors: (i) decreased shivering which results in less heat production, (ii) blunting of the peripheral heat retention mechanism, and (iii) a decrease in core body temperature. In longer operations, the decreased overall weight and percentage of fat results in physiological changes that affect heat retention. Most of this research comes from studies on Army rangers who are perhaps the prime example of people exposed to long-term SUSOPS.

In general, the physiologic changes that occur in the body must be taken into account when planning for SUSOPS. The impact of weather, exercise, and nutritional intake must be taken into account when assessing for operational requirements.

PHARMACOLOGICAL COUNTERMEASURES FOR SLEEP DEPRIVATION AND FATIGUE IN SUSTAINED TACTICAL OPERATIONS

Tactical SUSOPS may lead to sleep deprivation and fatigue due to alterations in sleep patterns and long periods of sleeplessness. Sleep deprivation has been shown to cause fatigue, impair cognitive function, slow decision making, and alter mood; all of which can potentially compromise a tactical mission. Although there is a lack of solid clinical trials directly assessing the effectiveness of drugs that counteract fatigue and sleeplessness on law enforcement tactical operators, conclusions may be drawn from studies looking at therapeutics for SUSOPS in the military and aviation literature. Medical personnel in support of SUSOPS have therapeutic options available to assist operators maintain their reaction time and decision making, which is critical for successful mission completion. This section will briefly review the medical options that may be utilized to battle fatigue-related problems.

In general, cognitive function and reaction times decrease 30% to 40% during the first night and 60% to 70% after two nights of sleep deprivation (SD), leading to operation ineffectiveness (7). Naps of 2 hours can recuperate performance levels, but may result in sleep inertia and cognitive slowing for up to 2 hours after napping. Full-length sleep periods are optimal but often not feasible due to operational requirements and lack of comfortable, quiet sleep environments

Stimulants/Alertness-Enhancing Drugs

Drugs capable of maintaining wakefulness have been utilized in the past and are a viable option in tactical SUSOPS. Ideally, such a drug would have the following characteristics: quick onset, minimal side effects (particularly in hot/cold environments), no interference with operator performance (e.g., judgment, confidence levels, target acquiring, engagement speed, marksmanship), nonaddicting, no disruption of normal sleep patterns, and no delay in sleep onset. Choosing a drug depends on length of task, anticipated hours of SD, and the operational environment. All of the below-mentioned stimulants may be thermogenic and cause a slight baseline rise in core temperature. This may increase risks for hyperthermia, especially in hot and humid conditions. Stimulants should not replace adequate work–rest cycles, but may be necessary for brief periods when SD is unavoidable. Traditionally, amphetamines have been used in past military conflicts, but caffeine and the newer drug modafinil are also therapeutic choices for SUSOPS environments.

Personnel providing medical oversight and supervision during SUSOPS should have primary control for the administration of any stimulant medication given to operators, excluding caffeine ingested in normal drink/food. One should consider the risks and benefits of any such drugs and, because the indications for modafinil and dexamphetamine in SUSOPS are considered off-label (not FDA approved), informed consent for voluntary use is highly recommended. Dextroamphetamine, caffeine, and modafinil all maintain alertness, improve cognitive function, and increase response speed during SD. A brief review of each drug will be discussed subsequently.

Amphetamines

Dextroamphetamine (Dexedrine) is the most commonly researched and prescribed amphetamine in sustained military and flight operations, with use in combat and air operations dating back to Vietnam. It is the only stimulant prescription authorized by U.S. Army and U.S. Air Force policies for combating fatigue. Doses of 10 mg have an average half-life of 10 hours and it is best utilized for long-term maintenance of alertness (up to 64 hours) (1).

Side effects include palpitations, tachycardia, elevated blood pressure, restlessness, anxiety, euphoria, and dryness of mouth. Concerns over subjects taking this medication include poor judgment from overconfidence and "amphetamine psychosis" (suspicion, psychosis, oversensitivity); however, there have been no documented cases of serious amphetamine-related problems or flight mishaps in U.S. Air Force personnel to date (2). It is important to remember that dextroamphetamine is a Schedule II drug with significant abuse potential and should be administered accordingly.

Caffeine

Caffeine is widely available nonprescription drug that has a long-standing history of safety, making it ideal if no medical control is available for SUSOPS. Side effects include palpitations, tachycardia, elevated blood pressure, restlessness, anxiety, frequent urination, and loss of fine motor control (12). Despite this, caffeine has been shown to aid target detection and engagement time during sustained attention operations under fatigued conditions, without affecting marksmanship performance (13). Caffeine in pill form is available in doses from 100 to 500 mg and has a half-life of about 5 hours. A brewed cup of coffee has 135 mg of caffeine, a 12-oz cola drink averages 44 mg, and caffeine gum has approximately 45 mg caffeine per piece. Tolerance in regular users may require higher doses and caffeine is best suited for short-term maintenance of alertness (up to 24 hours) (1). In addition, caffeine (particularly caffeine in gum or liquid form) may be helpful to offset sleep inertia after a nap period to quickly bring an operator to an acceptable level of functioning.

Modafinil

Modafinil (Provigil) is a stimulant initially developed for narcolepsy that has been recently studied for use in SUSOPS. Unlike amphetamines, it does not act on the central nervous system to maintain wakefulness. It may, therefore, allow sleep in break periods during missions when naps are feasible. For SD >24 hours, a 2-hour nap is recommended for anchored sleep, ideally at the circadian nadir of the second night. Modafinil is effective at maintaining wakefulness until that point and, like caffeine, can also be utilized after naps to decrease sleep inertia. Ideal dosing is 100 mg every 8 hours during SD and its half-life is approximately 10 to 12 hours (1). It appears to be non-addictive, does not result in physiologic tolerance, and is a Schedule IV drug.

Side effects are dose related but less common than amphetamines and caffeine. Headaches, palpitations, nausea and vomiting, elevated blood pressure, and anxiety are uncommonly reported. Modafinil does not appear to have other significant side effects, such as tremors or loss of fine motor skills, that may interfere with flight performance or target assimilation. Although a tendency for overconfidence was noted in one study utilizing 300 mg of modafinil (14), another study using lower doses showed no evidence of an overconfidence effect (15). Although not documented, modafinil may increase the risk for heat injuries during prolonged exercise in hot environments and this should be considered if administering this drug in such situations (11). One recent small study showed that shift workers had more difficulty falling asleep after taking 200 mg modafinil, contradicting earlier reports. Participants in this study, however, took the drug the morning after, not before, the night shift and this may have resulted in this unexpected finding (16).

Modafinil seems best suited for intermediate-term maintenance of alertness (up to 40 hours), but it lacks operational research studies at this point. Use of modafinil should be monitored closely and administered by medical personnel familiar with its side effects.

Sleep Promoting Agents

Naps and anchor sleep are ideal to combat the effects of fatigue and SD, and sleep periods are sometimes necessary in SUSOPS. Falling asleep in an SUSOPS environment can be difficult because of the sleep environment and excitement of the operation. Drugs capable of inducing sleep may be utilized in tactical SUSOPS and should ideally work quickly, not interfere with normal sleep patterns, be non-addicting, and allow for earlier-than-expected awakening. Three drugs, namely temazepam, zolpidem, and zaleplon, are commonly used in SUSOPS to allow for adequate sleep periods and have all been approved for operation use by the U.S. army and U.S. Air Force. All have different characteristics that permit medical personnel to tailor their use for specific scenarios. Various factors, such as medication onset and duration as well as desired onset and length of sleep period, will play into the decision to use one drug over the other. In certain situations, brief naps are preferred, whereas in other situations, longer sleep periods are appropriate. Knowledge of drug characteristics will allow the provider to choose an agent that will allow sleep, while preventing drug-induced hangover drowsiness during subsequent operations. Clear and precise warnings to the users of such medications should be given. These warning should include admonitions as to the very rapid onset, disinhibition, potential hangover drowsiness, and impaired state after taking such medications. In particular, specific directives against driving, cleaning weapons or having sensitive discussions after taking such medications are paramount for the tactical provider.

Zaleplon

Zaleplon (Sonata) is a very short acting agent that allows for sleep induction without prolonged effects. The usual dose is 5 to 10 mg and is a good choice for initiating very short naps (<3 hours postingestion) or sleep at an earlier-than-normal time. This also works well for an operator who desires to fall asleep early in anticipation of an early morning operation, without a drowsy feeling upon awakening. For eastward travelers, in it useful to combat jet lag if traveling through only 3 to 4 time zones by initiating sleep at earlier times than usual. Trials have not demonstrated hangover problems (1).

Zolpidem

Zolpidem (Ambien) initiates and maintains sleep for approximately 4 to 7 hours, making it ideal for sleep periods <8 hours. At doses of 5 to 10 mg it is ideal for longer naps, provided there is no need for early sleep termination that requires the operator to be functional immediately upon awakening. Side effects, withdrawal symptoms, and abuse potential are low to absent, and it has been proven to be safe and efficacious. For eastward travelers across three to nine time zones, zolpidem has a role in initiating and maintaining sleep for longer periods than zaleplon. It will last long enough (unlike zaleplon) until the normal sleep cycle begins, but will have worn off for an earlier-than-usual wake time. Zolpidem is known for a rapid onset of action and, therefore, users should be cautioned to take the medication immediately prior to lying down.

Temazepam

Temazepam (Restoril) has a longer half-life than the other agents (9 hours) and is best suited for longer sleep periods. It not only initiates sleep, but also maintains it for longer periods of time. In personnel working nights (such as with shift workers), sleep initiation is generally not a problem as long as he/she has not taken certain stimulants. Staying asleep is usually the problem, because of disruptions from the environment (noise, light, uncomfortable sleep area) and from normal daytime circadian rises in alertness. Temazepam allows for 8-hour sleep periods and is a good choice for temporarily augmenting the nighttime sleep of operators who westward travel across as many as nine time zones (1). Precaution must be taken to prevent awakening psychomotor sluggishness, because temazepam may cause sleep inertia hangover (17). Medical personnel should take into consideration both the duration of temazepam and the operational requirements before administering it to an operator.

PRATICAL ISSUES IN MISSION PLANNING

In addition to the physiologic effects of SUSOPS, there are other practical considerations beyond pharmacology, which must be addressed prior to team deployment. First, personal sanitation issues must be evaluated, especially for those individuals such as snipers who might have to be in one location for a very long period of time without the ability to move around at will. As such, containers for urination and defecation must be available for those individuals to dispose of waste during prolonged operations. One can also consider a commercial product to assist in channeling urine away from the body such as a condom catheter. There are a number of such products available right now for use by both men and women.

Teams must be prepared for significant alterations in temperature during SUSOPS. Not only will there be temperature changes throughout a 24-hour period with the rise and fall of the sun, operations over a number of days could present drastically different weather patterns. Planners must have both cold and warm weather gear, along with wet weather gear available during SUSOPS. Additionally, prolonged exposure to the sun could result in sunburn, which can affect thermoregulation, concentration, and mobility.

Hydration is an issue that must be considered by team planners for SUSOPS. There are a number of different ways to estimate water requirements in an exercising individual. One must remember that these are rough estimates, and aggressive early hydration is the norm in places like the Middle East. A rough estimate of the minimum water requirements per day is 35 mL/kg/day. Another way to look at it is 1 mL per calorie consumed. Both methods are going to give you a minimum water consumption of more than 2 L, and this needs to be taken into account when planning. Dehydration can rapidly reduce team effectiveness,

▶ **TABLE 18.1. Methods of Estimating Water Requirements.**

Body Weight	
For first 10 kg	100 mL/kg/24 hr
For second 10 kg	50 mL/kg/24 hr
For additional weight over 20 kg	20 mL/kg/24 hr
35 mL/kg body weight/day	
1 mL/kilocalorie consumed	

especially when mobility is a continued requirement (Table 18.1).

Nutrition is also important for SUSOPS. In the 3 to 5 days preceding a particularly strenuous operation, individuals should increase there carbohydrate intake in preparation for the increased workload. Approximatley 10 g/kg body weight per day is a rough estimate on what the carbohydrate intake should be during this period. During strenuous activity, liquid carbohydrate supplementation can be effective and should be at least 45 g/hour.

Sleep is also something that must be considered in SUSOPS. As previously reviewed, there are a number of pharmacologic options that can potentially extend the effectiveness of team members. However, it may be just as easy to work out work–rest cycles to maximize the team's prolonged capabilities. Team members should either nap for <30 minutes or approximately 3 hours in order to maximize the effectiveness of REM sleep and improve after-nap alertness.

Equipment can be effected by prolonged operations. For one, heavy equipment can fatigue the operator decreasing his overall effectiveness and hastening his return to the frontline. Also, if operations are in an austere environment, one can anticipate equipment malfunctions or breakage. This must be accounted for in terms of backup equipment; most SUSOPS will need some level of redundant equipment that can be easily distributed to member of the team.

Finally, stress can rapidly become an issue for team members involved in intense, SUSOPS. SD can make it more difficult for an individual to cope with prolonged stress, and underlying psychological profiles must be taken into account when assessing one's team members prior to deployment. Work–rest cycles should be employed during SUSOPS to ensure the team retains its effectiveness.

TAKE HOME POINTS

1. There is an increased risk of hypothermia over time in SUSOPS.
2. Certain drugs, such as modafinil and dextroamphetamine, can be helpful at maintaining alertness during SUSOPS.
3. Sleep aids, such as zolpidem, can assist in work–rest cycles, if appropriately utilized.
4. Preparation is critical to SUSOPS: issues such as personal hygiene, sleep, inclement weather, and nutrition must be considered ahead of time to maximize team effectiveness.

SUMMARY

Sustained and continuous operations require a significant amount of mission planning prior to team deployment. As the medical authority, one must have a good understanding of the physiologic mechanisms that come into play during SUSOPS. Additionally, it is important to be familiar with the various drugs than can be utilized during SUSOPS to maximize the effectiveness of team-members. One must have a good understanding of the practical aspects of mission planning that come into play. Hydration, nutrition, sanitation, and sleep schedules are all important factors in mission success.

REFERENCES

1. Caldwell JA, Caldwell JL. Fatigue in military aviation: an overview of US Military-approved pharmacological countermeasures. *Aviat Space Environ Med*. 2005;76(suppl):C39–C51.
2. Ahanson R, Lewko J, Campbell D, et al. Adaptation to night shifts and synchronization processes of night workers. *J Physiol Anthropol Appl Sci*. 2001;20:215–226.
3. Akerstedt T. Shift work and disturbed sleep / wakefulness. *Occup Med*. 2003;53:89–94.
4. Akerstedt T, Ficca G. Alertness-enhancing drugs as a countermeasure to fatigue in irregular work hours. *Chronobiol Int*. 1997;14:145–158.
5. Castellani JW, Stulz DA, Degroot DW, et al. Eighty-four hours of sustained operations alter thermoregulation during cold exposure. *Med Sci Sports Exerc*. 2003;35:175–181.
6. Buguet A, Moroz DE, Radomski MW. Modafinil-medical considerations for use in sustained operations. *Aviat Environ Med*. 2003;74:659–663.
7. Angus RB, Heslegrave RJ. Effects of sleep loss on sustained cognitive performance during a command and control simulation. *Behav Res Methods Instrum Comput*. 1985;17:55–67.
8. Baranski JV, Gil V, McLellan TM, et al. Effects of modafinil on cognitive performance during 40 hr of sleep deprivation in a warm environment. *Milit Psychol*. 2002;14:23–47.
9. Belenky G, Penetar DM, Thorne D, et al. The effects of sleep deprivation on performance during continuous combat operations. In: Marriot B, ed. *Food Components to Enhance Performance*. Washington: National Academy Press; 1994:127–135.
10. Belenky G, Wesensten N, Thorne Dr, et al. Patterns of performance degradation and restoration during sleep restriction and subsequent recovery: a sleep dose-response study. *J Sleep Res*. 2003;12:1–12.
11. Buguet A, Moroz DE, Radomski MW. Modafinil-medical considerations for use in sustained operations. *Aviat Space Environ Med*. 2003;74:659–663.
12. Committee on Military Nutrition Research, Institute of Medicine. *Caffeine for the Sustainment of Mental Task Performance: Formulation for Military Operations*. Washington: National Academy Press; 2002.
13. Gillingham RL, Keefe AA, Tikuisis P. Acute Caffeine Intake Before and After Fatiguing Exercise Improves Target Shooting Engagement Time. *Aviat Space Environ Med*. 2004:75:865–871.

14. Baranski JV, Pigeau RA. Self-monitoring cognitive performance during sleep deprivation: effects of Modafinil, D-amphetamine, and placebo. *J Sleep Res*. 1997;6:84–91.

15. Buguet A, Radomski MW, Moroz DE, eds. *Effects of Modafinil on Thermoregulation During Physical Exercise and Sleep Deprivation in a Hot Environment*. Toronto: Defense and Civil Institute of Environmental Medicine; 2000: ISBN 0-9688317-0-2.

16. Gill M, Haerich P, Westcott K, et al. Cognitive performance following modafinil versus placebo in sleep-deprived emergency physicians: a double-blind randomized crossover study. *Acad Emerg Med*. 2006;13:158–165.

17. Paul MA, Gray G, MacLellan M, et al. Sleep-inducing pharmaceuticals: a comparison of melatonin, Zaleplon, Zpiclone, and temazepam. *Aviat Space Environ Med*. 2004;75:512–519.

Lifts and Carries

W. Thomas Burnett

OBJECTIVES

After reading this section, the reader will be able to:

1. Recognize the importance of having multiple physical extraction techniques specific to the environment and resources available.
2. Understand the importance of remote assessment prior to rapid rescue.
3. Become familiar with several different extraction techniques for both the conscious and unconscious patient.

HISTORICAL PERSPECTIVE

At no time during an operation is the tactical medic more vulnerable than during the physical extraction of an injured patient. Carrying an injured patient from a hostile environment often leaves the rescuer without the benefit of self-protection and limits his mobility, reflexes, and visualization of his surroundings. It is for this reason that the medic must be familiar with multiple methods for transporting an injured patient. The medic must take into consideration the patient's condition, available resources, available manpower, and the immediate safety of the environment in which he will be operating. The ultimate goal is to provide rapid patient removal in the most reasonable manner while providing the greatest safety for both the medic and the victim.

Many situations require that a patient be removed from an unsafe region before any further medical treatment may be provided. The medic must be able to assess the scene and quickly determine how to best remove the patient to a zone where more definitive care may be safely initiated. Often, the patient assessment must occur from a remote distance because the medic does not have immediate access to the patient. A conscious patient may be able to assist with his own extraction, or the medic may be able to assist the patient to an area of increased visual concealment or physical cover. An unconscious patient must be assessed to determine which method of removal is safest and most appropriate. For example, the unconscious patient with a gunshot wound to the head and an active shooter in sight surely poses a much greater risk to the medic than benefit to the victim, but the unconscious patient that fell from a height would require a completely different extraction technique that is more appropriate to his injuries.

Above all, it is important to remember that the tactical environment is a dynamic scenario that requires the medic to adapt to the surroundings to choose the best rescue method based on available resources, manpower, scene security, and mechanism of injury.

PHILOSOPHY

The initial assessment of a casualty will dictate the method used to physically extract him from an austere environment. The mechanism of injury is the most important factor in determining the approach, rescue, and retreat technique for the casualty, but the medic must also consider the most reasonable and timely approach given the immediate threat and the condition of the casualty.

Immobilization of the cervical spine should be reserved for high speed motor vehicle collisions, falls from heights, or significant blunt or blast injuries. There is no indication for cervical spine immobilization for penetrating head or neck trauma or for falls from <1 to 2 meters unless there are neurological deficits or localized pain of the cervical spine. The average time for adequate cervical spine immobilization by a trained paramedic is five and a half minutes. Unless specifically indicated, unnecessary spinal immobilization will create a significant time delay that may place the casualty and the rescuer at risk for additional injury without providing additional benefit to the patient.

Tourniquets are rapidly employed to control life-threatening extremity hemorrhage prior to transport from the hot zone until the patient can be moved to a more secure environment and the wounds may be assessed further. The splinting of injured extremities should occur prior to the patient's extraction only if time and security permits safe application by the medic. With all transports, it is essential to guarantee that the patient's weapon is secured prior to any movement. Remember that an alert but partially immobile patient may still be able to provide additional firepower for a team during approach or retreat.

In situations where the patient is not physically accessible but is alert, the most appropriate initial rescue technique is to verbally direct the casualty to the nearest cover or concealment until the immediate threat is neutralized. Commercially available throw ropes can be deployed and clipped to the casualty's vest to physically assist a patient's movement a more secure location when direct approach is unsafe. It is important to note that the attachment points to the vest must be strong enough to drag the casualty. Attachment points on many vests are not strong enough for this task. The use of a web harness specific for this task may improve the ability to drag the casualty to safety. The nonalert casualty that cannot safely be approached requires the medic to observe the casualty from a distance (binoculars may be helpful) to perform remote assessment and determine the overall status of the patient. Important considerations include the survivability of the patient's wounds, the degree of patient movement, the quality of the patient's breathing, the estimated blood loss, the presence of obvious extremity injuries, and the overall color and appearance of the patient. Once these are noted, the medic will better understand how much assistance the patient can give to his own extraction and determine the resources and manpower required to provide the safest and most appropriate method of rescue.

When the decision is made to approach the patient, the medic must utilize all available resources. When faced with an active shooter and the casualty requires an open field approach where no cover or concealment is available, the goal is a rapid and safe retreat to a more secure environment. Diversionary tactics, such as the use of noise (flashbangs, sirens, bullhorns, and car alarms are all readily available), smoke, or cover fire, may distract or confuse an active shooter and provide additional security during such an approach. If they are available and time permits, shields and vehicles should always be utilized to provide additional cover during an open field approach with an active shooter.

LIFT AND CARRY TECHNIQUES

The type of extrication technique utilized depends on the available resources and manpower, the level of consciousness of the casualty and the amount of assistance he can offer and the security of the immediate surroundings. The ABCs of extraction dictate *Ambulation Before Carry*, if the casualty can assist with his own retreat it decreases

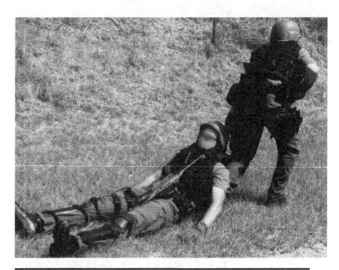

FIGURE 19.1. Collar or Loop Drag. (Photo by Rod Stegall.)

necessary resources and provides additional security during transport. Manual carries are utilized when a nonambulatory patient is in the hot zone and the patient must be rapidly moved to a region of higher security. They require the least resources and provide the quickest retreat but also often provide the lowest level of security during movement. The quickest and simplest method of casualty removal is the Collar or Loop Drag. This technique is rapidly deployed in the hot zone when the rescuer is in the immediate vicinity of the casualty and cover is very close. The rescuer simply grabs onto collar or loop of the patient's tactical vest and drags him to the nearest area of cover or increased security (Fig. 19.1). This is a rapid response tactic that is difficult to maintain for a moderate or long distance and assumes the casualty has a collar or loop to grasp.

The Fireman's Carry is another widely taught single rescuer technique; however, it has limited "real world" application due to the physical requirements and high profile of this carry. After raising the casualty to a standing position (Fig. 19.2), the rescuer faces the patient and grabs

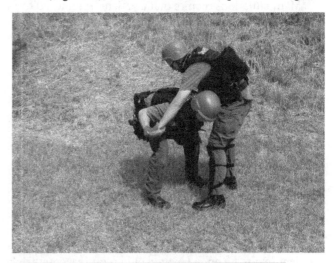

FIGURE 19.2. Fireman's Carry. (Photo by Rod Stegall.)

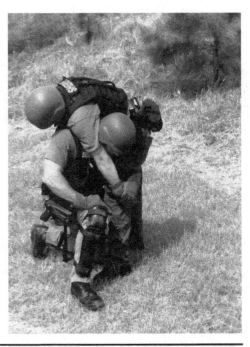

FIGURE 19.3. Fireman's Carry. (Photo by Rod Stegall.)

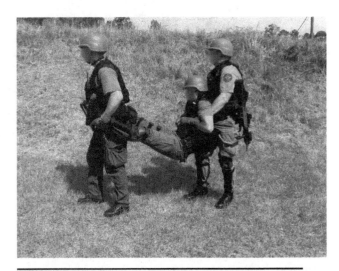

FIGURE 19.4. Fore-and-Aft Carry. (Photo by Rod Stegall.)

his wrist, lifting the arm overhead. The rescuer then bends at the waist and kneels while pulling the casualty over the rescuer's shoulders. The rescuer moves his other hand behind the patient's knees and grabs the patient's hand from behind the rescuer's neck. The rescuer places his free hand on his knee for support while slowly standing and adjusting the patient for proper weight distribution (Fig. 19.3). Although this technique can be utilized with a conscious or unconscious casualty for travel over a moderate distance, it's use is limited to a very strong rescuer in limited tactical conditions.

A third single rescuer technique is the Pack-Strap Carry. After raising the casualty to a standing position, the rescuer turns his back to the casualty's front and brings the patient's arms over the rescuer's shoulders. By bending slightly at the knees, the rescuer positions his shoulders under the casualty's arms and grasps his wrists. The rescuer bends forward and positions the casualty as high on his back as possible in order to distribute his weight equally on the rescuer's back while avoiding dragging the patient's feet on the ground. This technique can be used over moderate distances for a conscious or unconscious patient, but does not allow the rescuer to have use of either hand for security. Also, the Pack-Strap Carry should not be used for patients with obvious upper extremity fractures.

If two rescuers are available, the Fore-and-Aft Carry is the most useful technique for moving a patient. The taller rescuer locks his hands under the supine casualty's arms and around his chest. The shorter rescuer kneels between the casualty's legs while facing away from his head. The shorter rescuer then grasps behind the casualty's knees and both rescuers lift the patient off the ground (Fig 19.4). This

method can be rapidly utilized for moderate to long distances in a conscious or unconscious patient.

In an open field approach, additional security can be provided when a shield man and a rear guard are available. The four man stack is led by the shield man and approaches the casualty with the shield man moving slightly ahead of the patient. The middle two rescuers deploy the Fore-and-Aft Carry technique while turning to face the back of the rear guard. The stack then retreats with the rear guard now leading the team back to cover or increased security (Fig. 19.5).

There are many commercially available poled and poleless litters, SKEDs and Half-SKEDs, and other assist devices that allow from one to four rescuers to transport a

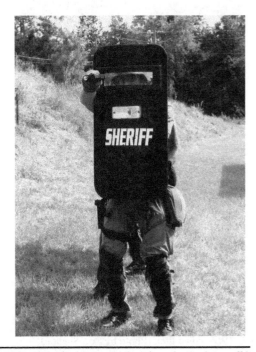

FIGURE 19.5. Shield approach. (Photo by Rod Stegall.)

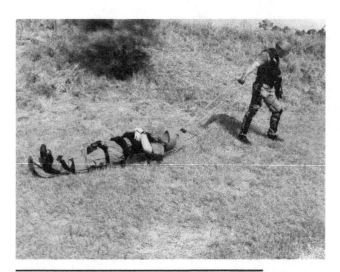

FIGURE 19.6. SKED liter. (Photo by Rod Stegall.)

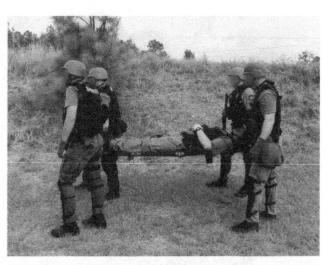

FIGURE 19.8. Four Person Carry with a poled liter. (Photo by Rod Stegall.)

patient over longer distances with relative ease and varied levels of security (Fig. 19.6). SKEDs can be used by one or two rescuers and allows the patient to rest on a full or half sized version in order to smoothly drag the casualty across moderate to longer distances. The full SKED may also be utilized for high-angle rescue.

The poled litter is one of the most stable and easiest method of transport over longer distances and can be carried by two to four rescuers (Figs. 19.7 and 19.8). Newer designs of liters are more compact and easier to transport when not in use; however, because of the rigid construction, it is not easily maneuverable when in a confined

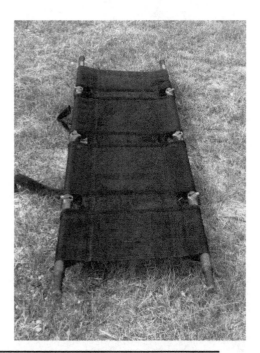

FIGURE 19.7. Poled liter. (Photo by Rod Stegall.)

space and may have limitations due to this. The poleless litter, however, offers many of the benefits of the poled litter but is lightweight and compact when folded and is very easily carried on the side of a tactical backpack for use in various scenarios. On the other hand, poleless liters do not distribute the casualty's weight evenly and can be very physically demanding for the rescuers that are carrying the torso. Additionally, the poleless liter tends to place the c-spine in significant flexion that could compromise the airway and limit c-spine immobilization (Fig. 19.9A). As experience has been gained in casualty care, new product lines have also been developed with a focus on high-threat extraction that allow rapid extraction using less effort, while still being able to provide a degree tactical cover (www.NARescue.com). The "Dragon Handle System" can be rapidly attached to the casualty by use of an extraction harness, drag strap or directly to the casualty. The casualty is then dragged to cover by one or two rescuers (Fig. 19.9B, C).The "Rat-Strap" attaches to the rescuers belt and allows for hands free extraction (Fig 19.9D).

With all methods of extraction, the medic must take advantage of cover and concealment and maintain a low profile when approaching the patient for assessment and utilize cover and concealment when available. The rescuer must always consider that it may be necessary to put the patient down in order to return fire and defend the patient and himself. Although the rapid extraction of the patient is important, it is more important for the rescuer not to become an additional casualty.

TAKE HOME POINTS

1. A relatively small percentage of injuries in the tactical environment necessitate cervical spine immobilization prior to rapid extraction.

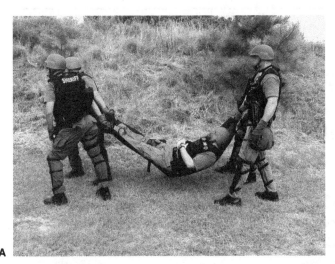
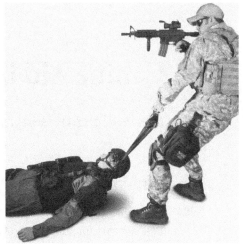
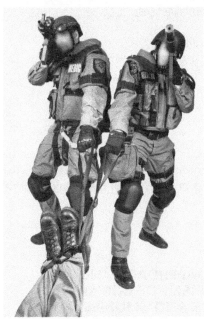
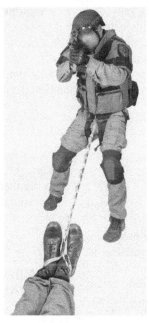

FIGURE 19.9. **(A)** Four Person carry with a Soft Liter. (Photo by Rod Stegall.) **(B)** Single Person Drag with a Dragon Handle System. **(C)** Two Person Drag with Dragon Handle System. **(D)** Single Person Drag with Rat-Strap.

2. It is important to evaluate the patient by using remote assessment when the patient is not immediately accessible and the casualty is unable to remove himself to cover or concealment.
3. Planning an organized approach and retreat provides the highest level of security available for the casualty and the rescuer.
4. Self-extraction of a casualty is preferable to assisted extraction when possible in the tactical environment.
5. Multiple techniques can be utilized to carry an immobile casualty to a more secure environment but must be weighed against the available manpower and resources and the level of rescuer safety each method offers.

SUMMARY

There is no *right* rescue method, but the *best* rescue method is the one most appropriate for the casualty based on the medic's overall assessment of the scenario.

It is essential that the medic quickly assess the patient's degree and mechanism of injury, the level of patient consciousness, the surrounding environment, and the immediate threats to safely choose the approach and physical extraction technique most appropriate for patient removal to a region of more definitive treatment while maintaining the highest level of security for the team.

Canine Aid in the Tactical EMS Setting

Benjamin Harrison and James Fudge

OBJECTIVES

After reading this section, the reader will be able to:

1. Contrast the basic approach to first aid and vital signs between canine and human patients.
2. Understand management principles for common environmental illnesses, wounds, and injuries in the canine patient.
3. Describe emergency interventions and procedures for the critically ill working dog in shock or cardiopulmonary arrest.
4. List medications that may be available with medical support for a tactical operation and understand their utility in treating canine patients.

HISTORICAL PERSPECTIVE AND OVERVIEW

The formal use of dogs in U.S. military operations dates back to the formation of the U.S. Army K-9 corps in 1942, and civilian law enforcement has been using police dogs for decades. The utilization of police dogs in tactical law enforcement environments is commonplace and the U.S. Police Canine Association was formed in 1968. Personnel providing primary medical oversight in tactical operations may also be called upon to provide first aid and basic trauma management of an injured animal. Most often these animals suffer environmental injuries, but working dogs may receive penetrating or blunt injuries in the line of duty and care generally follows the same basic trauma management protocols as for humans. The following chapter will provide a brief overview of basic first aid techniques and basic lifesaving care for a sick or injured police dog.

This chapter is written for trained medical emergency providers who should be able to apply most human emergency medicine skills to the working dog until it reaches definitive veterinary care. When serving as medical support for a tactical EMS unit that utilized K-9 units, it is imperative to create veterinary contacts and protocols for injured dogs ahead of time. With assistance from the veterinarian, create a canine first-aid kit that you will bring on operations. Knowledge of how and where to access emergency veterinarian care, especially after hours, is an important preparatory step that should be taken prior to

each mission. In addition, most dog handlers have been trained to administer first aid and are an invaluable asset to the medical provider when managing a sick or injured working dog.

GENERAL APPROACH AND MANAGEMENT OF COMMON ILLNESSES AND INJURIES

Approach/Handling a Sick or Injured Dog

Take care in approaching an injured animal. Even the gentlest dog may bite or struggle if in severe pain. First, have the K-9 handler attempt to muzzle the dog and/or restrain his head and neck before you approach, unless it is having fast or labored breathing. A firm, not tightly, placed makeshift muzzle using a rope or rolled bandage material can act as a restraint. A field expedient muzzle might restrain a large working dog somewhat, but an effectively muzzled dog can still be dangerous. Trusting implicitly a field expedient muzzle can easily result in injury to the care provider. It is preferable to rely on the handler to restrain his/her dog with a good muzzle. Ensure there is good, clear communication between the care provider and the handler throughout the entire treatment period. Speak in soothing tones and move slowly, trying to gain the dog's confidence as you treat it.

General Assessment

Normal vital signs for dogs include a rectal temperature of 101°F to 102°F, pulse rate of 80 to 120 bpm (larger dogs 60 to 80, young or small breeds 100 to 120 bpm), and respiratory rate of 14 to 16 (adult dogs), and 20 to 25 (young dogs). Mucous membranes of the gums are normally pink and capillary refill (checked in gum over canine tooth) is <1 second. Signs of shock may include: pale gums, dry lips, weak and rapid pulses, cool extremities, rapid respiratory rate, agitation, restlessness, and collapse. Dilated pupils, respiratory depression, capillary refill >4 seconds, white mucous membranes, and rectal temperature <98°F are all late signs of shock and impending cardiovascular collapse (1).

Heat Injuries

Dogs utilize the respiratory tract to dissipate heat and do not rely on their skin for heat regulation, as humans do. Excessive panting and labored breathing in a hot environment may mean a rise in core temperature and impending heat stroke. The high normal range of canine core temperatures are 102°F to 103°F, and hyperthermia is indicated by a core temperature of 105°F 110°F (2). Prevention of heat injuries in dogs may be prevented by providing adequate rest and plenty of water, especially during hot periods. Vomiting, collapse, ataxia, and red mucous membranes are ominous signs and should be acted upon immediately.

The priority in heat injury is to lower the core temperature as quickly as possible. This is most easily and effectively accomplished by completely dousing the dog in tepid (not ice cold) water and blowing air (preferably via a fan) over the dog. Convective heat loss in this manner is the most effective way to lower core temperature. A rectal temperature should be obtained and cooling measures should be stopped at approximately 103°F. Do not give antipyretics in heat injuries. Transport for further evaluation and treatment once the core temperature has been lowered (2).

Wound Management

Wounds should be referred to a veterinarian for definitive treatment. Hemorrhage control follows the same principles as for humans by applying direct pressure followed by elevation, pressure points, and tourniquets, if required. Pressure points in the leg can be found on the inside of the proximal portion of the fore and hind legs, as well as the underside of the base of the tail. Tourniquets are reserved for situations where bleeding is severe and not slowed by direct pressure or pressure points.

As in humans, delayed primary closure is a reasonable alternative to primary closure in the tactical environment.

Various factors, such as active bleeding or functional requirements, should drive decisions to close wounds primarily. If definitive veterinarian care is not available and repair is required, cleanse wounds in dogs as you would in humans with copious amounts of irrigation (3). Utilize anesthetics and nylon suture material to close gaping or bleeding wounds, but realize that the dog may chew or bite open the suture if it can reach the wound. Gently appose wounds, not typically closing wound edges as tightly as in people. Attempt to protect the wound and have the dog handlers supervise the dog to prevent the dog from reopening the wound. If the wound is clean, you can apply skin adhesives, using similar principles as in humans. Elizabethan collars are typically used on smaller animals and are generally not needed if the wound is closed and proper bandages applied.

Venomous Bites/Stings

Hymenoptera stings (bees, wasps, hornets) are common in dogs and should be treated symptomatically. Gently attempt to remove stingers with a flat hard surface and apply cool compresses. Benadryl, in doses of 1 to 2 mg/kg orally, can be given in addition to baking soda paste applied to the wounds.

Snakebites may occur to the working dog, often to the face or neck. Pit vipers are the most common snakebite in the United States, and the local effect of the venom may result in significant edema and even airway loss. Be prepared to place a surgical airway and aggressively treat shock with intravenous (IV) crystalloids in 20 to 25 mL/kg boluses to maintain adequate perfusion and blood pressure (see section on IV fluid therapy). Attempt to immobilize the bitten part and keep it below level of the heart. Constriction bands have not been proven to be effective and should be avoided in canine snakebites. Antihistamines are often given to dogs with snakebites but are an unproven standard of care. As in humans, the definitive treatment of venomous snake bites consists of antivenin therapy. Transport as soon as possible for antivenin if edema is progressing or for systemic signs of envenomation. Administer antivenin if it is available and there is a significant delay for transport to definitive veterinarian care. Dosing is weight based as with humans; a typical initial dose is 5 to 10 vials, depending on the severity of the envenomation. Start IV fluids and piggyback the antivenin in at a slow rate, watching the dog closely for signs of anaphylaxis (2).

Fractures

Gently restrain and muzzle an injured dog with an obvious extremity fracture. Unless grossly deformed, immobilize the limb in place and include the joint above and below the injury in the splint. Utilize rolled magazine, SAM splints, cardboard, wood, or other firm material to immobilize a fracture. Robert Jones bandages are ideal splints for dog extremity fractures, so check with the handler first to see if he is carrying one. If the dog is limping, assess for deformity or bony tenderness. If none are present, this may represent a strain or sprain. Apply ice, give a dose of buffered aspirin, and rest the dog. Persistent limping may require definitive evaluation to include radiographs. All suspected fractures as well as any significant injury should be evaluated by veterinary services for definitive management.

Multiple Trauma Mechanism of Injury

If the mechanism of injury is significant, such as if the dog was hit by a moving vehicle or sustained a fall from a height, it is important to consider the possibility of spinal cord injury and intracranial injury. Screening for spinal injury can be accomplished by noting movement of the extremities and noting the dog's withdrawal reaction to pinching the toe at the base of the nail taking care, because an injured and frightened dog may reflexively bite. Check for anal tone and level of consciousness. Document the level of consciousness by best response to AVPU (alert, responsive to verbal or pain, or unresponsive). Always have a working dog evaluated by a veterinarian as soon as possible with a significant mechanism of trauma.

ADVANCED LIFE SUPPORT AND EMERGENCY PROCEDURES

General Treatment for Shock

As with humans, attend to the "ABCs" when approaching a critically injured animal. Insure adequate ventilation and control life-threatening hemorrhage. In cold environments, cover the animal and place it on a warm object or blanket. If signs of shock are present in an injured dog, attempt IV-line access and infuse IV crystalloid.

Intravenous Access and Fluid Resuscitation

For mildly dehydrated dogs, subcutaneous injections of isotonic crystalloids (normal saline or lactated ringers) can be administered at 2 to 5 mL/kg. Multiple sites can be utilized in an aseptic manner, but it may take may take 6 to 8 hours for absorption and this is generally not appropriate for acute traumatic injuries. This practice has fallen out of favor and should be utilized only if you cannot obtain IV access and the patient is not in shock.

Infuse IV crystalloid (normal saline or lactated ringer's solution) in 10 to 15 mL/kg over 20 minutes for moderate dehydration, but no signs of shock. Lactated ringer's is the preferred crystalloid in dogs, but normal saline may be

utilized if that is all that is available. Infuse intravenous crystalloid, 20 to 25 mL/kg boluses, for signs of hypovolemic shock. Colloids, such as hetastarch, may also be infused if the dog is in hypovolemic shock; give 5 to 15 mL/kg boluses over 10 to 15 minutes in addition to crystalloids, or alone if that is the only IV fluids you have available. Repeat IV fluid boluses until the dog has signs of adequate reperfusion as evidenced by urine output (1 to 2 mL/kg/hour), improved mental status, and a mean arterial blood pressure of 80 to 90 mm Hg. A dog's blood volume is approximately 90 mL/kg and in shock states up to 2 to 3 times that volume may be required to restore cardiovascular parameters to acceptable levels (2,4).

IV access can be accomplished in the jugular vein or peripheral site, but this can prove challenging to the inexperienced provider due to a lack of knowledge of animal anatomy. For IV access in the foreleg, first shave a 2 to 3 inch band of hair just proximal to the distal leg joint (carpus) and clean with Betadine or chlorhexidine. Have one person stabilize the foreleg while the person placing the IV catheter straightens the leg beyond the joint. The cephalic vein is located anteromedial, above the joint. With the thumb, twist the flesh above the joint laterally. This exposes and stabilizes the vein, acting like a tourniquet. With a jabbing motion, insert the catheter into the vein. Canine skin is tougher to penetrate than in humans and veins tend to roll more. Utilize an 18-gauge × 2-inch catheter for large dogs and a 20-gauge × 2-inch catheter for medium-sized dogs.

Intraosseous (IO) access is a viable option for the critically injured dog. As with humans, any flat surface of a bone may be utilized; in dogs, it is most common to place IO lines in the trochanteric fossa in the femur or proximomedial tibia. Although pediatric IO lines may be adequate for young puppies, adult IO lines (such as the EZ-IO with drill) will be needed for older and larger dogs. Tape the catheter in around the entire leg circumference and place a rolled bandage or elastic bandage over the area to protect it from the animal. Unlike humans, this should not cut off the venous supply as long as the material isn't placed too tightly.

Cardiopulmonary Resuscitation in Dogs

Although cardiopulmonary resuscitation (CPR) is generally ineffective for traumatic cardiac arrests in animals and humans, it can be helpful in medical resuscitations and other environmental emergencies such as electrical injuries. To perform chest compressions, place the base of your hand just behind and above the foreleg elbow on the chest wall where the chest is at its widest. Compress about one-half the width of the thoracic cavity, or 1 to 2 inches in smaller dogs and 2 to 3 inches in larger dogs. To ventilate, close the dog's mouth firmly and wrap your hands around his snout, blowing forcefully into the nostrils. Be careful, because obtunded or unresponsive dogs may reflexively bite. Look for an appropriate chest rise; if ineffective, ensure that no air is escaping from the mouth and that you are blowing hard enough. Realize that ventilating in this manner is not very effective; therefore, it is better to place an endotracheal tube in the dog. In general, it is much easier to intubate a dog than a person.

Ideally, two people should perform CPR, because one person CPR is generally ineffective. If two people are performing CPR, the best ratio of cardiac compression to ventilation is 1:1, but the ratio for one-person CPR is 15:2. The size of the animal also dictates rates and position. For smaller dogs (<7 kg), a lateral recumbent position (side down) at a ventilatory and chest compression rate of 120 times per minute is ideal. For larger dogs (>7 kg), 80 to 100 times per minute suffices in the dorsal recumbent (back down) position, which may be difficult to achieve without a "V"-shaped trough. Open thoracotomy with open cardiac massage should only be initiated in cases of witnessed cardiac arrest after penetrating thoracoabdominal injury, as long as operative capabilities are available and ready nearby (2,5).

Emergency Drugs and Algorithms

A comprehensive discussion of emergency drugs in the injured animal is beyond the scope of this chapter; however, some basic concepts merit review. Dogs are more likely to act like children in shock pathophysiology with initial compensation followed by intractable hypotension if not treated appropriately. In general, providers can generally follow a similar treatment pathway in animals as found in human advanced cardiac and pediatric life support courses. Drug dosages should be weight based and follow indications as in ACLS/PALS. To treat bradycardia in dogs, it is appropriate for larger working dogs (>30 to 40 kg) to receive adult dosages of ACLS medications, such as epinephrine, atropine, or lidocaine (e.g., atropine at 0.02 mg/kg or 1 mg IV). Drugs may also be given via the endotracheal tube as in humans (usually 2 to 3 times the normal IV dose). In larger dogs, cardioversion and defibrillation attempts also follow similar doses as for humans (e.g., 100J, 200J, 360J for defibrillation). Use large amounts of gel on the contact (defibrillator paddles or pads) to ensure adequate contact with skin beneath a thick coat. Benzodiazepines (lorazepam or diazepam) can also be given in appropriate doses rectally, IV, or via the endotracheal tube for seizures or cocaine/sympathomimetic ingestions (5).

Advanced Airway Management

Dogs may require definitive airway management and adequate choices for induction drugs that are also utilized in humans include ketamine (10 mg/kg) with or without a benzodiazepine, such as midazolam (0.5 mg/kg) or valium (0.5 mg/kg). Succinylcholine at 0.22 mg/kg may be used as a paralytic for rapid sequence intubation. The basic approach to intubating a dog is to get the longest Miller (straight) laryngoscope blade available. In general, use endotracheal tubes 1 to 2 sizes larger than calculated for the dog's size, since their tracheas are larger than humans (e.g., a large working dog may require an 11.0 mm ETT, so use the largest ETT). Place the dog in a sternal position and wrap the tongue with gauze, grabbing the tip and pulling it out of the mouth. (Do this only after adequate sedation to avoid being bitten.) Depress the now-exposed epiglottis anteriorly and insert/check the endotracheal tube as you would in humans, securing it in place with rolled gauze.

Medications

Aspirin can cause gastric ulcers, which can be life threatening if ignored but which respond to withdrawal of the medication. It should be relatively safe to give an occasional dose for pain (10 mg/kg), but use enteric coated or buffered aspirin and do not give for extended periods if possible. The dose of acetaminophen for dogs is also 10 to 15 mg/kg and, although generally safe, it occasionally causes liver failure and death from dose-related effects. Ibuprofen and other NSAIDs have a narrow therapeutic window, and a recommended dose is 5 mg/kg/day, divided. Ulcer formation and renal failure may result, especially if given for more than several weeks (6). Morphine at higher doses than usually given for humans, 0.5 to 1.0 mg/kg, may be given IM, IV, or SQ for severe pain (2,7).

TAKE HOME POINTS

1. When compared with the adult humans, large working dogs have a higher baseline core temperature, but similar respiratory and pulse rate ranges.
2. In general, stabilize and treat most common environmental illnesses, traumatic wounds, and injuries in the canine patient as you would human patients in the prehospital setting.
3. Aggressively treat shock states with intravenous crystalloid fluids and follow basic human advanced cardiac life support principles in the canine patient in cardiopulmonary arrest.
4. In critical canine patients, administer drugs using weight-based dosages similar to those recommended in ACLS or PALS. The dose of parenteral morphine for very painful conditions is 5 to 10 times

higher in the canine patient compared with human dosages.

SUMMARY

This chapter is intended to give a brief overview of basic canine aid for the human medical element in a tactical operation. Prior coordination with the dog handler to identify the nearest veterinary support in a tactical operation is imperative. Whenever possible, seek immediate veterinary care for definitive treatment of a sick or injured dog. If immediate intervention is required before transport can be accomplished, this chapter can assist the medical provider care for the sick or injured dog in that rare instance.

REFERENCES

1. Bamburger M. *The Quick Guide to First Aid for Your Dog*. New York: Howell Book House; 1993.
2. Bistner SI, Ford RB. *Kirk and Bistner's Handbook of Veterinary Procedures & Emergency Treatment*. 6th ed. Philadelphia: WB Saunders; 1995.
3. Swaim SF, Henderson RA Jr. *Small Animal Wound Management*. 2nd ed. Baltimore: Williams & Wilkins; 1997.
4. Slatter DH. *Textbook of Small Animal Surgery*. Philadelphia: WB Saunders; 1985.
5. Ettinger SJ, Feldman ED. *Textbook of Veterinary Internal Medicine*. 4th ed. Philadelphia: WB Saunders; 1995.
6. Kore AM. Toxicology of nonsteroidal antiinflammatory drugs. *Vet Clin North Am*. 1990;20:419–429.
7. Kukanich B, Lascelles BDX, Papich MG. Pharmacokinetics of morphine and plasma concentrations of morphine-6-glucuronide following morphine administration to dogs. *J Vet Pharm Ther*. 2005;28:371–376.

Chapter 21

Tactical En Route Care

Robert T. Gerhardt

OBJECTIVES

After reading this section, the reader will be able to:

1. Discuss the history of tactical en route care.
2. Understand basic principles of planning, coordinating, and executing tactical en route care in the context of prehospital trauma life support (PHTLS) tactical combat casualty care.
3. Be aware of the limitations as well as potential complications that might be encountered in the en route care setting, along with countermeasures to mitigate them.

INTRODUCTION

Over the past century, a revolution in the resuscitative and definitive care of victims of conflict has taken place. In addition to the development of new surgical techniques, resuscitation strategies, pharmaceuticals, and other adjuncts, the military and contingency medicine communities have placed increasing emphasis upon the process of converting the victim into the patient: that is to say, medical evacuation and en route care of combat casualties. The term *en route care* is defined as "the care required to maintain the phase treatment initiated prior to evacuation and the sustainment of the patient's medical condition during evacuation" (1). The en route care process involves the medical treatment of injured and ill personnel, during evacuation between levels of care. This may occur at any point beginning with first response and ending with rehabilitative care, if needed.

In civilian EMS circles, air medical transport refers to the use of dedicated aircraft and medical crews, which provide critical care advanced life support or advanced life support (ALS) emergency care and transportation of trauma and medical emergency patients. This service may be provided either from accident sites (scene response) or from primary care centers to tertiary or definitive care (interfacility transfers). *Aeromedical evacuation* is the commonly applied, but technically inaccurate, term used by the U.S. military for what would otherwise pass as air medical transport (more precisely, "aeromedical" refers to the anatomical and physiological effects of flight on human systems). MEDEVAC, a contraction of the phrase "medical evacuation," is the U.S. Army's vernacular for both ground

and air medical transport and implies the employment of dedicated vehicles under control of the Army medical department (AMEDD), as well as en route medical care. CASEVAC refers to the process of transporting casualties by any available conveyance and generally implies that no skilled medical treatment is provided en route. *Prehospital care* is a term that encompasses the emergency care and transport of sick or injured persons in the out-of-hospital setting by varying levels of health care providers. Emergency medical services (EMS) systems are organized and integrated organizations employing air, ground, and even waterborne transport units, staffed by trained emergency medical care providers under the direction and license of a physician medical director, who provides pre- and interhospital care. Such systems are usually designated and regulated by state public health or emergency services authorities and are often integrated into regional trauma and cardiac care systems.

To be effective and sustainable, en route medical treatment rendered in the tactical setting of must simultaneously possess the following characteristics: efficacy, simplicity, and facility and tactical validity. Efficacy implies that the procedure or intervention has actually been proven to save lives. It must also be possible to perform such interventions quickly and easily, given rudimentary training and initial proctoring by a qualified instructor. Last, medical interventions in the combat setting should be able to be performed in a fashion that places the patient, the provider, and the transport element at minimal risk for additional injury and that facilitates the most rapid possible extraction from the line of fire. This latter consideration constitutes perhaps the most complicated aspect of en route combat casualty care, because the majority of published EMS literature to date pertains to civilian settings with well-developed health care systems and relatively short time-distance issues.

TRANSPORT CONSIDERATIONS

Time–Distance and Environment-Of-Care Issues

Traditionally, the primary tenet of en route care has been, "the treatment is speed." Although medical interventions both at the time of wounding and en route to definitive care have made their impacts, the transport time interval between point-of-wounding and definitive care remains a critical component in the survival of victims of conflict.

The U.S. military refers collectively to the effects of the operational milieu as METT-TC issues: namely, mission, equipment, terrain and weather, time, troops (both yours and your adversary's) and civilians on the battlefield (2). All of these factors possess the potential to impact, either positively or negatively, an evacuation plan. As such, the prudent en route care provider will, at minimum, be aware of these issues; at best, one will participate in the process of planning the mission with the express purpose of ensuring that medical expertise is integrated into the developing plan.

In the case of most tactical operations, no such formal fronts exist. In addition, hostile forces are divergent in terms of operational capability, mobility and adherence to the law of war (to date, none are formal signatories to the Geneva Conventions). Areas of responsibility (AOR) for allied combat arms and combat support units may be broad and deep, resulting in significantly greater distances required for evacuation. These increased distances coupled with the potentially compounding effects of rough terrain, inclement weather and a broader maneuver area for hostile forces, all conspire to increase the risks inherent in casualty evacuation and en route care. As such, the importance of tactical medical and casualty evacuation pre-planning has taken on a new sense of urgency.

Important time–distance considerations in casualty evacuation and en route care include:

1. Location, number and type of elements supported
2. Their organic medical support and evacuation assets
3. Location of echelon II and III CHS (combat health support) units in your respective AOR
4. Terrain features affecting your potential evacuation routes
5. Analysis of hostile forces locations, capabilities and limitations, and prior conduct toward noncombatant/medical units
6. United States or allied maneuver and support elements available to escort or otherwise assist the evacuation mission

7. Friendly evacuation assets available to you, including dedicated medical evacuation vehicles and aircraft, nonstandard vehicles, potential crew members, and nonmedical attendants
8. Your source of launch authority

METT-TC information forthcoming from the requesting unit is most readily obtained by receipt of a Standard MEDEVAC Request, usually composed in a nine-line format. An example of a standard MEDEVAC request appears in Table 21.1.

Once armed with this information, the evacuation planner may then determine whether casualties may be evacuated from supported units directly to higher-level care by single sorties or whether ambulance exchange points (AXP) may be required. In addition, rules of engagement and operational plans may be constructed for the employment of air medical and casualty evacuation assets, if available.

The decision whether to employ air medical evacuation appears initially simple in the sense that all immediate and urgent surgical casualties should be evacuated preferentially by air. The decision to employ air assets in the tactical environment is complicated by numerous issues, including the marked vulnerability of rotary wing aircraft to virtually any modern weapons system, including small arms. This danger is amplified in urban environments, where flight paths and LZ's often intersect closely with buildings and other structures, which may provide safe haven and a direct field of fire to hostile elements intending to engage the aircraft. A sobering thought to be considered by anyone requesting air medical evacuation is the possibility that their request may result not only in the loss of the casualty's life, but also those of the air crew in the event of a catastrophic aircraft mishap or combat loss.

Appropriate indications for air medical evacuation include the following:

1. Casualties meeting criteria for urgent evacuation (loss of life, limb, or eyesight within 2 hours)
2. Casualties meeting priority evacuation criteria, but for whom other means of evacuation will cause deterioration
3. Circumstances in which the organic medical capabilities of the supported unit have been rendered ineffective (mass casualty incident, medical element neutralized by hostile action)
4. Risk of loss of evacuation aircraft and air crew is considered manageable by launch authority

Medical Crew and Patient Safety

Casualty evacuation and en route care possess their own unique mission environment beyond that of the general setting of field operations. Thus, like other operational personnel, the en route care provider should conduct individual, crew and patient care precombat checks and

▶ **TABLE 21.1. Sample US/NATO Standard MEDEVAC Request.**

1. Location of LZ for casualty collection (eight-digit MGRS grid coordinates)
2. Radio frequency, call sign, and suffix of requesting element
3. Number of patients by precedence:

   A—Urgent
   B—Urgent Surgical
   C—Priority
   D—Routine
   E—Convenience

4. Special equipment required:

   A—None
   B—Hoist
   C—Extrication equipment
   D—Ventilator

5. Number of patients:

   A—Litter
   B—Ambulatory

6. Security at LZ/pick-up site:

   N—No enemy troops in area
   P—Possible enemy troops—approach with caution
   E—Enemy troops in area
   X—Enemy troops in area—armed escort required

7. Method of marking LZ/pick-up site:

   A—Panels (VS-17 or similar)
   B—Pyrotechnic
   C—Smoke
   D—None
   * Additional methods may be listed by local TACSOP

8. Casualty nationality and status:

   A—U.S. Military
   B—U.S. Civilian
   C—Non-U.S. military
   D—Non-U.S. civilian
   E—Enemy prisoner of war

9. NBC Conditions (use only if applicable):

   N—Nuclear
   B—Biological
   C—Chemical
   – IN PEACETIME, describe LZ terrain

inspections (PCC/PCI). In addition to standard field equipment, weapons, communications and other logistical considerations, the following unique concerns should be considered and addressed:

1. Have available copies of current professional licenses and certifications.
2. Dress in layers and bring additional warm clothing (temperature fluctuations may be extreme as a result of ambient weather vs. vehicle compartments, altitude, etc.).
3. Wear appropriate body and eye armor/protection, as well as a helmet, both for protection from hostile fire as well as accidental injury within the crew compartment of the evacuation vehicle.
4. Be prepared to furnish safety harness, hearing and eye protection, rain protection, and blankets to patients you transport.
5. Consider the use of hearing protection when practicable.
6. Carry multiple forms of personal identification.
7. Carry or have at hand standard precautions protective supplies.
8. In the air transport setting, consider avoiding the ingestion of gas-producing foods and beverages such as legumes, cruciferous vegetables, and carbonated drinks for the 8- to 12-hour period before anticipated flight or on-call status, if you are susceptible.
9. If you are susceptible to motion sickness, consider the use of approved anti-emetic agents (a trial is suggested prior to operational use in order to assess for side effects); nonpharmaceutical approaches that have been reported to possess some efficacy include: fixing gaze on the horizon or other distant object, accupressure bands applied to the wrists, and small meals high in simple carbohydrates. Perhaps the best remedy for motion sickness is acclimatization: the more often you ride in a vehicle or fly, the less likely you are to become motion-sick.

Patient Preparation

The basic precepts of care under fire include rapid extrication of both the casualty and provider from exposure to direct hostile fire, by the most expeditious means available. After this has been accomplished, more formal attempts at pre-evacuation packaging should be undertaken. Such preparations take on increasing importance at the AXP or in those patients who are being transferred from a forward resuscitative surgical element to a CSH. Such "intraoperative" patients will require more detailed preparation in order to ensure that their condition does not deteriorate en route.

Detailed checklists for preparation before, during and after evacuation missions are provided in Tables 21.2 to 21.5.

EN ROUTE CLINICAL CARE

Clinical "Show Stoppers"—Diagnosis and Treatment

As part of the predeparture patient assessment, or during the evacuation mission, en route care providers must

▶ **TABLE 21.2. Predeparture mission checklist.**

1. Assemble your team and gear
   a. Patient movement items (PMI)
   b. Pharmaceuticals
   c. Expendable supplies and IV fluids
   d. Oxygen
   e. Safety equipment
   f. Tactical, load-bearing equipment and armor
   g. Personal weapons, as appropriate
2. Coordinate with evacuation vehicle crew regarding:
   a. Prevailing weather conditions
   b. General route
   c. Tactical concerns
   d. Patient requirements (speed, flight ceilings, if applicable)
3. Communicate with sending unit/facility
4. Communicate with receiving unit/facility
5. Resources needed
6. Coordinate LZ or AXP location, crew pickup

be constantly vigilant for the presence or development of life-threatening conditions affecting the patients in their charge. Anticipation of these conditions, when followed by appropriate interventions may prevent deterioration prior to arrival at the next level of care.

The following sections will discuss the circumstances, diagnosis, and treatment of the more common life threats or "show stoppers," which the en route care provider may encounter.

Acute Airway Compromise

A secure airway with the concomitant ability to support ventilation is the primary requirement for patient survival. As such, the en route care provider must assure airway patency prior to evacuation; otherwise, one must be prepared to mitigate complications in what may be clearly a suboptimal transport environment.

▶ **TABLE 21.3. Patient On-site Reception Checklist.***

1. EXAMINE the patient.
2. BRIEF the patient, if possible.
3. SECURE IVs and other tubes, establish flow control (pressure bag and dial-a-flow device or infusion pump).
4. EMPTY fluid reservoirs and ATTACH vented bags for air travel.
5. LABEL, COIL, and SECURE all lines and wires
6. REPLACE air with sterile solution in all indwelling cuffs and balloons for air travel (crystalloid IV solutions are suggested).
7. ATTACH monitors and safety gear (ear plugs, straps, seatbelts).
8. SECURE the patient.
9. ADMINISTER transport medications and sedation if indicated.
10. TRANSFER oxygen and all devices to stretcher.
11. OBTAIN initial and serial vital signs.

*Performed if tactical circumstances permit.

▶ **TABLE 21.4. En Route Care Checklist.**

1. KNOW location of emergency gear.
2. COMMUNICATE with evacuation vehicle crew.
3. EXAMINE the patient (again).
4. MONITOR your oxygen tanks, IV flow rates.
5. AVOID snaring lines and wires.
6. OBSERVE monitors, reservoirs, patient.
7. USE standard precautions.
8. BOLSTER yourself when using sharp implements.
9. WEAR seat belts or retention straps.
10. SIT when you can.
11. PRACTICE sound and light discipline when possible.

The axiom, "when in doubt, intubate," is strongly recommended prior to evacuation. In circumstances where this is impossible or impractical, the provider's goal will shift toward attempting to prevent airway compromise while en route. Toward this end, access to continuous suction, nasopharyngeal (NPA) and oropharyngeal airways (OPA), bag-valve-mask apparatus or portable ventilators, supplemental oxygen, and related airway adjuncts should be confirmed. In addition, a laryngoscope with appropriate straight (Miller style) and curved (MacIntosh style) blades, assorted cuffed and uncuffed endotracheal tubes, tube stylets, and rescue airway devices such as tracheal-esophageal tubes (Combitube), the laryngeal mask airway (LMA) or a cricothyroidotomy kit should be available and in working order prior to departure.

Advanced airway maneuvers are at best a challenge in the transport environment. Cramped crew/patient compartments, tactical flight or ground maneuver, limited visibility, potentially hypoxic and combative patients, and the risk of hostile fire conspire to make such attempts undesirable except in the most critical circumstances. In the event that unanticipated airway compromise occurs to the transport patient, the provider may find rapid sequence intubation (RSI) to be a valuable tool in the re-establishment of a secure and patent airway. It should be noted, however, that RSI is in itself a procedure fraught with risk and should not be attempted by providers unless they are qualified to perform intubation and possess experience in the use and management of complications associated with intravenous (IV) paralytics, induction agents, and analgesics.

▶ **TABLE 21.5. Mission Destination Checklist.**

1. EXAMINE the patient (again).
2. REPORT patient information on final approach, if you can.
3. UNLOAD under direction of the flight crew.
4. AVOID snaring lines and wires.
5. SECURE weapons with evacuation vehicle crew (if any).
6. COMMUNICATE with receiving medical and nursing staffs.
7. DOCUMENT your care and leave a copy.
8. RECOVER your gear for return, as appropriate.
9. Have a SAFE trip home.

The goal of RSI is to facilitate endotracheal intubation in a rapid but semicontrolled manner before the patient experiences cardiopulmonary failure as a result of their injury or acute illness. Short-acting pharmacologic agents are preferred for RSI because, under ideal circumstances, the procedure is brief and in order to facilitate rescue maneuvers in the event of failure. In the en route care environment, RSI consists of five stages: preinduction preparation, induction, paralysis, intubation, and recovery. During preinduction, the patient is preoxygenated (if possible) using a nonrebreather mask set at an oxygen flow rate >10 lpm; RSI medications, intubation equipment, and adjuncts are prepared, and the patient is positioned in a manner that best facilitates successful laryngoscopy. Induction is then performed with the goal of placing the patient into a sedated or anesthetized state. A paralytic agent is then administered. After paralysis has been attained, laryngoscopic endotracheal intubation is performed, and artificial ventilation is commenced. During recovery, the airway is secured, the patient is reassessed, and sedative, analgesic and longer-acting paralytic agents may be administered as appropriate.

Induction should include both analgesia and sedation components. Pharmaceutical induction agents appropriate for use in RSI include etomidate, the combination of fentanyl and midazolam, and ketamine. Although longer acting and thus requiring greater post-RSI care, a combination of morphine and diazepam are effective and may be more readily accessible in the deployment environment. Etomidate is a particularly attractive agent in the setting of transport RSI, as it is short-acting, possesses both analgesic and sedative properties, and causes minimal impact on hemodynamics, even in the setting of hemorrhagic shock. As a dissociative agent, ketamine offers a viable alternative for RSI, conscious nasotracheal intubation and cricothyroidotomy, and field surgical procedures, such as amputation, due to its ease of administration (IV or IM), duration of action (up to 1 hour per dose), and minimal hemodynamic effect. Care should be exercised when ketamine is used due to the risk of emergence phenomena (paranoia and nightmares) and idiosyncratic reactions that may include bronchorrhea and transient hypertension. Emergence phenomena may be avoided either by reassuring conversation by the provider or by moderate dosages of benzodiazepines.

Alternatives to RSI in the setting of airway compromise in the conscious patient include nasotracheal intubation or surgical cricothyroidotomy. Although enjoying a recent yet short-lived resurgence in popularity, needle cricothyroidotomy with high-pressure trans-tracheal jet ventilation (HP-TJV) is not generally recommended. Although it may hold value as a temporizing maneuver in children (for whom surgical cricothyroidotomy is technically difficult), HPTJV requires special equipment, access to high-pressure oxygen delivery (in excess of 45 psi), and generally provides inadequate ventilation for adults beyond an initial period of 5 to 10 minutes.

Pneumothorax and Related Closed Space Gas Accumulation

Traumatic pneumothorax is a potentially life-threatening condition, and may rapidly progress to tension pneumothorax. The transport environment may further complicate this and similar clinical conditions where gas accumulates in an enclosed physiologic space, such as in the cases of pneumocephalus resulting from head or maxillofacial trauma, Eustachian disfunction and related barotrauma, ileus or pneumoperitoneum resulting from abdominal trauma, and circumstances involving indwelling inflated catheter cuffs. Such conditions are exacerbated particularly in the setting of air evacuation via nonpressurized aircraft, such as helicopters.

Boyle's law states that at a constant temperature, as ambient pressure decreases, the volume of a gas increases proportionally; in a practical sense, this means that a patient with a simple pneumothorax embarking by air transport is likely to develop a tension pneumothorax as the aircraft ascends to altitude. The same may be said for other trapped-gas states. As such, it is recommended that patient suspected or known to have such conditions receive decompression prior to transport, if practicable. If not, transportation by any conveyance should be planned and conducted via routes that minimize elevation risk as well as facilitate tactically sound evacuation. Although little scientific evidence exists in this area, a reasonable empirical guideline for transport of patients who are at risk for altitude-induced barotrauma is to avoid altitudes in excess of 5,000 feet above mean seal level (MSL), where possible. Given standard weather conditions, this ceiling would produce roughly a 17% decrease in pressure of an enclosed-space gas with a resulting volume increase of roughly 20%. In tactical circumstances where the baseline altitude already exceeds this guideline (such as in mountainous terrain), the evacuation team should bear in mind that any additional increase in altitude will produce even greater increases in gas volume, and eventually, pressure.

Clinically suspected tension pneumothorax is a clinical entity comprising an urgent-surgical state, requiring lifesaving intervention in the form of needle decompression followed by tube thoracostomy with suction as soon as practicable. Simple pneumothorax is difficult to diagnose without chest radiography, however clinical suspicion may provide sufficient impetus to perform needle thoracentesis. Clinical signs of tension pneumothorax include tachypnea, respiratory distress, hypotension, hypertympanic percussion and decreased air movement upon auscultation of the effected side, and palpable deviation of the trachea toward the contralateral side. It is advised that the provider palpate the trachea rather than merely visually inspect for deviation, because this is a late sign. Although tension pneumothorax may be accompanied by hypoxia as measured by transcutaneous pulse oximetry, lack of this sign should not be construed as excluding the diagnosis. Simple pneumothorax may present with little more than respirophasic chest pain and mild tachypnea; thus, the provider must maintain a high level of suspicion for this condition when the patient's history and mechanism of injury warrant it.

If tension pneumothorax is suspected, the en route care provider should consider needle decompression to be a reasonable diagnostic tool as well as an initial therapeutic maneuver, because the risk of inducing a small and clinically insignificant pneumothorax as a result of needle thoracentesis is far outweighed by the lifesaving benefit of definitive diagnosis and decompression if a tension pneumothorax is actually present. As always, such procedures should be conducted by qualified personnel who reasonably suspect this condition, and who are prepared to treat its complications.

Ideally, pneumothorax should be treated by tube thoracostomy prior to evacuation, particularly in the setting of air transport. If this is not practical, but pneumothorax is suspected while en route, needle thoracentesis should be performed, using a large bore (14-gauge or larger) Angiocath, which may be attached to a 3- to 5-mL syringe filled with 2 cc crystalloid solution, if desired. Anatomic landmarks are the superior surface of the second intercostal space, in the mid-clavicular line, of the affected side. Such a location maximizes the chance of accessing an apical pneumothorax while minimizing potential injury to the neurovascular bundle running along the inferior surface of each rib. Prior to puncture, this site should be cleansed with povidone iodine or an alcohol prep pad, at a minimum. After site preparation, and if circumstances permit, lidocaine 1% may be infiltrated subcutaneously at the site, followed by Angiocath insertion perpendicular to the skin surface to a depth of 5 cm, or until air is aspirated. In such a case, aspiration should continue until the patient's respirations become nonlabored or until no additional air may be aspirated. At this point, the needle may be withdrawn and a three-way stopcock and tube may be attached and secured with tape or suture. The latter field expedient device facilitates subsequent aspirations in the event that the pneumothorax reaccumulates prior to tube thoracostomy.

Other sources of transport-related barotrauma include: pneumocephalus or pneumoperitoneum resulting from penetrating trauma and subsequent occlusive dressing, eustachian tube dysfunction, and iatrogenic expansion of endotracheal and urethral catheter tube cuffs filled with air. Dressings covering puncture wounds should be checked periodically while en route and should be vented as clinically indicated. Tube and catheter cuffs should be filled with crystalloid solutions or sterile water prior to evacuation, obviating the risk of gas expansion.

Uncontrolled Hemorrhage and Hypovolemic Shock

Ideally, any accessible sites of controllable hemorrhage will be managed prior to arrival of the evacuation team. If not, standard direct pressure followed by pressure dressings should be placed. If these fail or if the tactical circumstances prohibit the time and exposure required of both the patient and provider for the application of direct pressure and elevation, then a tourniquet should be applied. If the tourniquet was placed primarily to facilitate tactical extrication, then it is advisable to place a pressure dressing on the wound site and attempt tourniquet release as soon as time and circumstances permit. If this attempt fails, the tourniquet should be reapplied and left on for the duration of the evacuation to next level of care.

Likewise, in the tactical setting, it is important that the en route care provider examine the patient both for forehead markings describing tourniquet placement, as well as to determine whether a tourniquet was placed but not recorded by the initial medical treatment provider. If one is found, an attempt should be made to determine the circumstances of its placement, and if for tactical extrication purposes, a trial removal strategy should be performed as described previously, preferably while en route.

Despite the previously reported incidence of 5% mortality from controllable extremity hemorrhage in past conflicts, the greatest challenge posed by hemorrhage to both the patient and provider in the current setting will likely result from either blunt or penetrating thoracoabdominal trauma or nontraumatic internal hemorrhage (3). Such casualties will not likely be stabilized until resuscitative surgical intervention is available to them. As such, perhaps the single most important intervention beyond basic life support is rapid transport to the nearest available element capable of providing such care.

While transport is undertaken, the en route care provider is advised to secure the patient on the stretcher in order to avoid additional injury due to motion. Then, attempt to prevent hypothermia and subsequent cold coagulopathy by keeping the patient warm. In the tactical transport setting, this is best accomplished using passive external means, such as blankets, vehicle heating systems, and room-temperature IV fluids. It is unlikely that warmed fluids may be delivered using standard IV tubing sets; however, it is advisable to avoid infusing frankly cold fluids, which may hasten hypothermia. Although patients without frank respiratory distress do not require high-flow oxygen, supplemental oxygen may offer an incremental benefit by increasing the partial pressure of dissolved oxygen in the plasma, perhaps resulting in improved tissue oxygenation. As such, supplemental oxygen to maintain a transcutaneous pulse-oximetry level of 100% is suggested, if available. IV access should be confirmed or established, preferably with two large-bore peripheral lines with heparin/saline locks. If the patient exhibits signs of shock and peripheral access is not obtainable, alternatives include external jugular venous cannulation, intraosseous devices and central venous cannulation. Recently, intraosseous infusion has undergone a renaissance with the development of facile administration kits, such as the Bone Injector Gun (which accesses the humeral head, anterior tibial plateau, or iliac crest) and the FAST-1 (which employs an auto-penetrating sternal device). Central venous access may be obtained by qualified personnel using the standard Seldinger technique or by field expedient means. The latter technique, which should be employed only under emergent circumstances, involves femoral venous access by means of a large bore peripheral IV catheter using femoral pulse and/or anatomical landmarks as guides.

Currently, the optimal type and volume of IV solution to employ in acute hemorrhagic shock is still a subject for debate. It would appear, however, that the limited evidence available points toward smaller volumes of hetastarch, hypertonic saline (HTS), plasma, or whole blood as being the most effective in terms of replacing intravascular volume, minimizing inappropriate immune response and cellular injury, and improving overall survival. Unfortunately, HTS solutions are not readily available commercially for use as intravascular volume replacement, whole blood and plasma are impractical, and effective artificial blood replacements are as yet to be discovered. Hetastarch, however, is currently being stocked in deployment settings. As such, the general consensus for treatment of uncontrolled hemorrhage is to use the minimal quantity of IV volume replacement required to maintain minimally-adequate tissue perfusion. Reasonable endpoints for this state include a palpable femoral pulse, a systolic blood pressure of 90 mm Hg, and improved mental status in nonhead injured patients. This state is best achieved through a 250- to 500-cc bolus of Hetastarch, followed by judicious isotonic crystalloid infusion, if needed. Lacking hetastarch or in the case of intra-osseous access (where hetastarch and HTS are currently not recommended), judicious use of IV crystalloid solution to maintain the aforementioned minimal adequate perfusion is recommended.

Recently, chitosan- and fibrin-based hemostatic dressings have been developed and fielded; however, definitive data regarding their efficacy, recommended usage, and limitations in human subjects are still forthcoming (4).

Dysbarism Patient Care

The term *dysbarism* refers to the pathological effects upon human systems exerted by decreased or increased ambient atmospheric pressure. This entity should be suspected in casualty care settings that involve underwater operations involving SCUBA, rebreather or mixed-gas breathing apparatus; rapid ascent to high altitude in nonpressurized aircraft or after rapid decompression; and in the setting of thermobaric or closed-space detonation of munitions (such as MOUT or combat vehicles).

Generally, dysbarism is subdivided into barotrauma, arterial gas embolism (AGE) and decompression illness (DCI). In addition, nitrogen narcosis and oxygen toxicity are conditions unique to the diving medicine setting, generally resolve with ascent to sea level, and as such, will not be addressed here. Barotrauma includes potentially any injury relating to the mechanical effects of trapped-gas expansion within the body.

AGE results most from the pulmonary over-pressure syndrome in which the victim undergoes traumatic injury to the pulmonary vascular bed as a result of rapid ascent without adequate exhalation. The combination of the entry of macroscopic gas bubbles into the pulmonary venous system (which translates rapidly into gas bubbles into the left atrium and ventricle and thus arterial system) coupled with Boyle's law (decreasing pressure causes a corresponding increase in volume given a near-constant temperature) results in potentially catastrophic cerebral, coronary, visceral, and extremity arterial occlusion.

DCI results when an individual breathing ambient air at a given depth or altitude ascends too rapidly, resulting in the macroscopic accumulation of nitrogen gas bubbles, which were previously in solution in the body tissues. These resulting and expanding bubbles may exert mechanical traumatic effects as well as biochemical and autoimmune damage to organs, soft tissues, bones, and joints, and may potentially cause death. DCI is classically divided into types I ("the bends") and II ("the chokes" or "the staggers"). As its eponym implies, DCI-I involves the extremities, joints and skin, primarily. DCI-II, which is the more serious clinical entity, involves the central nervous system (CNS), including brain and spinal cord, cardiopulmonary system, or the inner ear.

The definitive treatment of AGE or severe DCI involves hyperbaric therapy. Evacuation units and organic medical elements of operational units engaged in activities that risk dysbarism should include the identification, liaison, and transport preplanning for emergency hyperbaric chamber access. Ground evacuation routes should be selected that minimize ascent to elevation to the extent possible. Likewise, nonpressurized aircraft should attempt the lowest flight altitude that is possible given safety and tactical situation, to include near nap-of-earth flight, if practicable. Pressurized aircraft should avoid ascent over 8,000 feet, at which point sea level-equivalent cabin pressure becomes difficult to maintain.

En route care of dysbarism patients is primarily supportive. Basics include confirmation or establishment of a secure and patent airway, adequate oxygenation and ventilation, analgesics, and splinting of affected extremities.

Despite previous literature, no evidence exists to support transport either in the head-elevated or the head-depressed position. As such, it is recommended that patients with suspected dysbarism be transported either in the supine position, or in a similar position of comfort, unless other injuries are present and preclude such positioning. Supplemental high-flow oxygen is recommended, as it may hasten nitrogen washout in DCI cases. Limited evidence also suggests potential salutatory effects of aspirin (325 mg is suggested) and lidocaine (1 to 1.5 mg/kg IV) for suspected AGE or DCS-II. As the risks of these agents in otherwise healthy individuals are relatively low, both are suggested as potential adjuncts while en route to hyperbaric treatment. Current evidence, although limited, speaks against the use of glucocorticoids in the setting of DCS or AGE.

Head Injuries and Seizures

Both blunt and penetrating head injuries continue to be common occurrences in modern conflict, despite the advent of improved helmets. Associated concerns include airway injuries, eye or ear trauma, maxillofacial fractures, intracranial hemorrhage, infection, and seizures.

Multiple trauma patients with head injuries who are in shock should first receive stabilization aimed at airway control, adequate ventilation and oxygenation, and hemodynamic support to the level that adequate perfusion of the CNS and other vital systems are restored. In cases of head injury where the airway is not secure or in the event of inadequate ventilatory effort, rapid sequence intubation (RSI) is suggested prior to evacuation, if practicable. In such cases, current though limited evidence continues to support the use of prophylactic lidocaine (1 mg/kg IV) if the patient is not hypotensive (5,6). In addition, induction agents should be selected which possess both sedative and analgesic properties. Etomidate (0.3 mg/kg) is an ideal single-agent for induction, because it is short-acting, possesses analgesic and inductive properties, and has minimal negative hemodynamic effects. Alternative or follow-up agents include a combination of midazolam (0.1 mg/kg) and fentanyl (2 μg/kg). Vecuronium (0.1 mg/kg), a nondepolarizing neuromuscular blocking agent, is recommended as a paralytic, although care should be exercised due to its long effect life (30 to 50 minutes). After the airway has been secured, ventilation should be maintained with supplemental oxygen to maintain a pulse oximetry reading of 99%.

Patients with blunt head injuries may be at risk for coincidental cervical spine injury; thus, rigid cervical immobilization is recommended during transport. If signs of intracranial pressure elevation are present (deteriorating mental status in the absence of shock, dilated unilateral pupil, decorticate or decerebrate posture), mild hyperventilation is appropriate, although this procedure is best guided by arterial blood gas analysis for pCO$_2$ (ideal range 32 to 35 torr). If hemodynamically stable, the osmotic diuretic mannitol may be administered intravenously (0.5 to 1 mg/kg). An indwelling urinary catheter may facilitate patient care if mannitol is administered en route. As with patients with dysbarism and enclosed-space air collection, patients with suspected intracranial injury should be transported at the minimal possible altitude, and should be positioned either in the supine or 30-degree upward angle of bed, if clinically and tactically appropriate.

Seizure is a common complication of craniocerebral trauma, and may adversely impact outcome if left untreated. Seizures occurring in the setting of craniocerebral trauma should be controlled initially with lorazepam or diazepam administered intravenously (0.05 to 0.1 mg/kg). This dose may be repeated if necessary, with the warning that these agents may precipitate respiratory depression and hypotension. The patient should then receive a loading dose of Fosphenytoin (17 mg/kg IV infusion at 150 mg/min or IM) or phenytoin (17 mg/kg IV infusion given at a rate not to exceed 50 mg/min).

Transport of craniocerebral trauma patients should be conducted at maximum safe speed to the nearest available source of neurosurgical intervention.

Hypoglycemia

Blood glucose is the exclusive metabolic substrate for the brain, and plays a critical role in other biochemical processes. Glycogen, the storage form of glucose in the liver and muscle, is quickly depleted by stress, shock, injury, and environmental insults. This condition may be further exacerbated in glucose-intolerant individuals. Hypoglycemia, defined as blood glucose <55 mg/dL, may cause altered mental status, impaired metabolism, and may result ultimately in shock, coma, and death, if untreated.

Hypoglycemia should be suspected in combat casualties with altered mental status, even in the setting of head injury. This condition is readily diagnosed if a handheld glucometer is available. In cases of altered mental status in the absence of a glucometer, or if hypoglycemia is diagnosed, a 25 g dose of 50% dextrose (D50W) should be administered. If mental status improves, the dose may be repeated until blood glucose is returned to a level >60 mg/dL.

Hyperglycemic states have been associated with adverse outcomes in craniocerebral trauma, however if hypoglycemia cannot be excluded, a single dose of D50W is unlikely to cause frank hyperglycemia. As such, its trial administration is warranted, if available in the aforementioned circumstances.

Rhabdomyolysis and Acute Renal Failure

Rhabdomyolysis is a clinical entity which results from muscle injury (7). Although it may occur as a result of myotoxic chemical ingestion or myopathies, it is most commonly seen in the trauma setting resulting from the combination of excessive exertion with dehydration, or in crush injuries. This results in the release of myoglobin into the blood stream, with subsequent acute intrinsic renal failure (AIRF). In the setting of exertion with dehydration, rhabdomyolysis may be confounded by prerenal azotemia. Kidney damage is believed to result from two mechanisms: mechanical obstruction of nephrons by myoglobin, and by direct chemotoxic effects of myoglobin on nephrons and proximal tubules. When taken alone, rhabdomyolysis is usually self-limited and responds well to supportive care. In combat casualties, however, it may compound the effects of other injuries and lead to a multiple organ failure state, which has been linked to markedly increased risk for mortality.

While the diagnosis of rhabdomyolysis will not likely be made until the patient reaches level III CHS assets, it should be suspected in any casualty presenting in a hypovolemic state who has recently been under exertion (which describes a large proportion of the casualty population). In addition, delayed or long-distance evacuation may place the casualty at greater risk for development of this condition. An initial screening test for rhabdomyolysis includes the presence of "blood" on a urine chemical dipstick with the absence of erythrocytes on microscopic urinalysis, as both myoglobin and hemoglobin will render a positive urine chemical test. Serum and urine myoglobin is an unreliable marker for rhabdomyolysis, due to early blood stream clearance and variable concentration in the urine during the AIRF state. More reliable and definitive diagnosis may made when supranormal concentrations of creatine kinase (CK) are detected in the bloodstream, which may occur within 24 hours of injury, and may remain elevated for days following. The full syndrome is present when serum creatinine (the primary chemical marker for AIRF) also rises above normal concentrations. Hypocalcemia, oliguria, coagulopathy, and hyperkalemia may ensue, followed by deterioration and death if untreated.

To date, neither specific, outcome-based guidelines exist for the diagnosis of rhabdomyolysis nor for when it should be treated. As such, a suggested guideline for the diagnosis of clinically significant rhabdomyolysis might include the presence of serum CK levels in excess of 500 mg/dL, or a trend of rising CK levels coupled with rising serum creatinine, despite standard supportive care including adequate hydration.

The treatment of rhabdomyolysis begins with volume replacement. In the acute setting, this translates into adequate IV fluid resuscitation followed by oral rehydration solutions. While definitive clinical data are currently lacking which would allow specific recommendations, it would appear prudent to suggest that aggressive IV volume replacement be withheld until active sources of hemorrhage have been controlled. As such, initial en route care should include prudent IV fluid replacement to maintain adequate tissue perfusion, coupled with a transfer report advising the gaining CHS unit of the patient's status and suspected risk of rhabdomyolysis, if applicable. After hemostasis has been accomplished and normal hemodynamic status has been restored, copious administration of isotonic crystalloids are the fluid of choice for total-body fluid volume replacement. Care undertaken for postresuscitative surgical patients en route to level III CHS elements may thus include more aggressive fluid replacement as well as urinary output monitoring, as directed by the transferring physician. In such circumstances, placement of an indwelling urinary catheter with reservoir prior to evacuation will facilitate en route urine output monitoring. In cases of mild exertional rhabdomyolysis without organ system failure, most patients will recover with such supportive care.

While no well-controlled human studies exist, significant animal data supports the use of serum and urine alkalinization both for the clearance of myoglobin by increasing its solubility, as well as for its potential protective effect on nephrons. Like so many other aspects of this condition, the determination of when to alkalinize is still a subject of debate. It would be prudent, however, to consider early alkalinization in patients who manifest elevated serum creatinine in the presence of serum CK levels in excess of 1,000 or who have clinical histories and examinations strongly suspicious for rhabdomyolysis (i.e., a patient with a crush injury and brown-pigmented urine). Alkalinization may be achieved by an IV bolus of 1 to 1.5 mEq/kg of sodium bicarbonate (or 100 mEq for the average adult), which is followed by an IV infusion of normal bicarbonate that is initiated at a rate of 150 cc/hour and titrated by urine pH. D5-Normal bicarbonate solution may be prepared by injecting three standard 50 mEq ampules of sodium bicarbonate into 1 L of 5% dextrose in water (D5W). Initially, alkalinization should be confirmed by an arterial or venous pH approximating 7.5 with a corresponding urine pH over 6.5. After a steady state has been achieved, urine pH may be followed by chemical dipsticks.

Rhabdomyolysis with renal failure that does not respond to adequate hydration and alkalinization may benefit from hemodialysis with hemofiltration to remove myoglobin pigment. Progression to oliguric renal failure will require dialysis until recovery.

Respiratory Distress

Once a patent and secure airway has been established or confirmed, the next most critical component of en route care is the assurance of adequate ventilation and oxygenation. Naturally, respiratory distress is a direct threat to casualty survival, and its detection and treatment are paramount to the en route care provider.

The causes of acute respiratory distress are legion. They may include, alone or in combination, any of the following states: acute traumatic, mechanical or inflammatory airway obstruction; pneumothorax or hemothorax; pericardial effusion/tamponade; pulmonary embolism; congestive heart failure resulting in pulmonary edema; noncardiogenic pulmonary edema (NCPE) resulting from iatrogenic opioid overdose, near-drowning, acute respiratory distress syndrome or high altitude; chemical pneumonitis (CBRNE agents, inhalation of tactical smoke or volatile chemicals released during enclosed space fires in MOUT settings or combat vehicle extrication); infectious pneumonitis (community-acquired or CBRNE agent-induced); carbon monoxide inhalation or other toxicant-induced hemoglobinopathies; acute bronchospasm; and dysbarism-related bronchial or pulmonary injuries. The end result, however, is similar: impaired ventilation and oxygenation which will require intervention.

Initial signs and symptoms of acute respiratory distress include patient reports of difficulty breathing or "air hunger" (then sensation that one cannot breathe effectively); abnormal respiratory rate (presuming a normal range of 10 to 24 respirations per minute); observable or measurable decreases in air movement during inspiration or expiration; stridor or audible wheezing; visible scalene or intracostal muscle retractions, copious respiratory secretions with or without cough; cyanosis; wheezes, crackles or rhonchi on pulmonary auscultation; and hypoxemia as measured by transcutaneous pulse oximetry. Caution is advised when interpreting pulse oximeter data, because inaccuracies may result from peripheral vasoconstriction, improperly applied leads, and motion artifact. In addition, carbon monoxide toxicity will result in artificially elevated pulse oximetry measurements, unless the device contains a co-oximeter.

If respiratory distress is suspected, resuscitative care should be instituted and a reversible cause should be sought preferably before evacuation, or if necessary, while en route. Transport altitude should be limited to the extent possible. Supplemental oxygen should be administered with a goal of transcutaneous oxygen saturation of 99%. Inhaled B-2 adrenergic agonists, such as albuterol should be administered if wheezing or decreased air movement is present. Clinical signs of pulmonary edema may be treated with furosemide (0.5 to 1 mg/kg IV) and morphine (0.1 mg/kg), if hemodynamic status is stable and dehydration is not present. Suspected tension pneumothorax should be treated initially with needle decompression thoracostomy. Although there is no specific treatment available for pulmonary embolism en route, supportive care should be provided and receiving providers should be advised if this diagnosis is suspected.

If the patient exhibits signs of acute airway obstruction or respiratory failure, endotracheal intubation should be performed via direct laryngoscopy with Magill forceps available for foreign object removal, if discovered. If orotracheal intubation fails in this setting, emergent surgical cricothyroidotomy should be performed.

Infection Prophylaxis

The setting of conflict has been described arguably as an environment in which "dirt is dirtier" than in developed settings (8). Further, preliminary studies in animal models imply a significant benefit to early antibiotic administration for the prevention of soft tissue infections and sepsis in the setting of soft tissue penetrating trauma (9). Given these observations, and the limited risk of antibiotic administration to otherwise immunocompetent and antibiotic-naïve individuals without hypersensitivity to the agent administered, it is recommended that early antibiotic prophylaxis in the echelon I, II and en route care setting be administered.

If antibiotic prophylaxis is to be employed, the agent of choice would be simple to administer, effective over a broad spectrum of potential pathogens, be absorbed and reach bactericidal tissue concentrations rapidly, require once- or twice-daily administration, and be cost-effective. With the limited prospective data available, recommended agents that meet this profile include the quinolones levofloxacin (500 mg orally or IV once daily) or gatifloxacin (400 mg PO or IV once daily), and the third generation cephalosporin ceftriaxone (1 to 2 g IV or IM once daily). Ceftriaxone is considered superior to other cephalosporins in this case due to its ease of administration and single daily dosing, broad antimicrobial spectrum and rapid absorption, and minimal hypersensitivity profile.

Antibiotic prophylaxis is recommended for penetrating trauma of the thorax, abdomen, pelvis, neck, or extremities, and may be particularly useful in settings where transport to definitive care may be delayed due to weather, terrain or hostile action. Oral levofloxacin or gatifloxacin is suggested for casualties with an intact airway who are capable of ingesting solids and liquids. Ceftriaxone is recommended for casualties with altered mental status, shock, penetrating abdominal wounds or suspected acute abdomen, or in cases of known hypersensitivity to quinolones.

Pain and Analgesia

Despite decades of dogma to the contrary, numerous studies have demonstrated that the judicious use of analgesic agents does not significantly alter the physical examination or impede diagnosis (10). In addition, timely and adequate relief of pain is both a humane and often the only effective treatment that may be offered to a casualty awaiting or undergoing evacuation.

In the setting of mild, particularly musculoskeletal injuries, or for suspected renal or biliary colic, a trial of a nonsteroidal anti-inflammatory drugs (NSAIDs) (either ibuprofen 800 mg, or ketorolac 15 mg IV or 30 mg IM) is appropriate. For more severe wounds, or if NSAIDs fail to provide adequate relief, opioid analgesics provide definitive acute analgesia. Despite the advent of numerous alternative agents, morphine continues to be the most efficacious as well as cost-effective opioid analgesic. The appropriate initial dose is 0.1 to 0.2 mg/kg IM; the same initial dosage is appropriate for IV administration, but should be administered in aliquots of 2 to 4 mg until the patient reports adequate analgesic effect. In the appropriate settings, oral oxycodone or hydrocodone (5 mg usually formulated with 500 mg acetaminophen), one to two tablets administered every 4 to 6 hours or fentanyl transdermal patches (25 mcg—up to three may be applied) may be given. Although a relatively new development in deployment settings, the fentanyl patch is gaining acceptance due to steady-state analgesia for periods up to 72 hours, making this agent especially appropriate in settings where evacuation may be delayed, but adequate patient observation may be maintained.

Despite common practice, the majority of patients experiencing acute pain syndromes who receive adequate but judicious opioid analgesic dosages will not require continuous physiologic monitoring. If, larger opioid dosages are required for adequate analgesia or if there are signs or a suspicion of altered mental status, respiratory compromise, or shock, then the patient should be closely monitored during initial care and transport. In the event of iatrogenic overdosage of opioids, the provider may administer naloxone, an opioid antagonist, at a dosage of 0.2 to 2 mg IV or IM. This dosage may be repeated as necessary, but should be given judiciously, as complete opioid reversal will result in relapse of pain.

Anaphylaxis

Exposure to environmental agents, petroleum and other industrial chemicals, munitions, medications, and even latex medical equipment may precipitate an allergic hypersensitivity reaction. The worst example of this condition is anaphylactic shock, resulting from massive histamine release. This clinical entity may comprise bronchospasm, bronchorrhea, hypotension, urticaria, altered mental status and may culminate in cardiac arrest quickly followed by death. As such, it must be recognized and treated rapidly.

In the setting of the combat casualty, where hemorrhagic shock, respiratory distress, and altered mental status may already be present as consequences of initial wounding or accident, the en route care provider must maintain increased vigilance for anaphylaxis. When it occurs, the setting usually involves sudden clinical decompensation not readily explained by existing injuries, often accompanied by a rapidly developing pruritic, maculopapular, coalescent erythematous rash (urticaria). Caution is recommended, however, as urticaria does not always accompany anaphylactic shock.

En route care management of anaphylactic shock begins with assuring a secure airway and adequate ventilation. Subsequently, true anaphylactic shock should be treated with epinephrine. Commonly, it is administered as a 1:1,000 concentration in a dose of 0.3 cc subcutaneously. If IV access is established and the 1:10,000 IV dosage ampule is available, then epinephrine may be prepared and administered as a 1:100,000 unit dose by combining 1 cc of standard IV epinephrine with 9 cc of normal saline or lactated ringer's solution. This 1:100,000 unit dose may be administered in aliquots of 1 to 2 cc until adequate hemodynamic and respiratory status is restored.

In cases of initially-stabilized anaphylactic shock, or for milder presentations of acute allergic reactions, the histamine-1 antagonist diphenhydramine should be administered (1 mg/kg up to 50 mg, as an IV bolus over 2 minutes, or IM if IV access is not available). In addition, cimetidine (a histamine-2 receptor antagonist with histamine-1 side effects) should be administered if available (4 mg/kg up to 300 mg IV or IM), followed by methylprednisolone (1.5 mg/kg up to 125 mg IV or IM). In stabilized patients, oral prednisone 60 mg is an alternative.

Anaphylactic shock patients should be transported to the nearest available CHS level III facility capable of providing medical intensive care.

Carbon Monoxide and Other Inhalational Toxicants

Patients who sustained their injuries coincidental to a closed-space fire or tactical smoke use (MOUT or combat vehicle damage), or whose primary presentation is respiratory distress in such a setting, are at risk for intoxication by a host of inhaled chemicals. These agents include carbon monoxide, low-level cyanide, petrochemical vapors and tactical smokes. Noteworthy among these is concentrated white tactical smoke (as may be encountered in MOUT building-clearing operations), which when combined with humid environments or precipitation, may form a phosgenelike toxic gas. In addition, several CBRNE agents incite chemical pneumonitis, pulmonary edema or hemorrhage, or decreased erythrocyte oxygen-carrying capacity, all of which may cause an immediate life threat or complicate extant combat trauma.

Although the diagnosis of toxic chemical inhalation may not be made definitively until the patient reaches level III CHS assets, it should be suspected in any casualty with respiratory distress that is either unexplained or out-of-proportion to existing wounds. Signs and symptoms may include tachypnea, tachycardia, hypoxemia by pulse-oximeter, cyanosis, retractions, altered mental status, or agitation.

En route care interventions in this setting are limited, and begin with active airway and ventilatory support as needed. High flow oxygenation either by non-rebreather mask or endotracheal tube should be administered to optimize tissue oxygenation as well as to induce oxygen washout of toxic gasses (recall Dalton's law). If possible, an attempt may be made to determine to which type of agents that the patient may have been exposed. Expended munitions or intact shells, container ingredient labels, and HAZMAT data sheets maintained in some industrial facilities are examples of clues that may assist the provider in determining possible toxicants.

If a specific agent is suspected or identified, this information should be communicated to providers at the accepting CHS facility, preferably while en route, if possible. By doing so, the receiving facility may locate or otherwise obtain specific antidotes as applicable (cyanide treatment kits, nerve agent antidotes, etc.), prepare isolation facilities, and summon resuscitation teams.

Burn Patients

Traditionally, burns have composed a relatively small percentage of battlefield casualties, with the notable exceptions of MOUT operations and large-scale mechanized forces battles. In the current SASO environment, with its shift toward operations in urban areas, increased vulnerability to tactical aircraft and vehicles, and the resurgence in the use of incendiary devices as improvised munitions by hostile forces, burn treatment has returned to the fore.

Traditionally, militarily significant burn exposures have been grouped into three categories: thermal, chemical, and electrical. A significant hybrid of these categories is produced by thermobaric munitions, whose blast, heat, and violent barometric shock effects result in markedly increased lethality, as well as more severely injured survivors.

On first blush, it might appear that there is little to do for burn patients en route, beyond general supportive care. To the contrary, the risk of potentially long time intervals between initial injury and level III CHS, with the concomitant environmental and tactical exposures, warrants more in-depth initial and transport treatment, if practicable. In addition, burns often are complicated by trauma in the setting of the combat casualty. This forms a potentially deadly combination, as injury severity and subsequent mortality indices are increase significantly. The practical conclusion is that casualties with significant burns warrant aggressive treatment in the CHS I, II, and en route care phases.

Both diagnosis and therapeutic intervention for burn casualties is facilitated by an accurate field assessment of the depth, severity and expanse of the burned tissues. Although the reader is referred to appropriate texts for a detailed discussion of this topic, a brief review follows.

Burn expanse is described as percent of total body surface area (TBSA). A rapid and facile estimate of TBSA may be determined by using "the rule of nines." In adults, this rule assigns 9% TBSA each to the head and neck and to each upper extremity; 1 % to the perineum; and 18% each to the anterior trunk, posterior trunk, and to each lower extremity. In infants, an adjustment is made for the relatively large proportion of TBSA composed of the head; to whit, in infants, use 18% for head and neck, 1% for perineum, 18% each for anterior and posterior trunk, 9% for each upper extremity, and 14% for each lower extremity. A more accurate although time-consuming estimate employs the respective patient's palm surface area as a crude approximation of 1% TBSA.

Burn severity is generally defined by degrees. **First-degree** burns are composed of epithelial epidermal injury only. There is redness, pain, and tenderness to palpation, but no blisters or charring. **Second-degree** burns involve partial thickness skin injury and usually present with blisters, erythema, and severe pain. **Third-degree** burns involve full-thickness injury of the dermis and subcutaneous tissues. The burn appears charred, white, or leathery, and is usually insensate. Border areas may be erythematous and tender. **Fourth-degree** burns involve muscle, fascia, and bone.

Determination of depth (full- or partial-thickness) is best deferred to burn specialists equipped with special diagnostic methodologies, such as biopsy, ultrasound, and laser Doppler flowmetry.

En route care for the burn casualty commences, as always, with assuring or establishing a patent airway, adequate ventilation and oxygenation, and a hemodynamic state that supports adequate tissue perfusion. The latter becomes a paramount concern in casualties with significant burns, due both to insensible losses of fluids through the burned tissues as well as broader third-spacing of fluids as a result of the burn injury. These events conspire to decrease intravascular volume, potentially endangering vital organs and systems.

Airway burns should be treated as an emergent condition, due to the risk of sudden and massive upper airway edema, precipitating airway collapse that often becomes refractory to orotracheal intubation. They should, however, be differentiated from simple facial burns, which do not present an airway emergency. Signs of potential airway burn include a mechanism of enclosed-space fire or thermobaric blast; and physical signs including carbonaceous sputum, oro- or nasopharyneal burns, raspy voice, or stridor. Patients presenting with suspected airway burn should undergo RSI and endotracheal intubation as soon as possible prior to the actual development of airway compromise. In such cases, the provider should be prepared to perform cricothyroidotomy as a rescue maneuver if the orotracheal route fails.

Several formulas have been published for the calculation of fluid resuscitation volumes in burn settings. Although the optimal method for directing fluid resuscitation in burn patients is to maintain a minimum urine output of 35 cc/hour in adults (1 cc/kg/hour for children under 2 years and 0.5 cc/kg/hour for children), a reasonable guideline for the en route care provider to initiate would be 2 cc/kg estimated body weight multiplied by the estimated total body surface area of the burn, administered over the first 8-hour period. This constitutes the first half of the total burn resuscitation volume recommended by the Parkland Formula (with the remaining 2 cc/kg per percent of TBSA to be administered over the following 16-hour period) (11). It is important to note that burn patients will require this fluid volume simply for burn resuscitation; additional IV fluids will likely be required for replacement of acute traumatic injuries, normal requirements, and for replacement of additional insensible losses, such as that produced by tachypnea or dehydration state occurring prior to injury. Thus, for example, in the first 8-hour period, an 80-kg adult with a 30% TBSA second- and third-degree burn and a partially amputated arm, who was already dehydrated prior to evacuation and who has other injuries, may require 5,800 cc for burn resuscitation, 1,200 cc for normal maintenance, 2,000 cc for replacement of fluids lost by dehydration; and 1,000 cc or more due to an extremity hemorrhage controlled by a tourniquet. Given these infused volumes, as well as the requirement for monitoring urine output as a guide for further fluid administration, placement of an indwelling urinary catheter and reservoir should be placed at the first opportunity.

Optimal solution for initial IV volume replacement is lactated ringers (LR) solution; an alternative is normal saline, although this solution is associated with the risk of developing hyperchloremic metabolic acidosis due to the relatively large volumes required during resuscitation. In pediatric patients, LR with 5% dextrose (D5LR) is recommended due to the propensity for hypoglycemia due to metabolic stress.

Casualties being transported from near point-of-wounding who are victims of white phosphorous (WP), tar, napalm, or other volatile agents may require decontamination or neutralization of the offending agent prior to evacuation, if tactically feasible. The reason for this measure is to attempt to arrest the process of continued tissue damage. If possible, WP wounds should be immersed in water to mitigate continued burning; if available, a topical mixture of suspension of 5% sodium bicarbonate and 3% copper sulfate in 1% hydroxyethyl cellulose, should be applied. Tar burns should be flushed copiously with cold water until the tar hardens and is cool to the touch. Napalm and other petroleum/volatile liquid residues should be flushed with cool water until removed.

Additional en route care measures include the application of dry, sterile dressings or single large clean sheets to burned surfaces, keeping the patient warm, en route physiologic and urine-output monitoring, if practicable, and adequate analgesia. Opioids, such as morphine (0.1 to 0.2 mg/kg) for IV administration in cases of moderate to severe burns or oxy- or hydrocodone with acetaminophen (one or two 5/500 mg tablets) for minor burns are the most appropriate analgesics for use in this setting.

Patients with first-degree burns or second-degree burns of <10% TBSA not involving the head, perineum, or full-circumference of an extremity may be initially managed by level I CHS providers and returned to duty. Such patients with coincidental traumatic injury, or more severely burned patients, should be evacuated to higher level CHS for further evaluation and management.

Circumferential burns pose a greater risk to casualties in the form of potential vascular compromise due to the formation of an eschar. These lesions are charred, noncompliant band of burn tissue, and are often accompanied by underlying tissue edema and related extravascular extravasation of fluids. Third- and fourth-degree burn eschars that extend around the entire circumference of an extremity may induce a compartment-like syndrome culminating in vascular compromise, ischemia, and ultimately, loss of the extremity. Likewise, circumferential eschars of the trunk may cause life-threatening respiratory insufficiency resulting from severely degraded thoracic compliance during inspiration. Last, circumferential neck eschars may endanger the airway or cerebral circulation.

Emergency escharotomy in the en route care setting should be performed only as a last resort, primarily when signs of distal vascular compromise, altered mental status, or respiratory distress are present. The procedure is usually accomplished with a scalpel, although electrocautery devices are also effective if available. Neck escharotomy should be performed by incising the full-thickness of the eschar from sternal notch superiorly to the level of the chin. Escharotomy of the thorax is performed by making bilateral incisions along the anterior axillary lines extending from each respective clavicle to the level of the tenth ribs. Once completed, the vertical incisions should be connected by horizontal incisions extending across the anterior chest in order to form a free-floating square of eschar tissue with the intended result of improved thoracic compliance. Extremity eschars should be performed as longitudinal incisions on both the medial and lateral surfaces of the affected extremities, extending the full length of the eschar. If required, hand escharotomy may be performed by making the incision over the palmar crease through the constricting eschar. If the wrist is involved, the incision should be directed toward the ulnar side once crossing the wrist in order to avoid the superficial palmar arch vessels. Digital (fingers and toes) may be decompressed by making similar medial and lateral incisions to the level of the intrinsic muscle fascia.

Escharotomy performed several hours after initial injury may result in temporary reperfusion injuries, which present in a fashion closely resembling compartment syndromes. Thus, en route care providers who are transporting patients postecsharotomy should remain vigilant for recurrent signs of distal extremity ischemia, and should be prepared to perform fasciotomies if evacuation is delayed or expected to be long in duration.

Altered Mental Status & Combative Patients

The confused, agitated and in the worst case, the combative patient, may present an extreme challenge to the en route care crew. Perhaps more than in the case of other evacuation missions, the provider and vehicle crew members must take definitive and pre-emptive measures to assure both their safety as well as that of all patients transported, including those who are the focus of this discussion.

Early in the evaluation of the altered casualty, and in addition to searching and removing potential weapons, it is critical to rule-out hypoxia, hypoglycemia and obvious signs of craniocerebral trauma as etiologies. Hypoxia should be treated and reversed if possible. Hypoglycemia should be either ruled-out or presumptively treated. If craniocerebral trauma is suspected, initial stabilization should be instituted.

After reversible causes have been ruled-out or treated, the en route care provider must assess whether the casualty poses a safety threat in their current condition, whether restraints might be appropriate and effective, or whether chemical sedation may be indicated. Under such circumstances, it is suggested that the provider errs on the side of conservatism with regard to securing the patient prior to transport.

While still considered by some to be effective in specific in-patient settings, simple physical restraint of agitated or combative patients is not recommended in the evacuation setting. The reasons for this conclusion are multifactorial, and include concerns for vehicle instability and occupant safety presented by a thrashing patient; the risk posed by a combative patient who might slip their restraints while en route; and the difficulty of en route medical assessment of an uncooperative patient. As such, harnesses and straps are suggested only for securing compliant patients to their stretcher or other conveyances.

If the decision is taken to sedate an agitated or combative patient, it becomes incumbent upon the provider to redouble the en route monitoring of that patient, particularly with regard to airway patency, ventilatory effort and hemodynamic status. Physiologic monitors including pulse oximeter (oxygen saturation, heart rate) and ECG monitor (heart rate) should be augmented by physical diagnostic maneuvers, such as pulse checks (rate, strength,

and location), observation of chest movement with respiration, and examination of the oropharynx for pooled secretions (if not intubated). In such settings, placement of a nasopharyngeal airway (NPA) is advisable. Oropharyngeal airways (OPA) are not recommended due to risk of inducing the gag reflex with resulting vomiting and aspiration.

When selecting a sedation agent, the provider should consider duration and depth of sedation desired, comorbidities, known allergies, the setting of transportation, and what agents are available for use. In general, phenothiazines such as haloperidol and chlorpromazine are not recommended for the evacuation setting, due to their risk of inducing seizures, neuroleptic-malignant syndrome and extrapyramidal reactions. Agents such as lorazepam, diazepam, midazolam, ketamine, and diphenhydramine are acceptable agents for en route sedation. The mainstay benzodiazepines lorazepam (0.025 to 0.05 mg/kg IV or IM) and diazepam (0.05 to 0.1 mg/kg IV or IM) provide effective sedation and anxiolysis, and are readily available though routine supply channels. The shorter-acting but more potent midazolam (0.05 to 1 mg/kg IV, IM, or intranasal atomized) provides greater titratability. The dis-associative anesthetic ketamine (1 mg/kg IV or 3 mg/kg IM), although not typically used as a sedative agent, provides an alternative for rapid control of a combative patient without the risk of respiratory depression or hypotension. If used, care should be exercised due to potential side effects including bronchorrhea (treated with atropine or inhaled atrovent), transient hypertension and emergence nightmares. Lastly, the ubiquitous antihistamine diphenhydramine (1 mg/kg IV or IM) provides mild sedation and anti-emetic effects for most patients with minimal alteration in sensorium or physiologic parameters.

In the worst-case scenario, combative patients who may not be effectively restrained by reassurance by providers, physical restraints, or chemical sedation may require RSI, paralysis, and intubation prior to departure in order to ensure safe transport with the ability to perform necessary interventions. Although this is a rare instance, this approach remains a part of the en route care armamentarium.

SUMMARY

Tactical en route care is an emerging concept, borne-out of recent innovations in the forward projection of resuscitative surgery and other advanced life support care beyond the traditional combat hospital setting. Although it presents both unique challenges and new opportunities for its practitioners, and awaits prospective and evidence-based analyses of outcomes and systems development, this unique subdivision of air medical transport has the potential for explosive development in the coming decades.

REFERENCES

1. US Joint Chiefs of Staff, US Department of Defense. *Doctrine for Health Service Support in Joint Operations*. Washington: US Government Printing Office; 2001; Joint Publication 4-02.

2. US Department of Defense. *Dept of Defense Dictionary of Military and Associated Terms*. Washington, DC: Defense Technical Information Center; 2003; JP 1-02 [amended 5 September, 2003].

3. Bellamy RF. The cause of death in conventional land warfare: implications for casualty care research. *Milit Med*. 1984;149:55–62.

4. Pusateri AE, McCarthy SJ, Gregory KW, et al. Effect of chitosan-based hemostatic dressing on blood loss and survival in a model of severe venous hemorrhage and hepatic injury in swine. *J Trauma*. 2003;54:177–182.

5. Levitt MA, Dresden GM. The efficacy of esmolol versus lidocaine to attenuate the hemodynamic response to intubation in isolated head trauma patients. *Acad Emerg Med*. 2001;8:19–24.

6. Durrani M, Barwise JA, Johnson RF, et al. Intravenous chloroprocaine attenuates hemodynamic changes associated with direct laryngoscopy and tracheal intubation. *Anesth Analg*. 2000;90:1208–1212.

7. Bontempo LJ. *Rhabdomyolysis. Marx: Rosen's Emergency Medicine: Concepts and Clinical Practice*. 5th ed. Philadelphia: Mosby; 2002:1762–1770.

8. Mabry RL. *Personal communication*. Brooke Army Medical Center, Texas, 2001.

9. Mellor SG, Cooper GJ, Bowyer GW. Efficacy of delayed administration of benzylpenicillin in the control of infection in penetrating soft tissue injuries in war. *J Trauma*. 1996;40(suppl 3):S128-S134.

10. Ducharme J. Acute pain and pain control: state of the art [published correction appears in *Ann Emerg Med*. 2000;36:171]. *Ann Emerg Med*. 2000;35:592–603.

11. Edlich RF, Bailey TL, Bill TJ. *Thermal burns. Marx: Rosen's Emergency Medicine: Concepts and Clinical Practice*. 5th ed. St Louis: Mosby; 2002:801-13.

Chapter 22

Armored Vehicles in Rescue and Tactical Medical Operations

Robert T. Gerhardt

OBJECTIVES

After reading this section, the reader will be able to:

1. Discuss the history of armored vehicles
2. Understand when the use of armored rescue is appropriate
3. Describe common scenarios and rescue techniques that involve armored vehicles in tactical missions

Both military literature and the popular media abound with accounts of the successful use of armored tactical vehicles (ATVs) in the setting of conflict as well as equally compelling tales of what happened in their absence. Recent documentaries depicting the failed Mogadishu Raid of 1993, the North Hollywood Shootout of 1997, and the Sadr City Uprising of 2004 highlight the potential value of ATVs in both military and law enforcement operations in urbanized terrain, as well as the consequences of their absence. In the current geopolitical climate, the growing threat of domestic terrorist activity, civil unrest, and easy access to illegally acquired military-specification ordnance compels all organizations involved in the homeland security mission to evaluate potential threats and to consider the use of ATVs as one of many tools to mitigate them. As a natural outgrowth of such planning, tactical medical planners and providers should be familiar with the practical application of ATVs to their mission.

A BRIEF HISTORY AND BACKGROUND

Numerous historical references exist with regard to the use of armored conveyances in the ancient world, such as the Egyptian and Roman application of chariot warfare, Hannibal's employment of war elephants, and armored knights and chargers of the medieval period. The first recorded use of motorized ATVs in combat was in the First World War by the British Expeditionary Forces during the Battle of the Somme, in 1916. By the end of that war, the concept of employing ATVs in the setting of conflict was firmly established. Further doctrinal development of ATV strategy

and tactics by such historical figures as George Patton, Erwin Rommel, and Heinz Guderian served to integrate ATVs into combined arms operations. More recent experiences during the Arab-Israeli War of 1973 and Gulf Wars I and II have served to further cement the primacy of the ATV as a means of defeating both fixed fortifications and motorized threats and of delivering or extracting personnel in relative safety despite high-lethality environments. Thus, it is intuitive that ATVs were ripe for adaptation to civil sector use in tactical law enforcement and related homeland security operations.

While the development of armored ambulances has paralleled that of general purpose ATVs, the degree of progress and technical sophistication has been slower for the former. The subordinate nature of tactical medical support, lower funding priorities for medically related initiatives, and understandably higher emphasis on "tooth" versus "tail" innovation have contributed to the common practice of the adaptation of *armored fighting vehicles* into *armored rescue vehicles*, rather than de novo tactical medical vehicle designs.

ADAPTATION AND INNOVATION IN ARMORED VEHICLES FOR TACTICAL MEDICAL OPERATIONS

The preponderance of ATV designs used in tactical medical operations arises from one of three categories: (i) retrofitted military armored fighting vehicles (tracked and wheeled armored personnel carriers); (ii) modified or otherwise up-armored civilian vehicles (armored cars, limousines, sport-utility vehicle variants); or (iii) hybrid "ground-up"–designed urban tactical vehicles. Among these, the vast majority of tracked or otherwise heavily armored ATVs are acquired either on-loan or as property transfers to law enforcement organizations from the U.S. Department of Defense via various military surplus divesture programs. Wheeled vehicle types reflect greater variation, and their acquisition is largely a function of the respective organization's program budget, terrain analysis, and mission requirements. Examples of ATVs used in tactical medical operations, and their respective performance characteristics, are given in Appendix 1.

TACTICAL APPLICATIONS AND IMPLICATIONS

Potential functional uses for ATVs in tactical medicine and related applications are numerous and, to some extent, limited only by the planner's imagination. Common applications include (i) tactical team insertion, including medical elements; (ii) bystander/casualty rescue and tactical team extraction; (iii) use as a weapons platform (lethal or less-than-lethal); (iv) use as a communications platform for a hostage negotiator; (v) use as a CBRNE-hardened operational platform; (vi) use as a medical supply/logistical backhaul vehicle when returning from patient transport; (vii) use as a leader/medical officer reconnaissance platform; and (viii) use as the ultimate mobile incident command or mass casualty triage command post.

Given the myriad potential uses of ATVs and the likely finite resources available to the tactical commander, it is incumbent on the medical planner to integrate medical support or contingency plans requiring ATV usage into the overall mission planning process at the earliest possible point. Considerations during this planning phase include the anticipated number of medical operators to be transported; the type of mission to be executed, along with subordinate phases, if applicable; the anticipated most likely and worst-case casualty/patient transport requirements; the type of care that will be rendered; the evacuation destination and whether ambulance exchange points or helicopter landing zones will be employed; the estimated weight and volume requirements for medical and other rescue-related equipment to be employed by the medical team; and a plan for management and transport of CBRNE-contaminated casualties, if applicable.

Ideally, the medical element should be integrated into the full tactical team and well accustomed to the ATVs, equipment, and other crew members prior to an actual tactical mission. If this is not the case, it is strongly advised that the medical element utilize any available opportunity to become familiarized in the time prior to mission execution.

ARMORED TACTICAL VEHICLE MEDICAL CREW CONSIDERATIONS

When first "saddling-up" in an ATV, the medical operator will likely form two immediate impressions: a sense of greater security and the relatively cramped quarters of the crew compartment. In all but the most spacious ATVs, this sensation will be amplified after taking into account the impact of the confined space on the ability to transport and provide en route medical treatment to casualties/patients.

During the majority of the tactical mission, and certainly during movement phases, the designated vehicle commander and driver (sometimes the same) will have operational control of the vehicle. If operating as part of a convoy, medically designated vehicles are generally placed toward the center or near the trail segment, for both tactical and practical considerations. If it is operating as a single vehicle, the ATV's crew may be charged with several mission phases (e.g., covered movement of the team, reconnaissance and negotiation platform, breach element, fire coverage, casualty and team extraction). It is likely that the medical mission will play a subordinate role.

While preparing for and executing the mission, medical ATV crewmembers will have to cope with constraints placed by payload issues (personnel, patients, and equipment/supplies). Prior to mission execution, it is advisable that medical operators consider both most likely and most dangerous scenarios, and plan their immediate actions in response, so as to employ the greatest possible economy of movement, exposure, complexity, and equipment requirement. The depth of complexity of anticipated medical interventions should correspond proportionally to the tactical zone of operations and the time and distance constraints involved. In general, the principles described in the Tactical Combat Casualty Care (TCCC) module of the American College of Surgeons prehospital trauma life support (PHTLS) curriculum are advisable for application. To whit, medical procedures during the assault/extrication phases ("hot zone") are best limited to rapid and simple hemostatic maneuvers (such as tourniquet application) along with movement into the ATV. Once under the cover of the ATV, the medical operator may perform more complex assessment, emergent airway interventions, and needle chest decompression if required, along with intravenous access if practicable. En route care and follow-on management ("warm zone" and above) may involve pharmaceuticals (analgesics and antibiotics per protocol), splinting and immobilization, mitigation of environmental exposures, and decontamination if appropriate. Further evacuation to definitive care will likely be executed after patient exchange to a standard ground or air ambulance.

In addition to standard environmental threats, the potential for a vehicular fire must be considered when conducting ATV-based medical operations. Efforts at mitigating this threat are aimed primarily at prevention and early intervention. Tactical medical operators anticipating spending significant time in or around ATVs should seriously consider fire-resistant tactical uniforms and undergarments (such as Nomex), eye protection, gloves, helmets, and footwear. Fire-retardant blankets are useful for covering patients undergoing extrication. All crew members should be well versed in locating and employing onboard fire suppression systems. If the ATV is equipped with an onboard Halon or other automated, pressurized-gas fire extinguisher system, crew members should also familiarize themselves with standard vehicle egress instructions and postegress rally plans.

TACTICAL INGRESS/EGRESS DURING OPERATIONS

While the ATV crew commander/driver will likely assume the preponderance of responsibility for deciding where and under what circumstances the medical crew will mount, ride, and tactically egress the ATV, medical operators should be involved in this planning process. Ideally, and presuming the mission does not involve a "hasty" movement-to-contact, there will be sufficient time to consider the type and amount of equipment that the medical operators will require, including patient care and medical supplies, extrication or obstacle-clearing equipment, etc. In general, annexes to the medical mission (e.g., the requirement for forced entry/breach, complex extrications from rubble) are best managed by other tactical operators not charged primarily with medical care. In addition, contingency plans for non-medical-attendant assistance (such as litter bearers and security element) should be considered. In any case, and while weight and cubic volume issues are important, medical operators should approach tactical planning with a "worst-case/most-likely case scenario," and packing/loading should progress to the worst-case scenario as closely as is feasible.

In general, tactical employment of the ATV in medical operations results from the need for speed, cover (vertical as well as horizontal), and lift capability for both patients and treatment personnel. As such, both vehicular and dismounted routes-of-march should be selected and used with an eye toward tactically sound, maximally concealed and covered routes, but must be simultaneously integrated with any other ATVs being employed, as well as with static overwatching elements supporting the ATV patient-extrication mission.

Tactical ingress/egress of the ATV should occur as near to covering structures as possible; if the patient(s) is(are) located in an open, unprotected setting, multiple ATVs may be needed to provide a screen for the designated medical ATV, if they are available. In the event of single-vehicle operations, the medical ATV should be positioned in such a manner that the ingress/egress hatch is pointed in the position possessing the lowest threat posture at the time of arrival. While this observation might appear both intuitive and obvious to the reader, its importance cannot be overemphasized.

As the medical team egresses toward the patient(s), standard tactical movement-to-contact principles should be employed, with the anticipation that threat contact is likely, regardless of the presence of additional nonmedical operators. This "care-under-fire" phase should emphasize rapid but tactically valid movement to the patient and a balance between optimal patient packaging and minimal tactical exposure to hostile fire. As a practical matter, minimal medical intervention should be performed until the patient and tactical medical team are again under adequate cover, whether that be the ATV or temporarily in a fixed structure prior to final extraction.

After arrival back at the ATV, the patient(s) should be loaded as quickly and safely as practicable. If possible given the ATV's configuration, those patients requiring the highest level of care should be loaded last, to facilitate rapid unloading at the destination medical treatment facility or ambulance exchange point. It may be necessary, however, to load patients nondoctrinally based on the potential requirement for en route interventions, number of patients, etc.

SAFETY AND ENVIRONMENT-OF-CARE

While in proximity and once ensconced within the ATV, operators, passengers and patients will be subjected to a unique environment, which is not always benign. A well-worn axiom among ATV professional crew members is "the tank is designed to kill people, and it doesn't care who." To paraphrase, individuals operating in or around an ATV should pay close attention both to their own personal safety and to that of their colleagues and charges.

Specific issues that arise in this setting include climate control; lighting; noise; vibration; spatial disorientation; access to electric, water, and waste management capability; and the potential for blunt or even penetrating injuries due to the confined space and difficulty in anchoring oneself within an ATV crew compartment.

When onboard systems are available, the internal temperature should be modulated using them; if the ATV is so equipped, CBRNE air filtration systems might provide a dual benefit in that they often are capable of cooling or heating the air passing through them, thus providing some augmentation to onboard climate control systems if present.

Adequate lighting for en route care as well as standard vehicle operations may present a challenge, depending on the available onboard lighting systems. In addition, tactical constraints may necessitate subdued or color-filtered lighting, and the potential for operations using passive night vision enhancement devices must be considered in both the planning and the premission training phases. It is prudent for the tactical medical provider to plan to be self-sufficient with regard to lighting support, with the suggestion that personnel obtain and carry their own standard and filtered light sources and backups for use both within the ATV and while dismounted.

In addition to the enhancement of patient care and dismounted tactical operations, lighting devices often provide the most effective means of signaling the presence of dismounted personnel in proximity to an ATV, to mitigate the risk of accidental injury or death due to ATV-pedestrian collision. Dismount signaling as well as vehicle safety should, at the minimum, be discussed and, at best, be rehearsed by the ATV crew-dismount team, which naturally should include tactical medical personnel.

While operating within an ATV, occupants will likely be exposed to levels of noise, vibration, and spatial disorientation that rival those of some tactical aircraft. Thus, as the tactical situation permits, occupants should carry and employ hearing protection, helmets and body armor, field-expedient padding, or other appropriate insulative garments to mitigate this threat. Additionally, extra safety equipment should be carried if practicable for use by patients and passengers who may be transported.

While it is hoped that the ATV phase of tactical medical care will be brief, the requirement for electric power for medical and other equipment, as well as water (for drinking and decontamination) and potential biohazardous waste (body fluids) management capability, should be considered in the planning phase. In addition to these considerations, the real potential for blunt or even penetrating injuries resulting from unrestrained passenger impact on internal crew compartment structures will generally necessitate the continued wear of individual body armor and related protective equipment. Tactical medical personnel should also take whatever steps are available and practical to mitigate the risk of further injury to patients and other passengers during transport by employing available safety equipment, bolsters, restraints, and other field-expedient devices.

EN ROUTE CARE

Unlike the circumstances encountered in standard emergency medical service transports, tactical en route care in the setting of ATV operations is likely to be brief in duration and limited, due to time, space, and tactical constraints. Emphasis should be placed on urgent interventions required to prevent imminent death or irreversible harm. This topic is discussed in more depth in Chapter 21, on en route care.

APPENDIX 1. COMMONLY ENCOUNTERED ARMORED VEHICLES WITH POTENTIAL TACTICAL MEDICAL APPLICATIONS

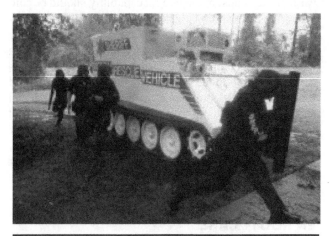

FIGURE 22.1. Modified M-577 armored personnel carrier, Lake County Sheriff Department, Ohio.

▎**TABLE 22.1.** **Specifications from Pinzgauer, Steyr-Diamler-Puch, Inc.**

No. of crew	2	2
Height	2 m	7 ft
Length	5.3 m	17 ft
Max. range	800 km	432 nm
Max. speed	120 kph	75 mph
Max. weight	5,000 kg	11,023 lb
No. of passengers	12	12
Payload	2,400 kg	5,291 lb
Service life	20 yr	20 yr
Span	1.8 m	6 ft
No. of wheels	6	6

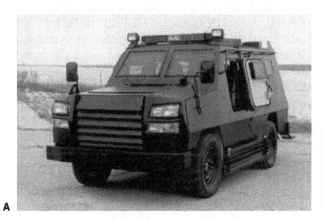

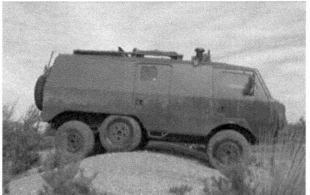

A   B

FIGURE 22.2. Peacekeeper tactical vehicles: Cadillac-Gage Inc. (**A**) and Pinzgauer, Steyr-Diamler-Puch, Inc. (**B**).

Psychological Effects and Management of Law Enforcement and Medical Providers in the Tactical Environment

James L. Greenstone and John G. McManus, Jr.

OBJECTIVES

After reading this section, the reader will be able to:

1. Discuss the concept of hostage and crisis negotiations.
2. Understand the role of the medical provider during a hostage or crisis situation.
3. Understand the role of law enforcement personnel during a hostage or crisis situation.
4. Discuss the basic errors made by medical and allied health personnel during a critical incident.
5. Discuss the psychological effects of a hostage or crisis situation.

HISTORICAL PERSPECTIVE AND PHILOSOPHY

Necessary to the effective management of both medical and law enforcement personnel in the hostage and barricaded environment is an understanding of the procedures utilized and skills available. Negotiations in these environments, to include medical facilities, are never "hit or miss" attempts. Serious skill development is required and effective team function is the rule.

Since the development of modern police hostage negotiations techniques in the 1970s, several typologies have been offered for categorizing hostage takers (1–8). For example, some frameworks are based on whether the perpetrator has a mental disorder or is a criminal (in some cases, including an additional category for terrorists); still others emphasize whether the victim is a stranger versus a family member. Negotiation strategies based on these categorizations are utilized by hostage negotiators in guiding their interventions. In recent years, conceptualizations of the hostage taker have been modified and restructured. The newer conceptualizations also include subjects in domestic crises (9–12). In all cases, an initial assessment and subsequent diagnostic profile is essential for defining the resolution strategies.

SYSTEMS AND ORGANIZATION

One accepted typology for discriminating among hostage takers involves two major categories and at least four subcategories (13–16). As reported in Table 23.1, Psychotic Disorders are distinguished from personality or character disorders. Psychotic Disorders are further divided into Paranoid Schizophrenia and Bipolar Disorder. Despite its absence from the *DSM-IV* (18), the term *manic-depression* has been retained as a useful working diagnosis for hostage negotiators (3). Generally, hostage negotiators have been confronted with the manic-depressive individual in the depressed state (3).

The typology presented is not intended to be exclusive or exhaustive. As with any attempt to understand human behavior, alterations are made as needed to improve procedures and results. Diagnostic and profiling skills are emphasized and expected. While not always achieved, precision is the goal in all instances.

Character Disorders are subdivided into the Inadequate Personality and the Antisocial Personality. Even though inadequate personality is not an accepted DSM-IV diagnosis (18), it has demonstrated usefulness in discriminating among hostage takers.

As shown in Table 23.1, field diagnoses inform negotiation strategies. For example, the approach effective with

▶ **TABLE 23.1. Issues and Concerns in the Tactical Environment.**

Police versus nonpolice
Negotiator versus nonnegotiator
SWAT versus non-SWAT
Knowledge versus skill
The police overlay to negotiation operations
Education versus training
Team member versus "hotdog"
Cooperation versus resistance
Police negotiations versus negotiations

▶ **TABLE 23.2. Roles of the Physician in the Tactical Environment.**

Profiling
Providing medicine across the barricade
Assessing threat for Negotiations Team
Making ongoing threat assessments
Making evaluations
Protecting the force
Participating in the think tank
Advising the Primary Negotiator
Functioning as Coach
Evaluating the intelligence of the hostage taker or barricaded person

the highly depressed and suicidal individual may prove much less useful with the psychotic or antisocial subject. Although there are still some who take the "shotgun" approach to negotiations, the more refined the diagnosis and understanding of the subject involved, the more accurate and precise the negotiation strategies can be. For instance, although problems sustaining effective work relationships are common to inadequate and antisocial personalities, knowing that the underlying difficulties are vastly different in these subjects can be very useful. The overwhelming nature of the work environment for the inadequate personality is quite different from a work environment in constant turmoil due to the actions of the antisocial subject. Whereas the former frequently quits the job, the latter often gets fired. Understanding such nuances may help to select strategies in negotiating with these individuals. For example, the inadequate personality may need the reassurance of the negotiator that he is doing the best that he can despite his sense of repeated failures. The antisocial personality may need to be approached with ego-enhancing statements that reinforce his self-concept. For instance, it might be suggested that it is the employer's fault, not the subject's, that he was fired.

Exceptions to the classifications in Table 23.1 are also seen in the field and are considered when training negotiators. Many who suffer from depression are not bipolar but are reacting to a specific loss in their life (*reactive depression*) or experiencing a unipolar Major Depression. Also, not all persons who commit crimes are antisocial as described above. Some petty criminals are prompted by their circumstances to take hostages to use as leverage against the police. For example, a subject surprised in the act of robbery may take a hostage to use as a shield. The primary motive may have been robbery, not hostage taking. Similar reactions may be seen in medical settings. Although not the prime motivation of a distraught patient, for example, taking a hostage or threatening suicide may be an atypical reaction to stress encountered by medical treatment or external circumstances. Additionally, diagnostic characteristics may overlap somewhat in profiling actual subjects, and negotiators should expect this (19–24).

It is necessary to understand that police negotiators have many and varied responsibilities, and the develop-

ment of perpetrator profiles is only one of several simultaneous responsibilities of the hostage negotiations team members. As differentiated from most other situations in which assessments are made, police negotiators operate as members of specially trained teams with both discrete and overlapping responsibilities (Table 23.2). The broad scope of their duties and responsibilities requires knowledge and abilities both unique to police and common to other negotiation situations. Moreover, an officer's specific role on the negotiations team may vary from one incident to another, depending on the characteristics of the situation, availability of other personnel, and preferences of the team leader.

The organization of a police negotiations team can take various forms. The model reported in Table 23.2 is widely used to address the core responsibilities of the hostage negotiations team. This basic structure can, and should, be modified to meet the needs of specific teams under special conditions, and within the confines of a specific police department. Nevertheless, some negotiations teams will define themselves differently than has been done here and may use other names for the different jobs performed. It may be important to note that the organization of negotiations teams in this country is under study, and current discussions suggest that direction is emerging that may impinge on the current structure. This may include revising the structure of the team and also the utilization of personnel. However, regardless of titles or structure, the goals will remain the same: to get everyone out safely.

A negotiations team may be comprised of as few as one or two members, particularly in small departments that cannot dedicate more to this function. Indeed, in some incidents, a smaller team can be as effective as a larger team. However, where possible, a team of at least five members is advantageous for distributing the different responsibilities. Some teams will utilize more negotiators as a function of the nature of the incident. For instance, an incident that lasts an extended period of time may require more personnel. A more complex terrorist incident may require more negotiators for input or for separate negotiations.

Within the framework of the five-person team, the Primary Negotiator assumes the major responsibility for interacting with the hostage taker or crisis victim. All other jobs on the team are devoted to supporting the role of this negotiator. The Secondary Negotiator is responsible for assisting the Primary Negotiator and for assuring that all intelligence information directed to the Primary is conveyed in a timely and efficient manner. This negotiator also monitors all negotiations and substitutes for the Primary as needed.

The Coach provides a third set of ears in the negotiations room, and this person may be utilized in various additional capacities at the request of the Primary Negotiator, for example, maintaining the negotiations log or conveying information to the Intelligence Coordinator or Team Leader. This third person may also be the Police Psychologist in departments providing such services. He or she monitors the stress level of the Primary Negotiator and the hostage taker, usually referred to as the subject, and is available to provide perspective and input.

The Intelligence Coordinator is the recipient, repository, and developer of intelligence information gathered during an incident. Such information may then be further developed into specific negotiations strategies to be used by the Primary Negotiator. This is the person who would normally be responsible for gathering the information needed for completing field diagnostic assessments. Because complete information about the subject is not usually available, the Intelligence Coordinator is responsible for inserting additional information as it becomes available. Logs and records are also maintained at this level. One of the most beneficial roles of medical professionals involved in these types of situations would be to assist the development and utilization of related intelligence. Please refer to Table 23.3.

The person in charge of the overall functions of the Negotiations Team is the Negotiations Team Leader. The Leader must ensure the efficient functioning of the team while at the same time being available to liaise with the other teams and elements of command that are involved. These may include the Special Weapons and Tactics Team and the Incident Command Staff. The overall efficiency of the Negotiations Team depends on how well this job is performed.

As with most crises, hostage crises seldom occur when you are expecting them and are rested and ready. Call-outs to sensitive and potentially deadly situations can occur at any time, and usually do. Table 23.3 describes the mul-

tiple facets of a typical police hostage or crisis situation. It also describes the polyphasic nature of police negotiations. However, it should be kept in mind that the procedures listed in the table may be modified depending on the specific situation. It should also be underscored that the intelligence function responsible for developing the data for diagnostic assessments is only one of many responsibilities assumed by members of the Negotiations Team. Successful management and resolution of any incident require global knowledge of the sequencing and the skills to perform at any level as the need arises. These requirements for broad knowledge, readiness for action, and flexibility clearly differentiate the hostage negotiations situation from most other negotiations situations and from most clinical situations.

THE MOST SERIOUS ERRORS MADE BY MEDICAL PERSONNEL IN A HOSTAGE NEGOTIATIONS SITUATION OR TACTICAL ENVIRONMENT

1. Failing to understand and to appreciate the level of training and skill attained by the police responders and, as a result, assuming that you know more than they do about resolving the situation at hand.
2. Not following instructions given by the police.
3. Trying to become involved in what is going on without a prior understanding of the situation.
4. Trying to take over the negotiations.
5. Not following instructions given by negotiators or tactical personnel.
6. Not responding to "yes or no" questions when speaking on the phone to the negotiator.
7. Trying to negotiate with the hostage taker or barricaded/suicidal subject.
8. Walking through police lines or perimeters in an attempt to access the hostage taker or hostages.
9. Not providing information to negotiators or to tactical personnel when queried.
10. Not understanding the advisory role of medical personnel in a hostage, barricade, suicide, or other tactical situation.
11. Delaying calling 911 or other police units after the situation begins.
12. Failing to evacuate patients in the area.
13. Attempting to disarm hostage takers or suicidal individual.
14. Failing to allow negotiators and tactical officers to handle the situation
15. Failing to obtain training for self and to train staff about procedures to be followed.
16. Failing to follow established procedures during the incident.

▶ **TABLE 23.3. Police Procedures and the Medical Professional.**

Police procedures are critical.

- Follow the procedures.
- Follow the procedures.
- Follow the procedures.

17. Attempting to appease the hostage taker.
18. Failing to understand the relationship between police procedures and police negotiations. This one will get you killed.
19. Failing to provide needed security of area prior to arrival of police.
20. Unnecessarily giving in to the threats of the hostage taker or barricaded person.
21. Failing to stay safe as the first priority.
22. Failing to understand the police negotiations process.
23. Making unsupportable assumptions.
24. Utilizing nonhelpful significant others in negotiations.
25. Failing to adequately screen significant others prior to consideration of putting them in contact with the hostage taker or barricaded subject.
26. Contradicting the police negotiator during negotiations.
27. Providing too much information.
28. Failing to understand and to recognize when negotiations are being degraded by inappropriate actions.
29. Failing to recognize when progress is made in negotiations.
30. More than one person's attempting to negotiate at the same time.
31. Failing to gather and to use intelligence information intelligently.
32. Not using a team approach to work the situation.
33. Rushing the negotiations process.
34. Failing to obtain proper practical training in the management of hostage and barricaded situations prior to functioning with a hostage negotiations team.
35. Failing to appreciate the tactical emergency medical roles of health care providers, including, for example, (a) providing medicine across the barricade, (b) assessing hostage takers, (c) assessing the threat, and (d) taking care of negotiators and tactical personnel.

TAKE-HOME POINTS

1. Medical and allied health professionals can be of valuable assistance to negotiators and to tactical personnel.
2. The role of medical and allied health professionals must be determined by police personnel and by the totality of the circumstances.
3. It is important that medical professionals be ready to assist as needed and as directed.
4. The more medical professionals understand what to expect, the more helpful they can be.
5. Medical professionals should be ready, be knowledgeable, be trained, and be careful.

SUMMARY

Finding one's self in the middle of a hostage situation or a suicidal crisis is not usually expected fare during the course of a normal day. Such a happening within one's professional setting may complicate matters even further. Appropriate and helpful responses may not be those learned in school or on television. These responses are based on a reservoir of experiences, trial-and-error learning, and psychological understandings of these particular events. The greater the understanding of these situations by health professionals, and the additional knowledge of their particular and unique role, the greater the likelihood of a life-sparing, successful resolution to the instant event.

REFERENCES

1. Fowler WR, Greenstone JL. Hostage negotiations for police. In: Corsini R, Auerbach AJ, eds. *Concise Encyclopedia of Psychology.* 2nd ed. New York: Wiley; 1998.
2. Greenstone JL. *The Elements of Police Hostage and Crisis Negotiations: Critical Incidents and How to Respond to Them.* New York: Haworth Press; 2005.
3. Greenstone JL. The role of tactical emergency medical support in hostage and crisis negotiations. *Prehosp Disaster Med.* 1998;13(2): 130–132.
4. Greenstone JL. *A Hostage Negotiations Team Training Manual for Small and Medium Size Police Departments.* Dallas, TX: Leviton & Greenstone; 1998.
5. Fuselier D, Van Zandt C, Lanceley FJ. The antisocial personality as a hostage taker. *J Police Sci Admin.* 1981;March:30–40.
6. McMains MJ, Mullins WC. *Crisis Negotiations: Managing Critical Incidents and Hostage Situations in Law Enforcement and Corrections.* Cincinnati, OH: Anderson; 1996.
7. Strentz T. The inadequate personality as a hostage taker. *J Police Sci Admin.* 1983;March:30–35.
8. Arieti S. Psychopathic personality: some views on its psychopathology and psychodynamics. *Comprehens Psychol.* 1963;4:301–312.
9. Fowler WR, Greenstone JL. *Crisis Intervention Compendium.* Littleton, MA: Copley; 1989.
10. Greenstone JL, Leviton S. *Elements of Crisis Intervention.* Pacific Grove, CA: Brooks/Cole; 1993.
11. Greenstone JL. Crisis intervention skills training for police negotiators in the 21st century. *J Police Crim Psychol.* 1993;10(1): 47–56.
12. McMains MJ, Lanceley FJ. The use of crisis intervention principles by police negotiators. *J Crisis Negot.* 1995;3(1):3–30.
13. Bolz F. *Hostage Cop.* New York: Rawson, Wade; 1979.
14. Cooper HHA. Negotiating with terrorists. *Int J Police Negot Crisis Manage.* 1997;Spring:1–8.
15. Fuselier GW. A practical overview of hostage negotiations. *FBI Law Enforce Bull.* 1981;June/July:2–5.
16. Hare RD. Psychopaths: new trends and research. *Harvard Ment Health Newslett.* 1995;September:1–5.
17. Strentz T. Law enforcement policy and ego defenses of the hostage. *FBI Law Enforce Bull.* 1979;April:10–13.
18. American Psychiatric Association. *Diagnostic and Statistical Manual of Mental Disorders.* 4th ed. Washington, DC: APA; 1994.
19. Biggs JR. Defusing hostage situations. *Police Chief.* 1987;May: 33–34.
20. Davis RC. Three prudent considerations for hostage negotiators. *Law Order.* 1987;September:54–57.
21. Dolan JT, Fuselier GD. A guide for first responders to hostage situations. *FBI Law Enforce Bull.* 1989;April:10–15.
22. Fuselier GW. What every negotiator would like his chief to know. *FBI Law Enforce Bull.* 1986;March:15–20.
23. Soskis DA, Van Zandt CR. Hostage negotiations: law enforcement's most effective non-lethal weapon. *FBI Manage Q.* 1986;Autumn: 15–21.
24. Wesselius CL. The anatomy of a hostage situation. *Behav Sci Law.* 1983;1(2):10–15.

Chapter 24

Tactical Pharmacology

Robert A. DeLorenzo

OBJECTIVES

After reading this section, the reader will be able to:

1. Understand the principals, limitations and precautions of prescription and over the counter medications in the tactical environment.
2. List the minimum essential components of a medication administration system for TEMS.
3. Discuss common prescription and over the counter medications encountered in the TEMS environment.
4. Understand the unique aspects of medication use and administration in a tactical medical system.
5. Understand the effects of certain medications on human performance.

Most of the medications in common use in prehospital care have application in the broad tactical sense (1). Familiar examples include epinephrine for cardiac arrest, albuterol for bronchoconstriction, and morphine for analgesia. Other medications, while infrequently used in emergency medical service (EMS), may in fact be quite useful given the unique and extreme circumstances encountered on tactical missions (2). Antibiotics for wound prophylaxis, acetaminophen for fever, and oil of clove for dental pain are examples of the latter category.

The tactical provider requires an understanding of the uses and limitations of a broad variety of medications, both prescription and nonprescription (over-the-counter [OTC]). The types and ranges of medications used will necessarily be dependent on the training and licensure of the provider (e.g., emergency medical technician, paramedic, physician). In all cases, the provider must be properly licensed and authorized to administer or dispense the medications described. All states and territories have specific laws and regulations governing dispensing and administration and the reader is encouraged to be familiar with them. Additionally, all nonphysician providers should use medications only in the context of effective and proactive medical direction. This chapter presumes a working knowledge of pharmacology and medication administration and is not intended as a substitute for standard texts on this topic.

PRINCIPALS

An effective program of medication use and administration for a tactical system requires several essential components (Table 24.1). Medical direction by a physician skilled and experienced in both EMS and tactical operations is the key to the success of any such program.

The components of a tactical medication program are similar to those in a typical community EMS system (1). However, the rigors of the tactical environment, remoteness of patients, and isolation of providers all require a degree of system robustness not frequently needed in ordinary EMS systems. Furthermore, if nonphysician providers will be using medications normally on the fringes (or even outside) of the traditional scope of prehospital practice, then a strong system is even more important.

Specific, written protocols must be in place, detailing the clinical conditions that may be treated with medications. The specific medication, indications, contraindications, dose, route, and so forth must be explicitly stated. Given the extreme and sometimes remote conditions encountered in tactical operations, a degree of flexibility and creativity will be required to allow the protocols to be effective (1). Special care must be taken to minimize the reliance on direct or online medical control when developing tactical medication protocols, as this form of communication is often difficult or impossible in the tactical setting.

▶ **TABLE 24.1. Minimum Essential Components of a Medication Administration Program for a Tactical Emergency Medical Service System.**

1. Strong medical direction
2. Clear scope of practice
3. Detailed written protocols
4. Quality assurance review

The medical director is also responsible for ensuring that all personnel authorized to administer medications have completed and remain current in their training.

No program of medical treatment is complete without a system to ensure provider quality, compliance, and performance and patient outcome. Quality assurance provides the data collection, analysis, and feedback necessary to improve provider and system performance and assure patient safety.

When choosing medications for use in the tactical setting, it is not sufficient to take the standard formulary for paramedic practice and adopt it en bloc for tactical use. Some standard prehospital medications may be inappropriate in the tactical setting, while others may need to be included. The overall goal is to establish a formulary that addresses the clinical problems likely encountered on tactical missions yet practical enough to administer in this setting. In general, there are several considerations (Table 24.2) in choosing to add a drug to the list of those available to the tactical medical provider.

Table 24.3 outlines potential drug categories and their use in each tactical zone. For the most part, medications are not indicated in the hot zone (1). The risk of provider and patient exposure to hostile fire is simply too great to justify any potential benefit medications may provide. Drug treatment is indicated in the warm zone but is generally limited to a few agents with high tactical value (e.g., narcotic analgesia) or time-sensitive requirements (e.g., prophylactic antibiotics). On occasion and when the

▶ **TABLE 24.2. Considerations Regarding Drugs for the Tactical Environment.**

1. Choose drugs to treat emergency medical condition likely to benefit from medication administration in tactical setting.
2. Avoid emergency medications unlikely to offer significant benefit in the tactical setting.
3. Choose over-the-counter drugs to treat uncomplicated symptoms likely to interfere with a team member's performance.
4. Avoid medications for treatment of a team member's symptoms that are likely to have unwanted side effects.
5. Choose drugs to provide prophylaxis for patients and team members against potential hazards in the tactical setting.
6. Choose drug types and dosage forms that are easiest and simplest to administer and are least demanding to monitor in terms of side effects.

▶ **TABLE 24.3. Potential Drug Categories with Particular Use in the Tactical Setting.**

Hot zone

■ Drugs not usually indicated

Warm zone

■ Opioid analgesics for severe pain
■ Cephalosporin antibiotics for severe penetrating trauma
■ Atropine and pralidoxime in acute nerve agent exposure
■ Nitrites and thiosulfates in acute cyanide exposure
■ Beta-adrenergic agents (nebulized) for acute riot control agent-induced bronchospasm
■ In limited circumstances, all usual prehospital medications may be appropriate.

Cold zone

■ All the above, plus all the usual prehospital medications
■ Selected nonprescription medications for certain acute symptoms
■ Selected prescription medications for certain acute symptoms (prescribed and administered by physician only)

tactical situation permits, other prehospital medications may also be administered in the warm zone. Once in the cold zone, all available prehospital medications may come into play, and in fact, the care of the patient is often transferred to the supporting EMS agency. Additionally, tactical providers may take advantage of selected nonprescription medications for the treatment of tactical team members acute minor symptoms (see Nonprescription [Over-the-Counter] Medications, discussed later in this Chapter).

EMERGENCY MEDICATIONS

In most tactical settings medications will play a small but potentially important role in the management of acute emergencies, particularly in the warm and cold zones. Depending on the circumstances, all the usual prehospital pharmacological armamentarium may find application in the tactical setting. Good medical and tactical judgment will determine the specific emergency medications appropriate for a given clinical and operational circumstance. In general, emergency drugs for the tactical setting should mitigate serious threats to health and should focus on the medical conditions anticipated in the field.

The management of cardiac arrest prearrest states can be problematic in the warm zone owing to the increased risk of hostile exposure for patient and provider when conducting intensive resuscitation. In most cases, the best course of action may be to move these and other critically ill or injured patients to the cold zone as expeditiously as possible, where full prehospital care can occur. If the benefits of warm-zone drug treatment outweigh the risks of a particular tactical setting, or if movement to the cold zone is impossible, then acute management to include all the usual prehospital medications may be justified.

In penetrating trauma (e.g., gunshot wound) medications play only an adjunctive role. Morphine (or equivalent opioid) for analgesia and a cephalosporin antibiotic are the primary parenteral agents (2). Intravenous (IV) or intramuscular morphine in small (2 to 4 mg or 0.05 to 0.10 mg/kg) increments is safe, effective, and humane, particularly if extraction and transport times are long. Higher doses of morphine are nearly as safe and even more effective, but vigilance is required to prevent dangerous side effects such as hypotension. Relief of suffering, not abolition of all pain, is the desired end point. Transmucosal fentanyl in the form of a "fentanyl lollipop" has been demonstrated to be an effective and safe form of analgesia that does not need to be administered parenterally. In less severe injury or pain, an oral analgesic such as acetaminophen may suffice. Nonsteroidal anti-inflammatory drugs such as ibuprofen have the theoretical disadvantage of dose-dependent platelet dysfunction, and may cause gastric irritation and therefore be less desirable. Cyclo-oxygenase-2 inhibitors such as valdecoxib and celecoxib initially held promise because they offered fewer platelet effects, however, postmarketing association with cardiovascular deaths has led to their withdrawal or restricted use.

While randomized controlled trials have not been performed in operational or even general prehospital settings, prophylactic antibiotics are routine hospital practice. Since time is clearly a factor in efficacy of prophylaxis, early administration in the field is a reasonable recommendation, particularly if the extraction and transport time exceeds 1 hour (1).

Prophylactic antibiotics, usually a first-generation cephalosporin such as cefazolin, are indicated in cases of significant gunshot wounds or other major penetrating trauma (3). A recent thought is to use oral doses of a fluoroquinolone, especially the third- and fourth-generation agents moxifloxacin and levofloxacin (4). The advantage here is the speed of administration (it can be self-administered) and low logistical footprint compared with storing and handling intravenous agents (4). Contraindications include unconsciousness and abdominal injury. Other emergency medications with particular application to tactical medicine include aerosolized beta-adrenergic agents, parenteral anticholinergics, oximes, nitrites, and thiosulfates. Albuterol or other inhaled beta-adrenergic agents may find use in the relief of riot control agent-induced bronchospasm and, also, as adjunctive therapy for certain industrial or terrorist-deployed chemicals such as chlorine and phosgene (5).

Atropine is the prototypical anticholinergic agent used in acute nerve agent exposure and, along with pralidoxime, forms the primary antidote against these highly lethal weapons of mass destruction (6). Thiosulfates and, possibly, nitrites form the current mainstay antidote for acute cyanide exposure, a rare but rapidly lethal threat in tactical operations (5). Given the rapidity with which cyanide acts, early administration of antidotes is imperative in any significant exposure. However, the frequent and potentially lethal hypotension and methemoglobinemia associated with nitrites limits their usefulness and the emerging approach to inhaled cyanide exposures abandons this drug in favor of IV sodium thiosulfate alone. Ingested cyanide toxicity may still benefit from nitrite therapy. In any case, impending approval of the cyanide antidote hydroxocobalamin may obviate the negative side effects of nitrite and thiosulfate agents (7).

In all cases, emergency drugs for anticipated use in the tactical setting should be shelf-stable, premixed, and, ideally, in unit-dose packages or prefilled syringes. It is difficult enough in the ordinary prehospital environment to calculate dosages, mix the drug, and draw up the correct amount. It is likely impossible to perform these functions under the threat of fire without seriously compromising performance or patient safety. Medical directors should work closely with tactical paramedics and organizational logistics support personnel to procure the types and forms of medications most suitable for the tactical environment.

PROPHYLACTIC MEDICATIONS

Certain prophylactic medications may have a special role in tactical medicine. By the nature of their mission, tactical officers have high exposure risk to certain chemical, biological, and radiological agents, particularly on missions involving threats of weapons of mass destruction (WMDs). If reliable intelligence indicates a particular WMD threat for which a prophylactic medication may afford some protection, then it is incumbent on the tactical medical director to evaluate this option.

The decision to prophylax a tactical team should always be made in the context of a medical benefit-risk assessment and must include the team leader or operations chief (5). Once the decision is made to offer prophylaxis, each team member should be informed of the indications, risks, and benefits of the prophylaxis. Declinations should be treated with respect and all should have the treatment or refusal recorded in the medical record.

Pyridostigmine is the prophylactic agent of choice against nerve agents. It increases the LD_{50} of soman (GD) by 50%, although it may not be effective for sarin (GB) or VX (8). The use of pyridostigmine for the treatment of myasthenia gravis and other neuromuscular disorders is well established and the accumulated medical experience with the drug is high. Side effects are common, afflicting up to 50% of individuals, and include dry mucous membranes and urinary retention. However, <1% of troops taking the drug during the Persian Gulf War (Operation Desert Storm/Shield) experienced side effects bothersome enough to warrant discontinuation of the medication (8). Lingering controversy over the role pyridostigmine may have played in the so-called Gulf War Syndrome remains, although multiple independent studies have failed to establish a link.

Ciprofloxacin and tetracyclines are the mainstay antibiotics for use in cases of certain biologic agents used as potential weapons of mass destruction (9). Treatment is most effective if begun 24 hours prior to exposure, however, the incubation periods of most biological agents is long and prophylaxis can usually be deferred 24 to 48 hours after exposure (when tentative threat identification has been accomplished).

Potassium iodide, available without a prescription, is a potential prophylactic adjunct in persons at risk of certain radiological exposures. Potassium iodide works by competitively inhibiting the uptake of iodine-131 by thyroid cells (10). Iodine-131 is the radioactive by-product of certain nuclear processes and is implicated in causing thyroid cancer in exposed individuals. The usual source of iodine-131 is the fission of transuranium elements and, thus, can only be expected in nuclear reactor accidents or in the fallout from nuclear detonations (5). Outside of these events, it is unlikely that a tactical team will encounter iodine-131 unless the operation involves a site storing the material (very uncommon) or a terrorist purposefully uses the material in a weapon. Table 24.4 identifies several WMD threats and the drugs used for prophylaxis.

Immunizations deserve special mention as a prophylactic strategy. Vaccines are generally the most reliable and effective means of protecting at-risk personnel. Periods of protection can range from many months to several years, thus affording long-term protection. However, the decision to vaccinate must be made well in advance, usually long before any specific threat is identified. Vaccines take at least 4 to 6 weeks to induce a host immunologic response, and in the case of the anthrax vaccine, several immunizations over a long period are required for full effect. Thus, any decision to vaccinate must be made as part of an organization's general or community threat assessment, and not as part of a response to any specific near-term threat.

▶ **TABLE 24.4. Selected Prophylactic Drugs Against Potential Weapons of Mass Destruction Threats.**

Threat	Drug
Nerve agent (primarily GD, soman)	Pyridostigmine
Anthrax	Ciprofloxacin or doxycycline
Plague	Tetracycline or doxycycline
Q fever	Tetracycline or doxycycline
Brucellosis	Doxycycline and rifampin
Tularemia	Tetracycline or doxycycline
Smallpox	Vaccinia immune globulin
Iodine-131	Potassium iodide

Any such plan must consider the willingness of the specific population to be immunized (11).

Complicating the issue of immunizations is the current lack of fresh stocks or adequate manufacturing capacity for many relevant vaccines. Smallpox vaccines are now in sufficient quantity (through dilution of the original, decades-old product) for use by larger segments of the population (12). The anthrax vaccine remains controversial for the military as court cases delay plans to vaccinate all troops (13). Currently, there are no national or specialty-specific recommendations for the immunization of first responders against potential biological terrorist threats.

Outside of WMD use, there is an interesting development in the use of prophylactic medications for use in tactical settings. Anecdotal reports from certain segments of the military special forces suggest a trend in using prophylactic antibiotics (usually oral fluoroquinolones) just prior to high-risk operations. The goal is to generate protective blood levels of antibiotic in case the operator gets shot. The practice is based on the theoretical advantage of preinjury antibiotic use in preventing serious infectious complications of penetrating wounds. Unfortunately, clinical studies weighing the safety and effectiveness of this approach are lacking.

NONPRESCRIPTION (OVER-THE-COUNTER) MEDICATIONS

Tactical team members suffer the same aches, pains, and minor ailments as the general public. The general public usually reaches for an OTC drug in the medicine cabinet or at the corner drugstore. The tactical officer on assignment, however, does not readily have this luxury. This forces the officer to choose between suffering the mild ailment (e.g., headache) or abandoning the mission and seeking relief to the rear of the scene (perhaps by visiting a pharmacy or local clinic).

Keeping tactical officers on the job and free of distracting aches and pains is a valuable medical service to the tactical commander and assures that maximal manpower can be applied to the missions. It is the rare tactical system that can afford to forward deploy a physician to every operation to care for such symptoms and dispense the correct OTC medication. Allowing the officers themselves to carry a variety OTC drugs is impractical and, if an officer does not appreciate the side effects, potentially dangerous. A compromise solution is to train and equip the on-scene tactical medic to dispense selected OTC drugs properly. By strictly limiting the formulary and indications, the medical director can control both the distracting symptoms and the drugs the officers are exposed to. In this fashion, two performance-reducing medical problems are mitigated.

The military has a long and rich tradition of authorizing combat medics to treat troops with OTC drugs, and

Proper training of medics
Strictly identified indications of relief of minor symptoms
Use of OTC drugs with a low incidence of side effects
Immediate physician referral for potentially significant symptoms
Dispense only to prescreened, physically fit officers
Accurate clinical record keeping
Physician review of all cases for quality assurance

OTC, over-the-counter.

increasingly, civilian agencies are exploring this expanded scope option (14). The keys to a successful tactical medic expanded scope program are listed in Table 24.5 and include proper training, detailed treatment protocols, and an effective quality assurance program (14). Medics must be well trained to discriminate between minor symptoms (e.g., minor headache) and potentially serious symptoms (e.g., worse headache, stiff neck, or fever) necessitating immediate physician referral (1). A mandatory physician review (within 24 hours) of all cases of medic-dispensed OTC drugs is prudent. The basics of pharmacology, medication administration, and side effects should be a part of the training program too.

The choice of which OTC medications to authorize should be based on the types of missions and the frequency of symptoms expected. Agencies that infrequently participate in lengthy or remote operations will need only two or three drugs on the formulary to manage leading symptoms. Agencies anticipating long or remote operations may desire an expanded list (Table 24.6). In all cases, medication safety, efficacy, and side effects should be considered. Some OTC drugs are not appropriate for tactical use owing to potential side effects (Table 24.7).

▶ **TABLE 24.6. Selected Over-the-counter Drugs with Potential Tactical Use by the Medic.**

Drug	Indication(s)
Ibuprofen	Headache, musculoskeletal aches and pains
Acetaminophen	Headache, musculoskeletal aches and pains
Pseudoephedrine	Nasal congestion and rhinorrhea
Phenylephrine, oxymetazoline spray	Nasal congestion and rhinorrhea
Loperamide	Diarrhea
Dextromethorphan	Cough
Oil of clove	Oral and dental pain
Throat lozenges	Scratchy throat
OTC H_2-blockers	Acid indigestion and heartburn
Ca, Al, and Mg antacids	Acid indigestion and heartburn

OTC, over-the-counter.

▶ **TABLE 24.7. Selected Over-the-counter Drugs Possibly Inappropriate for Tactical Use.**

Drug	Side Effect(s)
Aspirin	Prolonged bleeding time
Diphenhydramine and other sedating antihistamines	Drowsiness
Drugs with alcohol as a vehicle	Drowsiness, intoxication

DRUGS AND HUMAN PERFORMANCE

All medications, whether prescription or nonprescription, have side effects. In most cases, side effects are minor and of little direct consequence to the patient. However, in the case of the tactical officer armed with high-powered firearms and responsible for mission safety and success, even minor side effects can be disastrous when every physical and mental advantage is needed to overcome lethal adversaries.

The medical director and tactical medic have a special duty to advise officers and commanders of the potential risks of medication side effects and to devise a program to mitigate these risks. This includes prescription and nonprescription medications used by officers as well as caffeine, nicotine, alcohol, and illicit drugs that officers may be exposed to.

To effectively manage officer drug use and mitigate potential negative side effects, officers must report all uses. To ensure complete reporting, strict medical confidentiality must be maintained. The caveat, of course, is that if the officer is taking drugs incompatible with job performance (e.g., narcotics used by a vehicle driver), there must be a procedure to restrict duty. This policy should be clearly delineated and be fully compatible with state and federal privacy laws.

One of the best models available for developing a specific drug side-effect management program is found in civil aviation. The Federal Aviation Administration publishes a guideline on the use of OTC drugs, prescription drugs, caffeine, nicotine, and alcohol (15). Although the adaptation of guidelines designed for civil pilots is only imperfectly applicable to tactical officers, it is nonetheless a useful place to start. Other sources of information and guidelines on drugs and human performance include the American Medical Association and military aviation regulations (16–19). The former offer general guidance on the effects of alcohol and drugs primarily for the driving public, while the latter, extremely strict rules offer the ultimate in safety by limiting virtually all drugs that might affect performance. A review article classifies many drugs in terms of side effects (20).

It is impractical to list all medications and the potential side effects in this chapter. Instead, the medical director

▶ **TABLE 24.8. Side Effects of Some Common Over-the-counter Medications.**

Category	Medication	Side Effect(s)	Interactions

Pain relief and fever	Aspirin
	   Alka Seltzer, Bayer aspirin
		Ringing in ears, nausea, stomach
		   ulceration, hyperventilation
			Increased effect of blood thinners

	Acetaminophen
	   Tylenol
		Liver toxicity (at high doses or when
		   taken with excessive alcohol)	

	Ibuprofen Advil, Motrin, Nuprin	Upset stomach	Increased effect of blood thinners
	Naproxen Aleve, Anaprox	Upset stomach	Increased effect of blood thinners

Colds and flu	Antihistamines
	   Actifed, Dristan, Benadryl,
	   Drixoral, Cheracol-Plus, NyQuil,
	   Chlor-Trimeton, Sinarest,
	   Contac, Sinutab, Dimetapp
		Dizziness, impairments of
		   coordination, upset stomach,
		   thickening of bronchial secretions,
		   blurring of vision, decreased
		   sweating
			Increased sedative effect of other
			   medications and alcohol

	Decongestants
	   Afrin nasal spray,
	   Neo-Synephrine, Sine-Aid,
	   Sudafed
		Excessive stimulation, dizziness,
		   difficulty with urination, palpitations
			Aggravation of high blood pressure,
			   heart disease, and prostate
			   problems

	Cough suppressants
	   Benylin, Robitussin CF/DM,
	   Vicks Formula 44
		Drowsiness, blurred vision, difficulty
		   with urination, upset stomach
			Increased sedative effect of other
			   medications and alcohol

Bowel preparations	Laxatives
	   Correctol, Ex-Lax
		Unexpected bowel movement, rectal
		   itching	

	Antidiarrheals
	   Imodium A-D, Pepto-Bismol
		Drowsiness, impairment of
		   coordination, blurred vision, ringing
		   in ears (Pepto-Bismol)	

Appetite suppressants	Acutrim, Dexatrim	Excessive stimulation, dizziness,
		   palpitations, headaches
			Increased stimulatory effects of
			   decongestants; interference with
			   high-blood-pressure medications

Sleeping aids	Nytol, Sominex	(Contain antihistamines), prolonged
		   drowsiness, blurred vision
			Increased sedative effect of other
			   medications and alcohol

Stimulants	Caffeine
	   Coffee, tea, cola, caffeinated
	   soda pop, chocolate, No-Doz
		Excessive stimulation, tremors,
		   palpitations, headache
			Interference with
			   high-blood-pressure medications

Adapted from U.S. DOT. *Over the Counter Medications and Flying.* FAA Publ. No. AM-400-92/1. Oklahoma City, OK: U.S. Department of Transportation, Federal Aviation Administration; 1992.

should rely on the manufacturer's package insert or other suitable references (e.g., *Physicians' Desk Reference* [PDR], Medical Economics Co., Montvale, NJ) when judging new or unfamiliar drugs.

Table 24.8 details some side effects of common OTC preparations and it may be useful to share this information with tactical officers. In general, it is prudent to avoid engaging in high-risk missions until at least twice the usual dosing interval has elapsed. In other words, if the OTC drug labeling is "every 4–6 hours," then at least 12 hours should pass before the officer is cleared for high-risk duty (15). In some cases, physician judgment will dictate exceptions. Drugs with exceptional safety profiles (e.g., pseudoephedrine) and lacking in unacceptable side effects (e.g., drowsiness) may not require certain duty restrictions.

Of the OTC medications in common use, antihistamines represent the most prevalent risk. Many OTC antihistamines currently available cause some degree of unac-

ceptable drowsiness in at least some of the population (21). Unless the patient and tactical physician are both comfortable with the lack of apparent drowsiness in a particular case, it is best to avoid any of the sedating antihistamines during or preceding operational missions. A number of low-sedating or nonsedating antihistamines are now available and their use is preferred (22).

Many medications prescribed for acute conditions have undesirable side effects necessitating duty restriction. Chief among these are narcotic analgesics, which can cause significant drowsiness (23). One the other hand, most antibiotics are well tolerated and do not require duty modification. More complex are the myriad chronic medications that officers may be prescribed including antihypertensives, hypoglycemics, antidepressants, and anticonvulsants. Judging such patients' fitness for duty is as much about the medication as it is the underlying medical condition and, in any case, is beyond the scope of this chapter.

Needless to say, the tactical physician must be intimately familiar with the particular tactical officer's medical condition and medications and the specific demands of the job to properly make judgments of fitness for duty.

A few drugs deserve special mention because of their ubiquity and well-known effects on human performance. The negative effects of alcohol have been known for decades and all police agencies should have guidelines on its use (24). As a rule, alcohol should be prohibited within 8 to 12 hours of duty (longer for binge drinkers) and, in any case, should always be well below the legal limits for intoxication (typically 0.8 to 1.0 mg/dL) (18,25,26). Of note, commercial drivers must adhere to a level of 0.4 mg/dL (27). Tactical agencies may prudently adopt even more strict standards, approaching no detectable alcohol in the blood.

Nicotine and its most common vehicle, cigarette smoke, are not often considered for their acute affects on performance, but these have been documented (28). Of particular interest to the tactical environment is impaired night vision, decreased aerobic capacity, and increased susceptibility to frostbite.

Caffeine, while having fewer negative side effects than alcohol or nicotine, can, in large doses induce anxiety, palpitations, and tremors. Abstinence from caffeine as well as alcohol and nicotine can lead to various withdrawal symptoms, and the medical director must be alert for this possibility.

Pseudoephedrine has few side effects in low doses, namely, anxiety and palpitations. It does, however, interfere with heat tolerance, a major consideration for the tactical provider.

Illicit drugs such as cocaine, cannabis, amphetamines, barbiturates, and heroine are clearly incompatible with law enforcement in general and tactical operations in particular. Nonetheless, it is possible that some officers may succumb to this problem and the tactical physician is well advised to remain vigilant. Any credible evidence of acute consumption of illicit drugs is grounds for restricting all high-risk duty and driving based on medical grounds (28,29). Of course, drug treatment and legal consequence policies should be worked out well in advance and be clear and practical.

In selected cases, the judicious use of nonprescription drugs can be used to enhance human performance, at least temporarily. Caffeine and, occasionally, melatonin have been used to counteract the effects of fatigue, sleep deprivation, and circadian rhythm disruption (e.g., night shift). Caffeine, 4 mg/kg (or the equivalent in caffeinated beverages), may relieve drowsiness if taken before fatigue sets in (30). It appears less effective once fatigue occurs. In all cases, the effect is mild and not a substitute for adequate sleep. Melatonin is touted by some as effective for adjusting circadian rhythms, although study results are mixed (30). Effective doses likely are lower than the 1- to 10-mg forms available at most health food stores.

In highly selected cases, prescription performance enhancers may deserve consideration for combating fatigue or enforcing needed rest in prolonged missions (31). With the exception of modafinil (Provigil), practical experience is limited outside of the military, and the tactical physician must exercise a high degree of control and judgment when considering prescription medications to achieve desired effects. For improved alertness and avoidance of fatigue, solo U.S. Air Force pilots on long-distance flights are authorized to take dextroamphetamine (19). In a similar fashion, assuring needed crew rest in critical situations is accomplished with temazepam or zolpidem (19). Newer sleep agents including zaleplon and eszopiclone offer theoretical performance advantages but are not well studied in the population of interest. The relatively new drug modafinil, a nonamphetamine agent used to promote wakefulness, has lately gained acceptance in treating the effects of civilian shift-work sleep disorder and has also been studied by the aviation and military communities (32–35). For this reason, it may be the principal agent in those limited circumstances where tactical personnel are required to alter sleep cycles and reduce sleepiness because of pressing mission needs. It is important for officers to trial these drugs at least once prior to any critical mission use to ensure that side effects are acceptable.

All the prescription drugs mentioned are controlled substances and require impeccable record keeping, not to mention clinical judgment, in their use. To avoid any perception of impropriety, the tactical physician should limit this strategy to key team members, highly critical missions, and times when less dramatic strategies are impossible. Above all, the tactical physician should communicate to the tactical officer and commander the limited effectiveness and potential side effects of these drugs. There is no substitute for an effective rest and sleep management plan on prolonged operations.

TAKE-HOME POINTS

1. Medical direction is essential for a medication administration program for TEMS.
2. Providers must consider which medications are practical for use in the particular tactical setting and echelons of care.
3. Medications can alleviate or control annoying conditions or prevent disease.
4. Providers must consider the medications side effects and their effect on human performance in the tactical setting. Some common medications have side effects that are unacceptable for the tactical operator.
5. Providers must be trained and knowledgeable in medication uses, side effects and administration.
6. Judicious use of medications such as sleep aids, and stimulates can enhance human performance.

CONCLUSION

Medications and drugs offer the medic and physician powerful tools to solve specific tactical problems. Careful selection and judicious administration of selected emergency drugs can positively impact a number of critical medical problems likely encountered in tactical missions. Prophylactic medications can similarly prevent disease, while selected OTC drugs can control annoying and distracting symptoms. Equally important is knowledge of the side effects of drugs and medications, particularly those that may affect officer performance.

REFERENCES

1. De Lorenzo RA, Porter RS. *Tactical Emergency Care*. Upper Saddle River, NJ: Brady (Prentice Hall); 1999.
2. De Lorenzo RA. Improving combat casualty care and field medicine: focus on the military medic. *Milit Med*. 1997;162 (4):268–272.
3. Butler FK, Hagmann J, Butler FJ. Tactical combat casualty care in special operations. *Milit Med*. 1996;161 (Suppl 3):15.
4. Butler F, O'Connor K. Antibiotics in tactical combat casualty care 2002. *Milit Med*. 2003;168(11): 911–914.
5. De Lorenzo RA, Porter RS. *Weapons of Mass Destruction: Emergency Care*. Upper Saddle River, NJ: Brady (Prentice Hall); 2000.
6. Zajtchuk R, et al., eds). *Medical Aspects of Chemical and Biological Warfare*. Washington, DC: Department of the Army, Office of the Surgeon General; 1997.
7. Lam KK, Lau FL. An incident of hydrogen cyanide poisoning. *Am J Emerg Med*. 2000;18(2):172–175.
8. U.S. Army Medical Research Institute of Chemical Defense. *Medical Management of Chemical Casualties*. 2nd ed. Aberdeen Proving Ground, MD: U.S. Army Medical Research Institute of Chemical Defense; 1995.
9. Franz DR, et al. Clinical recognition and management of patients exposed to biological warfare agents. *JAMA*. 1997;278:399–411.
10. Zajtchuk R, et al., eds. *Medical Consequences of Nuclear Warfare*. Washington, DC: Department of the Army, Office of the Surgeon General; 1990.
11. Silk BJ, del Rio C, Ivansco LK, et al. Pre-event willingness to receive smallpox vaccine among physicians and public safety personnel. *South Med J*. 2005;98(9):876–882.
12. Arita I. Smallpox vaccine and its stockpile in 2005. *Lancet Infect Dis*. 2005;5(10):647–652.
13. Dyer O. US judge halts compulsory anthrax vaccination for soldiers. *BMJ*. 2004; 329(7474):1062.
14. De Lorenzo RA. Military medic: the original expanded scope EMS provider. *J Emerg Med Serv*. 1996;21(4):50–54.
15. U.S. Department of Transportation. *Over the Counter Medications and Flying*. FAA Publ. No. AM-400-92/1. Oklahoma City, OK: U.S. Department of Transportation, Federal Aviation Administration; 1992.
16. Lyznichi JM, Doege TC, Davis FR, et al. Sleepiness, driving, and motor vehicle crashes. Council on Scientific Affairs, American Medical Association. *JAMA*. 1998;279(23):1908–1913.
17. Consensus Development Panel, American Medical Association. Consensus report. Drug concentrations and driving impairment. *JAMA*. 1985;254(18):2618–2621.
18. Department of the Army. *Army Regulation 40-8, Temporary Flying Restrictions Due to Exogenous Factors*. Washington, DC: Department of the Army; 1976.
19. Department of the Air Force. *Air Force Instruction 48-123, Medical Examinations and Standards*. Washington, DC: Department of the Air Force; 2000.
20. Maes V, Grenez O, Charlier C, et al. Classification of medicines according to their influence on driving ability. *Acta Clin Belg*. 1999;1(Suppl):82–88.
21. Adelsberg BR. Sedation and performance issues in the treatment of allergic conditions. *Arch Intern Med*. 1997;157:494–500.
22. Weiler JM, Bloomfield JR, Woodworth GG, et al. Effect of fexofenadine, diphenhydramine, and alcohol on driving performance. *Ann Intern Med*. 2000;132(5):354–363.
23. Galski T, Williams JB, Ehle HT. Effects of opioids on driving ability. *J Pain Symptom Manage*. 2000;19(3):200–208.
24. Aksnes EG. Effects of small doses of alcohol upon performance in link trainer. *J Aviat Med*. 1954;25:680–683.
25. Mohler SR. Civil aviation medicine. In: De DeHart RL, Davis JL, eds. *Fundamentals of Aerospace Medicine*. Philadelphia: Lippincott Williams & Wilkins; 2005.
26. Landaver AA, Howat P. Low and moderate alcohol doses, psychomotor performance and perceived drowsiness. *Ergonomics*. 1983;26:647–657.
27. U.S. Department of Transportation, Federal Motor Carrier Safety Administration. *Commercial Driver's License Program. Regulations, Part 40: Drug & Alcohol Testing*. Washington, DC: U.S. Department of Transportation.
28. Rayman RB. Aircrew health care maintenance. In: DeHart RL, Davis JL, eds. *Fundamentals of Aerospace Medicine*. Philadelphia: Lippincott Williams & Wilkins; 2005.
29. Kruzthaler I, Hummer M, Miller C, et al. Effect of cannabis use on cognitive functions and driving ability. *J Clin Psychiatry*. 1999;60(6): 395–399.
30. Kuhn G. Circadian rhythm, shiftwork, and emergency medicine. *Ann Emerg Med*. 2001;37(1):88–98.
31. Wesensten NJ, Killgore WD, Balkin TJ. Performance and alertness effects of caffeine, dextroamphetamine, and modafinil during sleep deprivation. *J Sleep Res*. 2005;14(3):255–266.
32. Caldwell JA, Caldwell JL. Fatigue in military aviation: an overview of US military-approved pharmacological countermeasures. *Aviat Space Environ Med*. 2005;76 (Suppl 7):C39–C51.
33. Buguet A, Moroz DE, Radomski MW. Modafinil—medical considerations for use in sustained operations. *Aviat Space Environ Med*. 2003;74(6; Pt 1):659–663.
34. Czeisler CA, Walsh JK, Roth T, et al. U.S. Modafinil in Shift Work Sleep Disorder Study Group. Modafinil for excessive sleepiness associated with shift-work sleep disorder. *N Engl J Med*. 2005;353(5):476–486.
35. Westcott KJ. Modafinil, sleep deprivation, and cognitive function in military and medical settings. *Milit Med*. 2005;170 (4):333–335.

Administrative

Section Editor: JAMES A. PFAFF

Chapter 25

How to Set Up a Tactical Emergency Medical Service Program

Richard B. Schwartz and Navin K. Sharma

OBJECTIVES

After reading this section, the reader will be able to:

1. Identify the needs of a tactical emergency medical service (TEMS)
2. Discuss goals, missions, structure, and training for a TEMS program
3. Discuss the equipment and processes involved in setting up a TEMS program

"TEMS is a dynamic discipline that will continue to positively impact public safety, but with a knowledge and organizational base that will always be evolving based on the threats and missions before us, advances in scienceand technology, and last but not least, our imagination and passion to pursue excellence."

Richard H. Carmona
U.S. Surgeon General

Starting a tactical emergency medical service (TEMS) program can be a daunting task. However, with planning and proper acceptance from key partners, a successful program can be assured. There is no one best design for a TEMS program and each team must develop its program to meet its individual mission and resources. Historically civilian tactical teams have operated as a tactical unit without the unit's own direct medical support. In this system medical support of these units has consisted of calling 911 if there is an injury during training or callouts. A step up from this system is the notification of existing EMS services that an operation is taking place in a general area and a unit may or may not be stationed on the scene. This level of support may be inadequate in many TEMS settings. Over the past several decades there has been a trend toward the increased recognition of the need of integrated TEMS. Many professional and law enforcement agencies have recognized this need to have emergency medical care available at the scene of any incident involving police tactical operations (1). Despite this growing acceptance, there are still many tactical units without integrated medical support. A 1996 survey indicated that 78% of Special Weapons and Tactics (SWAT) teams did not have a medical director and that 23% did not have a medical preplan (2). These statistics have undoubtedly improved since 1996, however, when presented with the concept of TEMS there still may be resistance from both the law enforcement and the medical community during the early development of a TEMS team. This chapter helps provide a framework to assist in the initial development and sustainability of a TEMS program.

ESTABLISHING NEED

Identifying the need for TEMS and gaining acceptance from law enforcement command staff as well as the medical chain of command is a crucial first step in the process. Commanders should be made to recognize not only the critical nature of emergent medical care inside the perimeter but also the importance of medical threat assessment, preventive medicine, and the other aspects of TEMS in maximizing mission effectiveness. In fact, a greater amount of time is spent on these other activities than on actual combat/tactical casualty care (3). When properly briefed, commanders should understand the advantages of having an integrated TEMS program. Additionally, commanders should be aware of the potential economic consequences from liability incurred when falling below a standard of care (3). Assistance in this area can be obtained from a number of national, federal, and state organizations, including the International Tactical EMS Organization (www.items.org), the National Tactical Officers Association (www.ntoa.org), the Medical College of Georgia Center of Operational Medicine (www.mcgcom.com), and the Uniformed Services University's Casualty Care Research Center (www.ushuhs.mil/ccr/ccr.html). In areas where local physicians or the EMS community is not familiar with the TEMS concept, a similar education process may be necessary. Discussion with agencies that have TEMS programs and TEMS physicians on their staff would be an excellent start. The above-named support organizations can also be extremely helpful in helping local medical program directors (MPDs) network with their physician peers across the country with experience with TEMS units.

MISSION, GOALS, AND OBJECTIVES OF THE TACTICAL EMERGENCY MEDICAL SERVICE UNIT

The mission statement is a broad statement that defines the overall purpose of the program and why it exists. How this mission is to be accomplished can be defined by goals

---

Box 25.1. General Goals of Tactical Emergency Medical Services

- Enhance mission accomplishment
- Prepare medical threat assessment
- Monitor the medical effects of environmental conditions
- Reduce death, injury and illness, and related effects among team members, innocents, and perpetrators
- Reduce line-of-duty injury and disability
- Reduce lost work time
- Maintain good team morale
- Maintain team members' health and provide preventative medicine
- Coordinate with surrounding agencies and hospitals
- Decrease liability
- Possess basic forensic knowledge and crime scene preservation

Adapted from Marx J, Hockberger R, Walls R, eds. *Rosen's Emergency Medicine Concepts and Clinical Practice*. 6th ed. Philadelphia, PA: Mosby Elsevier; 2006.

---

and objectives for the unit. Broad goals of tactical medicine are listed in Box 25.1. These goals have expanded over the years. Initially TEMS providers focused only on the care and evacuation of the wounded; however, their role has expanded far beyond that and the majority of the effort of TEMS providers is now spent on health maintenance, preventive medicine, threat assessment, mission planning, and other aspects of TEMS (1,4).

Unit-specific goals can also be utilized. Objectives can be developed in the context of the unit's medical capability and the overall mission of the team in mind. For instance, if one is able to develop only a basic life support–level TEMS unit, then the objectives and expectations of the unit should match that level of medical expertise. Changes to the objectives would need to be made as the unit evolves to advanced life support standards or if the team takes on additional missions such as maritime operations.

STRUCTURE OF A TACTICAL EMERGENCY MEDICAL SYSTEM PROGRAM

The details of team composition and basic capabilities and equipment are covered in Chapter 1, however, it is important that essential elements be highlighted here, as the functioning of the TEMS program will depend on its structure. As indicated earlier, there is no best single structure for a TEMS program. In broad terms there are two basic structures: internal and external. Internal support refers to teams that have medical support that are both trained and certified medically and are sworn officers. External refers to teams that have medical support from other organizations, and they are generally not sworn officers (3). In reality there are advantages and disadvantages of both systems. Internal systems with experienced medical providers seem the most desirable, as the medical providers have unique training and certifications that give them credibility and the ability to work both medically and tactically. Officer safety issues, the use of force continuum, and general police tactics are second nature to this type of an internal support medical provider. However, this combination of an experienced medical provider who is also a full-time law enforcement officer is not as readily available to many jurisdictions as is the external structure counterpart. External teams are able to provide highly competent experienced medical providers but they do not have arrest powers and have limitations in the tactical environment. Despite the limitations of external teams, this is the model for the majority of tactical teams in the United States (3). There are teams of both organizational structures that function well, and a balance of medical and tactical skills is desirable.

How your team is established will depend on your available resources and local command structure. Team makeup is highly variable and, again, depends on your resources. Internal teams generally are made up of members with medical certifications at the EMT-B through EMT-P level. These programs will often have volunteer medical direction and oversight from a local physician familiar with TEMS. Several organizations have full-time physician support either as employees or under contract (5). This kind of arrangement is appealing and assures that the physician oversight is integrated with the tactical elements, as opposed to a volunteer arrangement, which may be less reliable. The MPD should meet the qualification standards for EMS medical directors established by the American College of Emergency Physicians and the National Association of EMS Physicians (6,7). Additionally, the MPD for a TEMS program should have TEMS-specific training and experience to most effectively provide medical oversight. Some tactical teams have been successful with physician/nurse TEMS programs. Some locations have even integrated TEMS support into graduate medical education programs (4).

The decision to arm or not to arm providers is often a controversial one, with strong opinions on both sides. With an internal team this is not an issue, as the medical providers are also sworn officers. This is highly appealing in the tactical environment, however, it may limit the medical skills of the providers as mentioned previously. Many external teams work successfully both with armed and with unarmed providers. If a decision is made to arm providers, it is accepted that the TEMS providers meet the same firearm qualifications as the other team members. Additionally, it is essential that the TEMS providers have documented training in the continuum of force. Obviously this process is much simpler with a sworn officer but many external teams have armed providers through a variety of processes. This issue will need to be addressed at the local level, as different jurisdictions have differing regulatory requirements.

Concerns over "role confusion" are often raised in discussions about arming TEMS providers (4,8). This concern appears to be primarily based on anecdote and not on documented accounts. Military Special Operations Medics and many civilian TEMS providers have functioned for decades armed and providing medical support for their teams without this confusion. In fact one of the core principles of TEMS is that the TEMS provider must address not only the medical problem but also the tactical situation in which that medical problem is taking place. For example, in a hostage situation a team is making entry and a team member is shot. When viewed from a pure medical standpoint the correct response would be for the element to hold and provide security while the team member is resuscitated and then complete the mission. This approach, however, will likely place the team and hostages at considerable risk and result in greater mortality and morbidity. For many teams the immediate action drill for this scenario would be to continue to neutralize the threat and, after the threat is eliminated, provide the care to the injured team member. This approach will likely improve the outcomes for the greatest number of hostages and team members. Having well-trained TEMS providers integrated into the team will avoid this confusion created by the potential conflicts between medical care and the tactical mission. Education of the tactical commanders on the importance of the TEMS provider as an integrated asset (whether integrated as an external or an internal team) will also help avoid this potential confusion. It should also be clear that the medic should not cover additional specialty duties in the tactical element. Like other specialty team members, such as the team leader, sniper, and breacher, the TEMS provider is a mission essential position and thus should not cover additional specialized duties (for example, sniper/medic).

CHAIN(S) OF COMMAND

Since TEMS operations involve supervision from two entities—the law enforcement command structure for tactical/police purposes and from the MPD's office for medical performance—they hence necessitate a double chain of command for the TEMS provider. This is similar to the bilateral command chain that fire-medics in fire service have to follow, that is, reporting to a fire command for fire tactics while following standing orders from their respective MPD for delivery of medical care inside the fire zone (9,10). A defined working relationship between these entities is essential for a well-functioning team. Most functioning teams meet this requirement through simple memoranda of understanding (MOU). Additionally, there are responsibilities to the MPD that the law enforcement agency should fulfill, and these should be addressed in the MOU between agencies. These responsibilities are summarized in Box 25.2.

EQUIPPING THE TEAM

The responsibility of equipping at team can be financially costly and should be addressed prospectively as the team is being established. For example, in 1997 it was estimated that the cost of properly equipping a TEMS provider on the Los Angeles County Sheriff's team was in excess of $6,000 (9). The equipment required for a TEMS provider will depend on two primary factors: the level of training of the provider and the role of the TEMS provider with the team. As noted, the TEMS provider should be dressed in the same agency uniform as the tactical team. This is important to avoid confusion and potential fratricide.

Protective equipment must also be available. The protective equipment required should include body armor as well as chemical protective equipment. Body armor comes in levels 1 to 4. As the number increases, so does the ballis-

tic protection. As a general rule, the degree of protection is increased as mobility and speed are decreased. A rule of thumb for the level of body armor is that at a minimum it should stop the rounds from the agency's own firearms. Additionally, ballistic protective helmets and eyewear are essential. Other protective equipment includes boots, gloves, and clothing as mandated by the environmental conditions. Chemical protective equipment should include an air-purifying respirator (APR) with an appropriate selected filter that will cover known radiological, chemical, and biological hazards. Personnel that utilize APRs must have a medical evaluation and be fit tested. The requirements that must be met to utilize APRs are given in the Code of Federal Regulations 1910.135. The team should also have the capability for "hasty decontamination" of team members who may inadvertently come in contact with hazardous materials. OSHA requires that emergency responders who may provide decontamination be trained to the First Responder Operations HAZMAT level, along with specific decontamination training. This training typically involves 20 to 40 h, depending on the course selected.

The medical equipment selected by the TEMS unit should be tailored to the training and experience of the medical providers and their role in the team. Many TEMS providers have a small "entry bag" for use when mobility is a major concern and a larger "aid bag" that can be used to augment the entry bag. The entry bag typically has very basic supplies that will be utilized during the "care under fire" phase and potentially in the "tactical field care" phase. Representative supplies include a tourniquet for uncontrolled extremity hemorrhage, simple airway devices such as a nasal airway, dressings (including hemostatic dressings such as the Hemconbandage), and a large-bore Angiocath for decompression of a tension pneumothorax. The larger aid bag contains a broader array of medical equipment and supplies that can be utilized to provide a higher level of care to the patient. The exact contents of the medical bags are skill- and experience-specific and should be tailored to your team's makeup. A frequently forgotten component of the aid bag is equipment to care for pediatric patients. Innocent children may be hostages or be injured in an operation, and this equipment is essential. Casualty evacuation equipment needs to be taken into account when developing your team. Various litters and stretchers exist to facilitate short patient transports, but consideration of dedicated vehicles for remote operations should be included in the planning.

TRAINING FOR TACTICAL EMERGENCY MEDICAL SERVICE PROVIDERS

The earliest program accessible to civilian law enforcement was the Counter Narcotics and Terrorism Operational Medical Support (CONTOMS) program. Today there are many TEMS training programs that provide training to multiple local, state, and federal agencies. Most civilian training programs have their roots in military medicine and follow many of the same principals. Many units in the Department of Defense have adopted a training doctrine called Tactical Combat Casualty Care (TCCC). The TCCC model focuses on three phases of tactical care: care under fire, tactical field care, and casualty evacuation (CASEVAC). The care under fire phase is the phase of care where the TEMS provider is under hostile fire. Medical care in this phase is limited to very simple procedures that are lifesaving, such as placement of a tourniquet for life-threatening hemorrhage. In this phase of care the suppression of enemy fire is the "best medicine."

Tactical field care is the phase when the TEMS provider is no longer under direct fire but a threat still exists. Tactical field care may involve transport of the casualty to a designated location for evacuation. In this phase, more advanced care can be provided, however, the tactical situation mandates practice variance from the noncombat scenario.

The last phase is the CASEVAC phase; here the casualty is evacuated from the battlefield to a higher echelon of care. Advanced medical providers and equipment may be prestationed for this phase of care. Advanced procedures such as endotracheal intubation and tube thoracostomy may be performed during transport. While these concepts were developed with a military model in mind, they apply to the medical support of civilian law enforcement as well. In fact the concepts of TCCC have been adopted by civilian training courses such as Pre-Hospital Trauma Life Support.

The majority of civilian TEMS training courses have now integrated the TCCC concepts into their training programs. One of the TCCC concepts that has transitioned to the civilian community is the concept of not limiting medical training to the medic. For example, the Medical College of Georgia has developed a series of courses called Tactical Operator Care (TOC) 1 to 3. These courses follow the TCCC concepts and apply them to the civilian environment. They were initially developed for training Federal Bureau of Investigation medical personnel but are now being offered for civilian law enforcement.

The TOC-1 course is a 2-day course for the agent/officer. The course focuses on self-aid, buddy aid, and medic assistance. Essential lifesaving skills such as hemorrhage control are taught to the operators. This course provides the agent with standardized medical kits and is taught in a hands-on scenario based model. The Tactical Operator Casualty Care (TOC-2) course is for the medic interested in becoming a TEMS provider. The course covers the essentials of TEMS including advanced procedure labs but also includes a day of instruction to become a TOC-1 instructor. This enables the TOC-2-trained medic to return to the unit and train and sustain the TOC-1 medical skills of his or her team. The Tactical Operator Critical

Casualty Care (TOC-3) course is an advanced course for the experienced TEMS provider who may need to provide care in remote areas. TOC-3 training can be tailored to the audience but includes live tissue resuscitation labs, cadaver procedure labs, and advanced tactical and medical simulation.

There are many factors involved in the selection of training for TEMS personnel. These factors include, but are not limited to, course availability, team mission, TEMS provider skill level, role of the TEMS provider on the team, and cost of training. While there are multiple courses available, some have limited availability due to lack of federal funding. While other courses may be available, their cost can be prohibitive. The training selected will depend a great deal on the skill level of your team members and the acceptable scope of practice for TEMS providers in your state. Specialty training may also be required, depending on your team's mission. For example, if your tactical team has a very active maritime program, then training in hyperbaric medicine and diving medical technician skills may be a worthwhile investment.

RECRUITMENT AND SELECTION PROCESS

A formalized recruitment process is important, as it will display a level of professionalism for the TEMS program and bring it on par with selection processes for other desired specialty units within law enforcement. This process can be handled entirely within the law enforcement agency (internal team) or can be a coordinated effort by the law enforcement agency and the affiliated medical agency. In either situation it is important to establish minimum criteria and a selection process. This process should be tailored to the individual agencies involved. An example of a formalized internal team qualification and selection process is one developed by the Vancouver, Washington, Police TEMS Unit, which has been shared with other agencies nationwide; it is outlined in Box 25.3 and 25.4 (10).

IDENTIFYING FUNDING SOURCES

A TEMS program can be an expensive venture. A pragmatic list of possible funding sources should be identified. Many TEMS teams come into existence with little to no official funding. However, working creatively with internal and external sources, units can function and flourish. Potential external funding sources for TEMS programs are listed in Box 25.5 (10).

Internal sources of funding may be found by virtue of expanding the team's services to other high-risk specialty units; TEMS operators can ride the coattails of their respective internal budgets. For instance, setting up a K9-Down Program within TEMS can **The SWAT Medic** help

Box 25.3. Example of Internal Team Member Qualifications: Qualifications for Vancouver, Washington, Police TEMS Unit

General Qualifications

- No at-fault driving-related traffic accidents within the past 2 years
- No firearms accidental discharges (ADs) within the past 2 years
- No other at-fault safety-related incidents within the past 2 years
- No sustained internal affairs investigations (IAs) within the past 2 years
- May have to pass a VPD background investigation if necessary (for non-VPD applicants)

Medical qualifications for this recruitment

- The SWAT Medic will be an EMT-Basic- or EMT-Paramedic-level trained officer and certified in the State of Washington to practice as such, or be able to gain reciprocity through the county MPD's office prior to being placed on the TEMS Unit.
- EMT-Basic-level experience must be a minimum of 1 year, and 2 years as an EMS/FIRE first responder. (Prior EMS or military-related EMS service will count.)
- Must be reasonably fit to perform medical duties under adverse conditions
- Must maintain Continuing Medical Education (CME) requirements as set forth by the County MPD
- Must be current in, Basic Trauma Life Support (BTLS) or Pre-Hospital Trauma Life Support (PHTLS) and Basic Life Support/CPR/AED certifications
- All SWAT Medics, irrespective of their levels, will be mandated to pass the appropriate County MPD's testing and qualifying exams (if they have not already done so).

Law enforcement qualifications

- Applicants must be in good standing with a Clark County law enforcement agency.
- Reserve Officers will have successfully completed the CCSO Reserve Academy and be current in their certification.
- All Officers shall be current with firearms qualifications and continually maintain that certification per their respective agency's policy.
- Must have a thorough understanding of the Use of Force Policy

Preferred qualifications

- All of the above, plus:
- A certification in a SWAT Medic School such as CONTOMS, the H&K TEMS course, or an approved Tactical EMS course
- Instructor ratings in
  - Basic Life Support (BLS: CPR + AED)
  - Advanced Cardiac Life Support (ACLS)
  - Pre-Hospital Trauma Life Support (PHTLS)
  - Basic Trauma Life Support (BTLS)
  - Pediatric Advanced Life Support (PALS)
- WA State Certified EMT-I instructor
- WA State Certified Paramedic with RN credentials

Essential knowledge and skills

- Tactical
  - Above-average officer safety skills
  - Proficiency in safe weapons handling
  - Knowledge in rendering safe weapon systems used by tactical team members
  - Knowledge of Department's force continuum guidelines
  - Knowledge of RCWs as related to Use of Force and Arrest
- Medical
  - Strong command of pre-hospital protocols and respective standing orders
  - Skills competency as set forth by the County MPD
  - Ability to facilitate Critical Incident Stress Debriefings (CISD)
  - Ability to assist in TEMS training

Essential abilities

- Work independently in absence of direct field supervision
- Have a clear understanding of Chain of Command issues
- Make decisions under extreme stress situations
- Deliver effective emergency medical support in varying environmental and logistical conditions
- Ability to operate medically and tactically under austere environments
- Execute and control emergency medical operations within the hot zone

---

Box 25.4. Selection process for Vancouver, Washington, Police TEMS Unit

■ For Reserve Officer/non-full-time law enforcement candidates: Submit a letter of recommendation from the candidate's medical supervisor (e.g., First-line Supervisor, Training Officer, etc.), in addition to the above.

■ Attend and pass a nonmedical oral board interview with a panel that is comprised of SWAT Commander, TEMS Team Leader, and a representative from the MPD's office.

■ Attend and pass a medical oral board interview with a panel of medical providers as approved by the MPD.

■ Pass SWAT Medical Program Director's standing orders exam for appropriate certification level. Candidates who have already taken and passed these exams, (e.g., currently practicing Clark County EMTs) do not have to retake this exam.

■ Pass a background investigation if required, for non-VPD applicants.

---

get assistance from the agency's K9 units. Assisting the local bomb squad on high-risk callouts would open doors with them. Justifying the need for TEMS coverage to Civil Disturbance Units (who often are larger teams than most SWAT units) would present the opportunity to tap into a portion of their budget; local drug task forces are yet

---

Box 25.5. Suggested External Funding Sources

■ Local area hospitals
■ Local businesses
■ Local EMS/fire agencies
■ State EMS grant processes
■ Federal grant processes
　■ Homeland Security
■ Major medical equipment manufacturers

---

another source of potential internal funding. TEMS providers should train with these units much the same as they would with SWAT. This not only allows for these other high-risk unit officers to see who we in TEMS are and what we can do for them, but also allows the development of professional bonds, much the same as has been traditionally done with SWAT. This will eventually result in a budget allowance for TEMS operational support being provided to these other high-risk units (10).

SUMMARY

The establishment of a TEMS program, while a difficult task, can be a successful endeavor if properly planned and developed. There are multiple existing models for TEMS programs and each model has advantages and disadvantages. Each agency must look at its mission and available resources and develop the TEMS program around them. Funding for TEMS programs is a significant hurdle for establishment of programs, and support for programs of this type should be encouraged at local, state, and federal levels.

REFERENCES

1. Schwartz R, McManus J, Orledge J. Tactical emergency medical support and urban search and rescue. In: Marx J, Hockberger R, Walls R, eds. *Rosen's Emergency Medicine Concepts and Clinical Practice.* 6th ed. Philadelphia: Mosby Elsevier; 2006.
2. Jones JS, Reese K, Kenepp G, et al. Into the fray: integration of emergency medical services and special weapons and tactics (SWAT) teams. *Prehosp Disast Med.* 1996;11(3):202–206.
3. Carmona RH. The history and evolution of tactical emergency medical support and its impact on public safety. *Topics Emerg Med.* 2003;25(4):277–281.
4. Vayer J, Schwartz R. Developing a tactical emergency medical support program. *Topics Emerg Med.* 2003;25(4):282–298.
5. Tang N, Fabbri W. Medical direction and integration with existing EMS infrastructure. *Topics Emerg Med.* 2003;25(4):326–332.
6. ACEP. Medical direction of pre-hospital emergency medical services. Policy Resource and Education Paper. Dallas, TX: American College of Emergency Physicians; 1992.
7. Alsonso-Serra H, Blanton D, O'Connor R. Physician medical direction in EMS (National Association of EMS Physicians Position Paper). *Prehosp Emerg Care.* 1998;2:153–157.
8. Integrated Force Health Protection (IFHP) Program. *Emergency Medical Technician-Tactical (EMT-T) Course Manual.* Bethesda, MD: Uniformed Services University of the Health Sciences; 2002.
9. Myers C. In the line of fire. *Emergency.* 1997; July:16–19.
10. Sharma NK. Vancouver (WA) police deploy SWAT-tactical EMS. *Tact Edge J.* 2000;Spring:35–38.

Chapter 26

Medical Control, Command, and Oversight

Jeremy N. Johnson and Bradley N. Younggren

OBJECTIVES

After reading this section, the reader will be able to:

1. Understand the historical perspective on how tactical medical oversight developed.
2. Understand and define the National Incident Management System (NIMS) and the Incident Command System (ICS) and how these entities can be utilized to improve medical control over a tactical scenario.
3. Consider and integrate contingencies into a tactical medical evacuation and extrication plan.

HISTORICAL PERSPECTIVE ON MEDICAL CONTROL

Medical control in its infancy existed on the battlefield of Napoleon's armies in the use of crude evacuation methods and treatment of wounded soldiers at or near the battlefield (1). Medical treatment, stabilization, evacuation, and control were further expanded during and after the Civil War (2), when in 1775 the Continental Congress authorized the creation of the first Army Hospital Department. With the development of ambulance units, evacuation routes, and basic front-line lifesaving care and the beginnings of the first fixed treatment centers staffed with doctors and nurses, the inception of what would be an early form of medical command control was initiated. A significant leap was made prior to the beginning of World War I, during which private intracity hospitals and hospital-based ambulances began to respond, transport, and care for patients under an ad hoc system that was largely separate from government control and oversight (3).

From a tactical standpoint, there were no formal centrally controlled forward medical units or organizations until World War I. In the 1950s and 1960s, following World Wars I and II, the United States initiated what could be considered an early National Response Plan (NRP) with air raid drills in preparation for the inevitable Russian ballistic missile strikes that never occurred. Since that time,

incident and disaster medical care have been primarily a local joint collaborative effort by both governmental and private organizations. At times, these interagency efforts have been ineffective on-scene, making it difficult to have appropriate utilization of medical resources (3).

Following September 11, 2001, the National Incident Management System (NIMS), the National Readiness Plan (NRP), the Federal Emergency Management Agency (FEMA), local Emergency Operation Plans (EOPs), and the Incident Command System (ICS) were either created or improved to address more effective interagency resource allocation and use (4).

At the city and county level, tactical emergency medical service (TEMS) members have been active, in very small numbers, since the mid- to late 1980s (2). As a result of events like September 11, 2001, Columbine, and other high-visibility mass casualty events, as well as the increased use of TEMS by police forces and the need for a centralized control of medical assets, the Special Weapons and Tactics (SWAT) Medical Commander has become a very important member of the ICS general staff (2,5). The importance of improved tactical incident medical control and planning is eloquently stated in the 1897 quote by Nicholas Senn, M.D., 49th President, American Medical Association: "The fate of the wounded rests in the hands of the one that applies the first dressing."

THE NATIONAL INCIDENT MANAGEMENT SYSTEM

NIMS was issued, by the President, on February 28, 2003, and directs all federal agencies and municipalities, through the Secretary of Homeland Security, to adopt a common incident response and action plan. Per FEMA document 501-1, "NIMS provides a consistent nationwide template to enable Federal, State, local and tribal governments and private-sector and nongovernmental organizations to work together effectively and efficiently to prepare for, prevent, respond to, and recover from domestic incidents, regardless of cause, size, or complexity, including acts of catastrophic terrorism" (4). NIMS is not a template for local states, governments, or municipalities to create an action plan for an isolated small incident but, rather, a framework and standardization of training, qualifications, planning, resource utilization, and communications to improve intercity, state, and federal coordination when large-scale national disasters occur (4,6–11).

Although NIMS is broader in scope and practice than most local incidents, a disaster of monumental proportions such as September 11, 2001, can happen at any time and anywhere. As such, the tactical medical commander needs to understand how to create a medical response plan that effectively coordinates with and integrates the utilization of national resources when needed. These include being proficient with and creating a medical response plan that fits within the NIMS and ICS framework and being adept at utilizing the Multi-Agency Coordination Systems when local medical needs are greater than local medical assets (12,13).

THE INCIDENT COMMAND SYSTEM

The ICS was developed in the 1970s to simplify the coordination of multiple agencies that may be involved in responding to a particular incident. It has been utilized in numerous scenarios, for example, the Columbine High School shootings. In a general sense, it creates a framework from which numerous agencies can understand how to appropriately interact and from whom directions should be taken (14,15). As such, this tested system provides agencies that have not had the opportunity to train together with a structure from which they can integrate. The command and organizational structure of the ICS is very complex and a significant amount of overlap exists among several agencies. For example, the tactical medical commander, as part of the ICS general staff, would interact with the liaison officer at the Incident Command (IC) headquarters for local, state, and national agency coordination. He or she would coordinate with the finance chief for potential medical claims, the logistics chief for the medical units and assets and establishment of supply points or resupply operations, and the operations chiefs for establishment of triage sites, staging areas, and air evacuations and coordination of TEMS with the team commander and task force leaders. However, even with this level of complexity, the established hierarchy of the ICS improves these interactions and interagency coordination (14).

Despite the numerous obstacles that existed during the Columbine incident, the agencies involved had a sound grasp of the ICS matrix. As a result, predefined command structures became secondary to the ICS, allowing for improved incident response and appropriate interagency coordination among police, firefighters, SWAT, EMS, and local hospitals, even though the majority of these agencies had previously never drilled or worked together. In a position statement following the event, it was suggested that while interagency drilling is important, it is more important to have a sound understanding of the ICS among all agencies and personnel responding to ensure appropriate resource utilization and successful incident resolution.

THE SPECIAL WEAPONS AND TACTICS TACTICAL MEDICAL COMMANDER

The SWAT tactical medical commander is part of the general staff of the ICS, reports to and advises the IC, and is responsible for every aspect of medical command, control, and oversight that occurs in the training, medical planning and execution phases, during and after a small- or large-scale incident, disaster, or terrorist act (14). As such, the medical commander, in the perfect situation, would be involved in the selection, training, and certification of all emergency medical personnel, would have total control over the treatment and evacuation assets on- and off-scene, and would have enough organic assets for casualty evacuation (CASEVAC) to local hospitals without having to use standard EMS. However, under the current system, there are no stand-alone SWAT TEMS systems that can handle more than an isolated small encounter before outside agency assistance is needed (2).

Command and Control Issues

The SWAT tactical medical commander is responsible for oversight of all communications related to the medical aspects for the tactical team, civilians, victims, integrated resources, and other outside agencies. However, to a large degree, much of the communication with outside agencies, such as ambulance services, fire departments, government agencies, and hospitals, is done per protocol via the ICS liaison (12,14,16).

The tactical medical commander is responsible for command and control of all organic and nonorganic medical assets in preparation for, during, and after an incident, and he or she is generally located at the IC headquarters (14).

Call signs and frequencies are preset by the IC headquarters and the tactical medical and operational plans determine who goes in and whether patients are treated on the scene or brought out to a predefined triage area, ambulance exchange point (AXPs), or waiting ambulances and EMS crews. Based on changing intelligence, additional assets can be activated as needed.

There are inherent issues with maintaining control over all medical assets. Per protocol, upon arrival to an incident, all medical and nonmedical assets should proceed to the IC headquarters for specific instructions and a mission brief (2,8,9,11,14–16). From this point on, any movements, change in allocation, release from duty, and transport of patients from the incident scene must come from the tactical medical commander. Once the entry team initiates its maneuver, the tactical medical commander is still in control but will be limited to remote care and command of the medical element (15). If available, the TEMS unit will operate under the command authority of the SWAT team commander and IC but will be following the established plans for evacuation, extrication, and zones of care. Thorough planning, training, rehearsals, and interagency agreements are the key to maintaining effective control on-scene (2,13,17).

When interagency coordination occurs, a central medical commander must maintain complete control but may do so through subordinate medical branch chiefs (11,14).

Training

As outlined by the ICS, small- to large-scale drills and training exercises are needed to ensure that all plans will function appropriately. Currently, large numbers of cities or governments do not have SWAT medical commanders, but there is an increasing number of TEMS units (18). Although there is currently no unified national standard on their training and certification, most follow the Committee on Tactical Combat Casualty Care (CoTCCC), Pre-Hospital Trauma Life Support (PHTLS), FEMA, NIMS, and ICS guidelines in their education (2,19). An initiative is currently underway to standardize TEMS training. This initiative is being lead by leading organizations in law inforcement, academics and industry (www.toccourse.com). For a SWAT medical commander, training with the local tactical incident response unit is imperative. In addition, planning, coordinating, and executing the medical aspects of exercises that involve small unit actions, as well as city-wide mass casualty incidents, ensure that issues with local interagency and state medical response, treatment, and evacuation have been fixed prior to a large incident that overloads local capacity (8,17).

Planning

Each incident will have unique risks for the police officers, EMS, fire department, civilians, victims, and assailants. It is therefore vital for the SWAT medical commander to be able to prepare and brief a plan to the IC that integrates medical risk assessments, treatment, and evacuation of all involved based on intelligence regarding the current threat (2). If an IC makes a plan without considering the medical assets, he or she may be unable to resolve the situation due to a lack of medical integration for evacuation or there may be an increased number of police, firefighter, or SWAT injuries due to tactical environmental exposures (17,20).

For example, if TEMS assets are available, the IC has the option of hot and warm zones of care versus full evacuation to waiting EMS. Zones of care are determined by the dangers that exist to the caregiver and patient, and the level of care that can be rendered in that environment. The "hot zone" is care rendered under fire and is based on a scoop-and-run theory. Treatment in the hot zone should be limited to stopping life-threatening bleeding and should not slow down evacuation or extrication to the warm zone. The "warm zone" is tactical field care that is given in temporary security. Basic life support and minimal trauma life support care can be given in this zone. The "cold zone" is equivalent to CASEVAC care, care given in the staging area, or care given while in transport to the medical treatment facility (2,17,19).

If there are multiple casualties that have significant injuries, the IC may opt for a more rapid breach or more lethal means of neutralizing the situation to save innocent lives (2,12,15). The tactical situation, number of assailants, and types of weapons all determine who enters with the SWAT team and is directly related to the type of injuries and the potential for casualties (2,17). If the area is not cleared or safe for EMS to enter, then either a TEMS asset needs to be used or patients need to be brought out to EMS services and the AXPs. The tactical medical commander and those responding to an incident will use AXPs when the distance is too far for the initial unit (i.e., TEMS should not leave the incident area) or it is too dangerous for standard EMS to initially pick up the casualties. An AXP not only is used for the transfer of casualties between ground evacuation platforms, but can be a location where the transfer of casualties occurs between a ground and an air evacuation platform. Normally an AXP is used for the transfer of patients between different types of platforms as opposed to transfer between like vehicles, but as mentioned, standard EMS will not be directly involved in a hostile rescue and the incident response area and there should be secondary and tertiary AXPs that can be occupied in anticipation of a moving incident like the one that occurred during the North Hollywood bank robbery in Los Angeles several years ago (22).

There are numerous planning factors that require consideration when determining whether an AXP is needed to support the ICS health support plan. The medical planners should analyze the casualty estimates, availability of evacuation assets, TEMS status, security, communications, road network, and time and distance between AXPs and receiving hospitals in determining if there is a need for an AXP (20,23). Planning for the use of an AXP must be done with the EMS assets that will support the medical evacuation plan.

Once the medical planner determines that there is a requirement for the use of AXPs, the medical planner and ambulance crews should examine and analyze the decision points to move or relocate an AXP (22). The medical planners need to determine what will trigger the decision to move the AXP, how it will happen, and what the signals are for it to occur. In any situation, the tactical medical commander will govern the shift based on intelligence from the IC.

Integration of Medical Assets

There are several levels of medical asset integration that the SWAT tactical medical commander must understand and have a working knowledge of. They include, but are not limited to, the TEMS members of the SWAT team, physicians, physician assistants, all available local, state, and regional ambulance companies, EMS, fire department paramedics, search and rescue, hospitals, trauma centers, pharmacies, coroners, and veterinary clinics. Although this process is daunting, it is not impossible and is made significantly easier by following the basic outline set forth by both the EOC and the ICS (2).

The SWAT tactical medical commander is responsible for ensuring the integration of local civilian assets into the operational plan prior to an actual event. These interagency standard operating procedures (SOPs) and agreements need to be prepared, presented, and signed, and formal training needs to be conducted to ensure that each agency understands its role in the event of their activation (2,8,13,16,17). In the case of doctors, reserve TEMS officers, and other medical personnel, a definitive plan needs to be in place for their activation, based not only on the current medical situation but also on the potential for further need.

A definitive plan for activation of a hazardous materials (HAZMAT) unit or local military unit with nuclear, chemical, and biological operating capabilities needs to be in place in the event of terrorist activity using these agents. When integrating private ambulance services into a medical response plan, an agreement needs to exist that allows for their continued use during an incident, to prevent a sudden loss of assets because of a predetermined time period or end point.

A significant number of large cities have Internet computerized hospital status programs that give real-time data on whether a hospital is green (accepting patients) or red (not accepting patients). Secondary systems exist separately or coexist for trauma designation or status. If such a system exists, then direction of patients by the tactical medical commander can be significantly more efficient. In the case of a mass casualty incident, prearrangements

need to be made with available hospitals to potentially take more patients than they ordinarily would.

Regardless of whether SOPs have been developed, a list or contact list of organizations, names, numbers, addresses, and e-mails needs to be created for every possible medical and nonmedical service that may be needed. This list is typically kept at the IC headquarters.

Contingency Planning

The need for contingency plans exists with every operation. As such, this section is designed to anticipate the many scenarios that a tactical medical commander may be in charge of. In doing so, the goal is to ensure that the mundane and obscure possibilities are not forgotten when planning for contingencies.

TEMS or no TEMS? What happens when your TEMS member is hurt (2)? How does the IC ensure mission progression if the SWAT team members are evacuating the injured? Do you risk evacuation by standard EMS when full security control has not been achieved (2,13,15,17)? A suspect has barricaded himself with explosives in a gas station that is next to a geriatric or retirement center. What do you do with all the medically needy? A child has been abducted. Do you have on-call pediatricians at the scene or do you rely on the basic pediatric advanced life-support (PALS) capabilities of the paramedics prior to transport to the hospital? The tactical medical commander may be activated for large-scale fires. Who is medically in charge on-scene, the tactical medical commander or the fire chief? A ferry has been taken by a suspect who is believed to have explosives onboard. There is a huge potential for a drowning rescue with numerous hostages from the ferry and the tactical medical commander is activated. Is the Coast Guard, Search and Rescue, or the tactical medical commander medically in charge on the scene? Can a patient who has been hastily decontaminated on-scene be safely transported to a local hospital without causing further injury to other medical personnel (2)?

This section is limitless. Each of these has special requirements that are generally covered in a broader sense by command, control and oversight, integration of medical assets, and interagency agreements as well as planning and logistical issues. To ensure that contingencies are appropriately addressed, one must consider all environmental, social, cultural, structural, and economical situations that exist within an area of operation (2,17,20,22,23).

Unique Issues for the Special Weapons and Tactics Medical Commander

There are potentially some unique relationships that could be factors for the acting SWAT medical commander. Most importantly, the role of the SWAT medical commander must remain just that. In other words, there will be instances where there are numerous other medical elements on the ground supporting an incident. In smaller operations, the SWAT medical commander might be the only medical supervisor on the ground and thus would also serve as the head of the overall medical unit. However, if there are other potential commanders on the ground, there will be instances where it is best for the SWAT medical commander to continue to focus on medical support for his or her team. This would leave some of the more general medical operations to another individual (2,14). This abdication does not imply that there would not be a reciprocal relationship between the two. Many times, the two individuals will find themselves working together, combining logistics with tactical support (2,11,14–16).

For the SWAT medical commander, there are a number of potential issues that must be addressed when creating or integrating into an ICS. First, one must expect the necessity of briefing the medical unit commander on the medical support requirements of the SWAT team. Specifically, the commander needs to know how many EMTs, paramedics, physician assistants, and/or physicians are on the ground in support of the SWAT team. The commander can use this information to integrate the SWAT team into the overall medical support plan.

Additionally, the concept of CASEVAC must be addressed, as that tends to involve many organizational components (2,8,9,21). Specifically, the tactical physician's SOP must be reviewed with the medical commander in order to come to an understanding of how CASEVAC is going to function during the operation.

OVERSIGHT/LIABILITY

An area of concern for physicians involved in the medical oversight of tactical units involves the liability that the individual incurs while providing medical support. This continues to be an area of intense discussion within tactical EMS and physician circles. There may be clear or implied liability incurred from supporting tactical missions by team members, hostages, civilian bystanders, or assailants (24). For example, during a tactical mission the assailant is detained, and during this process he suffers a fractured wrist. Do the medical assets provide medical support to this individual, or does the physician limit his or her role to medical planning, coordination with local EMS, and medical care of team members? Who decides whether an assailant or wounded officer is treated first? If the physician makes the decision to help in the medical management of an assailant or civilians at the scene, does that mean he or she automatically incurs liability in the medical outcome of these patients? This is a complex question that will vary from team to team based on physician preference and should be based on a thorough evaluation of state laws.

There are a few ways to ensure having malpractice coverage while functioning as the medical commander in tactical medicine operations. The medical commander might be able to get the supporting carrier of his or her primary practice to extend coverage to tactical operations, but this requires the commander to effectively carry liability coverage for risk incurred while acting in a role that is supporting a government or city agency, in a position that may not provide monetary compensation (25,26). This subjects the physician to significant personal and professional liability and would not be recommended unless no other options are available. Under the military medical system, medical personnel working under the auspices of the U.S. Government are covered by a general liability and comprehensive malpractice TORT that limits extraneous claims made against personal assets. This type of coverage is a preferred method for liability protection against suits that may be brought forth as a result of tactical medical operations. Another option is to have the state, city, or provincial government establish, finance, and carry a policy with a national insurance provider that covers any event requiring the activation of personnel or positions set forth in the ICS. The policy should also cover the medical personnel who respond, as long they have been activated by the ICS and local incident response plan, and as long as they are acting in an official capacity (27,28). If this is possible, it is important to get documentation in writing prior to going on missions, and any medical personnel are strongly discouraged from conducting tactical medical operations prior to the establishment of some form of liability coverage.

TAKE-HOME POINTS

1. The tactical medical commander should be an integral part of the ICS.
2. Planning should involve integration of all medical assets and possible contingencies.
3. The issues of oversight and liability should be addressed for all involved medical providers.

SUMMARY

The tactical medical commander should be fully integrated into the planning and execution of the mission. This requires a firm understanding of all elements for command and control as well as coordination of the available medical assets. Additionally, there should be contingency planning for all possible scenarios that may be encountered in the tactical scenario.

REFERENCES

1. Available at: www.pbs.org/empires/napoleon/n_war/soldier/page_1. html. Accessed December 2006.

2. Rinnert K, Hall W. Tactical emergency medical support. *Emerg Med Clin North Am.* 2002;20(4):929–952.
3. Available at: www.cs.amedd.army.mil/history/ele-milmed.html. Accessed December 2006.
4. U.S. Federal Emergency Management Administration (FEMA). *NIMS basic. Introduction and overview.* FEMA 501-1. 29 March 29 2006. Available at: www.fema.gov/pdf/nims/NIMS_basic_introduction_and_overview.pdf.
5. American College of Emergency Physicians. Tactical emergency medical support: policy statement. *Ann Emerg Med.* 2005;45(1):108.
6. U.S. Federal Emergency Management Administration (FEMA). *NIMS basic. The incident command system.* FEMA 501-B. 27 March 2006. Available at: www.fema.gov/pdf/nims/NIMS_basic_incident_command_system.pdf.
7. U.S. Federal Emergency Management Administration (FEMA). NIMS and the Incident Command System: NIMS ICS position paper. NIMS Integration Center. 23 November 2004. Available at: www.fema.gov/txt/emergency/nims/nims_ics_position_paper.txt.
8. U.S. Federal Emergency Management Administration (FEMA). State NIMS integration. Integrating the National Incident Management System into state emergency operations plans and standard operating procedures. Version 1. 8 September 2004. Available at: www.fema.gov/pdf/emergency/nims/eop-sop_state_online.pdf.
9. U.S. Federal Emergency Management Administration (FEMA). *NIMS basic. Resource management.* FEMA 501-4. 27 March 2006. Available at: www.fema.gov/pdf/nims/NIMS_basic_resource_management.pdf.
10. U.S. Federal Emergency Management Administration (FEMA). *NIMS basic. Preparedness.* FEMA 501-3. 27 March 2006. Available at: www.fema.gov/pdf/nims/NIMS_basic_preparedness.pdf.
11. U.S. Federal Emergency Management Administration (FEMA). *NIMS basic. Command management.* FEMA 501-2. 27 March 2006. Available at: www.fema.gov/pdf/nims/NIMS_basic_command_and_management.pdf.
12. Metro SWAT. *Standard Operating Procedures Manual, Version 1.* Bonney Lake, WA: Bonney Lake Police Department; 2004.
13. Mell HK, Sztajnkrycer MD. EMS response to Columbine: lessons learned. *Internet J Rescue Disaster Med.* 2005;5(1).
14. Irwin RL. The Incident Command System (ICS). In: Auf der Heide E, ed. *Disaster Response: Principles of Preparation and Coordination.* Atlanta, GA: Erik Auf der Heide; 1989. Available at: http://orgmail2.coe-dmha.org/dr/static.htm.
15. Barnes R, Blind R. Scene control policy. Kern County, CA: Emergency Medical Services Department; 2002.
16. Washington State Department of Health. West Region EMS & trauma care system plan. 13 May 2005. Available at: www.doh.wa.gov/hsqa/emstrauma/download/wrplan.pdf.
17. Department of the Army. *FM 8-43. Combat health support for Army Special Operations Forces.* Washington, DC: Department of the Army; 2000.
18. Carmona R. TEMS transitioning into the new millennium. *Tact Edge J* 2002;20(3):64–65.
19. Callaway DW. Tactical emergency medicine (TEMS). Available at: www.ncemsf.org/conf2006/presentations/callaway%20-%20tactical%20ems.pdf. Accessed 25 February 2006.
20. Department of the Army. *FM 8-42. Combat health support in stability operations and support operations.* Washington, DC: Department of the Army; 1997.
21. Department of the Army. *FM 8-10-6. Medical evacuation in a theater of operations. Tactics, techniques and procedures.* Washington, DC: Department of the Army; 2004.
22. Available at: http://harrymarnell.com/officer.htm. Accessed December 2006.
23. Department of the Army. *FM 8.55. Planning for health service support.* Washington, DC: Department of the Army; 1994.
24. Sztajnkrycer MD, Báez AA, Eberlein CM. Resident and faculty involvement in tactical emergency medical support: a survey of U.S. emergency medicine residency programs. *Internet J Rescue Disaster Med.* 2005;5(1).
25. Available at: www.nctma.net/user/NCTMA%20Newsletter,%20Fall%202005.pdf. Accessed December 2006.
26. Available at: www.legislature.mi.gov/(1lrhe5znoekd4y55wdnphk55)/mileg.aspx?page=getobject&objectname=2005-HB-5054&queryid=14530351. Accessed December 2006.
27. Available at: www.ileas.org/policies/tems.pdf. Accessed December 2006.
28. Available at: www.legislature.mi.gov/documents/2005-2006/publicact/pdf/2005-PA-0318.pdf. Accessed December 2006.

Chapter 27

Quality Assurance and Improvement

Peter J. Cuenca and James A. Pfaff

OBJECTIVES

After reading this section, the reader will be able to:

1. Define quality assurance and quality improvement
2. Discuss the necessary elements needed for successful emergency medicine services oversight

Quality assurance (QA) encompasses all actions taken to ensure that the standards and procedures of tactical prehospital emergency medical care are adhered to and the delivered services meet performance requirements set by an organization and its national certifying bodies. QA is executed by planned systematic activities ensuring that the organization's system performance conforms to its established technical and operational requirements (1). The goal of tactical emergency medical services (EMS) system quality improvement (QI) is to design and implement practical and efficient processes to measure and evaluate the quality of tactical emergency medical services leading to continuous and measurable improvements. QI occurs when new, previously unattained, levels of performance are achieved (2). For any tactical EMS organization to be successful, QA and QI must be integral components of the organizations routine operations. Successful QA and QI programs result in benchmarking outcomes and allowing the identification of best practices and the shaping of standards. Specific areas that must be covered in any successful EMS program include certification of skill set, oversight of training and medical care delivered, documentation of training, and integration of medical training within tactical operations, both exercise and real-world.

The first step of QA is ensuring that your tactical prehospital care providers are certified and licensed by your organization's recognized body, either a state agency and/or the National Registry of Emergency Medical Technicians (NREMT). This is sometimes dictated by the local area policy. Whether the system is composed of providers who are First Responders (FRs), Emergency Medical Technician—Basic (EMT-B)'s, Emergency Medical Technician—Intermediates (EMT-I), Paramedics (EMT-P), or any combination of these, certification and licensure, and their sustainment, are a must.

CERTIFICATION AND EDUCATION

Certification results after a professional organization has determined through written and/or hands-on examination that an individual is qualified to perform certain skills within, as in the case of the NREMT, a nationally recognized scope of practice. Licensure is granted by a state or other governmental entity that gives an individual the right to practice as an EMT in a specified area. This should already be done during the initial entry/processing of any individual to professional law enforcement/tactical operations organization, but it still deserves mention. After ensuring certification and licensure, it is imperative that time is planned in the training schedule to meet the medical sustainment training requirements of the tactical prehospital health care specialists. This may place a burden on the organization and individual operator, however, it is imperative that these individuals maintain a level of competency and credentialing that is recognized locally and/or nationally.

The Continuing Education Coordinating Board for Emergency Medical Services (CECBEMS) is the national accrediting body for EMS continuing education courses and course providers. It was chartered in 1992 by the following sponsoring organizations: American College of Emergency Physicians, National Registry of Emergency Medical Technicians, National Association of Emergency Medical Services Physicians, National Association of State EMS Directors, National Council of State Emergency Medical Services Training Coordinators, National Association of Emergency Medical Technicians, National Association of EMS Educators, and American College of Osteopathic Emergency Physicians. The purpose of CECBEMS is to develop and implement policies to standardize the review and approval of EMS continuing education (CE) activities. National standardization of the CE activity approval process for EMS personnel by CECBEMS has led toward nationwide improvement in the quality of the educational offerings. CECBEMS approval is required only for continuing education that is in a distributed learning format (online, video, journal articles, CD ROM programs). To meet National Registry requirements for nondistributed learning activities, the activity must be approved by either CECBEMS or the appropriate state EMS agency (3).

Training and CE are vital to the performance of EMS providers. Depending on the level of provider as well as the certification standards of the body under which the provider is licensed, the training and CE requirements for each provider will vary. However, regardless of the scope of practice and the requirements, training/CE should involve both didactic and practical components. The EMS medical director must be actively involved with the initial and sustainment training conducted within a particular system. In most systems, there is a training officer appointed by the director to run the daily operation of the training program. To gain legitimacy with field providers, the EMS director should be personally instructing and present when instruction is provided by EMS personnel/outside clinicians. Recruiting physicians from the receiving Emergency Department within their system will help to foster better communication and understanding with EMS providers. Medical directors should encourage medics within the system to become subject matter experts in specific areas of field care so they can serve as peer instructors.

MEDICAL OVERSIGHT

EMS medical oversight is defined as physician-directed prehospital emergency medical care. The EMS medical director assumes all medical and legal responsibility for the patient care administered by the prehospital provider. The prehospital personnel practice under the license of the medical director. Oversight of clinical skills occurs in several ways, indirect and direct. Direct medical oversight is online or immediate supervision of care. Indirect oversight is offline and can be further divided into prospective and retrospective phases. Providing medical oversight does not guarantee good medical care or patient outcome. Proactive medical oversight that performs regular assessments and in-depth reviews of all aspects of day-to-day operations will help to ensure that the prehospital emergency services delivered by its EMS system meet the current standard of emergency medical care (4). Some items that deserve specific attention from EMS medical directors are summarized in Table 27.1.

Although direct field supervision is the exception rather than the rule in most EMS systems, for an EMS system to

▶ **TABLE 27.1. Summary of Items that Deserve Specific Attention from EMS Medical Directors.**

- Monthly protocol review for adherence to the current medical standard of care, local law, medical administrative coding, and EMS policy
- Training, both medical and tactical operations
- Continuing education of all direct medical oversight personnel
- Direct field supervision of prehospital providers
- Required notification and communication by EMS providers to receiving hospitals
- Review of direct and indirect medical oversight patient records
- Review of patient outcomes
- Critique of in-the-field operations, both real-world and training exercises
- Protocol development and review
- Outcome analysis
- Reassessment after system changes are made

be successful, the medical director must have some direct field observation and supervision of care. The most effective quality management method available to the physician is direct observation in the field. This allows for real-time assessment, correction, and affirmation of provider clinical skills. Being in the field provides credibility for the medical director with the system providers. The medical director will have a better understanding of the adverse and austere conditions that the EMS providers often find themselves in. This understanding leads to better protocols and training for the system's providers.

PROTOCOL REVIEW

Monthly protocol review is vital to assuring the highest quality of clinical care for patients, in tactical EMS organizations and standard civilian organizations alike. When developing or reviewing protocols, medical directors must first consider the level of providers that operate within the system. Every protocol for the EMS system must be written specifically for each and every level of provider that exists within the system. Medical directors should consider reviewing the protocols of other surrounding EMS systems with similar capabilities as a starting point. Protocols need to be based on the current literature and recent research. The body of prehospital research available is limited but growing. There is a paucity of outcomes research for determining the best therapy for all EMS situations. For instance, even in the heavily researched area of cardiac arrest, it is not known how treatment protocols should differ for a 10-minute versus a 30-minute transport time. However, standards that exist in the literature should be adhered to. Medical directors should attempt to involve their providers as much as possible in clinical, outcomes, and systems research in EMS. New protocol development and implementation lends itself to this concept. EMS providers should be involved in protocol development and review. Also, the physicians at receiving facilities within an EMS system should be solicited for feedback regarding protocol development and performance. Their input can clarify situations in which EMS providers are inappropriately managing patients because of protocols.

Review of all patient run reports and patient outcomes is a requirement of all EMS systems. Someone within the organization should be performing this duty as the designated QA coordinator. The medical director of the system should have oversight and directly review all cases where protocols were not followed or there was a poor patient outcome. In addition, the medical director should conduct routine, random, and focused run reviews. The QA coordinator should be maintaining statistics on several key factors for each medic in the organization: (i) response time, (ii) scene time, (iii) transport time, (iv) number of attempted IVs, (v) number of attempted intubations, and (vi) number of traumatic resuscitations. In many cases, the run report may not adequately address the events of the call and whether there were issues in quality of care provided. Because of this, medical directors should active obtain information from other sources, including the law enforcement personnel involved, receiving facility staff, receiving facility physicians and nurses, and patients/patients' families.

EMERGENCY MEDICAL DISPATCH

The EMS communication responsibilities of a medical director include establishing and sustaining emergency medical dispatch (EMD) training for all dispatchers. Emergency medical dispatching involves the reception, evaluation, processing, and provision of dispatch life support and the management of requests for emergency medical assistance. Medical directors have the obligation of participating in ongoing evaluation and improvement of the EMD process. This process includes identifying the nature of the request, prioritizing the severity of the request, dispatching the necessary resources, providing medical aid and safety instructions to the callers, and coordinating the responding resources as needed. Medical directors should have oversight of the quality management program for EMD in their system.

TRAINING FOR QUALITY IMPROVEMENT

Civilian special tactics teams provide ready response to situations beyond the capabilities of normally equipped and trained law enforcement personnel. Police teams take mil-

itary tactics and hardware into high-risk situations that occur in their communities (5). Just as a military special operations unit includes a medical contingent in its operational package and planning, civilian special tactics teams must incorporate EMS personnel into the department's tactical operations. This is crucial for QI/QA to occur. Due to the nature of the missions, very dangerous conditions and unconventional hazards are commonplace for tactical law enforcement teams. However, the sole purpose of the special tactics teams is to minimize risk through training, teamwork, and preparedness. Therefore, it is imperative that special tactics organizations include medical support as a routine component of team training. Casualty play must be incorporated into every training event in order to exercise the capabilities in a realistic environment (6).

It is difficult to replicate the actual stresses, both mental and physical, that prehospital providers will experience. However, there are things that can be manipulated in training that will assure, refine, and improve combat casualty treatment reaction by your personnel. All training events should closely resemble the high-risk conditions to be expected on the tactical environment. All medical training should be done with the provider's full tactical load. Training should be conducted under both lighted and no-light conditions. Scenarios in which the primary medical provider is a casualty should be executed to determine if the proper level of cross-level training/buddy care is occurring. These events will demonstrate how personnel, skills sets, training, and equipment must be modified for maximum effectiveness.

There are no "standard courses" on which medical directors can base their training programs. Leaders must set up events based on the resources available and the training needs of their team members. As long as the training incorporates the elements mentioned above, it should be considered "standard." Also, it is important to ensure that the leaders of the organization understand medical care and how it relates to the mission. There should be scenarios in which leaders are faced with missions with limited or no medical support. Leaders should also be prepared to discuss tactical and medical actions after sustaining casualties. Leaders must make continual assessment of casualty status and requirements, medical assets available or lost, and the mission. Being fully prepared to adapt the execution of a mission with medical planning and possible casualty involvement should be an integral part of tactical and medical training and planning.

In every exercise/mission that occurs in both the civilian and the military areas, an after-action report (AAR) should be completed. This report includes a detailed, step-by-step review of all actions leading to the objective and at the objective, the medical support systems in place, and the actions that took place during the scenario. There should be a detailed summary of events, identified critical actions, failures, and procedures/tactics that need improvement. Specific attention should be paid to delivery of the right level of care at the right moment in the context of the tactical situation. This report should be done as soon as possible, while memories are fresh and details can be recalled. All parties involved, both tactical and medical, should meet again 24 to 48 hours after completing the mission to review the notes of the immediate AAR and reassess what was discussed. No AAR is useful if the lessons learned are not incorporated into improvements in the training and protocols of the tactical EMS system. Execution of lessons learned is a must.

TAKE-HOME POINTS

1. Providers should be certified and licensed by state and national accreditation agencies.
2. There should be ongoing review of all protocols and EMS runs.
3. QA/QI is a dynamic process that involves education, training, and skills improvement.

SUMMARY

QA encompasses a broad range of topics including training, supervision, protocol, and records review. In addition, there is the need for the critique and review of all field operations. Constant training and reevaluation are integral to the development and sustainment of an effective, well-run tactical emergency medicine system.

REFERENCES

1. U.S. Department of Transportation, National Highway Traffic Safety Administration. *A Leadership Guide to Quality Improvement for Emergency Medical Services (EMS) Systems.* Washington, DC: U.S. Department of Transportation; July 1997.
2. Swor RA. Quality assurance in EMS systems. *Emerg Med Clin North Am.* 1992;10(3):597–610.
3. Available at: http://www.cecbems.org/. Accessed March 15, 2006.
4. Krentz MJ. Medical accountability. *Emerg Med Clin North Am.* 1990;8(1):17–32.
5. Williams JJ, Westall D. SWAT and non-SWAT police officers and the use of force. *J Crim Just.* 2003;31(5):469–474.
6. Hall MT. Appendix P. The urban area during support mission case study: Mogadishu—Applying the Lessons Learned—Take 2. U.S. Army MOUT Training. Urban Operations Conference, March 23, 2000.

Chapter 28

Grant Funding for Tactical Operations

Richard V. King and Paul E. Moore

OBJECTIVES

After reading this section, the reader will be able to:

1. The importance of grant funding to tactical operations
2. The need to understand eligibility requirements
3. The role of the Internet in finding grant opportunities and applying for grants
4. Major sources of grant funding for tactical operations and law enforcement
5. Criteria used in judging effective grant proposals
6. How to compete effectively for grants

Grants are a major source of funding for tactical operations. Grant funds may be used to purchase needed equipment and for training and education, personnel, process, and infrastructure improvements, research, planning, and other purposes consistent with the intent of the grant. Applications may be solicited by the grantor in the form of a Request for Application (RFA) or Request for Proposal (RFP). Alternatively, a grant may be solicited by an individual or group who develops an idea and writes a proposal to request funding from a sponsor.

In the case of an RFP, the sponsor describes the intended purposes of the funding, the types of individuals or groups eligible to apply, and the required information that applicants must supply. Required information may include detailed descriptions of the applicant's plans, capabilities, accounting and control systems, inventory management, reports (specific information and times of reports), key deliverables, and budget required to accomplish the grant's objectives.

In an investigator-initiated proposal, an applicant identifies a need, develops a proposal, and submits it to a prospective grantor. The proposal may a simple one-page letter or a formal document including numerous details. In either case, essential information must be conveyed to assure the grantor that the applicant is eligible and capable of successful completion of the grant's objectives within a specified period of time.

Many grants provide funds as reimbursement. This means that the recipient must use its own financial resources initially and then submit expenses for reimbursement from the funding agency, typically on a monthly basis. Others may provide the funding up-front to allow the grantee more direct control over spending—some grantors even allow the grantee to earn interest on these funds.

Considering the time and effort involved, the tactical team should carefully consider whether it can commit the resources required not only to apply for the grant but, if the team receives the award, to manage the grant and accomplish the objectives. The team should only pursue a grant that they believe is a good fit with the team's purpose, mission, goals, and capability.

ELIGIBILITY REQUIREMENTS

Applicants must be certain that they are eligible to apply for the particular grant. Eligibility requirements are specified by the grant sponsors. The following is an example.

Any nonfederal agency chartered and empowered to enforce U.S. laws in the following jurisdictions: the United States, a State (or political subdivision) of the United States, or a Territory/possession (or political subdivision) of the United States, including:

- Local police
- Sheriffs
- State police
- County police (municipal police that operate on a countywide basis, e.g., Fairfax County, VA; Nassau County, NY)
- Native American tribal police
- Special police certified by the state
- Campus police certified by the state

A tactical medical team would qualify for these funds because of the law enforcement context of its duties and responsibilities.

THE ROLE OF THE INTERNET

Today the Internet is the primary tool for locating potential grant opportunities and submitting grant applications. It is also used by grantees to report on grant progress. An Internet search can quickly locate government agencies requesting grant applications as well as private foundations and other enterprises that wish to fund certain types of projects.

Web searches for government grant funding should include the Grants.gov (1) web site. At this site, one can search in a variety of ways, including by key word (such as Funding Opportunity Number [FON] or Catalog of Federal Domestic Assistance [CFDA] number), category (such as Law, Justice and Legal Services), agency (such as U.S. Department of Justice or Department of Homeland Security), or eligibility (such as state, county, city or township, and tribal governments).

More general searches can be accomplished using the various web search engines, such as Google (2) and others. Speed and efficiency in searching the web are dependent on one's choice of appropriate search terms, or key words. For example, one might try searching the web using terms such as *law enforcement grants* or *SWAT grants*. It is advisable to develop one's skills in using these search engines.

Grant seekers may find useful information at the National Criminal Justice Reference Service (NCJRS) web site, which is administered by the Department of Justice Office of Justice Programs (3). NCJRS is a "federally funded resource that provides justice and substance abuse information to support research, policy, and program development worldwide." It includes links to grants and funding opportunities.

MAJOR SOURCES OF GRANTS FOR TACTICAL TEAMS

There are many sources of grant funding, including government agencies (national, state, or local), the private sector, educational institutions, foundations, and international humanitarian organizations. Examples are:

- Department of Homeland Security (DHS)
- Department of Justice (DOJ)
- Department of Health and Human Services (DHHS)
- National Institutes of Health (NIH)
- Department of Energy (DOE)
- Department of Transportation (DOT)

- Department of Education (DOE)
- K–12 School Grant Funding
- The Robert Wood Johnson Foundation

Tactical medical teams should be particularly aware of funding through the DHS, DOJ, and DHHS. Major programs under each of these departments are described below.

Department of Homeland Security

The 2007 Homeland Security Grant Program (HSGP) allocated more than $1.6 billion in awards "to enhance the ability of states, territories, and urban areas to prepare for, prevent, and respond to terrorist attacks and other major disasters." HSGP funds can be used for "preparedness planning, equipment, training, exercises, management, and administration" in order to obtain resources critical to building and sustaining capabilities aligned with the Interim National Preparedness Goal and with State and Urban Area Homeland Security Strategies (4).

Urban Area Security Initiative Grant Program (UASI) funds address the unique planning, equipment, training, and exercise needs of high-threat, high-density urban areas, and assist them in building an enhanced and sustainable capacity to prevent, protect against, respond to, and recover from acts of terrorism.

The Law Enforcement Terrorism Prevention Program (LETPP) focuses on the prevention of terrorist attacks and provides law enforcement and public safety communities with funds to support the following activities: intelligence gathering and information sharing through enhancing/establishing fusion centers; hardening high-value targets; planning strategically; continuing to build interoperable communications; and collaborating with non-law enforcement partners, other government agencies, and the private sector.

Metropolitan Medical Response System (MMRS) funds support MMRS jurisdictions to "enhance and sustain an integrated, systematic mass casualty incident preparedness program that enables an effective response during the first crucial hours of an incident." The program prepares jurisdictions to respond to various mass casualty incidents, including "CBRNE, agricultural and epidemic outbreaks, natural disasters and large-scale hazardous materials incidents."

Several of the grants available through the HSGP provide funding for tactical team operations. Information about these programs can be viewed on the DHS's web site, including information about actual funding allocations to the various states (5). The State Homeland Security Grant Program supports the implementation of the State Homeland Security Strategy to address the identified planning, equipment, training, and exercise needs for acts of terrorism. In addition, it supports the implementation of the National Preparedness Goal, the National Incident Management System (NIMS), and the National Response Plan (NRP).

The Commercial Equipment Direct Assistance Program (CEDAP) (6) was created "to provide smaller law enforcement and emergency responder agencies with equipment items that will enhance and support regional response, mutual aid, and interoperability of responder equipment." The CEDAP is a DHS-funded program that provides "requested equipment directly to qualified selected applicants. CEDAP recipients also receive training and technical assistance on the equipment awarded to ensure that the devices are effectively used and properly maintained." The CEDAP targets smaller communities not currently eligible for funding from other DHS grants such as the Urban Areas Security Initiative grant program. Award decisions are made on the basis of need for the specific equipment and ability to use and maintain the equipment.

CEDAP funds may be used for equipment and training in five categories:

- Personal protective equipment
- Thermal imaging, night vision, and video surveillance tools
- Chemical and biological detection tools
- Information technology and risk management tools
- Interoperable communications equipment/technology

Department of Justice, Office of Justice Programs

The Edward Byrne Memorial Justice Assistance Grant (JAG) Program (7) is "the primary provider of federal criminal justice funding to state and local jurisdictions. JAG funds support all components of the criminal justice system, from multijurisdictional drug and gang task forces to crime prevention and domestic violence programs, courts, corrections, treatment, and justice information sharing initiatives." JAG funds can be used to pay for personnel, overtime, and equipment. Funds provided for the states can be used for statewide initiatives, technical assistance and training, and support for local and rural jurisdictions.

Community oriented policing services (COPS) methamphetamine (Meth) grants [8] have been awarded since 1998 to "help state and local law enforcement agencies reduce the production, distribution, and use of methamphetamine." These grants encourage recipients to develop partnerships with community leaders, local fire departments, drug courts, prosecutors, child protective services, treatment providers, and other law enforcement agencies "to create a coordinated response to methamphetamine proliferation." COPS grants have been used for "equipment, training, and personnel to improve intelligence-gathering capabilities, enforcement efforts, lab clean-up, training related to drug endangered children, and in the

prosecution of those who engage in methamphetamine-related crimes."

The majority of COPS funding has been awarded "directly to state and local law enforcement agencies to purchase officer safety equipment and supplies" and to provide training to first responders "who are combating the use and distribution of methamphetamine in jurisdictions across the United States."

The Bulletproof Vest Partnership (9) is a Department of Justice Bureau of Justice Assistance initiative that provides federal funds to support the purchase of bulletproof vests.

Department of Health and Human Services

The National Bioterrorism Hospital Preparedness Program (HBHPP) is intended to help hospitals, supporting health care systems, and partner organizations to prepare for and respond with coordinated, effective care to victims of public health emergencies, including terrorism. Priorities include improving surge capacity and decontamination capabilities, pharmaceutical supplies, training and education, drills, and exercises (10).

Other Grant Programs

Special Program Assistance for Needed Tactical Officer Assets (SPANTOA) (11) is a nongovernmental grants program specifically for tactical teams. It is intended to provide "important life saving equipment to SWAT/tactical teams that may otherwise not be able to obtain this equipment." All applicants are required to have a valid NTOA team membership to be eligible.

Tactical teams may also wish to investigate any funding or support opportunities available through the various equipment vendors, suppliers, and manufacturers with whom they do business. There also may be community or regional funding available for which they are qualified.

Medical personnel on the tactical teams should participate in the grant application process and help in expressing the team's needs and goals from a medical perspective. For example, the team seeks funding for training in the use of appropriate personal protective equipment to protect themselves in case of chemical, biological, radiological, nuclear, and explosive (CBRNE) events, or to learn how to administer antidotes.

THE STATE ADMINISTRATIVE AGENCY

State governments are eligible for funding under federal programs. The governor of each state has designated a State Administrative Agency (SAA) to apply for and administer the funds under the HSGP. The SAA is the only agency eligible to apply for HSGP funds and is responsible for obligating HSGP funds to local units of government and other designated recipients. In Texas, for example, the Governor of the State of Texas has designated the Governors Division of Emergency Management (GDEM) as the SAA to apply for and administer the funds under the HSGP (12).

The actual funding that goes to a state is determined by the specific grants applied for and received. For example, in Virginia, in fiscal year 2006, the Department of Criminal Justice Services' Law Enforcement Services Grants Unit administered 219 grants totaling $10,670,072 in federal funds and $1,087,834 in state funds [13]. These included:

- 65 Byrne Memorial Fund Grants: $2,428,726 in federal funds
- 20 Byrne Discretionary Anti-Gang Grants: $1,871,315 in federal funds
- 99 Law Enforcement Terrorism Prevention Grants: $6,370,031 in federal funds
- 35 School Resource Officer Incentive (Trust Fund) Grants: $1,087,834 in state funds

COMPETING EFFECTIVELY

Identifying and applying for grant funding should be an ongoing activity of the tactical team. Inevitably, some RFPs will be discovered only a short time before the application is due. Others may allow only a short time between announcement and due date. Often the odds of getting a grant on first application to a particular sponsor are low. The way to be successful, however, is to be vigilant in looking for appropriate grant opportunities.

Individuals, organizations, or agencies that apply for grants must thoroughly understand the requirements of the grant, as well as their own strengths and weaknesses. They must be able to articulate their mission, their inter- and intra-agency relationships, and their organization's niche in their community and in society as a whole. Furthermore, applicants should be knowledgeable about the sponsor, including prior awards granted and the types of organizations and projects that were funded. If possible, one should review successful past grant applications submitted to the sponsor.

It is not enough to have a good cause, to be thorough in completing the application, and to submit it prior to the specified deadline. Individuals or agencies must make a convincing case for why limited grant funding should be entrusted to them. In an RFP the sponsor will specify what information must be included in the application. The sponsor needs to know that the applicant has the individual, organizational, and system capabilities to be successful.

Applicants should clearly describe the current situation, the desired change or need, what they propose to do to meet this need, why outside funding is needed, and how it will be used. Include specific goals, milestones, time frames, and budgets, as well as any evidence—credible data and published literature—that supports your expressed point of view and proposed approach.

Grant reviewers may not be the same people who prepared the RFP. Often they are an ad hoc "peer" committee that scores each application based on specific criteria as described in the RFP and in guidance given to reviewers by the sponsor. Key criteria may include the match between the proposal and the mission and goals of the grantor, the potential impact of the proposed project, whether the proposal is unique and innovative, whether plans, time frames, and budgets are feasible, and whether the applicant seems capable (e.g., based on his or her position, letters of support, prior successes, previous publications, and notable accomplishments). Applicants help the reviewers, the sponsor, and themselves by providing information specifically to demonstrate their competence and capability—doing so may help increase the likelihood of receiving the award.

In any proposal the writing can be a critical determinant of whether a grant application is accepted or rejected. Writing should be clear and concise. A positive and professional tone should be used throughout the proposal. Pay attention to the language used in the RFP and in past successful grant applications. These may contain clues to guide your writing. The RFP may provide detailed guidance regarding the file format of the application and even the particular font types to be used. An agency that lacks the skills for and knowledge of grant writing may consider seeking assistance from a consultant who specializes in preparing grant applications.

Organizations seeking a grant and responding to an RFP need not apply as an individual agency or organization—they may combine resources and expertise with other individuals or organizations to present a more robust and comprehensive response. A partnership may allow more efficient use of grant resources and facilitate additional accomplishments for the public good. Two organizations that combine their resources and apply together may stand a better chance of being awarded the grant than if each were to compete separately. The tactical medical team might consider partnering with local hospitals, county and private, emergency medical services, and disaster response groups.

EFFECTIVENESS OF GRANT PROPOSALS

Grant reviewers of Homeland Security grants are now asked to evaluate the anticipated effectiveness of grant proposals in addressing stated national needs priorities (14). Applicants would be well advised to consider the following five criteria when writing their proposals.

1. Relevance (e.g., relationship to the national preparedness goal)
2. Regionalization (ability to communicate, plan, and collaborate across disciplines and jurisdictions)
3. Sustainability (including identifying means of funding the capability beyond the grant period)
4. Implementation approach (appropriate structures, resources, and tools in place to achieve results)
5. Impact (effectiveness of the implementation in reducing risks, threats, vulnerabilities, and consequences)

SUMMARY

Grants are an essential source of funding for the tactical medical team, therefore seeking grants should be an ongoing, core activity of the team. A wide variety of grants is available from federal and other sources. Information about grants can be found on the Internet and through one's SAA. A grant should be sought only if appropriate and closely aligned with the mission and goals of the team. Consider opportunities for partnering with other organizations when appropriate. Guidelines provided by grantors should be read carefully and followed precisely. Applicants should try to anticipate how grant reviewers will judge their proposal according to known criteria of effectiveness. Proposals should be concise but thorough, using a positive and professional tone. Assistance from experienced grant writers should be considered as an option, especially when internal grantsmanship skills are lacking and stakes are high. Do not be discouraged if a grant is not awarded on the first application. Persistence, over time, is the key to success in obtaining grant funding.

REFERENCES

Note: All web sites accessed June 2007.
1. Grants.gov. http://www.grants.gov.
2. Google. http://google.com.
3. National Criminal Justice Reference Service. http://www.ncjrs.gov.
4. U.S. Department of Homeland Security. http://www.ojp.usdoj.gov/odp/grants_hsgp.htm.
5. U.S. Department of Homeland Security. State contacts and grant award information. http://www.dhs.gov/xgovt/grants/index.shtm.
6. U.S. Department of Homeland Security. Commercial Equipment Direct Assistance Program. http://www.ojp.usdoj.gov/odp/docs/FY07_CEDAP_GUIDANCE.pdf.
7. U.S. Department of Justice. Edward Byrne Memorial Justice Assistance Grant Program. http://www.ojp.usdoj.gov/BJA/grant/07JAGLocalSol.pdf.
8. U.S. Department of Justice. Office of Community Oriented Policing Services. http://www.cops.usdoj.gov.
9. U.S. Department of Justice. Office of Justice Programs. http://www.ojp.usdoj.gov/bvpbasi/.
10. U.S. Department of Health and Human Services. Health Resources and Services Administration. http://www.hrsa.gov/bioterrorism.
11. Special Program Assistance for Needed Tactical Officer Assets. http://www.ntoa.org/grants.
12. North Central Texas Council of Governments. http://www.nctcog.org/ep/HSGP.
13. Virginia.gov. Department of Criminal Justice Services. http://www.dcjs.virginia.gov/cple/grants.
14. North Central Texas Council of Governments. http://www.nctcog.org/ep/UASI/HSGP_Effectiveness_Analysis_Fact_Sheet.pdf.

Chapter 29

Health Insurance Portability and Accountability Act (HIPAA) Impact on Tactical Emergency Medicine

Justin B. Williams and Annette Williams

OBJECTIVES

After reading this section, the reader will be able to:

1. Discuss the principles of privacy and confidentiality as they apply to the Health Insurance Portability and Accountability Act (HIPAA) and tactical emergency medicine.
2. Describe when protected health information may be released and what exceptions to HIPAA exist with regard to health care providers.
3. Delineate the special considerations law enforcement personnel are given under HIPAA with regard to protected health information.

The Health Insurance Portability and Accountability Act (HIPAA), is a recently enacted piece of federal legislation that places legal regulatory requirements on health care providers in all arenas of care, including tactical emergency medicine care. As a result, an intimate knowledge of its content, regulations, requirements, and potential consequences are mandatory for all health care providers.

HIPAA was passed into law in 1996 but, due to administrative obstacles and legal concerns, was not implemented fully until 2003. This legislation created legal obligations regarding "protected health information" (PHI), which up until this point had been addressed only in the oaths of health care providers and declarations/standards of national and international medical professional organizations. Creation of electronic health care transactions, especially involving third-party payer organizations such as medical insurance corporations, provided the impetus to provide legal protection for PHI.

Tactical emergency medicine operations are not exempt from these provisions. Health care provided in the course of health maintenance for tactical law enforcement personnel, as well as in the operational arena, falls under the auspices of HIPAA. Given the specialized nature of these health care situations, there exist special provisions under the law for health maintenance of both team members and subjects of law enforcement actions that are discussed here.

PRIVACY AND CONFIDENTIALITY

Privacy has been defined as the "right to be let alone," further described as freedom from exposure to, or intrusion by, others. There are three major categories described under the term privacy: physical privacy, informational privacy, and decisional privacy. Physical privacy describes the right to freedom from contact with others or exposure of one's body to others. Informational privacy relates to the prevention of disclosure of personal information, and decisional privacy reflects an ability to make and act on one's personal choices without interference from others or the state (1).

Confidentiality, while on the surface appearing to be nearly identical to privacy in meaning, specifically relates to informational privacy in that when information is deemed confidential, it is indicated that those who receive said information have a duty to protect it from disclosure to others who have no right to the information (1).

The principles of privacy and confidentiality are grounded in the fundamental moral principles of biomedical ethics: human dignity, autonomy, and beneficence. As it is commonly held that human beings are capable of making moral choices and acting on them, they are provided special status and, as such, demand dignity. The principle of autonomy follows in that without the ability to make choices independently, privacy and confidentiality are not possible. Beneficence, the dictum to "do good and avoid evil," provides the reasoning for institution of privacy and confidentiality in respect for the special status accorded human beings.

There exist four basic types of invasion of privacy (1).

1. "Unreasonable and highly offensive intrusion upon the seclusion of another"
2. "Unreasonable publicity given to another's private life"
3. "Appropriation of another's name or likeness"
4. "Publication that unreasonably places another in a false light before the public"

If a health care provider releases PHI without appropriate justification that results in harm to an individual, the provider is likely to be held accountable for damages. It is also possible that such an act could be deemed a malpractice offense, for it breaches the accepted professional standard of care.

HEALTH INSURANCE PORTABILITY AND ACCOUNTABILITY ACT REGULATION OVERVIEW

The main tenet of HIPAA requires health care providers and others with access to PHI to protect the confidentiality, integrity, and availability of PHI in any form, including written, oral, or electronic. These regulations apply to any person or entity that "furnishes, bills or is paid for health care in the normal course of business." This is commonly interpreted to include health care providers, hospitals, physicians' offices, employers, public health authorities, life insurers, and any other individual or organization with access to PHI. HIPAA mandates a "written notice of privacy practices" when practical to be provided to subjects before initiating evaluation and treatment (1). While this is not always practical in the operational environment, attempts to provide this outside the acute setting should be made.

Family members may be provided PHI with the "informal permission" of the patient, given to the health care provider. There exist exclusions to HIPAA, of which several are particularly germane to the tactical emergency medicine environment. There are 12 "national priority purposes" for which PHI may be released without the subject's prior written permission (2).

1. When required by law, statute, regulation, or court order
2. Judicial and administrative proceedings
3. Law enforcement purposes including criminal investigation and actions
4. Specialized governmental functions such as the military mission or correctional activities

5. Reporting of child abuse, elder abuse, incompetent adult abuse, and domestic violence (some states)
6. For the maintenance of public health activities, including reportable disease conditions, vital statistics, and adverse events
7. Health oversight activities such as audits and inspections
8. Disclosures about deceased persons to the coroner, medical examiner, or funeral directors
9. Organ, eye, and tissue donation
10. Some types of Institutional Review Board (IRB)-approved research
11. To avert a serious threat to the health or safety of a person or the public
12. Workmen's compensation claims

The penalties associated with HIPAA violations can be extreme. For wrongful disclosure of PHI, regardless of intent, there may be a fine of up to $5,000, with the possibility of 1 year of imprisonment. For disclosure of PHI under false pretenses, there can be a fine of up to $100,000 with 5 years of imprisonment possible. For disclosure for profit or with malice, a fine of $250,000 or 10 years of imprisonment is possible (1). The Office of Civil Right continues to actively investigate, and the Department of Justice to prosecute, reported HIPAA violations.

LAW ENFORCEMENT EXCEPTIONS

Law enforcement personnel are afforded special consideration under HIPAA. As described above, criminal investigations and judicial proceedings are excepted under HIPAA as national priority purposes. In standard practice, patients under investigation should be formally asked to provide permission to speak with police officers and other law enforcement personnel, but this is not mandatory in certain situations (1,3). Law enforcement personnel involved in collection of evidence, both physical and through interview, are excepted from PHI mandates from HIPAA. This applies to both actual and potential crime investigations.

Patients currently imprisoned in a correctional facility also do not have the same protections against PHI disclosure under HIPAA. A correctional facility is defined by the privacy final rule as "a prison, jail, reformatory, work farm, detention center, halfway house or any other similar institution designed for the confinement or rehabilitation of criminal offenders" (4). This exception also applies to individuals in transitional homes or psychiatric facilities that they are confined to for correctional reasons through the judicial system (3).

Initially, inmates should be asked for voluntary permission to share PHI with law enforcement personnel or corrections officers, but if this permission is not willingly given, then access to PHI is still allowed under HIPPA, if appropriate justification is provided. Patients under the custody of a law enforcement official may have PHI released, or release PHI without consent or notice, for (3,5):

1. Provision of health care to the individual
2. Health and safety of the individual or other inmates
3. Health and safety of the officers, employees, or others at the correctional institution
4. Health and safety of those transporting the individual
5. Law enforcement on the premises of the correctional institution
6. Administration and maintenance of the safety, security, and good order of the correctional institution

Correctional institutions may deny release of PHI to inmates without denial review in a few specific instances. Under the privacy final rule, disclosure could be denied if such disclosure could jeopardize the health, safety, security, custody, or rehabilitation of the individual or other inmates or the safety of any officer, employee, or other person at the institution (4). Even given this exception, a personal representative may be able to obtain PHI on the individual's behalf (4). When a prisoner or inmate is released from custody, all provisions for HIPAA are reinstated, and may not be revoked, regardless of the person's prior status, unless there is an active investigation ongoing.

In certain tactical emergency medicine settings, medical records for purposes of team member health and readiness are maintained. These records, with few exceptions, are covered by HIPAA (6). In the case of military or other uniformed federal government personnel, a practice of "profiling" may be maintained to provide a continual assessment of personnel readiness for the unit mission. In this case, the release of PHI is excepted from HIPAA. Whether similar restrictions apply to individual tactical law enforcement teams should be assessed in discussion with local and state authorities.

LEGAL EXCEPTIONS TO THE HEALTH INFORMATION PORTABILITY AND ACCOUNTABILITY ACT

HIPAA provides exceptions to its confidentiality regulatory standards in specific, non-law-enforcement situations. The Duty to Warn was established by a sentinel case, *Tarasoff v. the Regents of the University of California* (7). In this case a psychologist and supervising psychiatrist failed to warn a woman of the danger posed by their patient, although they were provided advanced warning of impending harm to the woman by the patient. This Duty to Warn has been a staple of common law for more than 30 years, and is an accepted breach of confidentiality under HIPAA.

Reportable medical conditions to public health authorities are also excepted under HIPAA. Examples of these include certain infectious diseases, bioterrorism agent exposure, child abuse, elder abuse, incompetent adult abuse, and injuries from knives, guns, or other deadly weapons (2). On a state-by-state basis, domestic violence may be a reportable condition, but this remains controversial in many localities.

Reporting of PHI to the guardians of minors and incompetent adults also falls outside the realm of HIPAA, with a few exceptions. Minors who have been emancipated in a court of law must provide independent consent for release of PHI to a third party. There are instances of "mature minors," for example, in the case of a pregnant minor, where she may be able to provide independent consent and decision-making authority for PHI disclosure for herself as well as her infant. There are also several medical conditions under which minors are allowed to seek independent medical consultation and are excepted from HIPAA, including seeking of contraception, substance abuse treatment, and sexually transmitted disease treatment (2).

The deceased, de facto, are provided special consideration under HIPAA, given that they are unable to consent to disclosure of PHI. Generally, disclosure of vital statistics is allowed, as well as disclosure of PHI to coroners, medical examiners, and funeral directors, without consent from family members or guardians.

Filming or recording of health care encounters is generally frowned on, unless it is performed for purposes of identification, diagnosis, or treatment of a patient. Should it be performed for other reasons, written consent must be obtained prior to display or use of the recording, and consent prior to capture of the recording is further recommended (1).

Media requests for information to health care providers should be met with suspicion. Many facilities and providers have a "no-comment" policy and allow all information disclosure to be handled by law enforcement personnel in a standard manner. Health care providers remain restricted by HIPAA from releasing information without consent unless previously described exceptions are met (1).

SUMMARY

HIPAA provides necessary enforcement potential for inappropriate violation of basic patient rights. Tactical emergency medicine, lying within the realm of law enforcement, is provided a few special exceptions to HIPAA but, in general, still falls under its regulatory authority. Thus, providers are still potentially subject to its consequences. Given the potentially high media exposure, as well as the particularly litigious nature of the subjects of tactical law enforcement, an intimate knowledge of this important new legislation is paramount for tactical emergency medicine providers.

REFERENCES

1. Moskop, JC, Marco CA, Larkin GL, et al. From Hippocrates to HIPAA: privacy and confidentiality in emergency medicine. Part I: Conceptual, moral and legal foundations. *Ann Emerg Med.* 2005;45(1):53–59, 60–67.
2. U.S. Department of Health and Human Services, Office for Civil Rights. Standards for privacy of individually identifiable health information; security standards for the protection of electronic protected health information; general administrative requirements including civil monetary penalties: procedures for investigations, imposition of penalties, and hearings. Regulation text. 45 CFR Parts 160 and 164. December 28, 2000, as amended: May 31, 2002, August 14, 2002, February 20, 2003, and April 17, 2003. Available at: http://www.hhs.gov/ocr/combinedregtext.pdf. Accessed September 13, 2006.
3. American College of Emergency Physicians. Law enforcement information gathering in the emergency department. ACEP policy statement, approved September 2003. Available at: http://www.acep.org/webportal/PracticeResources/PolicyStatements/ethics/LawEnforcementInformationGatheringintheED.htm. Accessed September 13, 2006.
4. U.S. Department of Health and Human Services, Office for Civil Rights. Summary of the HIPAA privacy rule. Available at: http://www.hhs.gov/ocr/privacysummary.pdf. Accessed September 13, 2006.
5. U.S. Department of Health and Human Services, Office for Civil Rights. HIPAA medical privacy—national standards to protect the privacy of personal health information. Available at: http://www. hhs.gov/ocr/hipaa/finalreg.html. Accessed September 13, 2006.
6. Rinnert KJ, Hall, WL. Tactical emergency medicine support. *Emerg Med Clin North Am.* 2002;20:929–952.
7. *Tarasoff v. Regents of the University of California.* 1976. 17 Cal.3d 425, 131 Cal. Rptr 14, 551 P.2d 334.

Performance of Research in the Combat and Tactical Settings

John G. McManus, Jr.

OBJECTIVES

After reading this section, the reader will be able to:

1. Describe the ethical considerations when conducting research in the tactical setting.
2. Define "human subjects" research and "Institutional Review Board."
3. Describe some of the rules and regulations that govern the conduct of research in the tactical environment.
4. Discuss research considerations when conducting research on "vulnerable" populations.
5. Describe some of the important scientific contributions that previous civilian and military research has made.

Before conducting any type of research, investigators must be familiar with and adhere to all legal and ethical obligations. Research investigators in both the civilian sector and military-related tactical environments hold an ethical obligation to allow potential participants input regarding actions that affect them. We summarize these motivations as being among those that ethicists call the principle of "respect for persons," which is essentially the acknowledgment of individual autonomy and protection of those with diminished autonomy (1). "Respect" is one of the three basic ethical principles (beneficence and justice being the others) defined by the Belmont Report (2). Prior to the publication of this report, there was great controversy surrounding human patient-oriented research and consent practices in both the civilian and the military communities in the United States.

Much of the previous medically related research conducted by the military has been surrounded by controversy. History is fraught with examples of "research" conducted in both civilian and military settings with questionable ethical principles. Some notable examples include (i) the Continental (subsequently United States) Army's use of compulsory variolation (exposing uninfected individuals to matter from smallpox lesions) on troops in an attempt to prevent the spread of smallpox during the American Revolution; (ii) the use of an experimental cholera vaccine on nonconsenting prisoners located in the

American-occupied Philippines during the Spanish American War, which resulted in 13 deaths (3); (iii) the infamous Tuskegee Syphilis Study, in which subjects were denied treatment and were misled even more after a diagnosis of secondary syphilis (4); and (iv) Axis power (Nazi Germany and Imperial Japan) experiments conducted during the Second World War (5).

Although these and other past military-sponsored research practices produced distrust toward federal medical institutions and the government in general, these events have been some of the most influential in shaping public perceptions of research and fostering the government's role in human subject's protection. Furthermore, these military experiments and subjects' experiences helped guide future regulations and rules that now serve to protect human subjects, both in the armed forces and in the civilian sector. In fact, at the conclusion of World War II, the Nuremberg Medical Trial became "the most important historical forum for questioning the permissible limits of human experimentation" (6). As a result the Nuremberg Code was established, based on ten points describing required elements for conducting research on humans (7). The Nuremberg Code was the first international standard for the conduct of research on human subjects and was affirmed in the United States in 1954 when the Army Surgeon General's Office issued a memorandum for human subject protection during research, becoming one of the first official documents to guide the conduct of human experimentation by military researchers (8). Currently there exist stringent regulations that must be followed to conduct research on soldiers and civilians on the battlefield and in tactical situations. This chapter serves merely as an introduction and brief overview of some of the terms and regulations that concern the conduction of research. Prior to beginning any type of research, the authors recommend seeking guidance from local authorities who govern the conduction of all animal and human research.

WHAT IS HUMAN SUBJECT RESEARCH?

Federal regulations define *research* as "a systematic investigation, including research development, testing and evaluation, designed to develop or contribute to generalizable knowledge." Studies that involve patient interviews, follow-up contact of patients to determine the effectiveness of a program or a treatment, chart review, analysis of computer-stored clinical and administrative data, and mailed questionnaires. Additionally, randomized trials of experimental drugs, devices, and procedures must be reviewed and approved by the Institutional Review Board (IRB) because there is contribution to generalizable knowledge.

Review of research involving human subjects is required by federal law. Federal laws and regulations regarding research on human subjects have specific requirements for IRB and study administration. To ensure that no ethical or legal violations occur during the conduction of research, the authors recommend that all human subject research, and all other activities that in part involve human subject research, regardless of sponsorship, must be reviewed and approved by an IRB prior to initiation. Human subject research is any research or clinical investigation that involves human subjects. Furthermore, investigators conducting human subject research must satisfy Department of Heath and Human Services (DHHS) regulations (45 Code of Federal Regulations [CFR] Part 46) and Food and Drug Administration (FDA) regulations (21 CFR Parts 50 and 56) regarding the protection of human subject research, as applicable before conduction of research. DHHS regulations define a human subject as a living individual about whom an investigator conducting research obtains (i) data through intervention or interaction with the individual or (ii) identifiable private information.

INSTITUTIONAL REVIEW BOARDS

An IRB is charged with protecting the rights and welfare of people involved in research and reviews plans for research involving human and animal subjects. Institutions

that accept research funding from the federal government must have an IRB to review all research involving human subjects (even if a given research project does not involve federal funds). The FDA and the Office of Protection from Research Risks (part of the National Institutes of Health) set the guidelines and regulations governing human subject research and IRBs.

An IRB is a committee, usually within a university or another organization, consisting of at least five members of varying backgrounds. An IRB must have at least one member who is a scientist and at least one member whose primary concerns are nonscientific. Additionally, there must be one member who is not otherwise affiliated with the institution (a community representative).The IRB reviews the proposals before a project is submitted to a funding agency to determine if the research project follows the ethical principles and federal regulations for the protection of human subjects. The IRB has the authority to approve, disapprove, or require modifications of these projects.

RULES AND REGULATIONS FOR CONDUCTING DEPARTMENT OF DEFENSE (MILITARY) RESEARCH

The foundation for the Department of Defense (DoD) rules and regulations governing the conduct of human subject research is primarily based on the regulations that govern all federally funded research. DoD regulations apply whether research is conducted on the battlefield, in a foreign theater of operations, or at medical treatment facilities in the United States. The first governmental regulations and policies were born out of previous abuses of research initially dating back to World War II and abuses of prisoners by Nazi doctors as previously described. The Nuremburg Code laid the foundation for research principles of informed consent, scientific merit, and minimized risks to research participants (5). The DoD, under Secretary of Defense Charles Wilson, adopted the Nuremburg Code in 1953 as its official policy for research. Further guidance on the conduct of research was provided by the 1964 Declaration of Helsinki, which addressed new issues regarding research with therapeutic intent, diminished competence, and formal oversight of research (9). However, due to continued abuses that were exemplified by the U.S. Public Health Service Tuskegee Natural History Syphilis Study, the federal government eventually took ownership of research protections (4). In 1974, the DHHS drafted the 45 CFR Part 46, Protection of Human Subjects, which governed human research protection. This policy was revised to include specific protections for pregnant women and fetuses (Subpart B), prisoners (Subpart C), and children (Subpart D). It was finally adopted by another 17 federal agencies including the DoD in 1991 and became known as "The Common Rule" (10). The Common

Rule incorporates the Belmont principles of beneficence, justice, and respect and requires that all human subject research be approved by an IRB before implementation of the study.

Despite the directive to the contrary, the DoD was also responsible for several flagrant research abuses such as administration of lysergic acid diethylamide (LSD) to soldiers and exposure of unconsenting populations to radiation. In 1972, prior to the establishment of 45 CFR Part 46, Congress inserted into appropriation bills the 10 USC §980 requirement for the DoD, entitled "Limitations on Use of Humans as Experimental Subjects." This code required the process of informed consent to be obtained in advance for all DoD-funded research. It states:

> Funds appropriated by the DoD may not be used for research involving a human being as an experimental subject unless 1) the informed consent of the subject is obtained in advance; or 2) in the case of research intended to be beneficial to the subject, the informed consent of the subject or a legal representative of the subject is obtained in advance. (11)

Amended three times by 1985, the most current version was amended in the 2002 Defense Appropriations Act to allow for an exceptional waiver by the Secretary of Defense of the advance informed consent process if a research project would (i) directly benefit subjects, (ii) advance the development of a medical product necessary to the military, and (iii) be carried out per all laws and regulations including those pertinent to the FDA. This change allowed the conduct of specific emergency research to be carried out under the provisions of the Emergency Research Consent Waiver, 61 Federal Register 51531–51533 (12). Legal interpretation of 10 USC §980 stipulates that, in cases where surrogate consent must be obtained, the IRB must determine if the research is intended to benefit all subjects. This interpretation has limited DoD participation in placebo-controlled studies or those that involve a standard-of-care arm, where surrogate consent is required and participants may not receive any direct benefit.

Human subject research by DoD agencies is also impacted by FDA regulations that govern investigational drugs and devices: 21 CFR Part 56 governs the function and responsibilities of the IRB reviewing and approving human studies including those involving investigational drugs, while 21 CFR Part 50 specifically addresses the requirements and elements of the informed consent process. DoD Directive 6200.2, "Use of Investigational New Drugs for Force Health Protection," establishes policy and assigns responsibility for compliance for the use of investigational new drugs for forced health protection and designates the Secretary of the Army as the DoD Executive Agent (13). Likewise, there are more specific regulations and directives governing DoD research that delineate unique issues to the DoD than the general Office of Human Research

Protections regulations. For example, 32 CFR Part 219, "Protection of Human Subjects," is the DoD version of the Common Rule. DoD Directive 3216.2, "Protection of Human Subjects and Adherence to Ethical Standards in DoD-Supported Research," was updated in December 2002 and provides changes from other federal regulations (14). DoD Directive 6000.8, "Funding and Administration of Clinical Investigation Programs," updates DoD policy and responsibilities regarding the administration and funding of clinical investigation programs at military medical and dental treatment facilities and the Uniformed Services University of the Health Sciences (15).

Within each branch of the military there are more service-specific regulations that govern different types of human subject research. The conduct of research within the Army Medical Research and Matériel Command is also governed by Army Regulation 70-25, "Use of Volunteers as Subjects of Research." This provides more specific restrictions on the recruitment, consent, and payment of volunteers to which the investigator must adhere during the conduct of the study (16). The conduct of research at any U.S. Army medical treatment facility is specifically governed by Army Regulation 40-38, "Clinical Investigation Program," that adheres to DoD, FDA, and Office of Human Research Protections federal regulations (17).

TACTICAL RESEARCH CONSIDERATIONS

As with combat research, there are several regulations and rules that apply to research conducted in the civilian environment. These regulations can be obtained at the DHHS Web site: http://www.hhs.gov/ohrp/. However, one topic worthy of discussion is research conducted on prisoners and detainees. The current military policy is that no research shall be conducted in the combat zone on detainees. However, in the civilian sector, certain types of research can be done on prisoners if the rules and regulations are followed and one obtains IRB approval. According to 45 CFR 46.303(c), a prisoner means any individual involuntarily confined or detained in a penal institution, including individuals detained in other facilities that provide alternatives to criminal prosecution or incarceration and individuals detained pending arraignment, trial, or sentencing. Finally, all research involving colleagues, victims, and medical personnel also require IRB approval.

CHALLENGES TO RESEARCH CONDUCTION

Research on the battlefield (whether its basic design is social, behavioral, or biomedical) and in civilian tactical situations presents a challenge to the entire research community and research process. The aim of medical care is to treat the wounded and either return them to duty or evacuate the severely injured to definitive care. Given the primary focus of tactical operations on mission accomplishment, coincidental human subject research by necessity is relegated to a subordinate role. Thus, development and implementation of either prospective studies requiring informed consent or retrospective studies of existing data require a very clear, well-defined protocol that can be conducted during the deployment time period but without compromise to the tactical mission. Concurrently, ethical considerations of conducting such research on the battlefield must be considered, to include the rights of research subjects, which are complicated by the traditional commander-subordinate role.

Military and tactical colleagues should be viewed as members of a vulnerable population and afforded the same protection as other vulnerable populations including minors, prisoners, and the economically disadvantaged. Clinical researchers desiring to conduct research in this setting must first develop an appropriate protocol, with the a priori conclusion that such research could not be replicated in a satisfactory manner in a domestic setting. Once such a protocol has been developed and its methodological and ethical validity confirmed by peer review, formal approval should be sought from the commanders of the units to be impacted by the proposed research and, subsequently, from the command element of the theater of operations to be studied. This command approval ensures that the proposed research can be conducted in a tactical environment without jeopardizing the mission and at the same time ensuring the integrity of the study.

Ensuring that the rights and welfare of subjects are protected, no matter where the study is conducted, is still the responsibility of an IRB. All services currently have an IRB that performs external review for combat research. Soldier-subjects should be afforded the same research protection as all other civilian research volunteers. Prospective research involving informed consent can be done only when the soldier-subject is able to provide his or her own written informed consent. The prohibition of 10 USC §980, with its intent-to-benefit clause, does not allow surrogate consent as an alternative to research on the battlefield.

SOLDIERS AS A VULNERABLE POPULATION

The performance of patient-oriented clinical research by the U.S. military also requires investigators to look at some of the ethical implications and the ability of soldiers to give informed consent. Because of the structure of the military environment, soldiers, in some circumstances, may be considered a "vulnerable population." In clinical research a vulnerable population is one that is unable to give in-

formed consent or is susceptible to coercion. The very nature and location of the soldier in combat (e.g., the battlefield) contributes to a sense of "vulnerability" and may also be a source of unintended coercion (18). At the best of times, during a combat situation, can informed consent be truly obtained? The mere stress of battle or a soldier's "eagerness to please" may not actually represent the ability of an individual to make a fair, informed decision. However, one could argue that the same concept applies to most trauma patients who are asked to participate in research. Are these patients any more "vulnerable" than soldiers?

Furthermore, because soldiers are told to obey all "lawful" orders from officers, they may feel compelled to obey "requests" from senior officials conducting research. To assure protection of the rights and welfare of military research subjects, the IRB may sometimes require an ombudsman to be present during the informed consent process. However, the ability of soldiers and their surrogates (legal representatives) to refuse some medical procedures is restricted (10). This regulation may be misinterpreted by soldiers and/or surrogates, resulting in confusion between a mandatory procedure (e.g., vaccinations) and medical research. The Army has revised the regulations covering medical subjects to prevent unintended coercion. Army regulation 40-38 states that soldier's commanders or supervisors may not be in the room during the consent process (17).

"Informed consent" research can be performed in an ethically legitimate fashion on today's battlefield if investigators can ensure that subjects are protected. Despite some controversy, the DoD and its investigators have an ethical responsibility for protecting its service members. Following the above policies and procedures as well as using appropriate research ethics will allow military investigators to ensure human subject protection.

TAKE-HOME POINTS

1. Research investigators in both the civilian sector and military-related tactical environments hold an ethical obligation to allow potential participants input into actions that affect them.
2. Currently, there exist stringent regulations that must be followed to conduct research on soldiers and civilians on the battlefield and in tactical situations.
3. The conduction of all research in the tactical setting should undergo review by an IRB.
4. Development and implementation of either prospective studies requiring informed consent or retrospective studies of existing data require a very clear, well-defined protocol that can be conducted during the deployment time period but without compromise to the tactical mission.

5. Military and tactical colleagues should be viewed as members of a vulnerable population and afforded the same protection as other vulnerable populations including minors, prisoners, and the economically disadvantaged.

CONCLUSION

The conduct of military and tactical medical research has and will serve as an important contribution to both the civilian and the military medical communities. Tactical research, when performed properly, is rewarding and aids in reducing morbidity and mortality on our battlefields. Furthermore, much of the research done in combat, in the past and today, has also been utilized in the civilian environment. The lessons of Vietnam and the development of trauma systems, the "golden hour," hemorrhage control products, and air medical services provide additional reminders of the mutual benefits gained by military and civilian practice. The role of medical research in the tactical setting continues to be diverse, conflicting, and disquieting at times, yet remains a pioneering and crucial part of modern medicine and national defense.

REFERENCES

1. Anderson AO. Medical ethics. Available at: http://www.geocities.com/artnscience/Med_Ethics.html. Accessed June 3, 2006.
2. National Commission for the Protection for Human Subjects of Biomedical, Behavioral Research. *The Belmont Report: Ethical Principles and Guidelines for the Protection of Human Subjects of Research.* DHEW Publication No. (OS) 78-0012. Washington, DC: U.S. Government Printing Office; 1979.
3. Chernin E. Richard Pearson Strong and the iatrogenic plague disaster in Bilibid Prison, Manila, 1906. *Rev Infect Dis*. 1989;11(6):996–1004.
4. White RM. The Tuskegee study of untreated syphilis revisited. *Lancet Infect Dis*. 2006;6(2):62–63.
5. Annas GJ, Grodin MA. *The Nazi Doctors and the Nuremberg Code: Human Rights in Human Experimentation.* Oxford: Oxford University Press; 1992.
6. Shuster E. Fifty years later: the significance of the Nuremberg Code. *N Engl J Med*. 1997;337:1436–1440.
7. Wilson Memorandum. February 23, 1953. From the Secretary of Defense to the Secretaries of the Army, Navy and Airforce. Available at: http://www. Accessed February 2006.
8. Lederer S. The Cold War and beyond: covert and deceptive American medical experimentation. In: Lounsbury DE, Bellamy RF, eds. *Textbook of Military Medicine: Military Medical Ethics*. Washington, DC: Office of the Surgeon General; 2003:527–528.
9. World Medical Organization. Declaration of Helsinki. *Br Med J*. 1996;313:1448–1449.
10. Protection of Human Subjects. 45 Code of Federal Regulations Part 46, Subpart A. Revised November 13, 2001 (effective December 13, 2002).
11. USC Title 10—Armed Forces, Subtitle A—General Military Law, Part II—Personnel, Chapter 49—Miscellaneous Prohibitions and Penalties §980. Limitation on use of humans as experimental subjects.
12. Amoroso PJ, Wenger LL. The human volunteer in military biomedical research. In: Beam TE, Sparacino LR, eds. *Military Medical Ethics. Vol. 2.* Washington, DC: Office of the Surgeon General, Department of the Army, and Borden Institute; 2003:563–603.
13. Department of Defense Directive 6200.2. Use of Investigational New Drugs for Force Health Protection. August 1, 2000.
14. Department of Defense Directive 3216.2. Protection of Human Subjects and Adherence to Ethical Standards in DoD-Supported Research. March 25, 2002.
15. Department of Defense Directive 6000.8. Funding and Administration of Clinical Investigation Programs. November 3, 1999.
16. Army Regulation 70-25. Use of Volunteers as Subjects of Research. Washington, DC: Department of the Army; January 25, 1990.
17. Army Regulation 40-38. Clinical Investigation Program; Headquarters. Washington, DC: Department of the Army; September 1, 1989.
18. Pape TL, Jaffe NO, Savage T, et al. Unresolved legal and ethical issues in research of adults with severe traumatic brain injury: analysis of ongoing protocol. *J Rehab Res Dev*. 2004;41(2):155–174.

Applied Concepts and Other Topics

Section Editor: MICHAEL W. PROCTOR

Chapter 31

Medical Implications and Planning for Riots and Mass Gatherings

Faith A. Dillard and Carl Menckhoff

OBJECTIVES

After reading this section, the reader will be able to:

1. As a tactical emergency medical services (TEMS) provider, describe the variables involved in preparing the medical care for a mass gathering
2. Describe the steps needed to plan for and implement medical care at a mass gathering
3. Discuss the special factors associated with different types of events
4. Discuss the world literature on mass gatherings

Mass gatherings are defined as planned events with large numbers of individuals gathered together in a specific area for a specific purpose. The number of people gathered may vary greatly, and although a mass gathering is classically defined as more than 1,000 people (1–4), the vast majority of mass gathering events far exceed this number.

In the United States alone, 165 million people attend NBA, NFL, and NCAA events every year (5,6), and with our ever-shrinking world we must now take into account a global perspective, in which we understand not only the epidemiology of an individual locality, but that of travelers and current worldwide health issues.

This chapter describes the myriad of factors that must be taken into account when planning and implementing medical care for a mass gathering and provides a step-by-step approach and timeline for setting up care for a future event. While the TEMS provider may not be directly involved with the medical planning for a mass gathering event, it is important to understand the principals involved and to be able to interface with the medical system that is in place for the mass gathering event.

Historical Perspective

The gathering of a large number of people together presents unique challenges for medical support, both logistically ands with regard to the wide variety of potential medical problems. For example, the density of the population at these events lends itself to the possibility of high numbers of victims in the event of a terrorist event as well as logistic difficulties in terms of triage, treatment, and transport. It is therefore important to have a well-prepared plan for all contingencies.

Since the dawn of history humans have gathered for pilgrimages, and fled en masse from famines, floods, and oppression in large numbers. Some of the earliest recorded include the biblical journey of Moses and the Israelites across the Egyptian desert and the first pilgrimage to Mecca in 628 AD, as Mohammed led 1,400 followers on the first Hajj (7). The Hajj has become the largest mass gathering in the world, with up to 4 million worshippers traveling to Mecca each year (8).

EVENT PLANNING

Event Planning Committee

The first step in the medical preparation for an event is to define and assemble the event planning committee. For a major event, this should occur at least a year prior to the event date (Table 31.1) and consist of the event coordinator, the medical director, EMS, venue public safety/security, fire protection, and law enforcement. The TEMS provider should take part in this planning process when possible. This early coordination is important for an effective response between the TEMS unit and the event medical staff. Having a good understanding of the Incident Command System (ICS) and having the event integrated into the local ICS is essential for mass gathering planning.

The event coordinator is responsible for coordinating the entire event (of which medical care is one part) and is often the key person in terms of logistical and financial support. The medical director is responsible for coordinating all aspects of medical care for the event, from triage and on-site first aid, to stabilization and transportation, to disaster planning. It is also the responsibility of the medical director to make sure that whatever plan is developed can be smoothly integrated into existing plans of EMS/fire/law enforcement/secret service or any other agency's preexisting plan. EMS plays a vital role in most mass gatherings and should be included in the planning for medical care from the start. While the traditional role of EMS is certainly useful, there are several studies (9–11) showing that protocols can be devised to expand their usual scope of practice to include a number of different treat and release scenarios. The roles of venue security and local law enforcement (including the TEMS team) need to be clearly defined. Crowd control, access to and egress from the event site, and the response to a terrorist incident are areas where they will have the lead role. How transfer of care occurs between the TEMS team and the event medicine team should also be addressed. The local fire service can supply information regarding the planned response to the event and should be made aware of any chemicals, pyrotechnics, or other fire hazards caused by the event (12). Many states, counties, municipalities, and local governments also have plans and legislation concerning mass gatherings. In planning for any event, these local and state guidelines should be sought out and integrated. In the event of a mass casualty incident (MCI), the roles of all of the various agencies involved need to be determined, with the medical director

TABLE 31.1. Timeline for Preparation.

Timeline	12 mo	10 mo	8 mo	6 mo	4 mo	3 mo	2 mo	1 mo	1 wk	1 d
Meet with event coordinator	X			X				X	X	
Define scope of event	X									
Assemble event planning committee	X	X								
Meet with planning committee		X	X							
Designate agency responsibilities	X			X		X		X	X	
Visit venue	X			X				X	X	X
Develop map of venue		X		X						
Designate medical director	X									
Develop plan for medical coverage			X	X						
Recruit volunteers	X	X	X	X	X	X	X	X	X	
Secure liability insurance				X						
Order uniforms/shirts					X					
Acquire communication system				X						
Test communication equipment				X					X	X
Acquire medical equipment & supplies			X	X	X	X	X	X	X	X
Set up for event									X	X

Adapted from Menckhoff CR, Shaw M. Mass gathering preparedness. In: Keyes DC, Burnstein JL, et al., eds. *Medical Response to Terrorism*. Philadelphia: Lippincott Williams & Wilkins, 2005:257–268, and Wetterhall SF, Coulombier DM, Herndon JM, et al. Medical care delivery at the 1996 Olympic Games. *JAMA*. 1998; 279(18):1463–1468.

negotiating a position within the command center. Local disaster preparedness plans may assist in planning and preparing for a mass gathering event, and some localities may request assistance from the Federal Disaster Medical Assistance Teams (DMAT) in their area. DMAT teams are often willing to participate, as the event also acts as training for their team.

Event Profiling

Profiling of the event itself is vital in planning for the necessary medical care. There is a myriad of variables that affect the volume of patients as well as the types of medical problems likely to be encountered. These, in turn, define the amount and type of staffing that will be needed.

Event Type

Certain types of events can be predicted to have a higher volume of patients. From a review of the literature over the last 35 years it is clear that an increase in the use of alcohol and drugs has a direct correlation with patient volume (5,13–16). It follows that events where this is more prevalent (primarily rock festivals, rock concerts, and raves) will have a higher medical usage rate (MUR). In one study of an outdoor venue hosting multiple events over a 5-year period, it was found that rock concerts had a 2.5 times increase in MURs over nonrock concerts (17).

Event type can also help predict injury type and severity. While the vast majority of patient encounters at any event are for minor complaints (18–20), some (usually high-kinetic energy) events have the potential for more severe injuries. In 1988, at an air show in Ramstein, Germany, an airplane fell into a patient enclosure, killing 45 and injuring more than 500 (21). Also in 1988, at the Three Rivers regatta, a formula 1 boat collided with the shore, injuring 24 spectators (22). At a rock concert in Washington, DC, in 1999 (23), the MUR was 82.9 patients per 10,000 people in attendance (PPTT), with injuries from mosh pits accounting for 37% of the encounters.

Weather

Changes in weather can greatly affect the number and types of patient encounters. In general, one should consider that extremes in temperature (especially heat) can lead to higher usage rate (5,24–27). At a 7-day AIDS bicycle ride in California in 1996 (28), temperatures reached 107°F one day, with 70% of cases seen being related to heat. Another study (29) calculated that for every increase in the heat index (heat and humidity) by 10°F, there was an increase of 3 PPTT. At a rock concert in Woodstock, New York, in 1994, however, there was rain followed by a drop in temperature of 30°F, which led to markedly increased usage rates of 143 PPTT (30,31). Similarly at a papal visit

in Colorado in 1993, temperatures dropped from 89°F during the day to 56°F at night and spectators who had been cooled with hoses during the day were shivering at night (32,33).

Crowd Size and Mobility

Calculated from a review of the world literature on mass gatherings from 1971 to 2006 (12,18,19,34,35), the average MUR at mass gatherings is 51 PPTT. Looking at events with <100,000 people per day, the MUR is 56 PPTT. A study of the Los Angeles Summer Olympics in 1984 (36–38) indicated that the highest MUR was at those events with mobile spectators and a crowd capacity of <30,000. While Michael and Barbera (39) found that as the number of people in attendance increased, the MUR decreased, it should be considered, however, that any venue, egress, or passageway where mobile crowd density may become critical (<5 ft^2 per person), stampede conditions may occur (40).

Duration

The effect of event duration has been a topic of much discussion in event medicine literature, and appears to have a mild direct correlation with MUR (5). This appears to be most prevalent at multiday events, as attendees become exhausted and incubation periods may elapse. At a 3-day outdoor music festival in England in 1989, insufficient water and toilets led to a gastroenteritis outbreak (41). This brings up the important aspect of syndromic surveillance. Today, modern mass gatherings must take into account and understand not only the epidemiology of their locality, but that of travelers and current worldwide health issues. The possibilities of bioterrorism must also be addressed as they pertain to large gatherings. The planners should have in place a method of surveillance and a plan to address multiple patient presentations of syndromes associated with agents that could be used by terrorists.

Indoors vs. Outdoors

This is important in a number of ways. Indoor events are not nearly as susceptible to the temperature and environmental issues discussed above. They are often much more problematic, however, in terms of egress in the event of an emergency. A careful plan must be devised to allow for access to patients within crowded stadiums and quick transportation when needed.

It should be noted that any event can be the target of terrorism, although high-profile events or those being attended by diplomats and other dignitaries should be considered to be at higher risk. At the 1972 Summer Olympics in Munich, 17 people were killed after eight Arab terrorists took Israeli athletes hostage. At the 1996 Summer Olympics in Atlanta, Georgia, the July 27 bombing killed 2 people and injured 110 (42–45). Events that have a high risk of a terrorist event should be given a high priority for coordination with the TEMS unit that may be responding.

Event Site

Outdoor events demand a number of special considerations. The topography of the land must be surveyed and accounted for in the event plans. Are there bodies of water that would predispose to drowning, areas that might allow for falls from height, wildlife that could cause harm (e.g., snakes, bees), or large areas without shade that might be problematic if it is hot and sunny? All these factors will help determine the types and quantities of patient encounters that may be expected. Indoor venues may have steep stairwells or seating, limited ingress and egress, or structural hazards.

Once the event site has been surveyed and the layout is known, decisions may be made regarding location of medical facilities. Plans should be made, in conjunction with internal security, for rapid access to and for patients. They should be made in conjunction with EMS and local law enforcement for rapid transportation to local hospitals. If air transport is a consideration, a landing area should be predesignated.

Staffing

Even the most languid event with the mildest weather will not be without illness and injury; therefore, the medical treatment plan should begin with a basic outline of how and where patients will be treated and who the providers will be. The level of care can include everything from Basic First Aid to Advanced Cardiac Life Support. Additionally, having staff trained in mass casualty care by certification in courses such as the American Medical Association's (AMA) Advanced Disaster Life Support (ADLS) is desirable.

Delivery of Care

First aid stations should be the minimum of care for any mass gathering. Preparation for these stations includes the following.

1. Supplies and equipment (basic EMS level versus advanced; spinal immobilization; cots, blankets; water/sports drinks; seating for medical staff) (Tables 31.2 and 31.3)
2. Station locations/placement (<5-min walk for any participant)
3. Signs and maps indicating locations of aid stations
4. Level of staffing and supplies must be addressed

5. Site safety: safe egress for the medical staff in a disaster situation as well as protection from stampeding crowds
6. Support of the aid stations during the event, such as restocking of supplies and support of the medical staff

Triage may be needed at the first aid stations, and caregivers should be prepared to prioritize care should the number of patients dictate.

Record keeping is a must, with a patient log to record all attendees requesting assistance. The minimum should be patient name and age, complaint, allergies, list of medical problems and medications, and vital signs, as well as including any treatment administered. An EMS record or hospital triage sheet may be all that is required.

An on-site clinic should be considered for events where the medical usage rate or acuity of patient presentations is expected to be high. This clinic should have ACLS capability and the ability to administer IV fluids. Also of importance is the location of the clinic in respect to transport of patients to a higher level of care and ambulance accessibility.

Roving teams of EMTs and paramedics are an effective way to deliver care to a large crowd as well as provide a level of medical surveillance. These teams should also include personnel certified in ACLS, and transportable ACLS equipment should be made ready and available. Individuals who may be unable to present without assistance to an aid station can be located and transported by these teams. They should be in constant contact with event managers via portable radios. Depending on the venue, planners should consider placing these teams on foot, bicycle, golf carts or other similar means of transport.

Security personnel may also be used for identifying persons in need of medical assistance and calling for medical teams or personnel. They may also be of great assistance in transporting patients to aid stations or ambulances.

Staging for all medical and aid stations should begin well before the event, as large crowds may hinder the staff from reaching their appointed sites.

Level of Care

Illness and injury at a mass gathering event can be evaluated and treated using multiple levels of health practitioners including physicians, nurses, paramedics, and emergency medical technicians (EMTs). The recommended level of staffing is 1 or 2 physicians for every 50,000 people attending the event and 2 paramedics (or 1 paramedic/EMT team) PPTT (46). Registered nurses may be substituted for paramedics or EMTs (1).

Physician oversight of a mass gathering event is essential. Whether medical direction is on-site or off-site, the physician(s) responsible should be instrumental in the

TABLE 31.2. Supply List.

Equipment and Supplies	Main Station	Secondary Station	Jump Bag
Stretchers or beds	X		
Portable suction	X	X	
Cardiac monitors/defibrillator	X		
AED	X	X	X
Oxygen	X	X	
Cooling fans	X		
Warming blanket	X		
Laryngoscope set	X	X	X
ET tubes 3.5–8.0	X	X	X
Oxygen supplies	X	X	X
Nebulizer sets	X	X	
Oral airways	X	X	X
Backup airway device	X	X	X
Ambu bags (adult & pediatric)	X	X	X
End tidal CO_2 detector	X	X	X
IV fluids: D5W, saline, LR	X	X	X
IV supplies	X	X	X
Bandages (Band-Aids, Kerlex, etc.)	X	X	X
Splinting material	X		
Suture—assorted	X		
Suture trays	X		
Steri-strips	X	X	
Irrigation saline	X	X	X
Sphygmomanometer	X	X	X
Stethoscope	X	X	X
Thoracostomy tray	X		
Spine boards	X	X	
Cervical collars	X	X	X
Golf carts	X	X	
Tables	X		
Jump bags	X	X	
Prescription pads	X		
Patient encounter forms	X	X	X
AMA forms	X	X	X
Glucose monitor	X	X	X
Handheld cautery	X		
Woods lamp	X		
Fluorescein strips	X		
Pulse-ox monitor	X		
Extra batteries	X		X
Clipboards	X	X	X
Epistaxis trays	X		
Cool packs	X	X	X
Otoscope	X		
Disaster triage tags	X	X	X
Pens	X	X	X
Pillows	X		
Ring cutter	X		
Coolers	X	X	
Soap	X	X	X
Sheets	X	X	
Eye irrigation	X	X	X
Oral rehydration fluids	X	X	
Suction tubing & tips	X	X	
Tape	X	X	X
Thermometer	X	X	
Towels	X	X	X
Pocket mask	X	X	X
IV poles	X	X	
Blankets	X	X	
Lock box for narcotics	X		

Adapted from Menckhoff CR, Shaw M. Mass gathering preparedness. In: Keyes DC, Burnstein JL, et al., eds. *Medical Response to Terrorism*. Philadelphia: Lippincott Williams & Wilkins, 2005:257–268, and Wetterhall SF, Coulombier DM, Herndon JM, et al. Medical care delivery at the 1996 Olympic Games. *JAMA*. 1998; 279(18):1463–1468.

▶ **TABLE 31.3.** Medication List.

Medication	Main Station	Secondary Station	Jump Bag
Aspirin	X	X	X
Tylenol	X	X	X
Motrin	X	X	X
Morphine	X		
1% lidocaine with & without epinephrine	X		
Maalox	X	X	
Benadryl (IV, PO, IM)	X	X	X
Epinephrine, 1:1,000 & 1:10,000	X	X	X
Topical antibiotic ointment	X	X	X
Phenergan (PO, IM, IV, PR)	X	X	
Prednisone (IV, PO)	X		
Albuterol (MDI & spacer)	X	X	X
1% hydrocortisone cream	X	X	X
Silver sulfadiazine	X		
Xeroform gauze	X		
Atropine	X	X	X
IV lidocaine	X	X	X
Sodium bicarbonate	X	X	X
Calcium chloride	X	X	X
Fosphenytoin	X		
Dopamine	X		
Furosemide	X		
Metoprolol	X		
Adenosine	X		
Insulin	X		
D50	X	X	X
Imodium	X	X	
Versed	X		
Valium	X		
Tetanus toxoid	X	X	
Activated charcoal	X		
Sunscreen	X	X	X
Sunburn lotion	X	X	X
Insect repellent	X	X	X

Adapted from Menckhoff CR, Shaw M. Mass gathering preparedness. In: Keyes DC, Burnstein JL, et al., eds. *Medical Response to Terrorism.* Philadelphia: Lippincott Williams & Wilkins, 2005:257–268, and Wetterhall SF, Coulombier DM, Herndon JM, et al. Medical care delivery at the 1996 Olympic Games. *JAMA.* 1998; 279(18):1463–1468.

planning phases of an event. While effective prehospital care can be administered by paramedics and EMTs, event analysis has found that having physicians present at mass gatherings decreases the EMS burden, with fewer hospital transports from the event (47). While on-site physicians may be considered expensive, the overall decreased impact on the health care system, including EMS transport capabilities, should be weighed. An event in Nigeria with more than 80,000 attendees was staffed by physicians alone, as no trained paramedics were available. Ninety percent of the patients presenting at that event were treated and released (48).

Extended protocols should be considered for EMS-level and nursing professionals, for instance: patients with minor complaints and injuries can be evaluated by paramedic and nursing providers and possibly be treated with nonprescription medications given that protocols have been put in place by the medical director of the event.

Transportation

Patient transport within the venue may be by foot, motorized cart, or stretcher. Personnel should all be supplied with maps of the venue and should be familiar with the location of key areas. Consideration of distances and routes of transport should be incorporated into event planning, with first aid stations placed in a manner in which they can be reached by attendees in a minimal amount of time but preserve the resources of the event staff. Distances and times by ground and air from the event to nearby hospitals should be calculated and transportation resources staged accordingly. Ambulance transportation is usually reserved for transport to hospitals, and event coordinators should have a clear understanding and plan for the utilization of local and public medical transport. If these resources are staged outside of the event or venue, a planned route and/or patient loading area should be addressed. Events that are secured where attendees have been screened and cleared will need planning for transport both inside and outside the secure area. Depending on the size of the area, there may be a need for ambulances and staff that have been screened and cleared to transport patients to the boundaries of the event for transfer to nonsecured ambulances. In smaller areas, motorized carts may suffice for transfer to the nonsecured ambulances for hospital transport.

Predicting the number of ambulances needed may not be straightforward. Whereas the MUR can be calculated using predictive modeling (49,50) or retrospective data from specific events (27,50), the number of patients transported to the hospital per thousand person in attendance (TTHR) has been found not to be as reliably predicted (50). Transport rates described in this article ranged from 0.03 to 0.07 TTHR. This roughly translates to actual patient transports of approximately 0.5 PPTT. Feldman, et al. describes an event where the transport rate was 0.6 patient PPTT (51). As described earlier, analysis of the type of event will more clearly define the expected need. Based on the studies described above, an expected transport rate of 1 patient PPTT should be a minimum in planning. Staging air transport may be costly and difficult, however, at some high-profile and secure events it may be a necessity.

Communications/Public Information

Communication and Information Management is generally operated under the Logistics Section Chief of the ICS and should ideally be planned and managed using ICS guidelines that will allow for coordination and information sharing between jurisdictions. Communications planning in an event should ideally begin operations long before a mass gathering event, ensuring that communications are functional, reliable, and robust enough for all eventualities. It may be necessary to distribute public information for attendees prior to the event regarding conditions such as weather, adverse conditions, and restrictions. Public information and consideration of press inquiries (possibly through a Public Information Officer) should continue through the event and mitigation phases.

Direct links to local authorities (fire, EMS, TEMS, police, public health) must be planned for and established. In addition, direct communications with nearby hospitals and the area base station may be needed. Agreements and plans should be established concerning communication of

▶ **TABLE 31.4. Resources.**

American College of Emergency Physicians. Provision of emergency medical care for crowds (55): www.acep.org/NR/rdonlyres/DCE46858-1F51-4225-B604-CAF476 CB5416/0/emscrowd.pdf

NAEMSP. Mass gathering medical care: the medical director's checklist (booklet)

NDMS web site: ndms.dhhs.gov

FEMA web site: www.fema.gov Special Events Contingency Planning Job Aids Manual—March 2005. www.training.fema.gov/EMIWEB/downloads/is15aSpecialEvents Planning-JAmanual.pdf

Red Cross web site: www.redcross.org

U.S. Department of Homeland Security web site: www.dhs.gov/dhspublic

CDC web site: www.cdc.gov

Local DMAT teams

Adapted from Menckhoff CR, Shaw M. Mass gathering preparedness. In: Keyes DC, Burnstein JL, et al., eds. *Medical Response to Terrorism.* Philadelphia: Lippincott Williams & Wilkins, 2005:257–268.

any event that will require interagency assistance or response.

Voice and Data Communications should be standardized between the ICS and local authorities. Redundancy should be considered for voice and data communications (analog or digital phone lines, emergency radio frequencies, cellular communication, and satellite communications). Assignments should be made for radio frequencies among groups including command, tactical, support, and transport groups (including ground-ground, ground-air, and air-air). Public address systems should be planned for using both voice and visual methods, if possible, to address crowds.

Finally, depending, again, on the complexity or sensitivity of the event or other factors such as national security (i.e., inaugural or political events), backup systems may need to be planned for. Power generators and mobile or replacement antennas can restore communications systems in the event of unforeseen complications in a mass gathering event.

ICS and Communications Training can be obtained free online through FEMA, at http://emilms.fema.gov/ (Table 31.4).

TAKE-HOME POINTS

1. When developing the medical plan for mass gathering events, one must anticipate the numbers of patients and types of injuries that may be seen, either by looking at the relevant variables or, if possible, by looking at the same event retrospectively (27,50).

2. TEMS units should coordinate with the medical planner for a mass gathering event before it takes place so an effective response can be planned.
3. The importance of a good system of communication should not be underestimated.
4. The TEMS team should be integrated into the disaster plan in case of a mass casualty incident.

SUMMARY

Every mass gathering has slightly different variables, thus no single plan can be applied to all events. With a systematic, organized approach, however, a plan for medical care can be devised for any event. TEMS planners should be involved with the medical planning for mass gathering events that they may be called on to respond to. Our goal as event medical organizers is to create a comprehensive plan for routine medical care, as well as disaster plans that can be implemented in the case of a mass casualty incident. Good preparation is the best way to ensure a medically uncomplicated event with minimal morbidity, where all involved are able to enjoy the experience.

REFERENCES

1. Sanders AB, Criss E, Steckl P, et al. An analysis of medical care at mass gatherings. *Ann Emerg Med*. 1986;15:515–519.
2. Rose WD, Larid SL, Prescott JE, et al. Emergency medical services for collegiate football games: a six and one-half year review. *Prehosp Dis Med*. 1992;7;157–159.
3. Parrillo S. Medical care of mass gatherings. In: Hogan D, Burstein JL, eds. *Disaster Medicine*. Philadelphia, PA: Lippincott Williams & Wilkins; 2002:274–278.
4. De Lorenzo RA. Mass gathering medicine: a review. *Prehosp Dis Med*. 1997;12:68–72.
5. Milsten AM, Maguire BJ, Bissell RA, et al. Mass-gathering medical care: a review of the literature. *Prehosp Dis Med*. 2002;17(3):151–162.
6. Grange JT, Baumann GW. The California 500: medical care at a NASCAR Winston cup race event. *Ann Emerg Med*. 1999;34(4):abstract.
7. Religion and ethics: Islam, history of the Hajj. Available at: http://www.bbc.co.uk/religion/religions/islam/practices/hajj_2.shtml. Accessed September 30, 2006.
8. Ambah FS. Saudi Arabia tries to create a safer Hajj. *Christian Science Monitor*. February 19, 2006.
9. Feldman MJ, Lukins JL, Verbeek PR, et al. Use of treat-and-release medical directives for paramedics at a mass gathering. *Prehosp Emerg Care*. 2005;9(2):213–217.
10. Lukins JL, Feldman MJ, Summers JA, et al. A paramedic-staffed medical rehydration unit at a mass gathering. *Prehosp Emerg Care*. 2004;8(4):411–416.
11. Salhanick SD, Sheahan W, Bazarian JJ. Use and analysis of field triage criteria for mass gatherings. *Prehosp Dis Med*. 2003;18(4):347–352.
12. Menckhoff CR, Shaw M. Mass gathering preparedness. In: Keyes DC, Burnstein JL, et al., eds. *Medical Response to Terrorism*. Philadelphia: Lippincott Williams & Wilkins, 2005:257–268.
13. Blandford AG, Obst CD, Dunlop HA. Glastonbury Fair: some medical aspects of a rock music festival. *Practitioner*. 1972;209:205–211.
14. Osler DC, Shapiro F, Shapiro S. Medical services at outdoor music festivals. *Clin Pediatr*. 1975;14(4):390–395.
15. Chapman KR, Carmichael, FJ, Goode JE. Medical services for outdoor rock music festivals. *Can Med Assoc J*. 1982;126:935.
16. Suy K, Gijsenbergh F, Baute L. Emergency medical assistance during a mass gathering. *Eur J Emerg Med*. 1999;6:249–254.
17. Grange JT, Green SM, Downs W. Concert medicine: spectrum of medical problems encountered at 405 major concerts. *Acad Emerg Med*. 1999;6(3):202–207.
18. Thierbach AR, Wolcke BB, Piepho T, et al. Medical support for children's mass gatherings. *Prehosp Dis Med*. 2003;18(1):14–19.
19. Varon J, Fromm RE, Chanin K, et al. Critical illness at mass gatherings is uncommon. *J Emerg Med*. 2003;25(4):409–413.
20. Chan SB, Quinn JE. Outcomes in EMS-transported attendees from events at a large indoor arena. *Prehosp Emerg Care*. 2003;7(3):332–335.
21. Seletz JM. Flugtag-88 (Ramstein air show disaster): an Army response to a MASCAL. *Milit Med*. 1990;155:152–155.
22. Vukmir RB, Paris PM. The Three Rivers Regatta accident: an EMS perspective. *Am J Emerg Med*. 1991;9(1):64–71.
23. Janchar T, Samaddar C, Milzman D. The mosh pit experience: emergency medical care for concert injuries. *Am J Emerg Med*. 2000;18(1):62–63.
24. Gordon D. The Pope's visit: mass gatherings and the EMS system. *EMS*. 1988;17(1):38–44.
25. Pons PT, Holland B, Alfrey E, et al. An advanced emergency medical care system at National Football League games. *Ann Emerg Med*. 1980;9(4):203–206.
26. Flabouris A, Bridgewater F. An analysis of demand for first-aid care at a major public event. *Prehosp Disast Med*. 1996;11(1):48–54.
27. Zeitz KM, Schneider D, Jarrett D, et al. Mass gathering events: retrospective analysis of patient presentations over seven years. *Prehosp Dis Med*. 2002;17(3):147–150.
28. Friedman LJ, Rodi SW, Krueger MA, et al. Medical care at the California AIDS ride 3: experiences in event medicine. *Ann Emerg Med*. 1998;31(2):219–223.
29. Perron AD, Brady WJ, Custalow CB, et al. Association of heat index and patient volume at a mass gathering event. *Prehosp Emerg Care*. 2005;9(1):49–52.
30. Dress JM, Horton EH, Florida R. Music, mud and medicine. Woodstock '94: a maniacal, musical, mass-casualty incident. *Emerg Med Serv*. 1995;24(1):21, 30–32.
31. Florida R, Goldfarb Z. Woodstock '94: peace, music and EMS. *J EMS*. 1994;19(12):45–50.
32. Paul HM. Mass casualty: Pope's Denver visit causes mega MCI. *J EMS*. 1993;18(11):64–68, 72–75.
33. Schulte D, Meade DM. The papal chase. The Pope's visit: a "mass" gathering. *EMS*. 1993;22(11):46–49, 65–75, 79.
34. Feldman MJ, Lukins JL, Verbeek RP, et al. Half-a-million strong: the emergency medical services response to a single-day, mass-gathering event. *Prehosp Dis Med*. 2004;19(4):287–296.
35. Morimura N, Katsumi A, Koido Y, et al. Analysis of patient load data from the 2002 FIFA World Cup Korea/Japan. *Prehosp Dis Med*. 2004;19(3):278–284.
36. Feiner B. EMS at the 1984 Olympics. *Emerg Med Serv*. 1984;13(2):16–19.
37. Baker WM, Simone BM, Niemann JT, et al. Special event medical care: The 1984 Los Angeles summer Olympics experience. *Ann Emerg Med*. 1986;15:185.
38. Weiss BP, Mascola L, Fannin SL. Public health at the 1984 summer Olympics: the LA county experience. *Am J Public Health*. 1988;78:686.
39. Michael JA, Barbera JA. Mass gathering medical care: a twenty-five year review. *Prehosp Dis Med*. 1997;12(4):305–312.
40. Fruin JJ. Causes and prevention of crowd disasters. *Student Activities Program*. 1981;48–53.
41. Chambers J, Guly H. The impact of a music festival on local health services. *Health Trends*. 1991;23(3):122–123.
42. Centers for Disease Control and Prevention—MMWR. Prevention and management of heat related illness among spectators and staff during the Olympic Games—Atlanta, 6–23 July 1996. *JAMA*. 1996;45(29):631–633.
43. Stiel D, Trethowan P, Vance N. Medical planning for the Sydney Olympic and Paralympic Games. *MJA*. 1997;167:593–594.
44. Ellis JM. EMS at the Olympics. *Emerg Med Serv*. 1996;53–55.
45. Wetterhall SF, Coulombier DM, Herndon JM, et al. Medical care delivery at the 1996 Olympic Games. *JAMA*. 1998; 279(18):1463–1468.

46. Parrillo SJ. EMS and mass gatherings. *EMedicine* 2006. Available at: http://www.emedicine.com/EMERG/topic812.htm. Accessed September 30, 2006.

47. Milsten AM. From start to finish: physician usefulness at mass gathering event. Available at: http://www2.acep.org/1,33863,0.html. Accessed September 13, 2006.

48. Olapade-Olaopa EO. On-site physicians at a major sporting event in Nigeria. Available at: http://pdm.medicine.wisc.edu/21-1%20PDFs/olapade.pdf. Accessed September 13, 2006.

49. Arbon P, Bridgewater FH, Smith C. Mass gathering medicine: a predictive model for patient presentation and transport rates. *Prehosp Dis Med.* 2001;16(3):150–158.

50. Zeitz KM, Zeitz CJ, Arbon P. Forecasting medical work at mass-gathering events: predictive model versus retrospective review. *Prehosp Dis Med.* 2005;(20)3:164–168.

51. Feldman MJ, Lukins JL, Burgess, RJ, et al. Use of treat-and-release medical directives for paramedics at a mass gathering. *Prehosp Emerg.* 2005;9(2):213–217.

The United States Department of Homeland Security

Michael W. Proctor

OBJECTIVES

After reading this section, the reader will be able to:

1. Understand the history of and need for the establishment of the Department of Homeland Security.
2. Describe the basics of the National Incident Management System and the National Response Plan.
3. Understand Homeland Security Presidential Directives 5 and 8.

The 21st century has brought many changes to the world, and in the United States we have witnessed many life-altering events in the infancy of the 21st century. Immediately prior to ushering in the new millennium the world readied for the potential threats of Y2K, and arguably perhaps we witnessed for the first time a change in the paradigm of preparedness. Globally, from the private sector to all levels of government, systems were inspected, processes were evaluated, and contingency planning occurred for the potential changes Y2K might bring. One might argue that the predicted problems associated with Y2K did not occur because they were blown out of proportion or that we actually adequately prepared for and corrected the potential pitfalls, and in reality this might be a debate with no conclusion. Just as the world breathed a sigh of relief and the pundits made the foregoing arguments, the events of September 11, 2001, altered the course of history and indeed the lives of the citizens of the world. As Americans we were made painfully aware that all of our planning efforts and contingency plans for disasters were woefully inadequate to meet the challenges of terrorism and weapons of mass effect.

Before September 11, 2001, our counterterrorism efforts, training, and education were piecemeal and overseen by a myriad of federal departments, including the Department of Defense (DoD), Department of Justice (DoJ), Department of Energy (DoE), Department of State (DoS), Department of Health and Human Services (DHHS), and Department of Agriculture (DoA), as well as the Federal Emergency Management Agency (FEMA), the Centers for Disease Control and Prevention (CDC), and a host of smaller agencies.

In 1996, Congress attempted to address some of the issues of preparation for weapons of mass effect (or many refer to them as weapons of mass destruction) with the passage of the Defense Against Weapons of Mass Destruction Act, more commonly known as the Nunn-Luger-Domenici Initiative. This bill recognized the lack of preparedness among first responders safely responding to acts of terrorism involving NBC (nuclear, biological, chemical) weapons and provided funding for the preparation of the 125 largest U.S. cities. The DoD was initially responsible for the delivery of this program and authorized to provide training and exercises to local jurisdictions in an effort to improve preparedness at the local level. The act also authorized the DHHS, through the Office of Emergency Preparedness (now the Assistant Secretary for Preparedness and Response; ASPR), to develop Metropolitan Medical Response Systems in local jurisdictions. At that time, the Office of Emergency Response was charged with oversight of the National Disaster Medical System and Disaster Medical Assistance Teams, which was transferred to FEMA after creation of the DHS, then transferred back to the ASPR in 2007. The Nunn-Luger-Domenici Initiative later turned it over to the DoJ's Office of Justice programs, more specifically the Office for Domestic Preparedness (ODP), which was later transferred to the DHS. The DHSS, through its Health Resources Service Agency (HRSA)'s Hospital Bioterrorism Program and the CDC, provided some funding and guidance for health care and public health in an effort to provide education and training concerning the effects of a weapon of mass effect.

HISTORY AND CREATION OF THE DEPARTMENT OF HOMELAND SECURITY

After the attacks on New York City and Washington, DC, in 2001, President George Walker Bush initially created the Office of Homeland Security within the White House and later, in 2002, called for the creation of a new federal department at the cabinet level to address the issues and concerns of homeland defense and hopefully consolidate and unify our nation's efforts to mitigate and respond to terrorist, naturally occurring, and man-made events. With strong congressional support, the DHS was created by the Department of Homeland Security Act of 2002. This act brought together 22 agencies relating to homeland defense/security that were formerly housed in the Departments of Agriculture, Commerce, Defense, Energy, Health and Human Services, Justice, Transportation, and Treasury or as independent entities. Agencies with functions relating to homeland security that were not included in the DHS were the Federal Bureau of Investigation (FBI), Central Intelligence Agency (CIA), and National Security Agency (NSA).

The creation of the DHS marked the largest and most encompassing restructuring of the executive branch since the creation of the DoD in 1947 (1947–1949). Former Governor Tom Ridge of Pennsylvania, who served as the first head of the White House Office of Homeland Security, was appointed the first Secretary of DHS on January 24, 2003. In March 2003 the involved agencies began the transfer to the newly created DHS, which became the third largest executive department in the federal government. The initial configuration of the DHS involved the creation of four major directorates: Border and Transportation Security, Emergency Preparedness and Response, Science and Technology, and Information Analysis and Infrastructure Protection (IAIP) (1).

The Border and Transportation Security Directorate

Mission

The mission of the Border and Transportation Security Directorate is to "develop and transition capabilities to improve the security of our nation's borders and transportation systems without impeding the flow of commerce and travelers" (2).

Strategic Objectives

- Prevent entry of terrorists, criminals, and illegal aliens
- Interdict terrorist instruments and contraband at the earliest opportunity

- Improve the security of U.S. transportation systems
- Facilitate flow of commerce and travelers: identify, disrupt, and dismantle entities that threaten the United States

Structure

The initial organizational structure of the Border and Transportation Security Directorate as created in 2002 brought together the major border security and transportation operations under one roof and included the following:

- U.S. Customs Service (from Department of the Treasury)
- Immigration and Naturalization Service (part; from DoJ)
- Federal Protective Service
- Transportation Security Administration (from DoT)
- Federal Law Enforcement Training Center (from Department of the Treasury)
- Animal and Plant Health Inspection Service (part; from DoA)
- Office for Domestic Preparedness (from DoJ)

The Emergency Preparedness and Response Directorate

Mission

This directorate is charged with preparing for and recovering from the consequences of catastrophes, both natural and man-made.

Specific Responsibilities

The directorate's oversight of the federal government's national response and recovery strategy includes the following responsibilities (3).

- Helping to ensure the preparedness of emergency response providers for terrorist attacks, major disasters, and other emergencies
- Establishing standards, conducting exercises and training, evaluating performance, and providing funds for the Nuclear Incident Response Team
- Providing the federal government's response to terrorist attacks and major disasters
- Aiding recovery from terrorist attacks and major disasters
- Working with other federal and nonfederal agencies to build a comprehensive national incident management system (NIMS)
- Consolidating existing federal government emergency response plans into a single, coordinated national response plan (NRP)
- Establishing comprehensive programs for developing interoperative communications technology and ensuring that emergency response providers acquire such technology

Structure

The initial organizational structure of The Emergency Preparedness and Response Directorate as created in 2002 included the following.

- FEMA
- Strategic National Stockpile and the National Disaster Medical System (from DHHS)
- Nuclear Incident Response Team (from DoE)
- Domestic Emergency Support Teams (from DoJ)
- National Domestic Preparedness Office (from FBI)

The Science and Technology Directorate

Mission

The Science and Technology Directorate, in partnership with the private sector, national laboratories, universities, and other government agencies (domestic and foreign), helps push the innovation envelope and drive the development and use of high technology in support of homeland security.

The directorate is focusing on enabling its customers—the DHS components—and their customers, including Border Patrol agents, Coast Guardsmen, airport baggage screeners, Federal Air Marshals, and state, local, and federal emergency responders, as well as the many other teams committed to the vital mission of securing the nation (4).

Specific Responsibilities

The main responsibilities of this directorate are as follows (3).

- Sponsoring research, development, and testing to improve current capabilities or invent new vaccines, antidotes, diagnostics, and therapies against biological and chemical warfare agents
- Coordinating the federal government's efforts to develop and implement scientific and technological countermeasures against catastrophic terrorism, including channeling the intellectual energy and extensive capacity of important scientific institutions, such as the national laboratories and academic institutions
- Conducting a national scientific research and development program to support the mission of the department, including developing national policy and coordinating the federal government's (nonmilitary) efforts to counter chemical, biological, radiological, or nuclear (CBRN) weapons or other emerging threats (likely to be done via agreements with DHHS)
- Establishing priorities and directing and supporting national research on, development of, and procurement of technology and systems for detecting, preventing, protecting against, and responding to ter-

rorist attacks using CBRN or related weapons and materials as well as preventing the importation of such weapons and materials into the United States
- Establishing guidelines for state and local efforts to develop and implement countermeasures in this area
- Promoting research and technology to develop sensors to detect chemical and biological weapons from production to deployment

Structure

The initial organizational structure of the Science and Technology Directorate as created in 2002 included the following.

- CBRN Countermeasures Programs (from DoE)
- Environmental Measurements Laboratory (from DoE)
- National BW Defense Analysis Center (from DoD)
- Plum Island Animal Disease Center (from DoA)

The Information Analysis and Infrastructure Protection Directorate

Mission

The IAIP Directorate coordinates capabilities for identifying, analyzing, and disseminating information on current and future threats, partnering with all intelligence-generating agencies. Its mission is to analyze intelligence and information from other agencies (including the CIA, FBI, DIA, and NSA) involving threats to homeland security and evaluate vulnerabilities in the nation's infrastructure.

Specific Responsibilities

The IAIP Directorate's specific responsibilities include the following (3).

- Receiving and analyzing law enforcement information, intelligence, and other information in order to detect and understand the nature and scope of potential terrorist threats to the United States and its allies
- Comprehensively assessing the vulnerabilities of key resources and critical infrastructures
- Integrating relevant information, intelligence analyses, and vulnerability assessments to identify protective priorities and support protective measures
- Developing a comprehensive national plan for securing key resources and critical infrastructures
- Taking or seeking to effect necessary measures to protect the nation's key resources and infrastructures (e.g., food, water, agriculture, and health and emergency services; energy sources and conduits; transportation; information and telecommunications systems; banking and finance; postal services; and other essential assets and systems)
- Administering the Homeland Security Advisory System, exercising primary responsibility for public

threat advisories as well as for provision of specific warning information and appropriate protective actions and countermeasures to state and local governments and the private sector

■ Reviewing, analyzing, and making recommendations for improvements in the policies and procedures governing the sharing of law enforcement, intelligence, and other information relating to homeland security within the federal government and between the federal government and state and local governments

Structure

The initial organizational structure of the IAIP Directorate as created in 2002 included the following:

■ Federal Computer Incident Response Center (from GSA)
■ National Communications System (from DoD)
■ National Infrastructure Protection Center (from FBI)
■ Energy Security and Assurance Program (from DoE)

Other Agencies

Other key agencies transferred to the DHS in 2002 include the Secret Service and the Coast Guard, which were allowed to remain intact and report directly to the Secretary of DHS. In addition, the Immigration and Naturalization Service adjudications and benefits programs report directly to the Deputy Secretary as the U.S. Citizenship and Immigration Services.

RESTRUCTURING AND REORGANIZATION OF THE DEPARTMENT OF HOMELAND SECURITY

Since the creation of the DHS and the transfer of the aforementioned agencies and entities in March 2003, the department has undergone restructuring and multiple reorganizations. On December 31, 2003, the DHS Office of Inspector General issued a management review identifying several major challenges and shortcomings of the newly created department (5). After the 2004 presidential elections Secretary Tom Ridge elected to step down and then federal judge Michael Chertoff was appointed by President Bush and confirmed by the U.S. Senate to lead the DHS.

It was in 2005, on Secretary Chertoff's watch, that the newly created and largely untested department faced its first major challenge of activation and response in one of the most significant hurricane seasons the United States has ever faced. Hurricanes Katrina and Rita proved to be a major test of the department, the NIMS, and the

NRP. The impact of Hurricane Katrina on the Gulf Coast of Alabama, Mississippi, and Louisiana, with the ensuing breakdown of the levee system and subsequent flooding of the city of New Orleans, illuminated many shortcomings of the DHS, NIMS, and NRP and the system in general. Arguably the most significant criticisms of the DHS followed the White House, U.S. House of Representatives, and U.S. Senate reports on Hurricane Katrina. The reader may access these reports by contacting the Government Printing Office (Superintendent of Documents, U.S. Government Printing Office, Stop SSOP, Washington, DC 20402-0001; bookstore.gpo.gov; toll free 1-866-512-1800) or via the Internet as follows:

■ U.S. Senate
Hurricane Katrina: A Nation Still Unprepared
Report of the Senate Committee on Homeland Security and Governmental Affairs, May 2006
http://www.gpoaccess.gov/serialset/creports/katrina nation.html
■ U.S. House of Representatives
A Failure of Initiative: Final Report of the Select Bipartisan Committee to Investigate the Preparation for and Response to Hurricane Katrina.
http://www.gpoaccess.gov/congress/index.html
■ The White House
The Federal Response to Hurricane Katrina: Lessons Learned
http://www.whitehouse.gov/reports/katrina-lessons-learned.pdf

The most significant restructuring and subsequent reorganization of the DHS followed the amendment of the Department of Homeland Security Act of 2002 by the second session of the 109th Congress in 2006 in a bill entitled The Post Katrina Emergency Management Reform Act of 2006. This bill became effective on January 1, 2007, with a completion date of March 31, 2007. The legislation brought about significant changes not only in the DHS but in the overall response system of the United States for the Stafford Act to military assistance in civilian response. Following the passage of The Post Katrina Emergency Management Reform Act of 2006, Secretary Chertoff issued a six-point agenda for the DHS incorporating many of the recommendations of the Post Katrina Reform Act (6). In addition, the Post Katrina Reform Act highlighted the need for a revision of the NRP, which currently is in draft.

HOMELAND SECURITY PRESIDENTIAL DIRECTIVES 5 AND 8

It is significant to mention in this chapter two significant Homeland Security Presidential Directives (HSPDs) that have a major bearing on the first response community at large. In 2003 President Bush issued HSPD-5 and HSPD-8, both significant in the organization and management of our nation's mitigation of, response to, and recovery after terrorist, naturally occurring, and man-made events. HSPD-5 directed the Secretary to establish a single, comprehensive national incident management system and administer a NRP. At first blush one might question why there was such a need for this directive, but historically until the issuance of HSPD-5 there was no uniform incident management system that spelled out and provided an outline for mitigation and response that linked the local response to the federal response. All levels of response, from local to state to federal, had formulated their own systems, which, as history has shown, proved many times to be in conflict and incongruent. The formation of the NIMS and the subsequent development of the NRP now provide a template and plan where the intent is for smooth integration of the state and federal response into the local response system.

Hurricanes Katrina and Rita revealed many flaws in the system and there has been slow assimilation of the NIMS and NRP into all levels of response, from local to federal. Hurricanes Katrina and Rita exposed the need for more rigorous adoption and utilization of the NIMS and NRP, and failures of all levels of response communities have been highlighted in all post-Katrina and post-Rita afteraction reports and evaluations. Implementation of the concept of all levels of response operating within the same framework, with common terms and communications, will be a great step forward in the way our nation trains for and responds to terrorist, naturally occurring, and man-made events. For further information on HSPD-5, the reader is referred to http://www.whitehouse.gov/news/releases/2003/02/20030228-9.html.

The companion directive to HSPD-5, also issued in 2003, is HSPD-8, which calls for the development of a National Preparedness Goal that

> will establish measurable readiness priorities and targets that appropriately balance the potential threat and magnitude of terrorist attacks, major disasters, and other emergencies with the resources required to prevent, respond to, and recover from them. It will also include readiness metrics and elements that support the national preparedness goal including standards for preparedness assessments and strategies, and a system for assessing the Nation's overall preparedness to respond to major events, especially those involving acts of terrorism. (7)

HSPD-8 also expanded the definition of the "first responder" beyond the traditional definition of law enforcement, fire service, and EMS to include, in addition to these three, emergency management, public health, health care/clinical care, public works, and other skilled support personnel (such as equipment operators) that provide immediate support services during prevention, response, and recovery operations (7). Also contained in this presidential directive are definitions of "major disaster," "major events," "emergencies," and "preparedness," as well as outlines and calls for processes to be developed to train, exercise, and measure preparedness (7).

CONCLUSION AND RELATIONSHIP TO TACTICAL EMERGENCY MEDICAL SERVICES

While tactical operations/medicine is not specifically mentioned in the development of the DHS or the accompanying documents and processes mentioned above, the inference is certainly there. Over the course of the past years we have seen an increase in the field of tactical operations and medicine as a result of our local, state, and federal law enforcement agencies' necessity not only to mitigate, deter, and respond to an increasing level of threat in our country but also to serve as the first-line response to terrorism and operations that occur outside of what we would term "daily activity." Law enforcement departments, especially tactical operations/medicine, are direct beneficiaries—or certainly should be—of the increased funding for equipment, training, and exercises made available by the creation of the DHS, NIMS, and NRP and the issuance of HSPD-5 and -8.

Certainly we only have to look at events of the first few months of 2007 to realize the importance of tactical operations and tactical medicine in the protection of our citizens and the response to terrorist events in our nation, be they domestic or international.

REFERENCES

1. Homeland Security. History: Who became part of the department? Available at: http://www.dhs.gov/xabout/history/editorial_0133.shtm (1 of 2). Accessed July 15, 2007.
2. Homeland Security: Portfolios: Border and Transportation Security. Available at: http://www.dhs.gov/xres/programs/editorial_0545.shtm. Accessed: July 26, 2007.
3. CIDRAP. Bioterrorism. Available at: http://www.cidrap.umn.edu/cidrap/content/bt/bioprep/planning/bt-prep-planning.html. Accessed July 26, 2007.
4. Homeland Security. Directorate for Science and Technology. Available at: http://www.dhs.gov/xabout/structure/editorial_0530.shtm Accessed: July 7, 2007.
5. Major Management Challenges Facing the Department of Homeland Security. December 31, 2003. Department of Homeland Security, Office of Inspector General, Washington, DC 20528. Accessed: July 15, 2007.
6. Homeland Security. Department 6-point agenda. Available at: http://www.dhs.gov/xabout/history/editorial_0646.shtm. Accessed: July 15, 2007.
7. Homeland Security Presidential Directive/HSPD-8. Available at: http://www.whitehouse.gov/news/releases/2003/12/20031217-6. html.

Chapter 33

VIP Protection and Care

Nelson Tang

OBJECTIVES

After reading this section, the reader will be able to:

1. Discuss the three different models used for protective EMS support
2. Define mobile protection
3. List possible medical missions related to VIP protective care

The protective mission exists whenever it is deemed appropriate or necessary to dedicate personnel and resources to the safety and physical well-being of an individual or group of individuals. Protection enshrouds these individuals, commonly referred to as "very important persons" (VIPs), in a conceptual envelope consisting of and supported by physical security enforcement, threat countermeasures, dynamic intelligence acquisition, and operational contingency preplanning. In the past decade, increasing emphasis has been placed on developing specialized emergency medical capabilities in support of protective operations.

BACKGROUND AND DEFINITIONS

Historically, protective methodologies were developed and utilized by law enforcement for the physical security of political leaders and high-ranking government officials, generically referred to as *protectees* or *principals*. Perhaps the most widely recognized example is that of the U.S. Secret Service and its protective mission serving the President and Vice President and their immediate families. Increasingly, the private sector has been similarly challenged to deploy protective measures for leaders of industry and commerce and popular sports and entertainment figures, as well as individuals of significant wealth and personal influence.

Within the protective arena, the enhancement of readiness for medical contingencies has gained recognition as an essential priority. Having immediate access to qualified and dedicated emergency medical resources for both the VIP protectee and, to a lesser extent, the personnel engaged in protection, or the *protective detail*, is consistent with the overall protective mission. The intrinsic medical assets dedicated to protection may be broadly deemed protective medicine. Protective medicine assets ideally serve dual functions, as both an evaluative adjunct for threat assessments and an immediate intervention mechanism in the event of medical contingencies.

The overriding principle that governs protective methodology is the single-minded focus on the security of the VIP or protectee. In fact, personnel involved in protection may be very simply separated into two distinct categories: those directly engaged in physical protection and those providing operational support. This basic concept may challenge conventional paradigms of the medical provider. Regardless of how experienced, advanced, or technically proficient the medical providers assigned to protection may be, they are nonetheless considered support personnel.

PROTECTEES

It is important to recognize that it is ultimately the VIPs or protectees that determine the level of protection, and similarly protective medical support, that is acceptable or desired. It may be generally true that protectees are often accepting of as much protection as may be offered to them, however, there exists the possibility that a particular VIP may elect to refuse some or all protection. Broad decision making and planning for protection must be in the context of protectee agreement and cooperation. It is further conceivable that protectees may specifically elect to minimize or dismiss entirely their medical support, potentially out of concerns for the public appearance of frailty or infirmity.

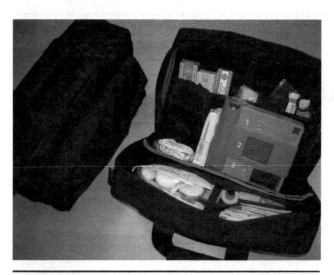

FIGURE 33.1. Medical gear deployed in support of the VIP protection mission may preferably be transported in smaller, more discrete bags so as minimize the suggestion of its contents. (Courtesy of the author.)

It is a generally advisable principle that medical personnel assigned to protection deploy and operate discretely, so as not to widely identify the nature or extent of their intended mission (Fig. 33.1).

Fundamentally, the actual medical care rendered to VIPs should not be expected to be intrinsically different from that afforded to the population at large, although certainly the scope and scale of available resources in some instances might be greater for such individuals. From generalized experience, it may appear that accessibility to both primary and specialist care is superior for the VIP, due to either their individual influence or the effectiveness of others acting on behalf of the VIP. Nevertheless, in the United States, access to appropriate and timely emergency care is considered universal and remains undifferentiated based on an individual's wealth, stature, or influence. Regardless of whether the clinical care sought is routine, urgent, or emergent, enhancing intrinsic medical capabilities may reduce the challenges posed to protective operations of getting care for a VIP.

MODELS OF PROTECTIVE MEDICAL SUPPORT

There exists a broad spectrum of emergency medical services (EMS) that may be deployed in support of protective operations. The manner in which these may be enlisted can be broadly categorized into three models of protective support. Each of these approaches has its intrinsic advantages and potential drawbacks. The selection of one versus another is a command decision of the highest order and must be commensurate with threat assessments and the overall level of protective support deemed necessary.

The most basic and easily configured level of support involves incorporating preexisting medical services and providers, on an ad hoc basis, into the protective environment (1). Examples are adding a local private or jurisdictional EMS to a traveling motorcade and arranging for medical providers to be either on-site or on-call at the location of an event attended by a protectee. This approach minimizes costs and requires little or no long-term intrinsic program maintenance. Potential disadvantages to be expected include medical providers lacking familiarity with law enforcement and protective operations, limited ability to conduct thorough background clearances of providers, and inconsistency of medical capabilities from venue to venue. The concerns for operational security (OPSEC) are elevated with these types of arrangements.

An intermediate model is one that incorporates some fixed medical capabilities into the protective operation itself in a longitudinal fashion. As an example, the agency or department responsible for protection may choose to employ or contract medical personnel and acquire EMS transport vehicles as intrinsic assets. This approach increases the degree of standing medical readiness and some capability, depending on levels of providers, for initial treatment, triage, and transport in the event of emergency medical contingencies. There are increased direct costs for this approach and it does relatively little to enhance the capability for primary care, preventive medicine, and advanced interventions and therapeutics.

The third and most proactive model of protective medical support involves the development of a comprehensive protective emergency medicine program. This includes qualified physician medical oversight, treatment and transport protocols, medical armamentarium appropriate for the protective environment and mission, and dedicated medical personnel trained and proficient in both emergency care and law enforcement operations. This approach parallels the development of emergency medical capabilities in support of the law enforcement tactical mission (2). Such vastly increased capability is costly, whether measured in terms of dollars, manpower, equipment, space, or administrative oversight. Nevertheless, depending on the need, it is arguably the most consistent with the fundamental mindset in the protection arena, which is directed toward maximal preparedness for potential contingencies.

MOBILE PROTECTION

When a protectee becomes mobile and leaves the relative security of a fixed location (one that has been appropriately cleared and secured by the protective detail), the potential exposure to threats is significantly increased. Whether traveling on foot or by vehicle, a protectee in motion may generally have fewer assets immediately available and yet

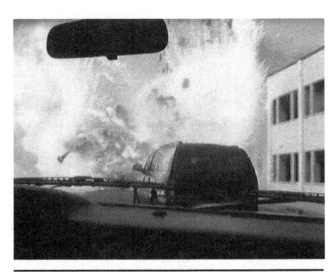

FIGURE 33.2. Mobile protectees are at greater risk for attack, even in the relative security of the motorcade. (Courtesy of the author.)

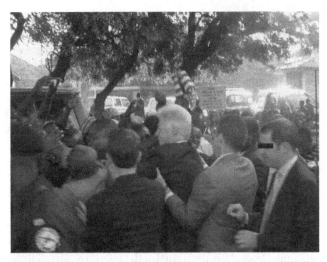

FIGURE 33.3. The protective detail maintains close physical proximity to the VIP and is extensively trained in the counter-measures to deploy in the event of a threat. (Courtesy of the author.)

be more susceptible to injury, environmental hazards, and attack (Fig. 33.2). The effective coordination of medical support in the mobile environment is similarly more complex.

The popular conceptualization of protection is frequently that of a group of security personnel standing or walking in close proximity to, and surrounding, the protectee. The assumption that a medical support provider belongs in the protective formation is erroneous and without practical basis. The medical provider must be considered an asset, one that is similarly endangered by threats on the formation.

The protective detail is uniquely and highly trained in countermeasures to deploy in the event of a physical threat to a protectee (Fig. 33.3). The emergency medical care provider possesses a different expertise and skills set. Further, the immediate actions to occur in such a scenario involve simultaneous neutralization of such threats as well as movement of the protectee out of the threat environment. All medical assessment and intervention requires some degree of time and physical space for effectiveness. Neither of these elements will be available in the event of a rapid evacuation or withdrawal. Instead, optimal strategic planning would place the medical assets in a location of close, but not immediate, proximity, with a capability to forward deploy in the event a threat is engaged or the detail moves without advance notice.

The caravan of motor vehicles in which a protectee travels is usually referred to as the *motorcade*, whether the number of vehicles is 2 or 20, and the vehicle transporting the protectee as the *limousine*. Traditionally, it is commonplace to see an ambulance, if utilized, toward the rear of the motorcade, with the ability and intent to bring this forward as needs arise. Ongoing research into protective methodology suggests that a civilian EMS ambulance is generally highly recognizable and may itself be a target in the event of an attack on the motorcade. Alternate vehicles with variable capacity for emergency patient transport may be considered and may have the advantage of lowered visibility and potentially greater mobility in variable terrains. Another strategy involves decentralizing medical assets in the motorcade in a systematic and coordinated manner such that not all resources and personnel are relegated to one particular vehicle.

HOSPITAL INTERFACE

The need for a VIP to seek care at a hospital or other treatment facility is problematic for the protective mission on many levels. Unless extensively preplanned, most such unanticipated visits mean that the health of the protectee is in question. Add to this mindset the complex logistics of transporting the VIP and transferring VIP care to a hospital environment and the concerns of protective personnel become elevated significantly.

In the United States, the general access point to hospitals is the emergency department, where the admixture of patients, health care providers, ancillary staff, visitors, and public safety personnel creates an outwardly chaotic environment in the best of circumstances. This is typically vastly different from what would be considered the ideal site security requirements for a VIP visit. Furthermore, the simple presence of the VIP can have an unintended, potentially deleterious, effect on the medical facility and staff themselves (3–6).

In high-level protective operations, the detail may have as one of its preplanning tasks the designation of specific hospitals or trauma centers that will be utilized in the eventuality of a VIP medical emergency. Assessment of an individual facility's medical capabilities and security attributes contributes to such determinations. If away from the base of operations, for example, during VIP travel, the detail may have protective personnel assigned to those facilities as liaisons throughout the duration of a VIP visit.

PROTECTIVE DETAIL CARE

Whether intended or not, medical support will generally be called on to render care to the individuals providing protection, specifically personnel of the protective detail itself. Particularly in the case of overseas deployments or other extended mobile operations, protective medical support must anticipate these needs and plan for additional personnel, equipment, and supplies to support this "sick call" need. As a basic force protection issue, the effectiveness of protective operations is critically dependent on the health and safety of its manpower. In the protection arena, very similarly to many law enforcement special operations, mission success is contingent on personnel who are fit, rested, hydrated, and appropriately managed for both routine and unexpected medical conditions.

As a rule, younger or less experienced protective detail personnel are typically less likely to seek advice or intervention for developing medical concerns. The consequence is that medical issues may be discovered at a relatively late stage of development. The relative inability to intervene early in this subgroup of the protective detail makes essential the need for vigilance and proactive interventions on the part of medical support personnel. Simple actions such as advocating hydration or ensuring safe food sources can significantly contribute to mission success by minimizing threats posed by performance degradation due to personnel illnesses.

INTERNATIONAL MISSIONS

When a VIP under protection travels internationally, the physical and medical risks are magnified tremendously. All of the existing baseline protective concerns remain, with the added potential complexities of diminished manpower and resources, unfamiliar environments, unstable or unfriendly geopolitical infrastructure, and underdeveloped local resources including emergency medical facilities, providers, and prehospital care. Even at the hospital level of care, local clinical practices and standards of care may be so dramatically different as to be considered unacceptable both for the VIP and for the protective detail itself (Fig. 33.4). Unfortunately, the decision making with

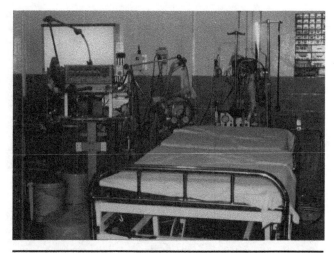

FIGURE 33.4. An intensive care unit in a foreign hospital demonstrates differences in standards of medical care that must be anticipated and addressed by the protective detail. (Courtesy of the author.)

regard to VIP travel must often be made independently of such concerns and it falls to the protective detail and its medical support to respond to and anticipate the potential consequences.

The potential lack of existing medical infrastructure in the international arena often means that the protective detail must travel with expanded intrinsic capabilities, often well beyond what might be deployed domestically. In terms of medical support, considerations must be given to the deployment of advanced medical providers including physicians and as much medical equipment and as many therapeutics as can be feasibly transported. This strategic planning is often made in the context of other security needs including communications equipment, vehicles, munitions, and augmented manpower. The allowances for increased medical support assets are often more easily accomplished in the setting of international missions.

INCIDENTAL CONTACTS AND BYSTANDER CARE

VIPs often associate with and travel in the company of large numbers of people. These may include friends, personal staff, administrative personnel, press, and media. Generally, these groups of individuals are not considered VIPs and are not afforded protection, including medical support. It is, however, not always reasonable to deny these individuals medical consultation or evaluation under routine circumstances. It should, nevertheless, be clearly understood that responding to such requests is not routine and decisions must be made on a case-by-case basis. It is sometimes the case that the VIP directs medical personnel to attend to an associate and such situations must be handled with tact and good judgment.

It is the inclination and training of emergency medical providers, as a rule, to render care whenever and wherever medical emergencies are encountered. In the pure protection arena, however, it must be understood and agreed on that all resources and efforts are to be directed to the VIP protectee (1). Personnel, equipment, supplies, and manpower intended to support protection must be reserved for protection. It would be considered unacceptable for such resources to be diverted to bystanders or anyone other than the protectee should a VIP emergency or need for evacuation arise. This conceptual potential conflict must be carefully considered and appropriate policies and procedures developed to ensure the clarity of the mission and the compliance of personnel.

TACTICAL SUPPORT

With the rapid evolution and advancement of civilian law enforcement tactical capabilities, there is without doubt the increasing opportunity to support protective operations. In some instances, the oversight of specific protective missions may actually fall to a particular agency's tactical unit or special operations branch. It is worthwhile to note, however, that a subtle but important distinction may exist between the roles of tactical elements supporting the VIP protection mission and those of general law enforcement operations. Although conventional tactics may tend to encourage stealth and coordination, tactical operators in the protective arena must be trained and prepared to rapidly engage emerging hostile elements both as a direct threat countermeasure and to afford an opportunity for protectee escape.

CONCLUSIONS

Historically developed by law enforcement for the protection of government and political leaders, the protective mission is increasingly being developed for a wide array of VIPs. The evolution of protective medicine in many ways parallels the enhancement of medical support for the law enforcement tactical mission. Strategic planning for medical support of protection requires a fundamental understanding of the mandates of protection, the protectees, models of protective medical support, and the complexities of providing protection in mobile, international, and potentially hostile environments.

REFERENCES

1. Maniscalco PM, Dolan NJ. Dignitary protection. *Emerg Med Serv.* 2002; 31(10):126–128.
2. Heck JJ, Pierluisi G. Law enforcement special operations medical support. *Prehosp Emerg Care.* 2001;5(4):403–406.
3. Smith MS, Shesser RF. The emergency care of the VIP patient. *N Engl J Med.* 1989;320(15):1421–1423.
4. Feuer EH, Karasu SR. A star-struck service: impact of the admission of a celebrity to an inpatient unit. *J Clin Psychiatry.* 1978;39(10):743–746.
5. Strange RE. The VIP with illness. *Milit Med.* 1980;145(7):473–475.
6. Mellick L. VIP patients should be treated differently. *ED Manage.* 2000;12(8):90–92.

Chapter 34

Canine Use in Tactical, and Search and Rescue Operations

Robert W. Deeds and Karen A. Deeds

OBJECTIVES

After reading this section, the reader will be able to:

1. Describe historical uses of canines related to tactical and medical operations
2. Describe the use of canines during tactical medical operations and mass casualty terrorism events
3. Discuss the selection and training methods used for canine use
4. Describe the limitations to canine team use in tactical medical operations

HISTORICAL AND CURRENT PERSPECTIVE

Canis familiaris, or the domestic dog, is defined as a highly variable domestic mammal closely related to the common wolf (1). Humans are believed to have begun canine domestication as early as 100,000 years ago. There are empirical genetic data to back this, however, written documentation outlining the use of canines is found to be inadequate, at best. The domestic dog is represented in sculpture, in Iraq, dating back to 6500 B.C., while bones in the United States date back to 8300 B.C. The dog's keen sense of smell and advanced ability to hear made it ideal to "work" as a sentry for potential threats. Because of the innate abilities the dog possessed, these functions developed as a natural obligation as its life intertwined with humans. If a dog was sleeping at the door of the home, it would surely alarm those within of any intruder. It was natural. Symbiotic relationships also prospered in both hunting and warfare. Royalty all over Europe are depicted in art and written word, throughout the Middle Ages and Renaissance, using dogs to hunt. Peasants, though not engaged in the same sporting hunts as their royal counterparts, often owned and trained smaller breeds to hunt small game, including rodents. As early as the Middle Ages, villagers used bloodhounds to hunt down and apprehend criminals. Carvings and statues in museums and temples in Assyria, Italy, and Britain depict dogs of war and their warrior handlers throughout the Middle Ages and the Renaissance. Doctors in ancient Corinth used dogs to assist in the determination of whether patients were alive or dead, using the simple wag of a tail as an alert.

In the United States, The American Canine Corp was started in Seminole War of 1835; this was the first canine corps in the country. Dogs were used as messengers, sentries, and trackers throughout the Civil War. In 1884, at Lechernich, near Berlin, the first training manual was written for military working dogs (MWDs). Germany and Belgium had police canine programs in many cities by the later part of the 1800s. In 1907, the New York City Police Department imported their first dogs from Belgium. With the advent of French Ring Sport in 1909, birth was given to many of the military and police training techniques we use today. In World War I, in using canines to locate wounded soldiers on the battlefield, the French further developed and organized training techniques for MWDs. By World War II, the majority of countries were utilizing dogs in the battlefield environment. By this time dogs were being used to assist in jobs such as sentry, messenger, search and rescue (SAR), patrol, and many others.

The first disaster dogs were trained in England during World War II to sift through the rubble after German bombing raids. By the 1960s, dogs were routinely being utilized in the United States to detect narcotics and explosives, and for patrol and tracking. Accelerant detection canines ("bomb dogs") were first used in the United States in 1986, by the Connecticut State Police.

A common, more modern, utilization of canines is in SAR operations (2). Most of the initial groundwork in SAR was done by law enforcement and the military. The Federal Emergency Management Agency (FEMA) has 28 Urban Search and Rescue (USAR) teams in various locations throughout the United States. These teams use four handler/canine teams on each deployment and are augmented by specialist and equipment for medical, heavy rescue, and technical search response. Volunteer SAR teams have developed across the United States. California Area Search and Rescue Dog Association (CARDA), started in 1976, is one of the largest and oldest in the United States. The growth of such volunteer teams has been nationwide, and currently approximately 125 certified teams exist. These volunteer teams provide local law enforcement (often in smaller municipalities) with skilled canine teams that otherwise would be cost-prohibitive.

CANINE USES IN TACTICAL MEDICAL OPERATIONS

Advancement of canine use in the tactical medical environment requires that a consistent and reliable performance is maintained in a productive, yet cost-effective manner. The uses of canines in the setting of terrorism events, mass casualty incidents, and other large-scale tactical operations or consequence management are many.

The use of trained canine teams to identify injured humans in the tactical setting may be beneficial to the overall medical management of the scene. Canine skills, such as detection of ongoing respiration, rafting of cells, and other innate abilities that still defy scientific explanation, may prove very beneficial in the most basic "triage," the identification of live victims, and extend the SAR functions dogs now perform.

Injured personnel and other victims may be positioned out of the immediate line of sight or positioned in a manner making even the most basic assessment of signs of life challenging. A canine's ability to rapidly distinguish live versus dead human beings in these potential settings is highly valuable. The ability of the canine to move with agility on varied surfaces may significantly increase the range of area accessible to the medical tactical team.

In the setting of a mass casualty incident, the use of canine skills to rapidly identify live but severely injured or unconscious victims may be a valuable patient assessment tool. This may be especially beneficial in the setting of multiple casualties with only a few tactical medical team members present such as may occur in remote or specialized tactical operations. The use of such "mass casualty dogs" in these scenarios may put fewer humans at risk.

CANINE SELECTION FOR USE IN TACTICAL MEDICAL ENVIRONMENTS

Skilled canine handlers and trainers are clearly a vital part of integrating canine teams into the tactical environment. Perhaps the most challenging aspect is identifying dogs that have the proper innate behavioral and physical traits. Many different skills and responses must be assessed when selecting and training a dog for use in a tactical medical environment (3). One of the first considerations is the reward system used to train the dog. The type of reward system used is important when training a dog for use in mass casualty tactical incidents. As a reward, toys are preferable over food. Food is commonly present in tactical mass casualty incidents, thus the use of food as a reward could potentially create confusion for the dog during an actual event. The ability of the dog to use a toy, rather than food, is only one of the challenges during the selection and screening portions of these dogs.

Does the dog have an adequate "prey drive" and "focus"? The dog's ability to maintain concentration and demonstrate a possessive nature toward the training aid (e.g., toy) are important traits predictive of success in the program. The refusal of the dog to release the toy easily, even when presented with distracting situations, is important. The demonstration of intense interest and a very energetic attitude toward training with the proper aids are signs of "high energy focus." These are highly desirable attributes and behavior qualities.

How long will the dog search for the training aid? An appropriate "hunt drive" is assessed by determining the quality and quantity of searching a dog will do for a hidden training aid. Tossing a training aid in high grass and delaying the release of the dog are examples of techniques used in assessing such hunt-based behavior.

Does the dog have the "nerve strength" or mental toughness to succeed in the anticipated tactical work environment? This behavioral trait is assessed by training the dog in environments with loud noises, under environmental challenges of heat and cold, daylight and darkness, and various surfaces, and for varying lengths of time.

Does the dog have the physical form and stature to accomplish success in the tactical mission environment? For the safety of the animal, it is important to evaluate whether a dog may be at significant risk or have a predisposition to chronic illness, orthopedic injuries, or vision challenges. The goal is simply to have a dog physically capable of working a long career.

Many of these behavioral and physical traits have been integrated in recognized screening programs used by professional handlers. The Disaster Canine Qualifying Screening is a good example of such integration. This particular tool is used by many FEMA USAR handlers. The screening document is available at the referenced disaster dog web site (2).

CANINE SKILLS TRAINING FOR USE IN TACTICAL MEDICAL ENVIRONMENTS

Defining the mission type and conditions are key elements in the effective use of canines in the tactical medical environment. Mission definition is vital to canine skills training. These dogs may be utilized in a forward position deemed unsafe for human medical team member entry. In this case, the handlers would need to have off-leash control, with both obedience and direction capabilities. For tactical use, the dogs would also have to be trained to use an appropriate alert when they find a live victim.

There are many examples of training programs for canines used in disasters. The program should be comprehensive, encompassing the key aspects of selection, training, and deployment. The purpose of training is to create default behaviors so that the dog functions instinctively, appropriately, and independently (3,4).

Training techniques vary, and their use must be determined by what phase of training you are in, the dog, and what you are trying to achieve. A common mistake that trainers make is limiting themselves to one type of training or a single technique. Effective training is often a mix of operant and classical conditioning.

Using adjunctive tools such as a "clicker," which is used to mark behavior, is also important. This is the same technique that trainers use to teach whales and dolphins at sea parks. It allows the animal to better understand the desired behavior requested of it. Later, after the dog knows the desired behavior, an appropriate amount of compulsion through traditional classical training or even the use of a remote training collar to enforce behavior can be utilized. For example, the tactical environment will necessitate that the handler is not always adjacent to the dog during working efforts. Therefore, a clicker may be utilized to mark the appropriate behavior, such as a bark, upon the dog's successfully identifying a live victim. In disaster canine training, this is referred to as a "focused bark indicating live human scent," or FBILHS (5).

Training canines is challenging. It requires that the trainer constantly move between canine instinct and canine control. There are many variations in technique application that facilitate success in canine training. A positive training environment that maintains the dog's excitement level will enhance performance at all levels of training (3–5).

LIMITATIONS TO CANINE USE IN TACTICAL MEDICAL OPERATIONS

There are limitations to the use of canines in the tactical medical response. An overview of these limitations would include environmental, physical, and financial considerations. In an environment where hazardous materials have been released, the use of canines may be significantly limited. This includes suspicion or known use of many chemical, biological, or radiological agents. If personal protection equipment is required for safe entry into the environment, then canine use is adversely impacted. Dogs trained for use in austere settings such as tactical and mass casualty scenes are not able to function effectively in most protective gear. The need for agility, balance, and traction for traversing terrain restricts these dogs even from using protective paw covers during operations. Particulate matter in the air and other airborne contaminants may significantly impair the canine's olfactory senses (6). This may prevent the dog from completing its mission due to failure to alert on the injured victims.

More commonly encountered environmental stresses can significantly impact use of canines in tactical medical operations. Extremes of temperature alone must be considered in the operational limitations of canines. For example, extreme heat may reduce the use of canines to only several minutes of intense activity between periods of rest and recuperation. The olfactory capabilities of a dog may be impacted by routine weather conditions such as wind and rain (6).

The cost of maintaining canine teams ready for immediate use during tactical medical operations may be the greatest limitation to consider. Financial considerations include team training, maintenance, veterinary care, deployment, recovery, and legal liability issues. Many other costs must be considered as well. For example, memoranda of understanding must be established with each proposed law enforcement agency and municipality. Joint training and exercise programs with each of these agencies are a significant financial consideration. Solutions to these costs of tactical use may include the model found in federal disaster dog handlers. Cost-effective canine teams may use contracted employees, independent contractors, volunteer organizations, and donations. Educating agencies and municipalities on the benefits of using canine teams in tactical medical operations is important in program creation and sustainment. Integration with existing canine teams, such as those involved in SAR, should be considered. The opportunity for dual-use integrated models may provide a cost-effective solution.

TAKE-HOME POINTS

1. Canines have unique innate traits that facilitate the identification of live victims.
2. A trained canine's ability to alert upon finding a live victim, especially a victim positioned out of the line of sight of the tactical medical providers, is a valuable "triage" tool.

3. The ability of the canine to move with agility on varied surfaces may significantly increase the range of area accessible to the medical tactical team.
4. Clear communication to canine handlers concerning the tactical medical scenarios likely to be encountered is one of the most important aspects of successful canine team operation.

SUMMARY

There is a substantial historic record of canine utilization that has laid the foundation for the expanding role of well-trained working dogs in tactical medical operations. This chapter has demonstrated current and suggested uses of these highly skilled canine teams during tactical medical operations and mass casualty events. Dog selection and training methods are critical elements to an effective canine tactical team. Limitations have been identified, which are an important decision-making component in strategic planning for successful canine team integration.

REFERENCES

1. Merriam-Webster Online Dictionary. Available at: http://www.merriam-webster.com/dictionary/dog. Accessed July 10, 2007.
2. FEMA disaster dog. Available at: http://www.disasterdog.org/forms.htm. Accessed April 10, 2006.
3. Pitts F, Engelbert L. The canine in disaster search and rescue. Available at: http://www.disasterdog.org/articles/disaster_dogs_101.htm. Accessed July 10, 2007.
4. Brownell D, Marsolais M, Hawn P. Disaster canine qualification screening, revision May 2002. Available at: http://www.disasterdog.org/forms/training/CanineScreeningV2.doc. Accessed July 10, 2007.
5. Hammond SM. *Training the Disaster Search Dog: A Dogwise Training Manual*. Wenatchee, WA: Dogwise; 2005.
6. http://www.disasterdog.org/articles/overview_of_canine_ofactory_system_oct2005.pdf. Accessed July 10, 2007.

Chapter 35

Tactical Emergency Medicine: Emerging Technologies for the Tactical Medical Provider

Stephen Brock Blankenship, Mark E. Gebhart, and Jason R. Pickett

OBJECTIVES

After reading this section, the reader will be able to:

1. Be familiar with recent technological advances that impact medicine in the tactical environment at the provider level.
2. Understand the role that these technologies may play in their particular system.
3. Understand the limitations of many of these technologies.
4. Balance the benefits of new technologies with the cost, probably impact, and drawbacks of technologies for use in tactical medicine.
5. Be aware of emerging advances that may play a future role in tactical emergency care.

Tactical emergency care is often viewed as an extension of basic trauma skills in the field of care in potentially hostile environments. Those who view tactical medicine this way may feel that bandages and intravenous fluid are the limits of needed medical skills and attention. Recent advances in technology clearly have helped decrease morbidity and mortality in today's operational environment. To be of great use, new technologies must meet the demands of the tactical environment and the care providers of varying skill levels who may be called on to use them. As a general rule, tools for tactical use must meet some of the requirements summarized in Table 35.1.

ADVANCES IN PATIENT ASSESSMENT

Amplified Stethoscopes

Though the stethoscope has been a tool of the medical provider since the 1800s, the biggest advance in this technology has come only recently, with the addition of electronic noise amplification. Some models have the ability to dampen ambient noise, to allow the listener to better hear desired lung sounds and heart sounds. The technology here operates on skills already possessed by medical providers at virtually every level. The key advantages posed by these scopes are the ability to improve transmission of important sounds while excluding others in the potentially noisy and hectic tactical environment. This becomes especially important considering that the medic may have been exposed to live gunfire and so may have a decreased ability to hear. Features such as the ability to record and play back sounds are probably of little utility to the tactical provider.

Ultrasound

Ultrasound is quickly becoming a standard of patient assessment in the emergency departments of the nation's hospitals. With the advent of battery-powered portable ultrasound units, this technology is now available to the field provider. Though its uses vary and are continually expanding, ultrasound for the tactical provider will likely be of greatest benefit for two principal functions: assessment of intraperitoneal blood and guidance for placement of central venous catheters. It has been used with some success in military deployments to Iraq (1) as well as onboard the International Space Station (2).

1. Assessment of intraperitoneal/pericardial blood. The Focused Assessment by Sonogram for Trauma, or FAST,

▶ TABLE 35.1. Requirements for Technology in the Tactical Setting.

Ruggedness. The adage, "If you take care of your gear, it will take care of you," is nowhere more appropriate than in the tactical setting. The tactical environment is notoriously hard on equipment. Proper care of any equipment is important, but this care cannot be a limitation to the operational effectiveness of the user.

Portability. Tactical care providers must often carry their medical equipment on their person, sometimes over great distances. Any equipment used for this purpose must be both lightweight and compact, or the user is likely to leave the equipment behind.

Ease of use. Tactical emergency care providers vary greatly in level of medical training. Technologies appropriate for the physician provider may not prove appropriate for the basic EMT or field medic. Any technology employed in the field must be applicable to the individual provider's level of training.

Speed of deployment. Tactical field care is performed expediently, often for reasons of personal safety or mission effectiveness. Any technology used for care in the field cannot be burdensome as far as the amount of time necessary to set it up and employ it.

Reliability. Any technology used in the field environment must be reliable, even under less-than-ideal conditions. If a device cannot be relied on to function at all times, it might as well be left behind.

Multipurpose use. The more purposes a device serves, the better suited it is to tactical care. Using devices that can perform multiple functions may enable the provider to lighten the load and leave behind other equipment that serves the same function.

exam has become a standard at many trauma centers nationwide. By using ultrasound to examine four areas, or "windows," the provider can assess the presence of significant intraperitoneal or pericardial blood requiring surgery in about 30 seconds, with a sensitivity of 77% to 81% and a specificity of 98% to 99% (3,4). A nonphysician provider, unfamiliar with the procedure, was able to perform the procedure with real-time online help from remote physicians in about 5 minutes (2).

2. Confirmation of endotracheal tube placement. Emerging evidence suggests that ultrasound of the lung may assist in assessment of intubated patients as an adjunct to confirm proper tube placement (5).

3. Placement of central and peripheral venous catheters. Studies have shown that ultrasound-guided procedures are more likely to be successful and less likely to result in arterial cannulation or pneumothorax (6,7).

4. Early recognition of shock. Ultrasound measurement of the inferior vena cava (IVC) may enable the tactical medical provider (TMP) to recognize and treat hypovolemic shock before acute changes in vital signs, mental status, or physical exam (8). The IVC correlates with volume status, shrinking in size as the preload decreases. This information may be useful to the TMP,

who must care for casualties over a longer period of time than the typical emergency medical services (EMS) provider.

5. Detection and assessment of fracture. Ultrasound can detect periosteal fluid collections, interruption or bulging of the cortex, or avulsion of bone. In the field environment, where x-rays are unavailable or require evacuation to a medical facility, ultrasound may provide the TMP with useful clinical information regarding the need for evacuation of a casualty. Fracture reduction may be urgently required in the field to reduce neurovascular compromise and prevent further injury to a fractured arm or leg. Ultrasound may guide the TMP in assessing the success of fracture reduction and visualization of bone alignment.

6. Detection of pneumothorax. Patients with even a small pneumothorax may develop a tension pneumothorax and rapidly deteriorate once they are under positive-pressure ventilation. Detection of pneumothorax may be difficult in high-noise environments, such as CASEVAC transports, battlefields, or chaotic civilian scenes. Ultrasound can be used to rapidly diagnose clinically significant pneumothorax at the bedside with 98% to 100% sensitivity, exceeding that of supine chest x-ray (9,10).

7. Detection of foreign bodies. Ultrasound may be used to detect foreign bodies in soft tissue that may have been introduced by shrapnel from explosive devices or fragmentation of bullets. Foreign bodies may be found in abscesses, removal of which will be necessary for the abscess to heal. Of particular interest are foreign bodies in the eye, which require immediate surgical intervention. Fragments or particles may be driven into the eye at a high velocity, going unnoticed by the victim. Likewise the puncture site may not be readily apparent on examination (11).

Vital Signs Monitoring

Trends in vital signs can be the TMP's first indication of trouble in patients who have suffered illness or internal injury. Automated monitoring of vital signs enables providers to care for multiple patients simultaneously, as they may be alerted to changes in patient condition without the need to be constantly at the bedside. Portable vital signs monitors have been in use in the hospital and air transport realms for decades. In the air transport setting, where auscultating lung sounds or blood pressures is severely limited by engine noise, these monitors are a necessity. Units typically used in this setting have utilized traditional methods of monitoring including electrocardiogram (ECG) leads, a noninvasive blood pressure cuff, and an oxygen saturation plethysmograph connected to the patient with wires. It is no surprise, therefore, that recent technology advances have sought to untangle us from the patient using wireless technology widely available in many cellular phone and home computer systems.

Vital signs monitoring systems currently available combine the ability to monitor multiple parameters in one compact device. Domestic air medical services have used various models for years with great success. Some models may have operating times of ≥8 hours on a single battery charge. More recent innovations bring connectivity to the field, which has been heretofore unavailable. The Welch-Allyn Propaq (12) series of monitors has been a staple of critical care transport for some time. Newer models have color screens for improved visual interpretation of vital signs, better visibility of warning alarms, and easier differentiation of waveforms.

Blood Pressure Measurement

Blood pressure in most settings is still measured by a non-invasive cuff that is periodically inflated to measure the systolic and diastolic pressures at intervals determined by the care provider. In critical care settings, it is often measured by a pressure transducer connected to a catheter placed in an artery. Recent advances in this area include a cuff that fits around the patient's wrist to monitor blood pressure noninvasively. The device measures impedance changes in the pulse wave and, therefore, can estimate the blood pressure continuously with each pulse. This potentially offers the advantage of ongoing monitoring without the need for arterial line placement and the potential risk of line infection and vessel damage.

Going Wireless

Vital signs monitoring systems available now or under development are making good use of wireless technology. Newer models are now wireless-capable, with the ability to transmit information from multiple monitors to a computer running an Ethernet local area network (LAN). This means that several of these monitors can be deployed quickly with a computer with wireless Ethernet, creating a central monitoring station where monitor alarms can be detected by care providers. Welch Allyn manufactures a field deployment kit that contains a laptop PC and multiple vitals monitoring stations in a rugged case for fast setup of emergency care environments in the field.

Such systems, which broadcast locally, can place the patient's vitals on a handheld personal digital assistant (PDA) carried by the TMP, allowing the provider to care for multiple patients and be aware of alarms without being at the patient's immediate bedside. Systems that are enabled on a wireless network may transmit vitals to a location far removed from the battlefield, allowing a medical provider (such as a physician) the ability to give real-time instructions via radio or other communication modality to the provider in the field.

What the Future Holds

The prototypical tactical wireless vitals monitoring system is LifeGuard, under development by NASA's Ames Astrobionics Team and Stanford University. The Crew Physiological Observation Device, or CPOD, is a battery-powered unit that utilizes Bluetooth technology to transmit ECG, pulse, respirations, and body position to a nearby computer. This computer can be linked remotely to a receiving station where data can be reviewed in real time by medical providers in virtually any location.

Units under development now include pills that patients can swallow, which provide real-time telemetry of pulse rate and oxygen content. Signals are read by a PDA device at the patient's side, which may then communicate with the TMP's computer station or PDA. While these have been tested in the laboratory, time will tell if they are reliable for field use in battlefield casualties.

None of the above devices are currently commercially available for tactical use, but they hold promise as future devices to enhance the TMP's ability to monitor patients, whether from 10 ft away or 10 miles up.

Smart Textiles

Of great interest to military commanders are clothing items with integrated vital signs monitoring. These devices (SmartShirts) have transducers woven into them for monitoring pulse and respiratory rate. An advantage of these systems is that they can be donned by tactical operators in preparation for a mission and commanders will therefore know exactly when an operator goes down and the operator's relative condition, to speed planning of evacuation. When the systems are operated remotely, commanders can use data from the sensors to steer a medic toward a wounded operator before the medic is even aware that an operator has gone down. In the acute-care environment, these shirts may free the patient from many of the wires required to monitor ECG, pulse, and respirations.

Pulse Oximetry

Pulse oximetry has been a staple of critical care for years, and has been used in prehospital care since the advent of portable battery-powered units. Pulse oximeters use a special light inside a probe that clips or tapes onto a finger, earlobe, nose, or toe to give real-time monitoring of pulse rate and oxygen saturation. The recent availability of a unit no more than an inch or two in any dimension makes this a viable option to be carried in the TMP's pack (13). There are also units available that combine pulse oximetry with end-tidal carbon dioxide ($EtCO_2$) detection (discussed on next page) or detection of carbon monoxide (CO).

End-Tidal Carbon Dioxide Monitoring

End-tidal capnography or capnometry is the measurement of carbon dioxide exhaled by a patient. It has been a standard of monitoring patient condition in the operating room since the late 1980s, and has recently spread to prehospital use as a means to confirm and monitor endotracheal tube placement. EtCO$_2$ monitoring has been found to have a significant impact on preventing misplaced endotracheal tubes in the prehospital setting (14–16). It may also be used during insertion of gastric tubes to detect inadvertent cannulation of the trachea (17).

End-tidal capnometry utilizes a clear plastic device that is placed between the endotracheal tube and the bag-valve-mask. A chemically treated paper membrane is displayed in the window of the device, which turns from purple to yellow in the presence of CO$_2$. When the endotracheal tube is properly placed in the trachea, this membrane will change color back and forth from purple to yellow with each ventilation.

Continuous EtCO$_2$ monitoring, or capnography, has become available with newer models of monitor/defibrillators as well as pulse oximeters. Unlike the chemical membrane CO$_2$ detectors, continuous monitors utilize an electronic sensor that is placed between the endotracheal tube and the bag-valve-mask. The patient may be continually monitored by means of a visual waveform on the screen that shows the level of CO$_2$ exhaled. The level is less important than the waveform, which should rise and fall with each ventilation.

Recently EtCO$_2$ has evolved as a means of rapid triage of disaster patients exposed to smoke or inhaled chemical agents such as cyanide. A device similar to a nasal oxygen cannula is now available to measure EtCO$_2$ in nonintubated patients. Within a few breaths, the capnometry waveform can give a reliable indicator of the patient's ventilatory status as well as the possibility of cellular poisoning by asphyxiants. EtCO$_2$ level has not been found to reliably correlate with arterial pCO$_2$ (18). It has been found to provide earlier warning to medical providers that a patient may be hypoventilating than pulse oximetry or respiratory rate (19,20).

Point-of-Care, or Bedside, Blood Testing

Bedside analysis, or point-of-care (POC) testing, utilizes portable electronic devices or chemical reagent strips for identification of enzymes, electrolytes, or substrates in blood or urine without the need to send the sample to a laboratory. Portable units now used at many hospitals have the ability to measure blood gasses, hematocrit, and electrolytes from one sample at the bedside within minutes. These rechargeable units are roughly the size of an eggplant and have the ability to print a small strip with lab results. To examine the utility of POC testing, it is important to know what tests are available and how they may fit into the scope of care of the TMP.

Glucose

Traditionally, blood glucose has been one of the most common field tests performed by this method. Electronic glucometers have become more accurate, faster, and easier to use than ever before, and their use is a skill mastered by the diabetic patient with little training. Chemical reagent strips are also available for use, and though less accurate, they give the provider a rough idea of the patient's blood glucose level. Hypoglycemia is a potentially serious and very treatable consequence of many diseases, from malnutrition to β-blocker overdose to sepsis.

Arterial Blood Gas

Arterial blood gas is sometimes used to guide care of patients with suspected respiratory distress or altered mental status. Measurements of pH, pO$_2$, pCO$_2$, a-A gradient, and base deficit are helpful for adjustment of ventilator parameters on ventilated patients. It is rarely, if ever, helpful in determining if a patient needs to be intubated or requires supplemental oxygen.

Hematocrit

The hematocrit is a measure of the percentage of blood that is comprised by red blood cells. In the absence of cyanide or CO poisoning, it gives a rough idea of the blood's oxygen-carrying capacity. After hemorrhage, fluid shifts into the vascular space from the tissue, diluting the remaining red blood cells and lowering the hematocrit. This value may guide the clinician in the decision to transfuse blood.

Electrolytes

Ions such as sodium, potassium, and chloride are tightly regulated in body systems, providing gradients that drive the machinery of many processes. Imbalances in these electrolytes, if severe, may be fatal. Dehydration may lead to derangement of sodium and chloride. Operators who rehydrate with plain water, without additional salt intake, may become hyponatremic, causing further symptoms and limiting operational effectiveness. Most worrisome among these electrolyte disturbances is hyperkalemia, which can rapidly be fatal without treatment. Burns and crush injury are potential causes of hyperkalemia that may be encountered in the tactical environment.

Cardiac Markers

Recent availability of POC testing of cardiac markers has opened wider debate about its utility in the field for triage of chest pain patients and for potential reduction of emergency department waiting times for patients who are undergoing a series of enzymes to rule out myocardial ischemia. For the typical civilian TMP, POC testing requires substantial cost, maintenance, and education, with little benefit. It is unlikely that blood test abnormalities will change care provided in the field or patient outcome. The possible exception to this is glucose testing, which can be effectively accomplished with chemical reagent strips or glucometers for very little cost, space, or weight.

Electrocardiogram

Portable ECG monitors that utilize a PDA as a platform for monitoring have recently become available for field use. These units have a small module that attaches to the PDA to interface with downloaded software. The ECG leads connect to this module for diagnosis and monitoring. Both 3-lead and 12-lead models are available for monitoring and diagnosis, respectively.

Infrascanner

An emerging technology uses an active infrared scanner for the detection of intracranial hemorrhage. Intracranial hemorrhage is a potentially devastating consequence of closed head injury, which, if untreated, may rapidly lead to death. Early detection may lead to earlier evacuation to a facility with neurosurgical expertise available. These units, currently under development, are portable and battery powered. The wireless probe for performance of the test interfaces with a PDA.

OPTICS FOR REMOTE ASSESSMENT

TMPs may be unable to directly access patients who may be injured or ill. Hostile fire or the potential aggravation of a hostage scenario may lead to increased numbers of patients and jeopardize a favorable outcome of the incident. The ability to assess patients before they can be treated may enable the provider to better anticipate resources required for treatment, extrication, or transport. Distance assessment may enable the provider to give appropriate medical advice to laypersons inside the barricade who may be able to access and treat the patient.

Distance assessment is limited, and a detailed survey of injuries and medical condition is not possible without components of tactile and auditory assessment. Some basic information, however, can expedite handling of patients once they can be accessed. There are several tools available to the TMP for distance assessment. These essentially boil down to optics of one sort or another. Though focused cardioid microphones are available for amplifying sounds from a specific area in the distance, virtually no useful information would be obtained.

Close Combat Optics

Though close combat optics have become standard issue to infantry in today's armed forces and many police tactical units, some are of no utility to the TMP for patient assessment, as they lack any magnification. Those that do have magnification may assist the TMP as a field expedient observation method.

Night Vision Equipment

The expense of night vision equipment, currently several thousand dollars per operator, makes this a technology limited to departments/units with large budgets. Night vision systems use cathode ray tubes to amplify ambient light to levels more easily detected by the human eye. These systems also expand the visual spectrum, making near-infrared light (which is normally invisible) part of the image seen by the viewer. The night vision user may use infrared illuminators, flashlight filters, and chemical light sticks to improve ambient illumination while remaining invisible to the enemy. These infrared markers can be worn by friendly personnel to reduce the possibility of friendly fire. Though the more modern units work very well in near-total darkness, all may benefit from an infrared illuminator for enhanced viewing.

Night vision devices generally come in three types: scopes, goggles, and cameras. Scopes can be handheld or mounted on a weapon. Goggles are usually helmet-mounted and may have a single or double objective lens. Cameras are connected to a screen for viewing, usually for monitoring or security purposes. Advances on the horizon in this field include "sensory fusion" scopes, which combine night vision with thermal infrared (discussed later), as well as panoramic night vision, which give a wider field of view than the 40 degrees common with current units.

Thermal Infrared Detection Systems

Infrared (IR) detection systems have enjoyed growing popularity among fire services and police services alike. Police departments often have IR detection systems mounted to helicopters for finding suspects over large areas. Fire departments have made use of the recent availability of handheld IR systems. These scopes, which typically consist of a "gun"-like detector and screen, have the ability to pick up radiant heat from live persons, hidden flame sources, and hot vehicle engines. They are not hampered by darkness, smoke, or fog, and do not require an illuminator. The technology is similar to that of night vision systems, but thermal imagers detect the shorter wavelengths of the IR spectrum. These wavelengths are emitted by objects due to atomic activity rather than reflected from outside sources. The more activity, the more IR that is emitted, and the brighter the image appears on the screen.

Fiber-optic Systems

Fiber-optic scopes are finding their way into more fields of use as technology improves. These systems use cables made of thin, flexible strands of glass or plastic to view objects from a perspective not normally attainable. Because of the properties of clear glass and plastic, light that meets the surface (interior or exterior) of the material will be reflected rather than passing through. In the fiber-optic cable, images that enter the strands at one end meet the long axis of the fiber at a tangent and will bounce off the inside of the glass fibers as it navigates down the cable around bends and turns. At the other end, where a viewing lens is fixed, the images meet the perpendicular ends of the strands and exit to be viewed through a lens. The objective end of the fiber-optic cable is affixed with a lens for viewing, depending on the purpose. Battery-powered units used for tactical observation will have a wide-angle objective lens to allow a wider field of view. Most of these units will have knobs that flex the tip of the fiber-optic cable in one direction or another, allowing the operator to look around. The use of fiber optics in tactical scenarios is well established. Tactical operators use fiber-optic scopes to peer through small cracks or holes in walls, floors, or ceilings to gather intelligence on room layouts, suspects, victims, weapons, and other useful information. They may be used to examine hiding places for evidence or hidden suspects without exposing the tactical team to hostile fire.

Fiber optics have been used in medicine for decades for pulmonary, surgical, urological, and gastrointestinal procedures. For the tactical medical operator, the use of fiber optics may soon move beyond remote patient assessment from behind a wall. Fiber-optic bronchoscopes are used by anesthesiologists, intensivists, ear, nose, and throat surgeons, and emergency physicians to examine the interior of the airway and facilitate difficult intubation. This could potentially lead to reliable, confirmed placement of endotracheal tubes with better confidence and, possibly, without the need for a laryngoscope.

Robots

With improved electronic viewing elements, video cameras are becoming smaller and less expensive to deploy in various applications. Video cameras mounted to explosive ordinance disposal (EOD) robots may provide the ability to look closely at patients from a distance. Models with sufficient power may be able to grasp and drag patients from the hot zone without endangering rescue personnel. These robots come at a price of several hundred thousand dollars and may be available through the EOD team or bomb squad. Refer to the manufacturer or training officer regarding the robot's capacity for dragging heavy objects, for example, bodies.

ADVANCES IN PATIENT TREATMENT

One-handed Tourniquets

Hemorrhage from an extremity is the most common preventable cause of death on the battlefield. Increased emphasis has been placed on training nonmedical operators in the application of a tourniquet to control bleeding. With recent wartime experience, several commercial tourniquets have become available that can be applied with one hand with little training (21). It has been recommended that all soldiers have a tourniquet on their person and readily available at all times for rapid use. Several studies have looked at the effectiveness of various tourniquet systems (22–25) (Table 35.2).

Intraosseous Access Devices

Intraosseous access has been a means of emergent infusion of medications and fluid in pediatrics for decades. Because of infants' soft bones, forceful insertion of a hollow metal needle can be accomplished with a lower probability of causing fracture. Recent availability of devices for intraosseous access in adults has garnered the interest of both the EMS and the special operations communities (29,30). Intraosseous devices can generally be placed within seconds, and their placement often requires less finesse than placement of a peripheral intravenous or central line. Some examples follow.

▶ **TABLE 35.2. Various Tourniquet Systems.**

Army One Handed Tourniquet (OHT; U.S. Army Medical Matériel Agency)
　The OHT consists of nylon webbing and D-rings; it creates tension when the provider pulls hard on one end of the webbing.

Combat Application Tourniquet (CAT; North American Rescue Products)
　The CAT consists of a nylon band with hook-and-loop closure and a plastic windlass and buckles.

Mechanical Advantage Tourniquet (MAT; Cybertech)
　The MAT consists of a padded band, a hook-and-loop closure, and a plastic rotating knob to increase tension.

Special Operations Forces Tactical Tourniquet (Tactical Medical Solutions) (25)
　This is similar in concept to the CAT, thought the windlass and buckles are metal instead of plastic.

Emergency and Military Tourniquet (EMT; Delfi Medical, Inc.) (26)
　The EMT consists of a wide band of material with an adjustable locking clamp. A bulb, similar to that found on a standard blood pressure cuff, is used to inflate the tourniquet once it is locked in place. The wider band and pneumatic inflator may cause less local tissue damage when applied and occlude arterial flow at low pressures (27,28).

FAST1

The FAST1 Intraosseous Infusion System (Pyng Medical Corp.) consists of a central needle for placement of an infusion catheter surrounded by several depth-finding needles to assist insertion into the sternum (31,32). The simple procedure consists of cleaning the site, placing a special adhesive dressing, inserting the catheter with the spring-loaded device, and placing a clear protective covering. The catheter is placed in the distal half of the sternum with one quick motion.

EZ-IO

The EZ-IO drill (Vidacare) is exactly what it sounds like: a drill that places a specially designed needle in the proximal medial tibia (33). The procedure is likewise simple, consisting of cleaning the insertion area, placing the catheter, and drilling the needle/catheter into the tibia or humerus. A depth gauge limits the insertion depth, reducing the chance of perforating both sides of the bone. The company also produces human-driven needles.

Bone Injection Gun

The Bone Injection Gun (BIG; WaisMed) (34) is a spring-loaded device that drives an intraosseous needle into the proximal tibia for infusion. This concept is similar to that of the FAST 1, which utilizes the sternum as an insertion point.

Hemostatic Dressings and Powders

Hemorrhage remains the leading preventable cause of death on the battlefield (35). Much media attention has been given to hemostatic powders (QuikClot, Trauma Dex, and Celox) and dressings (Hemcon) for battlefield use to enhance bleeding control in austere environments. Research on outcomes is ongoing and our clinical experience is growing, but these remain relatively new tools for the TMP. Each has its limitations, and use is still controversial among physicians who provide definitive care to battlefield casualties. Hemostatic agents are most effective at bleeding control when combined with standard wound management techniques such as direct pressure and application of tourniquets when appropriate.

QuikClot

This is a mineral powder that is applied to bleeding wounds that have failed bleeding control by other methods (36). The granules serve as a mineral "sieve," absorbing water to allow aggregation of blood cells (37). This product is issued as part of the individual first aid kit to U.S. Marine Corps units. QuikClot now comes in a vacuum-packed foil packet as well as a "sponge," which is a permeable sack containing the active powder to be applied to the wound. The sponge is applied to the wound as a whole rather than the contents being sprinkled into the wound like the powder. It is thought that QuikClot absorbs excess moisture at the wound site, enabling better aggregation of platelets and clotting factors and speeding clotting.

Chitosan Dressing

The chitosan dressing is a bandage made from shrimp shells that adheres to wounds in the presence of moisture and blood (38). The mechanisms for bleeding control are incompletely understood but include adhesion to tissues, attraction of circulating blood cells, and scavenging of nitric oxide with resultant vasospasm (39). The bandage can be removed by irrigation with saline or water when necessary. This bandage has become standard equipment in U.S. Army Ranger medic bags and vests.

Celox

Celox (chitosan powder) is another product recently tested for hemorrhage control. This is the effective ingredient of the chitosan dressing, but in powder form for application to deep wounds. The theoretical advantage of the powder is that it may be applied to deep wounds not readily accessible to a dressing and lacks the exothermic reaction that can be problematic with Quikclot administration.

Portable Ventilators

Invasive and noninvasive ventilation are staples of critical care in the emergency department and intensive care unit settings. Prolonged transport or care of patients who require definitive airway control with an endotracheal tube will require a dedicated provider to ventilate the patient by bag-valve-mask or a mechanical ventilator to take the provider's place. Ventilators in the hospital setting grow more sophisticated every year, smaller in size, with greater monitoring capabilities and the ability to modify more parameters in ventilation. Portable ventilators, though simpler in design, enable the provider to focus on other tasks while the patient is reliably ventilated (40).

One study found that oxygenation and ventilation of patients with head injury ventilated with a mechanical ventilator had suboptimal parameters when ventilated during prehospital EMS transport (42). Only 37% of patients in this study were "optimally" oxygenated and "adequately" ventilated, with unintentional hyperventilation being the most common derangement. The TMP, with limited capacity to perform arterial blood gases for adjustment of ventilator parameters, will have to pay close attention to the patient's condition and available monitors to stay ahead of potential consequences of improper ventilation.

Ventilators for use in the prehospital setting may be electrically powered, pneumatically powered, or both.

Pneumatically powered units have the advantage of not requiring charging or experiencing battery degradation. On the downside, unavailability of compressed oxygen or gas renders the unit useless. These units also consume gas for their own functioning, reducing the available oxygen supply. Electrically powered units have rechargeable or replaceable batteries to power controls and valves. The advantage of these units is more precise controls, a wider array of ventilator modes/functions, and generally more alarms to warn providers of potentially worrisome conditions. The following devices are of particular note:

Simplified Automated Ventilator (SAVE)

The SAVE is an extremely small (3.1 lbs) battery driven (5 hr run life) ventilator built for the tactical environment. The unit is self contained and utilizes a set volume (600 cc) and rate (10) with air pressure (38 cm H_2O) protection.

LSP Autovent 3000

The LSP Autovent 3000, a gas-powered unit, has only three dials, for control of respiratory rate, tidal volume, and pressure support. It lacks alarms or fine controls, but its simplicity makes it an attractive choice for tactical use for providers with limited ventilator experience.

Bird AVIAN

The Bird AVIAN ventilator is a system designed for critical care transport situations. It is a battery-powered unit with an electrically driven fan to maintain positive airway pressure. With several ventilator modes, warning indicators on a wide, bright backlit screen, and adjustable oxygen delivery, it offers great flexibility for patients during longer transports or prolonged ventilation in the field hospital environment. Its complexity and breadth of features are suited for providers very experienced in mechanical ventilation.

Bio-Med Devices CrossVent

Bio-Med Devices manufactures a ventilator that is more compact than many others. An oxygen-powered ventilator with few controls, it is a very basic model that may serve the most rudimentary function of automated ventilation. It lacks warning indicators for high pressure, and the ventilator modes are limited, but its portability and simplicity make it an attractive option for prehospital use.

Hartwell Medical Surevent

While there are many compact, lightweight ventilators available for prehospital use, there is one disposable model from Hartwell that deserves mention. The Surevent is a dis-posable ventilator unit for prehospital use. It is powered by a continuous oxygen source (regular O_2 tubing) and has controls for rate and peak inspiratory pressure only. The unit is decidedly low-tech; there are no alarms, no dynamic controls, and no adjustments made automatically by the unit. As such, the unit is less desirable than other units, particularly in environments where continuous observation of a patient is difficult. Close assessment and monitoring of patients is necessary to intervene in the case of pneumothorax, tube dislodgement, or acute decompensation. The unit's low cost and ease of use make it attractive as part of a disaster medical kit that may provide ventilation for multiple patients in a mass casualty situation.

ADVANCES IN PREVENTIVE CARE

Body Armor

With ever more stories in the media of body armor recalls, failed ballistic tests, and new armor materials certified and decertified by the National Institute of Justice (NIJ), and more choices on the market than ever before, the question of which body armor to choose for personal protection has become a daunting one. The military's decision to reimburse soldiers for the selection and purchase of their own body armor has opened up significant debates about quality control and how much oversight the sponsoring unit should have regarding the armor worn by its operators, a debate made more confusing by direct-to-consumer marketing by the armor companies.

Testing Body Armor

To understand body armor protection levels, it is important to know how the armor receives a protection rating. The standards of testing body armor have for years been set by the NIJ. The tests have historically consisted of test firing standardized loads of various calibers at test swatches of vest material, recording which penetrate the armor and which do not, and assigning a protection level in one of several categories. Certification levels of currently available armor are set as follows, in order of increasing protection.

It is important to know that the NIJ tests are essentially laboratory tests. It has been argued that these tests do not always realistically simulate real-world parameters of use. The NIJ uses a test distance of 16 ft, although 50% of U.S. law enforcement officers are shot within a distance of 0 to 5 ft (42), and 30% are contact shots where the muzzle of the weapon is held against the officer's body and fired.

New FBI Body Armor Testing Standard

The FBI has released its new testing system for ballistic armor which is a quantum leap ahead of previous testing standards. All armor tested must first meet NIJ standards for ballistic protection. Key points are the testing of multiple hits to a single panel, hits to the edges of the panel, the use of more lifelike ballistic gelatin to back the armor, and test shots fired against the armor when it is cold, hot, wet, or dry. It also includes contact shots fired against the vest. The data provided by these new tests will provide information on armor performance in conditions similar to expected use.

Soft Body Armor

These vests are made of woven or laminate materials sewn together in layers. These vests are lightweight, flexible, and often more comfortable than rigid or "plate" body armor. They offer protection from threat levels lower than plate armor does in return for increased mobility and less strain on the operator. Materials available in soft armor fall into two categories: woven and laminate.

Woven Material

Kevlar and Twaron are the chief woven materials used in soft armor. Strong and lightweight, Kevlar has been the material of choice for body armor since the 1980s. Its resistance to heat (it is also used in straps for firefighters' air packs) and moisture makes it a reliable choice for armor. With proper care, woven Kevlar vests provide excellent protection even beyond their expiration dates. Twaron is marketed as a more lightweight fiber than Kevlar.

Laminate Material

Instead of being woven, laminates have a ballistic fiber enclosed in a plastic covering with fiber strands oriented perpendicular to each other for strength. Fibers used in this type of laminate include Kevlar and Spectra, and they go under trade names like GoldFlex and Spectra Shield. Laminates offer more flexibility and a lighter weight for higher listed protection. One serious flaw in laminates, however, is that the fibers tend to migrate in areas where the armor is creased as it is worn. This results in reduced protection at these flex points. Laminates also have less heat resistance than woven materials. Contact shots are problematic for laminates, which melt from the heat of a contact shot, allow the fibers to migrate aside, and offer less protection from this threat. Peeling, delamination, separation, and creases are all problems with laminates that may leave the user unknowingly vulnerable to threats the armor is rated to stop.

Hard Body Armor

Also referred to as "plate" armor, hard body armor consists of a rigid plate in a carrier. These plates offer higher threat protection than many types of soft armor and offer unpar-

alleled protection from stab wounds. Hits sustained by this type of armor cause significantly less blunt force trauma to the wearer. "Stand-alone" plates do not need to be combined with soft body armor to meet their rated level of protection. Plates may be armor "inserts" that, when combined with soft armor (as in the military's BALCS-SPEAR), meet a rated threat. This protection comes at the cost of mobility, as the armor is quite heavy compared with soft armor. Plates may be made as inserts to be combined with soft armor, allowing the wearer flexibility in protection and mobility with a lighter-weight package. Three main materials are currently available for use.

Ceramic Plate: SAPI, eSAPI, and BALCS-SPEARS

This armor is a ceramic plate that offers up to level IV protection in a heavy rigid package. The advantage of this armor is its ballistic protection, which is greater than that of most other armor. Drawbacks include its weight and brittleness. Even routine use and handling may result in chips and cracks, and 10% to 15% of these armor plates are rendered unusable after a typical tour of duty on deployment. Cracks will typically form after two hits on this armor, necessitating replacement. Some plates may be backed by laminate material such as Spectra to further spread the force from a hit.

Compressed Laminates: Dyneema and Spectra

The problems that plague laminate materials in soft body armor are less prevalent in hard body armor. These plates are manufactured from compressed laminate materials such as Spectra Shield. Since the armor does not flex, it is not prone to fiber migration. The chief advantage of this armor is its reduced weight, which is roughly half that of its ceramic counterparts. It is also more durable under real-world use and will not chip, although the edges may fray. The ballistic protection offered by currently available plates is slightly less than that of the ceramics, being rated at or above level III but not quite at level IV.

Mars Steel

These plates are made of a molded 5-mm-thick steel plate. They offer advantages in that they are durable, do not crack, and come at a substantially reduced cost (~$200 a plate). These plates will not stop true armor piercing rounds or very hot rifle loads.

"Flexible" Hard Body Armor

One manufacturer, Pinnacle Armor, has developed a proprietary armor under the trade name Dragon Skin that is billed as the first flexible armor offering the kind of protection offered by plate armor. This armor, currently rated by the NIJ at level III, consists of rows of overlapping ballistic ceramic disks in a flexible carrier. The armor is heavy, 16 to 24 lb, depending on extra panels such as neck, shoulder, and groin protection, but offers some flexibility to conform to the user. The manufacturer claims that this armor's chief advantage is its ability to absorb multiple hits, in excess of 10 to 15 shots from an AK-47 rifle. Another potential attraction is the ability to have "gapless" protection from rifle fire in all areas that are covered by the vest. This protection comes at a price; the vests that provide gapless NIJ level IV rifle coverage weigh in at more than 40 pounds. There are some potential issues with penetration of oblique hits to the armor once it is heated (such as in the back of a Humvee in an operational area), which may allow the disks to shift more than normal. This could potentially lead to "gaps" in protection that the wearer is not aware of. In US Army tests, the Dragon Skin armor failed to meet expectations of protection from rated threats.

Hybrid: Steel + Laminate

One type of armor under development is comprised of a steel plate bonded to a laminate material like Dyneema. The plates are not substantially different in function than other solid armor plates currently available. This armor is still experimental but offers the theoretical advantage over other available armor plates of being able to sustain multiple hits.

Metal Matrix + Ceramic

The next generation of hard body armor may include a metal matrix composite in a ceramic plate to improve durability of the ceramic. This would help rectify the potential drawback of ceramic plates in their tendency to chip or crack under routine use.

Shear Thickening Fluid

A new concept in armor currently under development is the use of a liquid that is flexible under normal use, but becomes stiff when moved at high velocity by a projectile. Proposed applications include combining with traditional armor materials to supplement strength or stand-alone use. Although it is still in development, it has shown promise, particularly in protection from low velocity impacts from sharp objects, an area where traditional soft armor tends to be weaker.

Eye Protection

Substantial operational experience now exists to reinforce the importance of proper eye protection on the battlefield. A misplaced grain of sand can temporarily destroy an operator's depth perception, while a piece of shrapnel may end the operator's tactical operational career. While little has

changed in this field in years, it is important to know what features are available when selecting protective eyewear.

1. Single versus double lenses
2. Interchangeable lenses
3. Padded seats
4. Ultraviolet protection
5. Laser protection
6. Prescription inserts
7. Interface with night vision equipment

Hearing Protection

The noise of the battlefield, whether from gunfire, engines, helicopter operations, explosives, or distraction devices, poses a serious threat to the auditory health of the operator. Exposure to noise levels above 130 dB for as little as 2 minutes may cause permanent hearing damage. The report of a high-powered rifle may produce noises as loud as 150 to 175 dB, only a few of which may cause permanent hearing damage.

Hearing protection has moved beyond simple earplugs and earmuffs. Dynamic hearing protection includes devices that muffle loud noises but amplify quieter noises to enhance the wearer's ability to hear them. The resultant effect is that the operator can hear important noises on the field of operations yet be protected from loud incidental noises such as gunshots, explosions, and loud engines.

Dynamic hearing protection comes in several forms. The least expensive are noise-activated earplugs with non-electronic valves that close when exposed to louder noises. These plugs do not provide amplification of ambient noise but allow the wearer to hear almost normally in the absence of loud noise.

The type of dynamic hearing protection probably most familiar to avid shooters is the earmuff with noise enhancement technology. Simply, this consists of microphones affixed to the headset that amplify ambient noise inside the headset. This allows the wearer to hear ambient noise with normal or enhanced ability, yet enjoy protection from dangerous noise levels. For operators in environments that have even higher noise levels, the protection offered by these muffs can be increased by wearing earplugs underneath the muffs. With amplification, the wearer will hear ambient noise through the earplugs unimpeded. Models are available now that fit under helmets for tactical use.

A variation on the above is noise-enhanced earmuffs, which connect to communications systems such as radios or vehicle-mounted communications. These allow the wearer to communicate by way of a compatible two-way communication system. The most compact dynamic hearing protection systems are electronic systems that fit in or just behind the ear much like a hearing aid. These can provide ambient noise amplification yet still provide up to 29 dB of noise reduction. These devices range in price from $100 to nearly $1,000 for the highest-end systems. A very few will interface with two-way radios with standard minijack microphone connectors.

All operators and others who are likely to be exposed to the loud noises of the tactical environment should wear ear protection in training and in operations.

Fabrics for Heat Management

Wars in the Middle East have brought to the forefront of preventive medicine heat management to avoid casualties in hot environments. Fabrics that keep the wearer cool are of great importance to warriors who fight in warm environments with body armor and heavy loads. Polyester blends, available under brand names such as UnderArmour, Nike DriFit, and Invista CoolMax, offer instant moisture-wicking and rapid evaporation to speed cooling. Some concern has been raised about the flammability of such fabrics and their tendency to melt to the wearer under extremely high heat, and as a result they have been banned from issue to the U.S. Marine Corps. The U.S. Army bans the use of these synthetics for combat crew members of armor and similar transport units because of increased risk of flash fire in these vehicles. Body armor and external tactical uniforms may provide some protection from the dangers of flash fire to polyester base layers. Flashover fire has become an ever more present danger in urban and rural areas of the United States as clandestine drug labs increase in prevalence in all areas of the country. TMPs who have the option should evaluate the use of heat management fabrics by team members and make recommendations based on threats commonly faced by the team.

Fabrics to Prevent Heat Loss

Fabrics to preserve heat have become lighter, more comfortable, and more versatile than ever. Layers of polyester-blend technical fabric help conserve heat in cold environments while preserving mobility and wicking moisture from the wearer. Available in various weights and weaves, these fabrics range from a vanishingly thin base layer to thick fleeces that trap air next to the body, shutting in heat and shutting out wind. Many are waterproof and windproof, owing to outer shells or weaves to shed the elements while remaining breathable. An added advantage is that these fabrics tend to occupy minimal volumes when vacuum packed, enabling operators to carry extra in the eventuality that they find the weather colder than anticipated.

ADVANCES IN WARRIOR KNOWLEDGE

Personal Digital Assistant-based Learning

With the ever-expanding number of PDAs available, software becomes increasingly available to fit roles in medical care. These devices are compact and lightweight, though ones that are truly durable enough for field environments are few and far between. Still, with proper packing and care, a PDA may serve the TMP both on and off the field of care. Rugged versions from manufacturers such as Itronix, Rugged Notebooks, and Micronics have added brawn and durability compared to conventional models. Commercially available rugged cases may add additional protection against shock, impact, and water.

Field References

Some of the first software programs available for the PDA were medical titles for quick reference by medical providers of all levels. Some available titles that may be of interest are the *U.S. Army Special Operations Forces Medical Handbook* and clinical references such as Skyscape's *The 5-Minute Clinical Consult*.

Language References

While the list of available titles continues to grow, the TMP should browse available titles (many available from Palm.com). PDAs used in the field environment should be protected as much as possible from impact and water. Several hard cases are available in plastic orand metal to provide protection from direct impact and shock. For water protection, the TMP should consider placing the PDA inside a plastic bag for use.

Learning

During downtimes, the PDA is handy as a tool for improving one's knowledge base through a variety of programs. Palm-based testing and subject review may be accomplished through available question banks or questions assembled by instructors that may be downloaded to the PDA and answered at leisure. Some studies have shown good results with teaching procedures utilizing the PDA format. TMPs as well as instructors should consider the PDA as a means to improve knowledge during times or in places where carrying a textbook would be burdensome or impractical.

PDA-based references and teaching aids are expanding in availability and utility. While the references themselves may not be anything new or unavailable in other formats, the portability and convenience offered by the PDA make reference and learning by this method more conducive to those with limited spare time or who find their spare time in unusual places. The TMP may find that these resources enable continuous improvement of core knowledge and skills in preparation for or during field use.

Telemedicine

The concept of real-time consultation of expert medical authority is nothing new. Early versions of cardiac monitors included the capability to transmit ECG strips to a physician at a waiting hospital. With the emergence of 12-lead ECG as a viable prehospital technology, substantial time has been gained in the invasive treatment of acute myocardial infarction after transmission to a base hospital. Current examples include remote consultation of specialists from tertiary centers when patients cannot be evacuated immediately to higher levels of care. Medicine aboard the International Space Station is done with substantial real-time guidance through video and audio feedback from physicians on the ground. Commercial airlines, sensing a possible benefit to passengers out of reach of medical care, have contracted with services on the ground providing physicians who may give medical direction via radio to providers in the air, and some have installed portable telemedicine terminals that can transmit vital signs and audio feedback to these physicians (43).

Few advances have made telemedicine more practical to the TMP. Field providers who initiate care at the site of injury are not likely to benefit from telemedicine. Providers in environments where definitive care is not accessible or transfer of the patient is impractical may find consultation with physicians or specialists at other stations helpful. Video communication may allow physicians or specialists to demonstrate a procedure to field providers in remote locations. This is the one advantage of this technology over audio communication. It is doubtful that video input from the field will be of great use to the physician, as visual diagnosis of conditions, even in hospitals, is rare. For providers who work in field environments with limited lab capabilities, the ability to transmit a photomicrograph of a microscope slide may be considered.

Despite advances in ease of use and price of video conferencing, for the near-future most telemedicine will take place by phone, radio, or computer chat or e-mail. The latter should not be discounted; the ability to seek consultation from online references is widely used, even at urban hospitals.

ADVANCES ON THE HORIZON

Future advances in technology will bring better medicine through the hands of the providers who know how to use them.

Implantable Medical Chips

Controversial as it may be, a chip implanted into a patient that contains his or her medical information may provide lifesaving cues to medical providers about the patient's medical history, as well as appropriate identification and contact information. Privacy concerns cast a shadow over this particular technology; otherwise would-be adapters are hesitant to make this information accessible to anyone by a quick scan, without the patient's knowledge.

Ongoing Monitoring

Real-time telemetry of vital signs and other information, through the use of SmartShirts or similar technology, may assist the TMP in the future by reducing the time to recognition of illness or injury. Potentially TMPs may be aware of worrisome changes in patients before they can cry out for help or even before the illness reaches a critical point. The SmartShirts discussed above have been postulated as one means of seamless monitoring of battlefield personnel.

Blood Clotting Technology

An "ultrasound tourniquet," which potentially has the ability to augment clotting of deep tissue structures utilizing ultrasounds, is currently being developed by the Defense Advanced Research Projects Agency (DARPA) for field use. In theory, the ultrasound waves, many times more than used for diagnostic ultrasound, will lead to clotting of bleeding vessels below the surface of an extremity while not promoting clotting in intact vessels.

SUMMARY

Technology has a role in the hands of the properly trained TMP, though which technologies apply are specific to the provider and the operating environment. Ultimately these technologies, if not to treat or protect the patient, serve to augment the TMP's decision-making capacity. To avoid the "geek factor" and the resultant waste of money on devices of little practical value, TMPs must realistically appraise the environment in which they will be working and select technologies that provide the greatest benefit. Judicious selection of equipment will yield the greatest use while limiting excess combat load.

ACKNOWLEDGEMENT

The authors would like to thank Dr. Brock Blankenship, Dr. John Wightman, Karl Masters, Dr. Gary Roberts, and Joyce Grube for their assistance and insight for this chapter.

REFERENCES

1. Brooks AJ, Price V, Simms M. FAST on operational military deployment. *Emerg Med J.* 2005;22(4):263–265.
2. Sargsyan AE, Hamilton DR, Jones JA, et al. FAST at MACH 20: clinical ultrasound aboard the International Space Station. *J Trauma.* 2005;58(1):35–39.
3. Kirkpatrick AW, Sirois M, Laupland KB, et al. Prospective evaluation of hand-held focused abdominal sonography for trauma (FAST) in blunt abdominal trauma. *Can J Surg.* 2005;48(6):453–460.
4. Soundappan SV, Holland AJ, Cass DT, et al. Diagnostic accuracy of surgeon-performed focused abdominal sonography (FAST) in blunt paediatric trauma. *Injury.* 2005;36(8):970–975.

5. Chun R, Kirkpatrick AW, Sirois M, et al. Where's the tube? Evaluation of hand-held ultrasound in confirming endotracheal tube placement. *Prehosp Dis Med.* 2004;19(4):366–369.
6. Hind D, Calvert N, McWilliams R, et al. Ultrasonic locating devices for central venous cannulation: meta-analysis. *BMJ.* 2003;327(7411):361.
7. Hatfield A, Bodenham A. Portable ultrasound for difficult central venous access. *Br J Anaesth.* 1999;82(6):822–826.
8. Yanagawa Y, Nishi K, Sakamoto T, et al. Early diagnosis of hypovolemic shock by sonographic measurement of inferior vena cava in trauma patients. *J Trauma.* 2005;58(4):825–829.
9. Blaivas M, Lyon M, Duggal S. A prospective comparison of supine chest radiography and bedside ultrasound for the diagnosis of traumatic pneumothorax. *Acad Emerg Med.* 2005;12(9):844–849.
10. Rowan KR, Kirkpatrick AW, Liu D, et al. Traumatic pneumothorax detection with thoracic US: correlation with chest radiography and CT—initial experience. *Radiology.* 2002;225(1):210–214.
11. Wong DT, Giavedoni L. Foreign body, intraocular. eMedicine.com.
12. Welch Allyn. Manufacturer's database.
13. Nonin Corp. Manufacturer's database.
14. Davis DP, Fisher R, Buono C, et al. Predictors of intubation success and therapeutic value of paramedic airway management in a large, urban EMS system. *Prehosp Emerg Care.* 2006;10(3):356-362.
15. Singh S, Allen WD Jr, Venkataraman ST, et al. Utility of a novel quantitative handheld microstream capnometer during transport of critically ill children. *Am J Emerg Med.* 2006;24(3):302–307.
16. Silvestri S, Ralls GA, Krauss B, et al. The effectiveness of out-of-hospital use of continuous end-tidal carbon dioxide monitoring on the rate of unrecognized misplaced intubation within a regional emergency medical services system. *Ann Emerg Med.* 2005;45(5):497–503.
17. Burns SM, Carpenter R, Blevins C, et al. Detection of inadvertent airway intubation during gastric tube insertion: capnography versus a colorimetric carbon dioxide detector. *Am J Crit Care.* 2006;15(2):188–195.
18. Belpomme V, Ricard-Hibon A, Devoir C, et al. Correlation of arterial PCO_2 and $PETCO_2$ in prehospital controlled ventilation. *Am J Emerg Med.* 2005;23(7):852–859.
19. Miner JR, Heegaard W, Plummer D. End-tidal carbon dioxide monitoring during procedural sedation. *Acad Emerg Med.* 2002;9(4):275–280.
20. Kober A, Schubert B, Bertalanffy P, et al. Capnography in non-tracheally intubated emergency patients as an additional tool in pulse oximetry for prehospital monitoring of respiration. *Anesth Analg.* 2004;98(1):206–210.
21. Lakstein D, Blumenfeld A, Sokolov T, et al. Tourniquets for hemorrhage control on the battlefield: a 4-year accumulated experience. *J Trauma.* 2003;54 (Suppl 5):S221–S225.
22. Walters TJ, Wenke JC, Kauvar DS, et al. Effectiveness of self-applied tourniquets in human volunteers. *Prehosp Emerg Care.* 2005;9(4):416–422.
23. Calkins D, Snow C, Costello M, et al. Evaluation of possible battlefield tourniquet systems for the far-forward setting. *Milit Med.* 2000;165(5):379–384.
24. Wenke JC, Walters TJ, Greydanus DJ, et al. Physiological evaluation of the U.S. Army one-handed tourniquet. *Milit Med.* 2005;170(9):776–781.
25. Tactical Medical Solutions, LLC. Manufacturer's database.
26. Delfi Medical. Manufacturer's database.
27. Graham B, Breault MJ, McEwen JA, et al. Occlusion of arterial flow in the extremities at subsystolic pressures through the use of wide tourniquet cuffs. *Clin Orthop Relat Res.* 1993;(286):257–261.
28. Crenshaw AG, Hargens AR, Gershuni DH, et al. Wide tourniquet cuffs more effective at lower inflation pressures. *Acta Orthop Scand.* 1988;59(4):447–451.
29. Waisman M, Waisman D. Bone marrow infusion in adults. *J Trauma.* 1997;42(2):288–293.
30. Calkins MD, Fitzgerald G, Bentley TB, et al. Intraosseous infusion devices: a comparison for potential use in special operations. *J Trauma.* 2000;48(6):1068–1074.
31. Pyng Medical. Manufacturer's database.
32. Macnab A, Christenson J, Findlay J, et al. A new system for sternal intraosseous infusion in adults. *Prehosp Emerg Care.* 2000;4(2):173–177.
33. Vidacare Corp. Manufacturer's database.
34. WaisMed Corp. Manufacturer's database.
35. Committee on Fluid Resuscitation for Combat Casualties. *Fluid resuscitation: state of the science for treating combat casualties and civilian injuries.* Report of the Institute of Medicine. Washington, DC: National Academy Press; 1999:1–7.
36. Z-Medica. Manufacturer's database.
37. Alam HB, Uy GB, Miller U, et al. Comparative analysis of hemostatic agents in a swine model of lethal groin injury. *J Trauma.* 2003;54:1077–1082.
38. Hemorrhage Control Technologies. Manufacturer's database.
39. Alam HB, Burris D, DaCorta JA. Hemorrhage control on the battlefield: role of new hemostatic agents. *Milit Med.* 2005;170(1):63.
40. Rola P. Air transport and ventilators: a review. Special Projects, McGill University. Available at: http://sprojects.mmi.mcgill.ca/heart/pages/man000104r1.html.
41. Helm M, Hauke J, Lampl L. A prospective study of the quality of prehospital emergency ventilation in patients with severe head injury. *Br J Anaesth.* 2002;88(3):345–349.
42. Federal Bureau of Investigation. Uniform Crime Reporting Authority. *Law Enforcement Officers Killed and Assaulted in the Line of Duty.* Washington, DC: FBI; 2003.
43. Remote Diagnostics Technologies, Ltd. Press release.

Testifying in a Legal Proceeding

Jerry R. DeMaio

OBJECTIVES

After reading this section, the reader will be able to:

1. Know the situations in which a tactical emergency medical provider may be required to give testimony in a legal setting
2. Understand the most important items and procedures to remember when preparing to testify
3. Understand the basic principles of what to do and not to do when testifying in a legal proceeding

As a medical professional involved in tactical operations, there is a strong chance that you will be called on to provide testimony in a legal setting. For instance, if you are providing support to a law enforcement team on a raid or an arrest, you might be asked to testify about the medical condition or injuries sustained by the suspect, victims, or officers—this may be true whether you treat the individuals on the scene or at an emergency department. If an operation involves the transfer of a detainee or prisoner, you might be called on to testify about the subject's treatment or medical condition while in custody, or about the subject's health or treatment during the transfer, especially if the subject claims that he or she was mistreated. There is also a chance that you may be asked to testify in a nonmedical capacity about what you saw, heard, or experienced during an operation or during your response to a scene. In any of these situations, knowing what to look for and how to prepare for your testimony will make you a more confident and effective witness.

This chapter outlines some of the basics of providing testimony in a legal setting. The chapter is intended not to make you an expert on the legal rules of procedure or evidence, but to give you the basic principles to help you learn what to look for on the scene, how to work with the lawyer to prepare for your testimony, and what to expect when you are on the stand, with the ultimate goal that you will be an effective witness in any legal proceeding in which you are called to testify. This chapter will not prepare you for every possible situation. Each case will involve different issues, every lawyer you work with will have unique idiosyncrasies, and every court will have slightly different procedures, so you will have to work out the details with

the lawyer in each case. The concepts in this chapter, however, should be generally applicable. Testifying in court is a challenging experience for anyone, but with proper preparation, it does not have to be a painful one.

This chapter is written as if you will be a witness for the government in a criminal case, but be aware that that is not the only situation where you may be called to testify, even if the situation was one where you were directly working for or supporting a law enforcement agency. Depending on the circumstances, you might be called as a witness by the defendant in a criminal case or in a civil case. Remember that, despite the differences in the type of case, the same basic principles will apply to your role as a witness.

TESTIFYING IN COURT: AN OVERVIEW

If you are providing medical support to a police or other law enforcement agency, it is likely that, if you are called to testify, it will be in some portion of a criminal case, although it is possible that your testimony may be needed for other types of cases. Although the basics of testifying are generally the same regardless of the type of case, it is helpful to know a little about each type. In a criminal proceeding, as you are probably aware, the government brings charges against a defendant, whom the government has reason to believe has violated a criminal law. Most criminal cases are brought in a state court, but some criminal cases, including many fraud cases, weapons cases, drug cases, and national security cases, may be brought in U.S. federal court. The procedures in the two types of courts will vary slightly, but the basic structure of the case should the same.

A civil case involves one party suing another party for some sort of relief, often monetary damages; the U.S. or a state government may be a party. One example of a civil case where you may be called to testify is a lawsuit where a suspect is suing an agency for a violation of his or her civil rights, such as mistreatment during arrest or detention. You may also be involved in a special kind of civil proceeding known as a habeas corpus proceeding, in which a defendant in custody, usually criminal, challenges the government's constitutional basis for detention.

A third type of proceeding you may be involved in is an administrative proceeding, run by an administrative agency rather than a judicial court. A common example is an immigration case, where the government might be attempting to remove or deport someone from the country. Many aspects of these proceedings look like a criminal case, but they do not involve a violation of the criminal law and will not result in jail or prison time for the defendant.

Stages of the Proceeding

Unlike what happens on television, cases do not resolve themselves in 60 minutes. Depending on its seriousness and complexity, a criminal case may take weeks, months, or even years to resolve. In most cases, however, the basic stages are predictable. Several of these stages might require your testimony, and it is helpful to be familiar with them and their relationship to the case as a whole, because as the purposes of the hearings change, the scope and content of your testimony will often change as well. Knowing the basic procedural structure will also help you communicate with the lawyers and understand where your testimony will fit into the overall case.

Pretrial

A criminal case normally starts with an arrest, culminates in a trial, and, if the defendant is convicted, ends with sentencing (sentencing may also be followed by an appeal, but this chapter does not deal with appeals, as you will rarely, if ever be called to testify during the appellate process). However, to reach those milestones, many things must happen in between. After a defendant is arrested and detained, a series of hearings will take place quickly, normally within the first few days after the arrest. Defendants will normally have an "initial appearance" or "arraignment" where they are informed of the charges against them and appointed a lawyer if they do not have one and cannot afford one. There may also be a "probable cause hearing" or "preliminary hearing" to determine if there is sufficient evidence to proceed to trial. Additionally, a "detention hearing" may be held to determine what restrictions the defendant will

be under while waiting for trial. In a detention hearing the judge will weigh factors such as whether the defendant is dangerous to the community and if there is a risk that the defendant will not show up for court if released, to determine whether the defendant will be in jail, will be on some sort of electronic monitoring, or must post bail (or none of these) before trial. Depending on the court, some or all of these events may be part of the same hearing. These initial hearings usually involve very few, if any, witnesses. Often a single police officer or agent will testify, but depending on the court and the judge, other testimony, including medical testimony, may be required.

In addition to the initial hearings, the court will often hold a series of other hearings prior to trial to resolve issues that must be decided before the trial can begin. Some of these hearings may be referred to as "evidentiary hearings," "suppression hearings," or simply "pretrial hearings." Many pretrial hearings involve procedural issues that will only involve each side's lawyers, but for some hearings, the court may require testimony from witnesses. If you give testimony at such a hearing, it will normally be heard by a judge, not a jury. The issues at pretrial hearings where your testimony may be required will often include whether a certain piece of evidence will be admissible at trial or whether the prosecution has violated the constitution or any laws that would prevent them from continuing the case. Be aware that if you testify at a pretrial hearing, you may need to testify again at trial.

Trial

The trial is the portion of the case with which you are probably most familiar. At a criminal trial, evidence is presented by the government in an attempt to prove that the defendant committed the crimes with which he or she is charged. The defendant may present evidence to attempt to counter or discredit the government's theory of the case or may present evidence justifying the commitment of the crime (such as a "self-defense" argument). The defendant is not obliged to present evidence at all, and may choose not to, relying only on argument to poke holes in the government's theory of the case. The evidence at trial may be heard either by a judge or by a jury, who will then decide if the defendant is guilty of the charged crimes. If you are called to testify, it is very likely that it will be during the trial phase of the case.

Sentencing/Disposition

The final phase that you should be aware of is the sentencing or disposition of the case. In a criminal case, the sentencing hearing will take place sometime after a defendant has been found by either a jury or a judge to be guilty of a crime. Normally, the judge will assess factors such as the nature of the crime, the defendant's role in the crime, the defendant's criminal history, and other factors to determine an appropriate sentence. Again, depending on the court and the nature of the crime, your testimony may be required. If the crime is one where the jurisdiction authorizes the death penalty, the sentencing phase may look very similar to the trial, be tried in front of a jury, and require testimony.

Your Role

In any stage of the case, you may be called on to testify in one of several roles. In the medical field, you are probably most familiar with the use of a physician or other medical professional as an expert witness. This is a witness who normally does not have firsthand knowledge of the events of the case but, because of special knowledge, training, or education, is allowed to give an opinion about some issue to help educate the judge and jury. If you participate in a tactical operation as a medical professional, and you are asked to testify, there is a strong chance that you will be asked to give your professional medical opinion about something that happened. If that is the case, you must be prepared not only to give your opinion, but to be able to explain the basis of that opinion, including what facts you used and the analytical method by which you reached your conclusion.

Depending on the circumstances of the case and your role in it, you may also be called on to testify as a "fact witness," or as some combination of a fact witness and an expert witness. A fact witness is someone who has personal knowledge of a relevant fact in the case, such as an eyewitness to a crime, or a coconspirator testifying against a former colleague. If you have taken part in a prisoner transfer, for instance, you might have observed the prisoner's actions or heard comments he or she made outside of your medical evaluation or treatment. If what you saw or heard is relevant to the case, you might be asked to testify as a fact witness about it in addition to your medical testimony.

Whatever your role in testifying, it is important to remember where you fit into the overall picture. It is easy to want to try to win the case for "your side." It is also easy to plan on sitting back and only answering the questions you are asked. Ideally, your role falls between these two—the case is not yours to win or lose, but you are not merely a passive player. Your goal should be to give complete and truthful testimony, and honest opinions, with regard to your portion of the case, regardless of which side calls you. As a fact witness, you will be providing an important piece of the puzzle of what happened. As an expert witness, you will be imparting your specialized knowledge to the judge and jury so that they can make a fully informed decision. In either case, your complete and honest testimony will be essential to the proper functioning of the justice system.

PREPARING FOR TESTIMONY AT THE SCENE

When you know that you will be providing support to a tactical situation, it is never too early to start thinking about having to testify. The most important things to remember at this point are observing as much as you can and documenting extensively and thoroughly. Some things to remember are as follows.

- *Observe the scene*. Make a mental picture of the scene. Learn the layout of the building, vehicle, or area well enough that you could draw a map or picture again if you were asked to. If you have the opportunity to review a map or diagram of the area, do so. Do your best to remember where people were and what they were doing.
- *Listen*. One of the most important parts of observation entails listening, particularly to conversations or spontaneous outbursts. If the situation is appropriate, pay attention to what the suspects are saying. If you take a medical history or conduct a physical examination of anyone involved, make written notes of both medical and nonmedical statements made. If you write down something that is a direct quote, put the statement in quotation marks in your report.
- *Think of events through both a medical and a nonmedical filter*. Given your medical training, this will not always be easy, but remember that you might be called as a fact witness as well as an expert witness. Statements made during a physical examination of a subject that are irrelevant to the medical diagnosis or treatment may be relevant to other issues in the case.
- *Document, document, document*. Good documentation is absolutely essential to providing good testimony. Although at the scene you think you are not going to forget what happened, the chances are that in the time between the event and your testimony, you will forget parts of it. Good, thorough documentation will help you refresh your memory when you are testifying or preparing to testify, and will bolster your credibility if the testimony of what you remember is consistent with the notes you took at the scene. With regard to medical issues, document everything: both what you see and what you don't. Draw diagrams when appropriate—note, particularly, any injuries, marks, or scars. Do not try to make judgments about leaving what is unimportant, since you do not know what may be important later at a legal proceeding.
- *Look at your documentation with a critical eye*. Remember that whatever you document will be analyzed in court later. The old saw holds true: If you didn't document it, you didn't do it. And on the stand, if you try to claim that you did something or saw something that is not documented, you will be held to account for why it is not. Opposing counsel will portray any mistakes

or omissions as carelessness that should be imparted to your entire testimony. Any inconsistencies between your documentation and your testimony will be exploited. It is, therefore, crucial that you document accurately and thoroughly.

GETTING READY TO TESTIFY

If it becomes clear that you will be asked to be a witness, you will enter what is sometimes called the "witness preparation" phase. This is the most important phase of giving testimony, because it will take the raw material of what happened at the scene and will develop it into a form that can be presented effectively in a legal proceeding. This phase is *not* about "shaping" your testimony to fit a certain theory of the case. Rather, during this phase you should be working with the prosecutor to review what happened at the scene as you best remember it, discussing the strengths and weakness of your testimony, exploring the medical basis for any opinions, and becoming comfortable with getting on the stand to testify.

Working with lawyers is always challenging—they speak a different language and often approach problems differently than most people are accustomed to. Your inclination may be to defer to the lawyer when it comes to testifying, but you must remember that the preparation process is a two-way street. Although the prosecutor needs to prepare you for taking the stand, you must also prepare the prosecutor for your testimony. Lawyers are not medical professionals and, in fact, may know very little about medicine, so you have an obligation to help educate them about your own expertise, the relevant common medical practices in your field, and your professional opinion as it relates to the case. This includes educating the prosecutor about both the strengths and the weaknesses of your opinion and your potential testimony. With patience and cooperation, both you and the attorney will be better prepared when you take the stand.

Preparing for Direct Examination

When you take the stand to testify, the first part of your testimony will be "direct examination." In this phase, you will tell the story of what happened in response to open-ended questions from the prosecutor. As with all testimony, you will be under oath, and you will be expected to tell the truth. Here are some tips on preparing for your direct testimony:

■ When meeting with the prosecutor, *determine the essential points that you must communicate to the jury or the court*. To do this, there must be a meeting of the minds between you and the prosecutor: you know what happened at the scene, what your medical examination un-

covered, and what your medical opinions are, whereas the prosecutor knows what elements need to be proven in the case. To determine the key points of testimony, you must discover where these two bodies of knowledge overlap and where they are at odds. Determining the essential points of your testimony will help you keep your testimony focused on those issues relevant to the case, and will help you recognize opportunities to make those points on both direct and cross-examination.

■ *Be familiar with each side's theory of the case.* This goes hand-in-hand with determining your essential points. If, for instance, a defendant is claiming that he was beaten into giving a confession, you can make sure to communicate to the court what findings you made that were consistent or inconsistent with the defendant's claims as opposed to spending time on medical findings or opinions that do not relate to what either side is trying to prove.

■ *Become familiar with the questions that the prosecutor will ask.* Likewise, the prosecutor should become familiar with the answers you are going to give. This does not mean memorizing every question and answer, but nothing that happens on direct examination should come as a surprise to either you or the prosecutor.

■ If your testimony is going to be technical, *discuss with the prosecutor methods of defining medical and technical terms so the judge and jurors can understand.* Remember that the judge and jury will probably not have much medical background. You must figure out a way to illustrate or simplify any particularly difficult or complex medical concepts so the judge or the average juror can understand them and how they affect the case. Recognize that this may include procedures and terminology that are completely obvious or basic to you, as a medical professional.

■ *Review all documents that you are going to use during your testimony or that you expect might be used at the proceeding.* Make sure you are familiar with the content of any document or exhibit that you are going to be using or that you will be asked to identify. Occasionally the prosecutor will want you to identify or authenticate a document that will go into evidence. In such a case, the prosecutor will probably expect you to answer a series of foundational questions—prerequisite facts that need to be attested to before the document can be admitted by the court into evidence. Review these questions with the prosecutor.

Preparing for Cross-examination

Cross-examination is the defense attorney's opportunity to ask you questions, and is probably the most difficult part of giving testimony. Because hearings and trials in the United States are adversarial, the defendant's lawyer is allowed to attempt to discredit any witness put on by the government.

This normally means asking leading questions—usually yes-or-no questions—to get the witness to admit facts that are detrimental to the other side.

It is highly unlikely that your testimony will be without flaws or weaknesses. The best approach to weaknesses in your testimony is to confront the issues, to admit the differences, to provide reasons for the differences to the extent that you can, and not to get defensive. Often, the prosecutor can "soften the blow" by asking you about flaws in your testimony on direct examination—this will give you a chance to explain the deficiency in a less confrontational setting, rather than letting the defense attorney bring it up first. Having the prosecutor address a weakness decreases the "shock" value to the judge and jury and makes it clear that the prosecutor is not trying to hide something.

When preparing for cross-examination, review the following areas that may be open to attack by the opposing attorney. In each of these areas, devote some time to thinking about how you will respond when these questions are asked, and discuss these issues with the prosecutor. Note that what follows is not an exhaustive list, but it does contain some of the areas most often used to discredit a witness on cross-examination. You may want to ask the prosecutor to practice a "mock cross" with questions that can be expected from the opposing attorney.

1. *Expect your background and experience to be challenged.* This has the potential to be one of the most uncomfortable areas on cross-examination. Remember the following points.
   a. Expect that the defense attorney will know everything about your training, background, and experience relevant to the subject of your testimony, and has searched for your name and background on the Internet. If you are testifying as an expert witness, you will most likely have to provide a curriculum vitae (CV) to the prosecutor, who will be required to give a copy to the defense attorney. Anything in your background that might reflect negatively on your testimony should be made known to the prosecutor during preparation.
   b. If you are in a profession that is licensed, assume that the defense attorney has reviewed the status of your license and any disciplinary action that may have been taken against you.
   c. Be prepared to answer any questions that might suggest you are biased toward a certain outcome in the case—for example, this might include your past or present employment (Are you working for the government or under a government contract?) or activity in political or advocacy organizations, particularly if those organizations have taken positions that are relevant to the outcome in the case.
   d. Assume that the defense attorney will be familiar with any past testimony you have given. This in-

cludes the types of cases in which you have testified, how often you have testified for the government or defense, how many times you have made a certain diagnosis, and any specific testimony you have given. Make sure the prosecutor is aware of every past instance where you have given testimony in a legal proceeding.

2. *Expect the facts and assumptions underlying your opinion to be challenged.* This is an area that is ripe for attack during cross-examination. Some things to keep in mind during preparation are as follows:
   a. Attacks on the facts may start with attacks on your own perception: How was the weather that day? Was there smoke or haze around? Did you have a mask on that limited your vision? Were there loud noises in the background that might have prevented you from hearing the conversation?
   b. Think of any facts about the situation or patient that you do not know but that could have been helpful in reaching a conclusion—you may be asked about them. Similarly, think about important facts that, given your contact with the patient in question, you never could have known. What questions did you forget to ask the patient? What questions did the patient refuse to answer? Was the patient unconscious or in a state where he or she could not answer?
   c. Did you misread or misinterpret any data? Additionally are your recollection and the data from the event accurate in the first place? Here is one area where making detailed, accurate documentation at the scene, including diagrams if necessary, will help stem a line of questioning.

3. *Expect any medical or scientific theory or technique you apply to be challenged, as well as how you applied that theory or technique to reach your conclusion.* The extent to which this area gets attacked will usually depend on how well established the theory or technique is. To be prepared for these lines of questioning:
   a. For whatever the situation was, be prepared to explain what the standard practice is, and in what situations you would deviate from this practice. Expect any deviation from the standard practice to be questioned.
   b. Know the limitations of any theory or technique you use, both in general and in the specific case.
   c. Be familiar with the leading treatises and articles on the theory or technique, as well as any texts or articles that are critical of the technique. Often in cross-examination, you will be confronted with passages from textbooks or articles that recommend a course of action different from the one you used: be prepared to address those.

4. *Expect to be asked about your preparation.* On cross-examination, you invariably will be asked, "Isn't it true that you met with the prosecutor before this case? And

isn't it true that she went over the questions she was going to ask you?" The cross-examiner will attempt to suggest that you rehearsed your testimony with the prosecutor beforehand, or that the prosecutor told you what to say. The simplest and most direct response to this is that the testimony you are giving is the truth as you know it.

Resolve Any Logistical Issues

Finally, do not forget to make sure the logistical aspects of your testimony are taken care of:.

- Provide the prosecutor with an updated copy of your CV.
- Provide the prosecutor with copies of any notes or reports that you prepared in relation to the case.
- Resolve any issues regarding exhibits, including any exhibits that you are expected to prepare or bring to the trial.
- Work with the prosecutor to prepare any visual aids, such as large displays that are easier for the jury to see or computer presentations. If you are going to use any visual aids during trial, coordinate their use with the prosecutor beforehand.
- Coordinate your schedule of appearance, including travel and lodging arrangements.
- Finally, if possible, visit the courtroom where the hearing or trial will take place. The prosecutor, an employee of the prosecutor's office, or an employee of the court should be able to coordinate a time to allow you to see the courtroom and explain how it will be set up on the day of your testimony. This will be very helpful to get an idea of how the hearing will work without the stress of having everyone there.

Preparation is vital to developing a case and will be critical to having a good experience on the witness stand. If you feel uncomfortable or unprepared, ask the lawyer for more preparation time.

TAKING THE STAND

This is where the rubber meets the road. If you are not used to speaking in public, taking the stand in a criminal case can be an intimidating experience. If you are well prepared, however, your time on the stand may be rigorous but will ultimately be rewarding. If you are unprepared, it will be difficult not only for you, but also for the lawyers, judge, and jury. The most important things to remember when taking the stand are to think about your answers and relax as much as you possibly can.

As mentioned previously, you will give your testimony in several discrete portions. First is the direct examination, where you will tell your story in response to open-ended questions by the prosecutor. The direct examination will be followed by a cross-examination by the defense attorney, who will try to attack or discredit information that was brought out on direct examination. Once cross-examination is done, the court may allow the prosecutor to conduct "redirect examination." This will allow the prosecutor to ask you to address or explain issues raised on cross-examination. Sometimes, the judge will also allow "recross-examination," to allow the defense attorney to address issues raised in redirect examination. In theory these rebuttals can go on indefinitely, each addressing narrower issues that were raised in the previous examination, but rarely will it be allowed to go past recross.

General Guidelines for Testifying

The bulk of your preparation should be done before you get to court. You should be comfortable with your testimony and know what questions to expect from the prosecution and the defense. However, there are a few things to remember when you are on the stand.

- *First and foremost, you must tell the truth.* Before you testify, you will take an oath to tell the truth. Every fact that is, to the best of your knowledge, true should be admitted. Do not be concerned about whether the fact will help or hurt "your side" of the case.
- *Be aware of your appearance.* Dress conservatively and professionally, so the jury will concentrate on your testimony rather than on what you are wearing. Be aware that jurors will be in the public areas in and around the court; they may see you outside of the courtroom and draw impressions from those encounters. Do not discuss the case with anyone you do not know, and do not discuss the case with any other witnesses while waiting for your turn to testify.
- *Speak slowly and clearly.* This serves a number of purposes. First, the judge, jury, and lawyers all need to hear your answers. Additionally, the court reporter is taking down every word you say for the record, which may be used in further legal proceedings. Do not nod your head for a yes-or-no answer. Be prepared to spell complex, technical, or foreign words. Do not use jargon or technical terms without explaining them.
- *Do your best to direct your answers to the fact-finder.* If you are testifying in a jury trial, talk to the jury. If you are testifying in a hearing before the judge, address the judge.
- *Stop instantly when the judge interrupts you* or when an attorney objects to a question. Wait for the judge to tell you to continue.

On Direct Examination

- *Relax.* If you are prepared, direct examination is the easiest part of testifying. This is your story. In your discussions with the prosecutor, you should be familiar with what is going to be asked and what the answers are going to be.

- *Use your own words.* Do not try to memorize your testimony; it will sound rehearsed and unconvincing. Prior to testifying, go over the subject matter of your testimony in your own mind, then answer the questions as naturally as you can.
- *If you don't know the answer to a question, say you don't know.* Do not make up an answer or speculate as to what the answer might be.
- *If you do not remember something, say you do not remember.* If you cannot remember a key point, the prosecutor should be prepared to help refresh your memory with your report or notes. If you know what would help refresh your memory, tell the prosecutor what it is.
- *Do not exaggerate.* Do not make overbroad statements that you may later have to correct or explain. Be careful about saying "always" or "never."
- *Answer only the question you are asked, and then stop.* Listen carefully to each question, and ask to have it repeated if necessary. Do not answer without thinking. Explain your answer if necessary but do not volunteer information not actually asked for. If you realize that an answer you gave was not correct, correct it immediately. This applies to cross-examination as well.

On Cross-Examination

- *Relax, but stay on your toes.* Cross-examination is designed to be frustrating to the witness. The basic purpose of cross-examination is to raise doubts about the reliability or accuracy of your testimony. Do not get angry if you feel that your good faith or truthfulness is being questioned during cross-examination: that is part of the defense attorney's job.
- *Listen carefully to the questions.* During cross-examination, the attorney will ask you leading questions—questions that suggest the response that the attorney wants. In essence, the attorney will be telling the story, and will expect you to go along with it. Usually, the attorney will expect you to answer "yes" or "no" to the questions: avoid the automatic urge to say "yes" reflexively to any question asked. If the answer is "no," or if it needs an explanation, say so. Do not allow an attorney to put words in your mouth. Often, the judge will allow you to explain your answer. If not, saying that you need to explain will signal to the prosecutor to ask you a follow-up question on redirect examination.
- *Do not take things personally.* It is the defense attorney's job to point out holes and shortcomings in your testimony. It is also the defense attorney's job to point out

where you might be biased or inaccurate. Recognize this for what it is, and do not take personal offense.

- *Do not argue with the attorney.*
- *Do not look to the judge or to the prosecutor for assistance when you are being questioned by defense counsel.* If the judge interrupts, or if the prosecutor objects to the defense attorney's question, do not answer. If neither of those things happens, then you are on your own and you must answer the question asked.
- *Absolutely, positively, DO NOT LOSE YOUR TEMPER.* If you get angry, you will appear to the jury to be unstable or nonobjective. Always be courteous, even if the lawyer questioning you is not.

TAKE-HOME POINTS

1. Observe and document accurately and thoroughly at the scene.
2. Prepare until you are comfortable.
3. When you get on the stand, relax.
4. On direct examination, tell the story in your words, in a way the judge and jury can understand.
5. On cross-examination, listen to the questions, answer what is asked, and avoid the urge to argue or lose your temper.

SUMMARY

Testifying at a legal proceeding can be a challenging experience. It is not something you are used to doing on a daily basis, and your actions and opinions will be questioned and challenged, giving the whole process the possibility of being uncomfortable. If, however, you take the time at the scene and before your testimony to prepare yourself, and you work with the lawyers to familiarize yourself with the procedures, you will gain self-confidence and improve your performance. When you are on the stand, you will be able to relax, listen to the questions, and answer them with assurance.

REFERENCES

1. American Academy of Emergency Medicine. Position statement on ethical expert conduct and testimony. October 24, 2005. Available at: http://www.aaem.org/positionstatements/ethicalexpert.shtml.
2. Federal Rules of Evidence. Rules 601–615 (Witnesses) and 701–706 (Opinions and Expert Testimony).
3. Kahn L, Feldstern D. How to succeed as an expert witness. *Profiles DNA.* 1998;2(2):9–11.
4. Mauet TA. *Trial Techniques.* 6th ed. New York: Wolters Kluwer/Aspen; 2002.
5. Moses R. Expert witnesses in criminal cases, 2001. Available at: http://criminaldefense.homestead.com/experts.html.

Chapter 37

Applied Concepts: Public Policy and Other Considerations

Eric S. Weinstein and F. Mastrianni

OBJECTIVES

After reading this section, the reader will be able to:

1. List TEMS issues and topics relevant to public policy, legislative actions, and other considerations.
2. Describe the utilization of TEMS during all-hazards disasters that involve displaced populations impacting public policy and public opinion.
3. Review means to gather constituents to address and direct public policy to establish and support TEMS.

HISTORICAL PERSPECTIVE

Issues identified and published position statements important to tactical emergency medical support (TEMS) can historically be identified in many well-known organizations. These include the National Tactical Officers Association (NTOA) (1), American College of Emergency Physicians (ACEP) (2), National Association of EMS Physicians (NAEMSP) (3) and other professional associations that have issued policy statements. Statements such as these helped to shape the early public policy of TEMS.

INTRODUCTION

Public opinion and public policy are important considerations in TEMS future. The impression of the lay public and legislators needs to be accurate regarding TEMS. Highly visible to these key groups are media-based images of specialized law enforcement teams, both civilian and military, engaged against criminals and enemies of our nation. However, the supporting medical assets safely ensconced far from the threat of injury or concealed as one of the responding officers are practically invisible to the same key groups.

Public policy regarding the utilization of specially trained law enforcement personnel required locally for forced entry, warrant service, hostage negotiations, and other missions different than the routine has been well established. The public policy regarding TEMS as an integral team member in these specialized law enforcement operations is less well established. For example, funding provided for specialized operations may be wrongly assumed by the lay public and legislators to include provision for sufficient TEMS during these operations. The reality is that TEMS-specific funding is often not adequately provided and, in some situations, is actually being reduced. This is creating a public policy concern of supply and demand.

The supply of appropriately selected, trained, and maintained TEMS personnel may not be able to meet the demand of the specialized teams and operations they are designed to support. It is important that appropriate emphasis on the medical support of missions be recognized and maintained.

This and related complexities of TEMS must be appreciated by jurisdictional administrators (JA). The maturing of communications and detailed operational guidelines between law enforcement agencies are vital relationships being established to meet such important TEMS issues. Every TEMS provider can play an important role in establishing the proper public policy.

LEGISLATIVE INITIATIVES

The role of the jurisdictional authorities may be described as to protect the law enforcement officers that protect the citizens through TEMS (4). The law enforcement agency officer-in-charge, through careful review and interpretation of on-going intelligence, risk analysis, and after-action reports, is charged with determining the assets required to meet the daily challenges encountered. For some missions, the use of a special operations unit (e.g., a SWAT team) may be the most effective and the safest. This established need for a SWAT team may or may not include TEMS in the jurisdictional law enforcement.

Funding is an important determining factor in the inclusion of TEMS. For those jurisdictions unable to financially maintain or physically staff a SWAT team, law enforcement mutual aid agreements commonly permit regionalization of SWATs to assist local law enforcement with the complex missions beyond their capabilities.

Mutual aid agreements can identify a TEMS unit that will travel out of their jurisdiction to another in tandem with their SWAT team. This requires advanced deliberations that created the logistics and communications to incorporate a paramedic with a weapon or to perform advanced prehospital medical procedures in the local jurisdiction (5). The local law enforcement officer-in-charge and the incoming SWAT team's officer-in-charge will have to arrange for local assets if the mutual aid SWAT-TEMS is unable to travel with the SWAT team due to staffing shortages or the unfortunate limitations inherent in mutual aid agreements between prehospital care agencies or cross-jurisdiction practices of prehospital care.

The mutual aid model of providing such TEMS support has limitations. Some states and regions in somee states do not permit out-of-county or out-of-jurisdiction prehospital care personnel to, in essence, work within that county or jurisdiction without specific protocols, policies, and procedures, especially when a paramedic may be armed. Mutual aid agreements between law enforcement agencies may be separate and distinct from those between prehospital care agencies. This distinction should be flushed out and addressed through dialogue and research of the existing jurisdiction Scope of Practice statutes and the regulations of the TEMS prehospital care providers. Adjustments to these statutes or regulations may have to occur before the advancement of jurisdiction policies, procedures, and protocols to permit out-of-jurisdiction TEMS to be able to interface with indigenous prehospital care (6).

One example of a roadblock to appropriate incorporation of TEMS involved a lack of physician support of TEMS in Illinois due to malpractice fears. On September 29, 2004, the Illinois Law Enforcement Alarm System (ILEAS), composed of the majority of law enforcement agencies statewide, approved a resolution to support the TEMS inclusion into the E.M.S. Act. The ILEAS was facing the growing threat of methamphetamine labs and increased awareness and subsequent development of local law enforcement capabilities of terrorist threats. Their

commanders astutely determined that medical care of tactical teams was being delayed inappropriately. Their conclusion was that this care can be provided only by TEMS medics, but EMS protocols forbade EMS system members to enter the inner perimeter of an incident until the scene was safe and the mission had ended. Appropriately, they recognized that TEMS, a subspecialty of emergency medicine, would provide maximum protection. However, in Illinois, physicians would not volunteer their services because of the fear of medical malpractice liability. The ILEAS and the Illinois Department of Health (IDPH) created a TEMS taskforce, establishing a TEMS/EMS region with standardization of TEMS through state sponsorship and certification, which allowed TEMS physicians to receive limited medical indemnification through the EMS Act (7). On January 20, 2006, Illinois State Senator Dan Cronin introduced SB 2968 to the Illinois General Assembly, amending the Good Samaritan Act for various health care providers who provide volunteer TEMS services. As of April 4, 2006, both Illinois Houses passed the revised bill that amends the Good Samaritan Act, providing immunity from civil damages for EMT and first responders, as those terms are defined in the Emergency Medical Services (EMS) Systems Act (in addition to law enforcement officers and firemen), who provide emergency care in good faith without fee or compensation (instead of only without fee) (8).

Legislative issues regarding the weapon-carrying allowance of TEMS are an important issue. If the JA and law enforcement agency's officer-in-charge determine that for their SWAT to be successful TEMS is required, a key element to be decided is if the TEMS members will be armed (9). The legislative authority hurdles involved, including new statutes required to permit a paramedic to carry a weapon, may be significant.

Public policy and related legislative issues are also found in the types and amounts of education and training TEMS providers receive. The degree of law enforcement and SWAT specific training for each TEMS member resides with the SWAT officer-in-charge in coordination with the TEMS officer-in-charge. Standard paramedic and EMT training programs do not incorporate the rigorous physical, emotional, and intellectual decision-making components necessary for TEMS members. Again, this may require jurisdiction legislators to add statutes to accept prehospital care providers into programs with some level of security clearance for initial and subsequent maintenance education and training programs. A related example of this issue is found in Georgia.

On July 1, 2006, Chapter 5 of Title 35 of the Official Code of Georgia Annotated was amended to provide the Georgia Public Safety Training Center for emergency medical personnel beyond the previous limitation of only state and local law enforcement officers (10). Jurisdictions may choose to cross certify specially trained and certified emergency medical tactical technicians (EMT-Ts) as reserve police officers and tactically trained for inner perimeter and entry cell operations (11).

Employment-related human resource departments play an important role in the success of TEMS programs. The selection of the TEMS duties, responsibilities, training, and inherent risks are often the responsibility of this department. The budgeting for these additional requirements for an effective TEMS incorporated with the SWAT is dependent on the jurisdiction, as some law enforcement agencies may have a separate human resources department or be part of a larger, more comprehensive jurisdiction system. TEMS-related special operations requirements and skills may overlap with other pre-established human resource policies. Local advanced prehospital special operations may be established based on the inherent risks to include hazardous materials and technical rescue such as rope/high-angle, swift water, trench, and mountain rescue. However, TEMS is a distinct discipline (12).

TEMS INVOLVING DISPLACED POPULATIONS

The lack of forced or mandatory evacuation in the face of Hurricane Katrina is well documented, with volumes of disparate reports recommending guidelines and protocols for local Emergency Management Offices to incorporate. A SWAT team should have no operational mission with an orderly evacuation, issued in a timely manner, following the regional hurricane plan (13). One can imagine neighborhoods or population clusters that may not heed the prudent advice of local Emergency Management who wish to stay in the face of a predictable calamity. A news report from South Carolina summed it up in this quote: "If they won't go, the lawmen typically take down their names and phone numbers to notify next of kin in case something bad happens" (14). These individuals can then choose their own destiny with a clear understanding that they are on their own; once conditions deteriorate, there will likely be no rescue until more favorable conditions return. In an example from Georgia, policy and regulations have been established defining voluntary and mandatory evacuations during hurricane conditions (15).

Under evacuation conditions, especially after an official emergency order or proclamation has been declared, SWAT and TEMS activation should be anticipated. The Order or Proclamation is filed with the Emergency Management Agency in line of succession, county, state, or federal (16). TEMS may have to assist a SWAT deployment assigned to evacuate a jail, prison, or other facility at risk for civil unrest due to understaffing as the dynamics of the evacuation unfold or other unforeseen factors. This could be a prolonged operation, similar to a hostage situation or other more typical law enforcement SWAT deployment.

Public policy related to TEMS should reflect the many possible disaster scenarios with likelihood of TEMS utilization. If an evacuation is declared based on a suspected or known act of terrorism, a SWAT team providing force protection with TEMS support may have to evacuate a population at risk immediately. An industrial accident, such as weather or a naturally occurring disaster, may similarly trigger an immediate evacuation through tempting terrain or circumstances that may best be served by a SWAT that require TEMS to provide a show of force to dissuade looters, vandals, or those wishing to settle an old score in what may appear to be a lawless period.

A jurisdiction emergency management agency may not have resources to evacuate at-risk populations in the immediacy of the disaster and may require a SWAT for assistance, with TEMS resources to lend their expertise not only for their SWAT but other non-law enforcement participants. Specific duties may be to provide transitional guarding of pharmaceutical and other supplies stored on site, pending a more stable law enforcement contingent previously arranged under a more orderly evacuation.

This may also be encountered in the management of disabled populations. In 1992, the City of Frederick, Maryland reached an agreement with the U.S. Department of Justice to implement its community evacuation plans to enable those with impairments or other disabilities to safely self-evacuate or be evacuated by others. Identifying this population and addressing accessible transportation are important (17). The role of specialized law enforcement personnel and TEMS may provide assistance to this population. Coordinated exercises with local emergency management, fire, and other rescue agencies, routinely scheduled to review and then improve the evacuation plans, are suggested (18).

Plans describing the inclusion of specialized law enforcement personnel, including TEMS members, during disasters are important. Regulations and standards describing the importance of plans pertaining to hospitals, infirmaries, community residential care facilities, and other similar centers require a sheltering plan, transportation plan, and staffing plan for relocated patients or residents are well known (19,20). The flooding after the 2005 Hurricane Katrina that lead to the disruption of Lake Pontchatrain levees caught health care facilities unprepared to maintain bare minimum operations without resupply of personnel or materials, power or water, or for the looters that came seeking known repositories of necessities left unguarded. Swift water rescue and tactical force protection units from local jurisdictions and those that deployed were assisted by various Federal Law Enforcement Tactical Medical Programs following Hurricane Katrina (20).

CONVERGENT VOLUNTEERISM

Unsolicited medical personnel may volunteer at a SWAT operation, to assist the rescue, triage, and field treatment of victims or scene responders. This could be at a school, hospital, place of business, or other facility with a law enforcement presence beyond typical law enforcement supporting fire/rescue/EMS incident command. Specifically, if this may have been the result of suspected terrorists or industrial sabotage, SWAT assets may be required to best address the dynamic operation. Certain locations may require more force protection assets during the operation with the deployment of a SWAT team to integrate with the ongoing operation in mission specific instances. The joint position paper of the National Association of EMS Physicians (NAEMSP) and the American College of Emergency Physicians (ACEP) believe an organized approach is needed for the utilization of unsolicited volunteers in advance (21).

The added criminal, terrorist, or violent nature of an incident requiring a SWAT team escalates the requirement for heightened security at the perimeter of the incident, regardless of etiology. The TEMS Medical Director led-planned assets will have to be deployed to funnel these volunteers through an onsite rapid credentialing process, which will not only validate prehospital care responsibilities to reduce the chance of inappropriate clinical care but some security clearance to reduce the chance of further terrorism, contamination, or destruction of forensic evidence (i.e., keeping the bad guys away from the scene) (22). Through the use of the Incident Management System, the on-scene medical director, depending on jurisdiction either Fire/Rescue/EMS or the TEMS, will send a request for more assistance. The option to use volunteers already assembled, to call for more volunteers through a planned process involving local media, or through planned mutual aid agreements will be discussed. The Incident Manager has the ultimate authority to decipher credible requests for assistance through appropriate Incident Management principles as incorporated into the jurisdiction plans. The Incident Manager will similarly have the authority to send urgent dispatches to the media to modify or stop any further requests for help (20). Accountability is the most vital aspect of incorporating unsolicited volunteers and may require unforeseen resources that may distract and compromise the primary mission (23).

Preplanning includes a briefing of the command and control structure on-scene, specific to the clinical mission, available resources, patient care protocols, and applicable safety procedures that may include issuance of personal protective equipment. A clear understanding of the roles and responsibilities of the jurisdiction authority liabilities, available food and personal hygiene assets, and other relevant human resource policies and procedures designed for volunteers (19). Safety of all responders, those trained and equipped for the response, as well as these volunteers is paramount and with the dynamics of an incident complicated by the need for a SWAT with TEMS. The TEMS medical director must be aware that the convergence of volunteers not familiar with local accountability measures in an austere environment, lacking communication training and equipment may place these volunteers on the other side of the equation—once a responder, now a victim (20).

Evaluation of Resources

On occasion, just asking questions about a topic is enough impetus to influence public policy or to bring constituents together to identify areas of improvement. The West Virginia Office of Emergency Medical Services conducted a survey on TEMS, which was released July 31, 2006 (24). This survey, even with its limitations, was a good way to learn about TEMS in West Virginia by asking three simple questions: (i) Is there a SWAT, ERT or SRT team? (ii) Do they have medical resources, EMT-B or EMT-P, on the team? and (iii) If not, would they be interested in a training program? The survey was sent to more than 200 law enforcement agencies, from West Virginia State Police, county sheriff departments, and local police departments. The percentage of responding agencies is not surprising, with 20/55 (36%) of sheriffs and 48/171 (20%) of police providing significant data. The state police did not respond, but this was not considered to be a hindrance to interpreting available information (24).

The responding agencies included 42% of sheriff departments and 23% of police departments featuring a SWAT, ERT or SRT. However, 17% of the sheriff and 35% of police departments had medically trained EMT-B or paramedics on their teams, with some agencies that did respond to the survey leaving this question blank. The third question results speak to a lack of appreciation of a medical component to a SWAT, ERT, or SRT, with 46% of the responding sheriff departments not even answering the question and 19% not interested in a training program. Responding police departments were supportive of training (42% vs. 35%), but 23% did not answer the question (24).

Public policy, where the public constituents are the line officers, command, and control staff, as well as administrative and government staff can be influenced by addressing the comments provided. Most of the comments highlighted the small size of departments preventing the creation of a team. The need to have medical assets contained within the team was noted. As always, liability issues, perceived or real, were noted to be an inhibiting factor and determining the reality of these issues should be a result of this survey before any large scale effort to introduce, maintain, and advance TEMS in West Virginia and any jurisdiction has to address liability concerns (24).

TAKE HOME POINTS

1. All TEMS members should have a clear understanding of the public policy and related legislative guidelines in their region that impact TEMS operations, including such areas as weapons use, training and education, and human resource departments.
2. The inclusion of TEMS in the policy, regulations, and plans governing regional disaster response is important, as TEMS members skill in rescue, evacuation, and law enforcement medical support are valuable to the at-risk community.
3. Statistically based inquiries, such as a simple survey, as well as formal research initiatives may provide valuable information that can impact existing or forming TEMS teams, raise public and peer awareness of TEMS related issues, and provide important discussion points for a successful TEMS program.

CONCLUSION

TEMS is an evolving subspecialty of emergency medicine, with a separate spectrum of clinical research contributing to TEMS best practices incorporated into the design of dynamic policies and procedures. The TEMS practitioner must remain abreast of controversies, problems, and pitfalls of TEMS, as well as other aspects of emergency medicine with application to TEMS to continue the growth and sophistication of what the Second Annual TEMS Conference Attendees had only dreamed in 1989 (25). Public policy can and should be used to beg the question of creating a TEMS involving all constituents: citizens, law enforcement and allied health care personnel, jurisdiction administrators, and local government.

REFERENCES

1. Rasumoff D, Carmona RH. National Tactical Officers Association. Position statement on the inclusion of physicians in tactical law enforcement operations in the USA. *Tactical Edge Journal*. 1994;12(2):77–86.
2. ACEP Position Statement, June 2004. Tactical Emergency Medical Support. Available at: http://acep.org/webportal/PracticeResources/PolicyStatements/ems/TacticalEmergencyMedicalSupport.htm.
3. Heck JJ, Pierluisi G, et al. NAEMSP Position Statement:Law Enforcement Special Operations Medical Support. *Prehosp Emerg Care*. 2001;5(2):403–406.
4. Carmona RH, Rasumoff D. Essentials of Tactical Emergency Medical Support. *Tactical Edge Journal*. 1990;8(3)54–56.
5. New York State Department of Health. EMS Mutual Aid Planning Guidelines. Available at: http://www.health.state.ny.us/nysdoh/ems/policy/89-02.htm. Accessed October 19, 2007.
6. Commonwealth of Pennsylvania. Report to the Senate of the Commonwealth of Pennsylvania. Available at: http://www.swarthmorepa.

7. Illinois Law Enforcement Alarm System. Resolution to Support the Tactical Emergency Medical Support for Inclusion into the E.M.S. Act. Available at: http://www.ileas.org/policies/tems.pdf. Accessed October 17, 2007.
8. Illinois General Assembly. Bill Status of SB2968. Available at: http://www.ilga.gov/legislation/BillStatus.asp?DocNum=2968&GAID=8&DocTypeID=SB&LegId=24086&SessionID=50. Accessed October 19, 2007.
9. Carmona RH. Controversies in Tactical Emergency Medical Support. *Top Emerg Med*. 2003;25(4):342–343.
10. Georgia General Assembly. Senate Bill 581. Available at: http://www.legis.state.ga.us/legis/2005_06/fulltext/sb581.htm. Accessed October 19, 2007.
11. An example available at: http://www.tampagov.net/dept_fire/rescue_division/general_info/tactical_medical_response_team.asp
12. Charleston County, South Carolina. Employee Information. Available at: http://www.charlestoncounty.org/index2.asp?p=/departments/ems/employeeinfo.htm. Accessed October 19, 2007.
13. South Carolina Emergency Management Division. South Carolina Model Executive Order. Available at: http://www.scemd.org/Plans/index/.html. Accessed October 19, 2007.
14. Eric Connor. Beaufort County officials "cocked and ready to go." Savannah Morning News. August 25, 1998. Available at: http://www.savannahnow.com/stories/082598/CMNbeaufort.html. Accessed August 10, 2004.
15. Chatham Emergency Management Agency. Emergency Support Function (ESF) # 16 Evacuation. Available at: http://cema.chathamcounty.org/eop/esf16.htm. Accessed August 10, 2004.
16. City of Myrtle Beach Local Government Page. Basic Disaster Plan: Emergency Preparations. Available at http://www.cityofmyrtlebeach.com/disasterplans.html. Accessed August 10, 2004.
17. United States Department of Justice. Settlement Agreement between the United States of America and City of Fredrick, Maryland under the Americans with Disabilities Act. DJ 204-35-245. Available at: http://www.usdoj.gov/crt/ada/fredericksa.htm. Accessed August 10, 2004.
18. Batiste LC, Loy B. Job Accommodation Network Employers' Guide to Including Employees with Disabilities in Emergency Evacuation Plans. Job Accommodation Network Web site. Available at: http://janweb.icdi.wvu.edu/media/emergency.html. Accessed August 10, 2004.
19. South Carolina Department of Health and Environmental Control. Emergency Orders 8/13/1996 and 8/30/2004. Available at: http://www.scdhec.gov/hr/pdfs/licen/licgen/hleo.pdf. Accessed August 10, 2004 and September 21, 2005.
20. Davis JD, Tang N. Efficacy of a Federal Law Enforcement Tactical Medical Program following a catastrophic natural disaster: The DHS ICE SRT response to Hurricane Katrina. *Prehosp Emerg Care*. 2006;10(2):173–179.
21. Asaeda G, et al. Unsolicited medical personnel volunteering at disaster scenes: A joint position paper from the National Association of EMS Physicians and the American College of Emergency Physicians. *Prehosp Emerg Care*. 2003;7(1):147–148.
22. Cone DC, Weir SD, Bogucki S. Convergent volunteerism. *Ann Emerg Med*. 2003;41(4):459–460.
23. Milsten AM. Managing volunteers and donations. In: Ciottone G, ed. *Disaster Medicine*. Philadelphia: Mosby; 2006:242–244.
24. Whitaker A. *Tactical EMS Survey*. West Virginia EMS System Department of Health and Human Resources Bureau of Public Health Office of Emergency Medical Services. Available at: http://www.wvochs.org/shared/content/ems/pdfs/tactical%20ems%20survey%2020080806.pdf. Accessed October 19, 2007.
25. Carmona R, Brennan K. Review of the National Conference on Tactical Emergency Medical Support. *Tactical Edge Journal*. 1990;8(3):7–11.

org/government/documents/senatereport60_000.pdf. Accessed October 19, 2007.

Chapter 38

Applied Concepts: Public Relations

Eric S. Weinstein and William F. Mastrianni

OBJECTIVES

After reading this section, the reader will be able to:

1. To appreciate the similarities of all Public Information Officers using the Incident Management System.
2. To incorporate military security measures in civilian tactical emergency medical services (TEMS) operations.
3. To work with the media to help them help TEMS operations.

INTRODUCTION

The statement, "Keep the media off everybody's rear and make sure we look good," found under the heading "Public Information Officer Duties" in *The EMS Incident Management System* (1), paints a partial description of the TEMS liaison to the media, the public, and jurisdiction administrators and government officials. The added layer of criminal or terrorist acts requiring the intervention of a special weapons and tactics (SWAT) team and thus a tactical emergency medical service (TEMS) unit piques the interest of attorneys, business, and commercial interests as well as civilians, local and afar. The added sophistication of a TEMS Public Information Officer (PIO) to know and understand the activities of a SWAT team enriches the opportunities to appease the appetite of the audiences noted above, as well as further the objectives of the SWAT and TEMS teams in the community. An Incident Manager will determine the location, scope and scheduling of debriefings under the auspices of the PIO. In the dynamics of a SWAT action, the PIO may have to operate under predetermined policy and procedures to assure accurate dissemination of information in the context of operational security and other considerations. Frequent scheduled debriefings, with instructions for late-breaking intermittent information discussions, as well as computer links, handouts, graphs, diagrams, and any other factual information to assist the reporters, will only lend credibility to the PIO but reduce the unauthorized forays that may jeopardize the reporter and crew who venture into harm's way (1) (Table 38.1).

The TEMS PIO may wear many hats, including any number of administrative posts with the TEMS, law en-

forcement, or EMS/fire/rescue agency; other PIO responsibilities within a specific agency; or even a position within the county administrative structure separate and distinct from any response, field, or prehospital care agency. This chapter addresses unique aspects of the duties and responsibilities of the TEMS PIO, not only for useful knowledge synergy, for those wearing multiple PIO or other hats, but as a distinct discipline for all governmental PIOs to utilize during a SWAT operation. There are volumes of public information and relations guides, which have led to mountains of policies and procedures for law enforcement and fire/rescue/EMS agencies, emergency management offices, and jurisdiction administrators to follow as they stand before camera lights speaking into a host of microphones with the backdrop of the incident still unfolding (2). SWAT PIOs have their gold books of pearls to remember and pitfalls to avoid when ambushed or presented with confounding questions. An adaptation of all of these trials and tribulations, improved after a retrospective analysis of how the PIO could have or should have presented their organization and the information with more alacrity and poise, is the challenge of the TEMS designer. Department of Defense Directive 5122.5, issued by the Secretary of Defense for Public Affairs (ASD[PA]), September 27, 2000, adds the complexity of military activities.

The position of TEMS PIO shares similar duties with others in industry, business, politics, public service, and athletics. Above all, the TEMS PIO is the internal and external face and voice of the agency, fully aware of the agency's policies, procedures, and relationships with constituents. The responsibility to ensure a free flow of information bound only by operational security, jurisdiction, and agency policy in today's 24/7 instantaneous news

▶ **TABLE 38.1. Pitfalls of Managing Public Information.**

- Failing to bring in experts
- Avoid using complex language or jargon
- Avoid arguing, fighting, or losing your temper
- Do not predict
- It is okay to say, "I do not know"
- Failing to show empathy
- Lying, clouding the truth, or covering up
- Not responding quickly
- Not responding at all
- Failing to practice emergency communication

Adapted from Dilling et al. Public information management. Ciottone G, ed. *Disaster Medicine*. Philadelphia: Mosby Elsevier; 2006:128–129.

coverage is not only challenging but potentially lifesaving. Auf der Heide's editorial in the *Annals of Emergency Medicine* (3) espouses how an attentive TEMS PIO can positively affect the media's initial desire to help victims and the responders of an incident requiring SWAT deployment requiring TEMS. The TEMS PIO should work closely with all local media to follow a mutual plan of action to reduce confusion at the scene by communicating all the factual information available as the dynamics of the incident unfold; limit interference with operations, ranging from traffic avoidance, reduction in cell phone usage, and specific responses of volunteers if any are required; family rendezvous points; and where to find information to permit the response agencies the most appropriate freedom to attend to the mission at hand (3) (Table 38.2).

The Incident Management System will guide duties and responsibilities tailored to the specifics of the TEMS agencies' operational guidelines. Configurations of different TEMS agencies may place the TEMS PIO duties under the auspices of the jurisdiction administrator, law enforcement agency charged with SWAT, fire/rescue/EMS, or

▶ **TABLE 38.2. Duties of the TEMS Public Information Officer.**

- Internal SWAT, Fire/Rescue/EMS information exchange
- Community relations, public service announcements, recruiting
- News media relations as a factual resource for incidents or issues unrelated to the jurisdiction
- Point of Contact for all jurisdiction and mutual aid response incidents or issues
- Written, video, audio, and internet communication
- Training and incident multimedia recording
- Liaison with other branches of local, regional, and state health care delivery assets
- Active participant in any professional organizations representing TEMS PIOs
- Assist TEMS officers in the development of operational policies and procedures
- Maintain professionals standards of PIOs through continuing education

a separate entity within the jurisdiction. Therefore it is paramount that the TEMS officer-in-charge work closely with the non-TEMS PIO who may not be as facile or familiar with the specifics of TEMS or SWAT teams. Information can be made available, specifically if covered under the Freedom of Information Act and not confidential regarding personnel or jeopardizing operational security (3). Significant adjustments to the data set employed by the non-TEMS PIO may include an adaptation of the Department of Defense Principles of Combat Coverage. This includes the principles of open, if not transparent, information exchange, which may be different from a non-TEMS practitioner's awareness of operational security and may require a more detailed briefing for each mission or operation under the direction of the SWAT and/or TEMS officer-in-charge. Journalists who request and receive permission through proper channels to gain access to either the warm or the hot zone (see previous chapters) will be credentialed after a security clearance and abide by set rules established and clearly communicated to protect SWAT and TEMS personnel and their operations. Any violation of these rules may result in sanctions ranging from reduction in access to expulsion from that specific operation and future operations. Embedded journalists are discussed in more detail later, with applications of some of those provisions to other types of journalists. While acting as a liaison, the non-TEMS PIO should not interfere with operations while permitting the journalists access to operations cleared by the SWAT and/or TEMS officer-in-charge. All efforts should be made to facilitate the timely transmission of journalists' reports as long as mission or operational security is not jeopardized, like light and sound discipline (3).

MEDIA RELATIONS, USE OF THE MEDIA POOL, AND THE CNN EFFECT

The military media pool was established to limit the total number of journalists while providing sufficient coverage for any organization that requested privileges, out of economy of scale as well as security considerations. This can be applied to SWAT/TEMS operations, specifically if these are long-running (hostage standoff), involve dignitaries (presidential visit), are high-profile political (political party national conventions) or government conferences (G8 Summit) or athletic events (World Series), or are industrial accidents requiring specific special operations for rescue and recovery. This may not be standard in local jurisdictions, or even have been considered in the past, but remains in the TEMS PIO armamentarium for utilization. Journalists from local, state, national, and international organizations, as well as freelancers, will approach the scene of an incident at different times and from different locations. Scene security should have a clear plan of action to remove journalists who were either on-scene before the incident and remained or managed to evade deploying scene security. The TEMS PIO and/or the on-scene PIO, in concert with the on-scene Incident Manager, should establish a media representative venue, at least initially safely located, with easy access and sufficient power, if not unaffected by the incident; then, if possible, on-scene assets can be utilized for this location, for example, a generator. If a hardened facility is not available, the on-scene assets can be utilized, such as a tent or some type of shelter, if available. It is difficult to establish one plan for on-scene media relations, since each incident will not be the same. As plans evolve, review the literature available, in a retrospective manner, to learn how to tailor plans to guide future incident media relations (4).

Cunning on-scene SWAT officers have utilized local media resources to facilitate hostage negotiations and rescue efforts and to communicate, transmit, or send information back to a command and control location. Communication between SWAT/TEMS personnel on-scene in zones and between zones during the dynamics of an operation may be hampered by limited electrical power, poor visual access, reduced communication through jammed cell towers, damaged infrastructure, weather, background sound or noise levels, and lack of interoperable communication equipment among responding mutual aid organizations, agencies, or units. Media ethics and standards balanced with the desire to capture and report the incident as an observer should be considered when approaching a journalist to assist in operations. Reimbursement for damaged equipment should be assured and reinforced as soon as possible by a signed agreement. A detailed discussion of what materials may be retained or transmitted by the journalist for the journalist's use must occur to protect the integrity of the operation's security, confidential information of SWAT/TEMS personnel, and any legal proceedings afterward. The First Amendment protections may not apply if the journalist's equipment has been usurped by operations.

Belknap has detailed how the "CNN effect" can be utilized during military operations to gather intelligence (5). Livingston's formal definition of the CNN effect attributed the media's ability as "1) a *policy agenda-setting agent*, 2) an *impediment* to the achievement of desired policy goals, and 3) an *accelerant* to policy decision making" (6; italics in original). Given the quasi-military SWAT actions and sophisticated prehospital care of a TEMS unit, traditional and nontraditional media will seek innovative ways to get their information via advanced technology. Information exchange can foster the objectives of both the SWAT/TEMS units and the broadcasters without interrupting the development of policy, during an action and future operations, or impeding the goals set by the SWAT leader.

EMBEDDED JOURNALISTS

Scholars argue that Homer's *Iliad* set the tone for future war correspondence some 400 years after the Tro-

jan War (7). Jean Froussart chronicled the medieval 100 Years War most notably, traveling with Edward the Black Prince in 1367 during his campaign at Castile in Spain (8). A. R. Ward brought the horrors of Antietam to the American public with vivid drawings accompanying painstaking prose in the October 11, 1862, *Harper's Weekly* (9). The direct reporting of military conflict is not without peril. Ernie Pyle is perhaps one of the most notable correspondents in World War II to die in combat (10). The Reporters Without Borders report released March 20, 2006, tallies the 86 journalists killed and 38 kidnapped during the 3 years of the Iraqi War (11). The decision to embed journalists within a TEMS unit must weigh the risk of a high-profile civilian nonteam member injury or death versus the community relations benefit.

The unclassified Department of Defense report, "Public Affairs Guidance (PAG) on Embedding Media during Possible Future Operations/Deployments in the U.S. Central Command's (CENTCOM) Area of Responsibility," can be adapted for use in other unified command areas of responsibility (12). A SWAT/TEMS team can adapt this policy to shape public perception of the delivery of medical care at the scene of any incident involving tactical operations (13). Just as the Department of Defense strives to tell a factual story of military operations to reduce distortions that can affect the desired outcome of peace and security, a SWAT team desires to correctly portray the efforts of the TEMS specially trained prehospital care personnel under extreme conditions (13). The embedded journalists within a TEMS unit should be prepared for more than the usual "ride-along." The similarities of spending the shift or operation alongside the unit members enjoying the tedium of waiting for action, the detailed explanation of the preparation of mission-specific supplies and equipment, and the mental exercise of visualization of the appropriate sequence of clinical care end with the threat of violence and donning of personal protective equipment like their battlefield colleagues in Iraq (13). There will be a balance among operational security, media access, and the risk analysis of placing the journalist in harm's way (13). This balance will extend to the discussion of the specific SWAT tactical operations, the supporting TEMS activities, and the protection of any intelligence gathered to protect the legal ramifications of the police action.

Media representatives can be selected based on specific community relations goals, which may include assuring the public that SWAT members and citizens involved in a SWAT operation will have state-of-the art on-scene clinical care, to act as a recruiting advertisement or a well-intended signal to jurisdiction legislators to learn more about TEMS in nonexistent or underserved law enforcement communities. Global information may trigger a request from local media through usual inquiries fielded by either fire/EMS or law enforcement or even jurisdiction emergency management. The responsibility of accepting and fulfilling these requests falls under the duties of the

SWAT (and, in some instances, the TEMS) PIO. An inquiry form should be developed fitting the specific configuration of the TEMS relationship with SWAT (13). A waiver or release of liability created by jurisdiction legal representation is a necessity reflecting the risks (12). The SWAT mission or operational commander manages and determines specific assignments for embedded journalists. Embed authority may be delegated to subordinates such as the TEMS commander or the specific TEMS unit crew chief at the discretion of the SWAT mission or operational commander. This will be determined and communicated at the debriefing (13).

Journalists usually will not be permitted to utilize their own vehicles for liability and operation security, while space on TEMS vehicles will be made available as long as the mission specific needs are met and all TEMS members and potential patients will not be compromised. The journalists have to realize that they are responsible for transferring, transporting, and maintaining their equipment (13). During the debriefing journalists will gain an understanding that SWAT/TEMS communication equipment incorporated into the operation or mission can be adapted for use by the journalists if this is requested in the initial debriefing, during the actual operation, or after the operation. However, the operation or mission commander has final approval for these requests, which may be rescinded as necessary. Real-time transmission parameters are set in the debriefing and may similarly be curtailed if this is felt to jeopardize any component. Likewise, the journalists' embedded communication equipment may be utilized in the midst of the operation as a resource to accomplish the SWAT mission even if the intention is to record TEMS operations. The data collected by the journalist is protected under certain legal and ethical standards, though an agreement can be reached for the TEMS' request for after-action review, incorporation into training or process improvement, and even recruiting purposes (13). Data or information captured during the dynamics of the operation not initially covered or reviewed in the debriefing will be addressed in a specific "Release of Information" procedure, which will adhere to a short time frame for immediate, if not shortly thereafter, decision by the SWAT commander (13). Elements of the journalist's involvement will be reviewed in the debriefing as part of the explanation, listing the limitation of access to operational security and confidential personnel information (13).

SWAT commanders will ensure that journalists are provided with every opportunity to observe TEMS activities, although their personal safety has to be weighed in light of potential escalation of the unknown operational risks (13). The safety of all concerned is paramount; if at any time any member of the TEMS or SWAT team believes that journalists are unable to withstand the rigorous conditions or the stability of the operation is in question, the SWAT or TEMS officer charged with embed authority may restrict, limit, or withhold current or future access to operations (13). A journalist may become a casualty, and all efforts will be made to attend to his or her needs, balanced with the overall dynamic situation. Embedded journalists may terminate their tenure at any time but must understand that their travel from the current location to a location that is more favorable for their departure may not occur in a timely manner as dictated by the dynamic of the operation (13). If the SWAT commander has advance intelligence of a biological weapons release, there may be consideration to require the journalist to receive advance immunization or chemoprophylaxis through a negotiated process between the involved SWAT team and the journalist (13). Personal protective equipment may be required and it is the responsibility of the embed authority to prepare the journalist for the experience through appropriate debriefing, practice, and oversight (13). Specific identification will be issued for each operation within the Incident Management System for accountability purposes, such as fire departments, as well as to assure operational security. Background checks may be required for certain operations and can be adjudicated in advance.

OPERATIONAL SECURITY AND THE HEALTH INSURANCE PORTABILITY AND ACCOUNTABILITY ACT

With almost-immediate and pervasive professional media present at any and all law enforcement operations of remotely more than routine scale, combined with civilians with handheld digital cameras, Internet video feeds created in an instant, and ubiquitous cell phone cameras, called to the scene by lights and sirens, even before the operational gear can be unloaded, the reporting begins. TEMS personnel that come from law enforcement ranks receive training that protects operational security, while personnel that come from fire/rescue/EMS ranks are schooled in the Health Insurance Portability and Accountability Act (HIPAA) regulations. HIPAA regulations help to protect both protected human information (PHI) and actionable medical information (AMI) (14). Similarly to military operations, terrorists, criminals, and other perpetrators can use real-time medical intelligence gleaned from television, the Internet, and other sources to aid their efforts. The controlled release of injuries of alleged perpetrators, civilians caught in the action, law enforcement, and other government response agencies must be paramount to reduce the transmission of sensitive information. HIPAA applies to any and all injured patients: the good guys and the bad guys regardless. This does not end when the operation ceases, since AMI data can be obtained from hospital, morgue, and other sources, under the purview of the PIO of the law enforcement lead agency or jurisdiction administrator. Reporting of war dead has been a dreaded

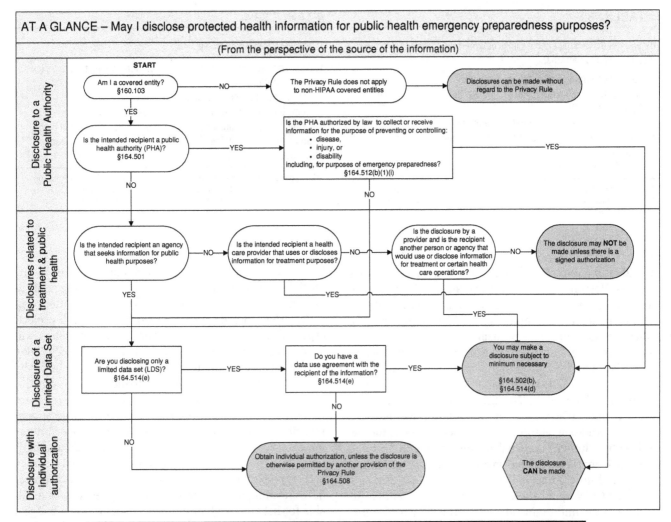

FIGURE 38.1. At a glance. May I disclose protected health information for public health emergency preparedness purposes? From at a glance: May I disclose protected health information for public health emergency preparedness purposes? U.S. Department of Health and Human Services Web site. Available at: http://www.hhs.gov/ocr/hipaa/decisiontool/EmergencyPrepDisclose.pdf. Accessed September 12, 2007.

consequence of military activities for centuries; in the past this news took days or months to travel from the war area to the hometowns of the dead. Now this can occur almost instantly, without regard to the emotional well-being of the families or friends of the injured or deceased (Fig. 38.1) (15).

HIPAA, passed in 1996, protects individuals' health information held by "covered entities" (16). A TEMS PIO discussing injuries must be careful not to release any information that can be linked to a specific individual—speaking only in broad terms such as numbers and types of injuries and, in certain cases not even discussing gender or age—to prevent the release of any data that might enable cunning media investigators to identify the injured person(s). A TEMS action to attend to injured does establish the unit as a Public Health Entity (PHE), as is any fire/rescue/EMS

unit in a non-TEMS function. Since the media is not a public health authority, no release of public health information is permitted without a specific discussion and a signed release, which, in the circumstances of a TEMS action, is unlikely to have been completed by any of the injured (17). A simple web-based interactive decision tool was released by the Department of Homeland Security in conjunction with the Department of Health and Human Services Office for Civil Rights to help guide a PHE with regard to patients with a disability in Emergency Preparedness and Recovery. Though not specifically designed for a TEMS action, this tool is a useful aid for a TEMS PIO (18) (Table 38.3).

A TEMS PIO may be called on to discuss the application of devices, strategies, and equipment used by a SWAT team or other search and rescue team (SRT). This may require factual experts available in the community or

▶ **TABLE 38.3.**

Be wary of discussing specific links between the following and resulting wound patterns:

1. Defined wounding and subduing methods
2. Injuries sustained while wearing defined Personal Protective Equipment (PPE)
3. Injuries sustained while in defined vehicles
4. Specific ballistic agents and the resulting failure of PPE or vehicles
5. Specific rescue and extrication techniques

Adapted from Policy 05-018. Release of actionable medical information policy memorandom. Department of the army. Headquarters U.S. Army Command. Fort Sam Houston, TX. December 2, 2005. p.5.7.f.c.

▶ **TABLE 38.4.**

TEMS Medical Research will:

1. Adhere to specific agency and jurisdiction administrative policy and procedure
2. Follow standard professional guidelines
3. Contribute to the general knowledge base
4. Draw logical conclusions or provide valuable information that does not negatively impact the SWAT, SRT, or agency mission
5. Respect all provisions of HIPPA

Adapted from Policy 05-018. Release of actionable medical information policy memorandum. Department of the army. Headquarters. U.S. Army Command. Fort Sam Houston, TX. December 2, 2005. 5.9.h.2.

provided by the manufacturer, the supplier, or other sources. Restraint use and subsequent injuries of the restrained are frequent sources of media coverage. Ballistics and nonballistic techniques in civilian populations are other examples of topics of media curiosity; with proper preparation the TEMS PIO can help the community to appreciate the dedication and commitment of local law enforcement to adhere to minimal force protection to get the job done safely. The TASER is a conducted electrical weapon (CEW) that is available for use by public and private law enforcement in widespread venues as well as by criminals and civilians for protection, through the black market. A basic investigation was published that found no cardiac, cellular, or other damage after a standard CEW application (19). Use of the scientific literature is an important adjunct to the TEMS PIO discussion, even if this may require consultation with the TEMS physician providing medical direction or other medical resources.

The TEMS PIO may be called on to create and discuss specific data linking casualties or injuries that occurred from a specific single action of a SWAT team or other SRT, from a combination of actions or from specific units within a SWAT team or SRT in defense of a policy, procedure, technique, or equipment, before a legal proceeding, such as an internal investigation, or before the jurisdiction administrator. Actionable information that maintains operational security will have to be tailored to the audience and may require assistance from operational officers as well as department legal representation. Information that may not be released includes photos that reveal operational equipment, strategy, and techniques through interpretation of the injuries sustained by those in the photos. All photos released must be reviewed through a department review process as well as HIPPA guidelines to protect the public health information of the individual, as well as in good taste to respect the injured and dead (20) (Table 38.4).

Good science is an important facet of all clinical medical care, practiced by all allied health care providers, in the

field and in the hospital. It is paramount that a TEMS PIO participate in clinical research, again, respecting applicable agency and jurisdiction as well as sound scientific principles. The esprit de corps created by a research project, especially one that involves local health care providers, will garner recognition for all involved. The TEMS PIO may not be facile with the terminology or the content of the project but, nonetheless, will have to monitor the activities and any subsequent publication and submissions to assure that mission-specific details do not jeopardize operational security or violate any HIPPA provisions. Opportunities may present that require review of action injury and mortality logs that must first undergo scrutiny for relevancy and to respect the above standards. New theory, procedures, techniques, equipment, and supplies may be available for field testing that may stretch operational budgets and provide the necessary publicity to advance the TEMS unit within the agency and jurisdictional administration. The TEMS PIO will work in concert with the officers or investigators to assure appropriateness and reporting accuracy.

CONCLUSION

The responsibility to accurately portray the duties of a TEMS agency falls on every member of the agency, from secretary to chief, from line officer to procurement head. A TEMS unit is an extension of a SWAT unit; operational security and the safety of all concerned require tight lips not to sink ships. All media broadcasters, traditional and nontraditional, should be considered at every juncture of communication: design, implementation, operations, and review of TEMS activities. Indeed they are the friends of a SWAT/TEMS unit, cultivated and enriched by a PIO who appreciates their needs as well as those of the SWAT/TEMS unit, through study of business and political "spin doctors" and ongoing discussions with all constituents who clamor for information.

REFERENCES

1. Christen H, Maniscalco PM. *The EMS Incident Management System*. Saddle River, NJ: Prentice-Hall; 1998:33–34.

2. Crisis and risk communication. Air War College Web site. Available at: http://www.au.af.mil/au/awc/awcgate/awcmedia.htm#crisiscomm. Accessed September 12, 2007.

3. Auf der Heide E. Convergence behavior in disasters. *Ann Emerg Med*. 2003;41(4):463–466.

4. Mordan J. Press pools, prior restraint and the Persian Gulf War. *Air & Space Power Chronicles Online Journal*. June 6, 1999. Available at: http://www.airpower.au.af.mil/airchronicles/cc/mordan.html. Accessed September 12, 2007.

5. Belknap M. The CNN effect: strategic enabler or operational risk. USAWC Strategic Report. Carlisle Barracks, PA: U.S. Army War College; March 30, 2001. Available at: http://www.au.af.mil/au/awc/awcgate/army-usawc/cnn-belknap.pdf. Accessed September 12, 2007.

6. Livingston, S. Research Paper R-18, Clarifying the CNN effect: an examination of media effects according to type of military intervention. Accessed on October 4, 2007 at http://www.ksg.harvard.edu/presspol/research_publications/papers/research_papers/R18.pdf. Harvard University; June 1997.

7. Basics of Homer's Iliad and Odyssey. Available at: http://www.necessaryprose.com/homerbasics.htm. Accessed September 12, 2007.

8. Larry Gormley. Jean Froissart - medieval war correspondent? eHistory Web sit. Available at: http://ehistory.osu.edu/World/articles/ArticleView.cfm?AID=3. Accessed September 12, 2007.

9. Louisville evacuation. The Civil War Web site. Available at: http://www.sonofthesouth.net/leefoundation/civil-war/1862/october/louisville-scare.htm. Accessed September 12, 2007.

10. The wartime columns of Ernie Pyle. Indiana University School of Journalism Web site. Available at: http://www.journalism.indiana.edu/news/erniepyle/. Accessed September 12, 2007.

11. Slaughter in Iraq. Reporters without Borders Web site. Available at: http://www.rsf.org/IMG/pdf/Survey_RSF_Iraq_06.pdf. Accessed September 12, 2007.

12. Public affairs guidance (PAG) in embedding media during possible future operations/deployments in the U.S. Central Commands (CENTCOM) area of responsibility (AOR). U.S. Department of Defense Web site. Available at: http://www.defenselink.mil/news/feb2003/d20030228pag.pdf. Accessed September 12, 2007.

13. Heiskell LE, Carmona RH. Tactical emergency medical services: an emerging subspecialty of emergency medicine. *Ann Emerg Med*. 1994;23(4):778–785.

14. Policy 05-018. Release of actionable medical information policy memorandum. Department of the Army. Headquarters. Fort Sam Houston, TX: United States Army Command; December 2005.

15. At a glance: May I disclose protected health information for public health emergency preparedness purposes? U.S. Department of Health and Human Services Web site. Available at: http://www.hhs.gov/ocr/hipaa/decisiontool/EmergencyPrepDisclose.pdf. Accessed September 12, 2007.

16. Policy 05-018.p.8.f.i.

17. HIPPA privacy rule: Disclosures for emergency preparedness. U.S. Department of Health and Human Services Web site. Available at: http://www.hhs.gov/ocr/hipaa/decisiontool/. Accessed September 12, 2007.

18. HHS announces new HIPPA privacy decision tool for emergency preparedness planning. U.S. Department of Health and Human Services Web site. Available at: http://www.hhs.gov/news/press/2006pres/20060705a.html. Accessed September 12, 2007.

19. Ho JD, et al. Cardiovascular and physiologic effects of conducted electrical weapon discharge in resting adults. *Acad Emerg Med*. 2006;13(6):589–595.

20. Policy 05-018.p.8.f.h. Department of the Army: Office of the Surgeon General. Release of actionable medical information policy information, OTSG/MEDCOM Policy Memo 05-018. Accessed at http://www.wramc.amedd.army.mil/departments/dci/Downloads/Protocol%20Templates/Publication/MEDCOM%20Policy%20Memo%202005-018_12-02-05.pdf on October 4, 2007; Washington, December 2005.

CBRNE and Public Health

Section Editor: KELLY R. KLEIN

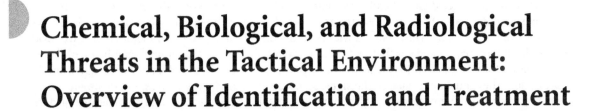

Chemical, Biological, and Radiological Threats in the Tactical Environment: Overview of Identification and Treatment

Kelly R. Klein, Richard V. King, Phillip Carmona, and Greene Shepherd

OBJECTIVES

After reading this section, the reader will be able to:

1. Hazardous material exposure risks for tactical operators.
2. The history of the use of hazardous materials as weapons.
3. Recognition of chemical, biological, or radiological contamination.
4. Field treatments and operational decision making for team members who have been contaminated.

HISTORICAL PERSPECTIVE

Many of the weapons that today would be classified as chemical, biological, or radiological agents have been used for more than 3,000 years. As early as 1000 B.C. the Chinese used arsenical smokes in warfare and throughout history. In 1346, the Tartars catapulted plague-infected bodies and heads over castle walls during the siege at Kaffa. The British Army is reported to have distributed blankets used by smallpox patients to Native Americans in the late 18th century. The modern use of chemical weapons began during World War I when the Germans soldiers used chlorine gas against the French during the second battle of Ypres, which prompted retaliation and escalation by all sides, including the French, British, and Americans. There were approximately 1,300,000 casualties, including 90,000 deaths on both sides, primarily from blister agents and choking agents. This new form of warfare brought about changes in decontamination procedures and improved protective equipment, which are discussed in Chapters 40 and 41 (1–3).

INTRODUCTION

Hazardous materials represent a complex and significant danger during tactical operations. The objectives of a tactical operation can be disrupted by even a single team member's becoming contaminated with a hazardous material. Tactical medical providers are challenged with not only providing care but also making assessments about mission viability.

A hazardous material is defined as any substance that poses a substantial risk to the health or safety of individuals or the environment when improperly handled, stored, transported, or disposed (1). The specific risks are dependent on the quantity and concentration of the substance exposure and the physical, chemical, or infectious characteristics of the material. The exposure may be due to an unintentionally contaminated environment or be the result of an act of aggression. Environmental contamination may be due to waste products such as from methamphetamine manufacture or due to unintentional releases caused by accidents or collateral damage. Hazardous substances also have the potential to be used as unconventional weapons. This, coupled with current concerns about terrorism, indicates that tactical medics must be prepared for more than the typical environmental contamination; they must be trained in the signs, symptoms, and treatments of chemical, radiological, and biological weapons.

Since conventional weapons, that is, lead projectiles and explosives, are a tactical team's most common threat, chemical, biological, and radiological threats might seem unlikely and not be in the tactical medic's forethought. However, the use of these agents is an unfortunate but enduring reality. Acts of chemical, biological, or radiological terrorism are infrequent but have had very high visibility and a marked psychological impact. Extremists such as Iraqi insurgents, the Japanese Aum Shinrykio cult, and even government leaders such as Saddam Hussein have demonstrated willingness to develop and use these agents as well as conventional weapons to make their point (4–6). These weapons can be used to attack offensively, threaten for negotiations, create public chaos, divert response resources, or facilitate escape. Alternatively, law enforcement agencies may use incapacitating chemicals as riot control agents. An example of this occurred in October 2002 when Russian forces used a fentanyl derivative to end a hostage situation in a theater (7). Unfortunately, this event resulted in several unintentional deaths among the hostages.

The tactical medic must be prepared to recognize when these agents are present, identify exposed personnel, and provide necessary field treatment, all the while protecting oneself and one's team. Agents that rapidly kill or incapacitate are most likely to prevent the team from completing its mission so the tactical medic must be familiar with the effects of nerve agents, cyanides, choking agents, vesicants, and incapacitating agents. Agents with delayed onset, such as radioactive material, biologics, may not interfere with short missions but will require postevent decontamination and observation or quarantine.

This chapter provides an overview of the more serious chemical, biological, and radiological threats that the tactical medic may encounter. It focuses on recognition of exposure field treatment options and appropriate operational responses. Extraction and casualty transport are covered in other parts of the book.

SIGNS AND SYMPTOMS: IDENTIFYING EXPOSURE

In some cases your team may have intelligence about threats that will allow increased awareness and use of protective equipment at the start of the mission. During an operation you will need to constantly assess the situation for possible threats. Your team may carry chemical and/or radiological sensors. There is a variety of sensors available and many factors must be considered regarding their use (8). Chemicals can be identified with detection papers or air sampling devices. Radiation detection devices such as survey meters and dosimeters are discussed further in Chapters 40 and 41. The use of detection equipment requires training and maintenance programs. In the absence of good intelligence or detection equipment, presenting signs and symptoms will be your indicator that a team member has been contaminated.

Clinical identification of a chemical, biological, or radiological agent exposure is performed by assessing the signs and symptoms of those exposed as well as taking a good history. The history should always include when the signs and symptoms started and whether an odor was present at the scene. Depending on what the patient was exposed to, the onset of signs and symptoms will vary. For example, chemicals will primarily be quick-acting (minutes to hours), whereas biological agents may take days to weeks to manifest signs and symptoms, and radiological agents can take weeks to months for signs and symptoms to appear. Although an odor may not be a sensitive indicator due to the high level of olfactory variability in people, it may, when noted, still be a valuable clue as to agent presence and identification.

CHEMICAL AGENTS

Signs and Symptoms

Quick-Acting Chemical Agents

Depending on the amount and route of exposure, chemicals tend to act quickly, causing local or systemic

▶ **TABLE 39.1. Chemical Agents.**

Agent	Signs and Symptoms	Onset of Action	Persistence
Vesicant/blister agents	Blisters, erythema, pain	Seconds to hours	Persistent
Nerve agent	Seizures, shortness of breath, vomiting, diarrhea, miosis[a]	Seconds to minutes	Volatile (GB) Persistent (VX)
Choking agents	Wheezing, pulmonary edema	Seconds to minutes	Volatile
Cyanides	Shortness of breath without cyanosis, seizures	Seconds to minutes	Volatile

[a]Miosis: pinpoint pupils. Toxidrome for severe exposure is SLUDGEM: salivation, lacrimation, urination, defecation, gastrointestinal distress, emesis, miosis.

symptoms within seconds to hours (see Table 39.1). They can cause damage through skin contact, inhalation, or ingestion. Protection from chemical agents relies on the use of appropriate personal protection equipment with chemical filter masks and skin barriers. The chemical's physical and pharmacological properties determine what risk the chemical poses. Chemicals that evaporate quickly or are volatile present a respiratory risk and chemicals that are persistent or oily may get on clothing and equipment and present a contact risk that might outlast the initial contact, so decontamination is extremely important. Always prenotify the hospital when bringing in a patient suspected of chemical contamination and notify them if any decontamination has already been performed.

Seizures

If the patient is experiencing seizures, always check for hypoglycemia and determine if the patient has a history of seizures or if there was recent head trauma. With the patient not in a bright light, check the patient's pupils; if the patient's pupils are pinpoint (miosis), the chemical agent is likely to be one that affects the central nervous system. The most likely chemical group is acetylcholinesesterase inhibitors: nerve agents or a class of pesticide called an organophosphate. However, it could be an opioid incapacitating agent. Enlarged pupils may indicate the use of BZ or some other antimuscarinic incapacitating agent, but these generally do not cause seizures. If, however, pupils are normal or slightly dilated, and if the patient was in an enclosed space without good ventilation or airway protection, then the patient might have been exposed to cyanide. All personnel need to immediately move to fresh air upwind of the area and patients need to be treated according to the severity of their signs and symptoms (Table 39.1). If there is intelligence that suggests the team may be exposed to a nerve agent, particularly soman, pretreatment with pyridostigmine has been recommended but not been proven to be efficacious (9).

Nausea and Vomiting

If you or your team members are exhibiting pinpoint pupils, nausea, and vomiting, this could again be due to an

exposure to an acetylcholinesterase inhibitor, that is, nerve agent or organophosphate. Move upwind, decontaminate, and treat appropriately (Fig. 39.1). However, if pupils are *not* pinpoint but team members are having nausea and vomiting, this could indicate another type of exposure such as high-dose radiation or low levels of phosgene vapor. Move out of the area to an upwind location, decontaminate your team members, and take them to the emergency department (ED) for further evaluation. Be sure to alert the ED staff that this could have been a chemical exposure and that the patient has already been decontaminated (you should make sure that your team member's weapon has been secured prior to arrival at the hospital). Do not be surprised if the ED chooses to decontaminate the patient again.

Skin Burning and Blistering

Most of the time, blister/vesicant agents are *persistent* in the environment. They are oily in consistency so they remain in the environment for a long time, as well as on skin, clothing, and equipment (6). Until washed off, they continue to be a contact hazard for the patient as well as

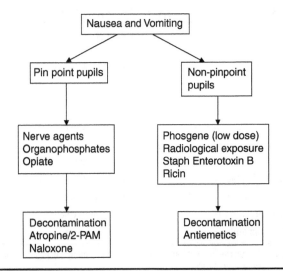

FIGURE 39.1. Nausea and vomiting algorithm for unknown exposure.

for the tactical and health care team. Furthermore, if the chemical has been aerosolized or is *volatile* by nature, then it is a risk to the respiratory tract and the eyes. It is important to realize that the time from contact to symptoms depends on the chemical itself. Mustard is insidious and has a gradual presentation of signs and symptoms, but some agents, such as lewisite, phosgene oxime, and T-2 mycotoxin, rapidly produce burning and blistering of exposed skin. The burning sensation can lead to team members' panic and the removal of their protective equipment as they rush to get rid of the burning sensation. This would cause them to be susceptible to a more significant injury through inhalation. If there is intelligence that suggests the team may be exposed to mustard vapor, pretreatment with *N*-acetylcysteine for 3 to 30 hours pre-exposure has been recommended but, again, not proven effective in human subjects (10) (Fig. 39.2 and Table 39.2).

Shortness of Breath and/or Wheezing

If your team members complain of shortness of breath, move them immediately into fresh air, then perform a check of their airway and breathing, without forgetting to check their pupils. If pupils are pinpoint, this could indicate an acetylcholinesterase inhibitor or possibly an aerosolized opiate incapacitator, such as fentanyl derivatives.

If the pupils are dilated and the patient continues to be in respiratory distress, with signs of bronchoconstriction or wheezing, administer bronchodilators. If the patient is not wheezing and complaining of not being able to breathe, consider the use of cyanide antidotes (cyanide antidote kit or hydroxocobalamin). Determine whether anyone noticed any odors in the room, which might be able to help identify the agent; an odor of fresh-mown hay

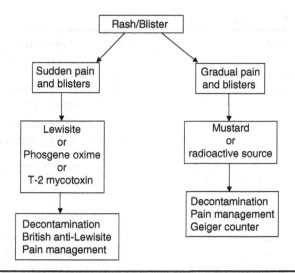

FIGURE 39.2. Rash/blister algorithm for unknown exposure.

could indicate phosgene, which can cause noncardiogenic pulmonary edema; a faint odor of almonds could indicate cyanide; and a garlic, mustard odor might indicate the vesicant mustard (Table 39.2 and Fig. 39.3).

Slower-Acting Chemical Agents: Minutes to Hours

Shortness of Breath and/or Wheezing

If, after exposure to a vapor, team members present with shortness of breath and mild wheezing, these could be early signs of noncardiogenic pulmonary edema from phosgene. If wheezing is not a sign and your team member is generally weak, complains of double vision (diploplia),

▶ **TABLE 39.2. Category A Biological Agents.**

Agent	Signs and Symptoms	Onset of Action	Treatment	Contagious
Smallpox[a]	High fever and b-b pellet lesions	Days	Supportive; vaccine for all who have been in contact but who are not yet symptomatic	Highly
Tularemia (rabbit fever)	Fever, cough, skin lesions	Days	Antibiotics	No
Viral hemorrhagic fever	High fever, petechia, bleeding from gums	Days	Supportive care	Highly
Pneumonic plague	Fever, bloody sputum	Days	Antibiotics	Yes
Bubonic plague	Fever, painful lymph nodes	Days	Antibiotics	No
Pulmonary anthrax	Fever, cough, bloody sputum	Days	Antibiotics	No
Cutaneous anthrax	Black, painless, eschar	Days	Antibiotics	No

[a]Depending on the public health department, quarantine will probably be instituted for those who have been exposed but are not yet symptomatic

From Darling RG, Catlett CL, Huebner KD, et al. Threats in bioterrorism. I: CDC category A agents. *Emerg Med Clin North Am.* 2002;20(2):273–309, with permission.

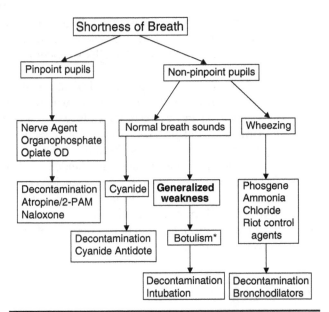

FIGURE 39.3. Shortness of breath algorithm for unknown exposure. *The weakness is descending in nature. It generally begins as double vision, difficulty speaking, and difficulty swallowing. This is followed by generalized muscle weakness and respiratory arrest due to the inability to control intercostal and other respiratory muscles.

and has difficulty breathing, this could indicate botulinum toxin, which can cause a descending paralysis. Check for facial drooping, a loss of facial wrinkles, difficulty making words (dysphonia), and difficulty swallowing.

Skin Burning and Blistering

The timing of when blisters and skin redness appear, and the location of the blisters, is important for agent identification, which might help with treatment. If the blisters appeared on the same day as the event and are found on areas of the body that were not exposed, the agent could be the vesicant/blister agent mustard. If the burning and blistering is immediate, then the chemical could be an industrial acid or base, or it could be from one of the military agents lewisite or phosgene oxime. However, if the signs and symptoms appear days after the mission, you should obtain a complete history of events leading up to the symptoms, as they could be due to exposure to a radioactive source. For example, during the mission the symptomatic person might have picked up a radioactive object and put it in a pocket over the site of the rash/burn (Fig. 39.3).

Treatment of Chemical Exposure

Nerve Agents and Organophosphates

Treat team members who are exposed to acetylcholinesterase inhibitors, that is, nerve agents or organophos-

phates, by administering atropine, pralidoxime, and, in the case of seizures or altered mental status, a benzodiazepine such as diazepam or midazolam. These treatments are available in prefilled autoinjectors designed for field use. In 2006 the U.S. Food and Drug Administration approved a binary autoinjector containing atropine and pralidoxime for civilian use that is similar to the military's Mark II kit. The atropine will dry up the secretions; the pralidoxime stops the localized muscle fasciculations (twitching) and will prevent "aging" of the offensive chemical agent so it does not become permanently bound to the receptor; and the benzodiazepine stops the seizures. The number of autoinjectors used on the symptomatic patient depends on the severity of the signs and symptoms exhibited. The more severe the patient, the greater the number of autoinjectors that should be administered in the field.

If you have been treating a team member with suspected nerve agent exposure who has not been decontaminated, and you are feeling slightly short of breath or having difficulty seeing, then you should administer one autoinjector kit to yourself and to other team members who are slightly symptomatic. Make sure you are wearing appropriate personal protection equipment and decontaminate your patient. Any team member who has received an autoinjector, even for a false alarm, should be evaluated at the ED. It is very important to decontaminate all team members and equipment, the hospital must be notified in advance whether or not a thorough decontamination has taken place, and the team should suggest that the hospital set up and decontaminate the patients prior to their coming in to the ED so as to protect the ED and staff.

Symptomatic Cyanide Exposure

The mainstay of treatment of potential cyanide exposure is removing the patient from continued exposure and providing oxygen. Symptomatic exposure to cyanide may require the use of a cyanide antidote. There are two antidotes available. A three-part kit (butyl nitrite, sodium nitrite, and sodium thiosulfate) has been used in the United States since the 1950s. The first two parts are nitrites, used as temporizing measures to help displace the cyanide from its binding sites and will cause hypoxemia in the form of methemoglobin. The third part is thiosulfate, which allows the cyanide to be secreted harmlessly in the urine and is the definitive treatment for a patient with symptomatic cyanide intoxication. You should familiarize yourself with the components of the kit prior to using it, as it contains multiple components.

Hydroxocobalamin was recently approved for use in the United States but has been used by the French fire service for many years for the treatment of symptomatic patients with cyanide poisonings from fires. Hydroxocobalamin is a precursor of vitamin B-12. It binds to the cyanide in the body, creating cyanocobalamin, which can then be harmlessly secreted in the urine. Unlike nitrites it does not reduce the oxygen carrying capacity. The main side effect of this drug is reddening of the skin and urine.

Botulism Intoxication

This toxin comes from the *Botulinum* bacterium. If aerosolized and respired, it can cause paralysis of all skeletal muscles including those that control respiration. These patients will complain of double vision, difficulty swallowing, difficulty speaking, and drooping eyes (11). Additionally, there will be generalized weakness with eventual respiration compromise. There is no field antidote and patients need to be taken to a hospital with an intensive care unit. There is an antitoxin available only through the Centers of Disease Control, however, there is a strict protocol for ordering it and for its release, and you must go through local public health first. Poison control (1-800-222-1222), your toxicologist, or your local bioterrorism coordinator should be able to assist you with the proper procedures.

BIOLOGICAL OR RADIOLOGICAL EXPOSURE

Signs and Symptoms

Delayed Signs and Symptoms

When nonspecific signs and symptoms of general malaise, hair loss, vomiting, or rash start days to weeks after an exposure, you should consider that the causative agent may be biological or radiological (11). It will be important to elicit a history not only from your sick team members, but also from their families, for several reasons: if the cause is biological, the history obtained from family members could help determine whether the agent is contagious; if the cause is radiological, it will be necessary to evaluate and follow family members for long-term effects of the radioactive material exposure. Additionally, there are many weaponized biological agents such as tularemia and anthrax that can mimic influenza (Table 39.2) (11). Check with local pubic health or hospitals to see if there are clusters of people with similar symptoms, or anyone with unusually severe symptoms, or if this "flu" is virulent and occurring at an unusual time of the year.

Cough with Fever

As stated above, the majority of weaponized biological agent infections will present with influenzalike symptoms (Fig. 39.5). It is important to take a good history of your symptomatic team members. You should ask about the

health of their close contacts, as this will give a good indication of whether this is a contagious agent and, if so, how virulent the agent is (smallpox, pneumonic plague).

An indicator of contagion for a biological agent is hemoptysis (blood in the sputum). This is seen with several contagious biological agents: pneumonic plague, tuberculosis, and viral hemorrhagic fever (Ebola). Cough without bloody sputum is less contagious. Examples include tularemia (rabbit fever), influenza, anthrax, glanders, and Q fever. If you feel that a team member has suspicious signs and symptoms and that this might be contagious, make sure you alert the ED prior to arrival, so they can prepare a negative-pressure room and can put on appropriate personal protection equipment.

Rash with Fever

Typically, a rash caused by a biological weapon will be accompanied by a high fever (Fig. 39.4). Aside from taking a detailed history, consider the location of the rash on the body. Does it affect the palms and soles of the feet? Is it painful to the touch? Is it isolated or systemic? For example, smallpox begins with a prodromal high fever, followed by lesions in the mouth, followed by a generalized vesicular rash, which is more concentrated on the extremities and head. The lesions are all at the same stage of development and are hard and painful to the touch. Cutaneous anthrax lesions are black and edematous but not painful. However, if the lesions are painful, they could be bubonic plague or cutaneous tularemia.

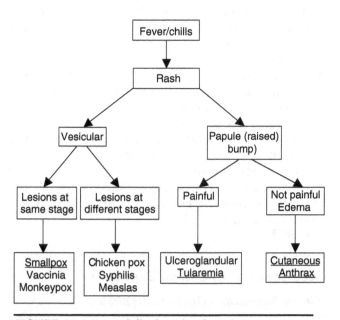

FIGURE 39.4. Fever/chills algorithm for unknown exposure.

▶ **TABLE 39.3. Radiation Exposure.**

Dose	Is Patient Radioactive?[a]	Signs and Symptoms	Onset of Action	Treatment
Local	Yes, possibly	Erythema, blistering, pain	Hours to days	Decontamination, radiation officer
Internal	Yes	Nausea, vomiting, anorexia, diarrhea	Hours to days	Decontamination, radiation officer, chelating agents, potassium iodine
Whole body	No	Nausea, vomiting, anorexia, diarrhea	Hours to days	Decontamination, radiation officer

[a]The use of a Geiger counter is useful for external contamination. More than 90% of the radioactive contamination will dissipate after clothing removal, showering, and hair washing. Internal contamination from inhalation, incorporation through wounds, and ingestion is much more serious but has never been shown to be harmful to the first responder or first receiver.

Rash without Fever

Look at the rash itself. Is it generally distributed over the body? If the rash is confined to one area of the body, especially just under a pocket, you should consider that this was caused by a radioactive source (Table 39.3). In the history, determine if the team member picked up any object from the scene and put it into a pocket next to the affected area of the skin. Also, generalized malaise with nausea and occasional vomiting can be an indication of radiation exposure (Table 39.3).

Swollen Lymph Nodes

If a team member presents with swollen lymph nodes in the groin, neck, or axilla, you should perform an examination to see if there is a bite or an infection distally. Bite sites should be examined to see if they are painful to the touch. Additionally, you should ask about what the team member was doing the previous week, as this may provide relevant information about possible sources. For example, had this individual been hunting and skinning rabbits? If so, this could be tularemia. Or was this person in New Mexico with others who are now complaining of similar symptoms? If so, this could be bubonic plague or Hanta virus. Tularemia, bubonic plague, and Hanta virus are not contagious (Tables 39.2 and 39.3).

Treatment of Exposure to Biological or Radiological Agents

Depending on the agent and level of contagion, one of the most important treatments is good nursing care. Bacterial infections like anthrax and plague can be treated with antibiotics. Viral infections like smallpox and viral hemorrhagic fever do not have a definitive treatment. Botulinum toxin is treated with respiratory support; it can be treated with botulinum antitoxin available through the local health department, which will request it from the Centers for Disease Control.

TAKE-HOME POINTS

1. Recognition of clinical signs and symptoms that are suggestive of exposure to a chemical, biological, or radiological agent exposure is an expected skill of the tactical medic.
2. Utilization of appropriate levels of hazardous material exposure personal protective equipment and decontamination methods is an important skill for the tactical medic.
3. Knowledge of time to onset of symptoms and signs, as well as level of functional incapacity likely, after exposure to hazardous materials is important to the tactical medic. Failure to know this will jeopardize all the tactical operators as well as mission completion.

SUMMARY

Throughout recorded history, hazardous materials have been used as weapons. For the tactical medic, an encounter with hazardous materials release may occur in conjunction with other commonly encountered scenarios such as those involving risk of blast or penetrating trauma. Therefore, the tactical medic not only must be prepared to deal with blast and penetrating injuries, but must be able to recognize the signs and symptoms of biological, chemical, and radiological injury and treat them appropriately (Table 39.4). The potential encounter with such hazardous materials clearly demonstrates the importance of appropriate knowledge of and skill in utilization of personal protective equipment and decontamination methods.

▌**TABLE 39.4. Chemical Agents and Adult Treatment.**

Chemical Agent	Treatment	Indication	Adult Dose
Nerve agent	Atropine	Various signs and symptoms of SLUDGEM	2 mg IVP or IM every 2 min until signs and symptoms resolve *or* IM autoinjectors[a]
	Pralodoxime	Various signs and symptoms of SLUDGEM, especially the nicotinic effects	600–900 mg over 15–30 min IV or IM, may be repeated once *or* IM autoinjectors[a]
	Diazepam	Only for seizures	5–10 mg IVP every 5–10 min for seizure control *or* IM autoinjectors[a]
Vesicant	Pain medication	Pain	Per protocols
	British antilewisite	Only if vesicant is known to be lewisite	Per protocols
Choking agent	Bronchodilators	Dyspnea, wheezing, pulmonary edema	β_2-Agonist inhaler or injection based on symptoms
Cyanide (blood agent)	Amyl nitrate	Temporizing measure: severe dyspnea or seizures.	One ampoule inhaled for 30 s, may be repeated every 3–5 min until definitive treatment; causes methemoblobinemia, and caution should be taken when used in hypotensive or hypoxic patients
	Sodium nitrate	Temporizing measure: severe dyspnea or seizures	300 mg IV over 15–30 min; causes methemoblobinemia, and caution should be taken when used in hypotensive or hypoxic patients
	Sodium thiosulfate	Definitive treatment: severe dyspnea or seizures	12.5 g IV over 20–30 min
	or Hydroxocobolamine	Definitive treatment: severe dyspnea or seizures	5 g IV over 15 min; repeat every 15 min as needed

Note. All of these exposures require evaluation in the hospital setting. Symptomatic team members as well as all medical field contacts should go through dry and wet decontamination before transport inside a treatment facility.

[a]Autoinjectors for acetylcholinesterase inhibitors contain 2 mg of atropine, 600 mg of pralidoxime (2-PAM), or 10 mg of diazepam. Depending on the severity of the signs and symptoms, up to three kits can be used per severely symptomatic team member.

Data from Refs. 12–15.

REFERENCES

1. USDHHS. *Hazardous Substances Emergency Events Surveillance, Annual Report 2003.* Washington, DC: U.S. Department of Health and Human Services, Agency for Toxic Substances and Disease Registry; 2003.
2. Smart JK. History of chemical and biological warfare: an American perspective. In: Sidell F, Takafuji E, Franz D, eds. *Medical Aspects of Chemical and Biological Warfare.* Bethesda, MD: Office of the Surgeon General, U.S. Army; 1997:11–47.
3. Urbanetti JS. Toxic Inhalational Injury. In: Sidell F, Takafuji E, Franz D, eds. *Medical Aspects of Chemical and Biological Warfare.* Bethesda, MD: Office of the Surgeon General, U.S. Army; 1997:247–270.
4. Brulliard K. Chlorine blasts kill 8; 6 troops also die in Iraq. *Washington Post*, March 18, 2007:sect 20.
5. Okumura T, Takasu N, Ishimatsu S, et al. Report on 640 victims of the Tokyo subway sarin attack. *Ann Emerg Med.* 1996;28(2):129–135.
6. Sidell FR, Urbanetti JS, Smith WJ, et al. Vesicants. In: Zajtchuk R, ed. *Medical Aspects of Chemical and Biological Warfare.* Bethesda, MD: Office of the Surgeon General, U.S. Army; 1997:197–228.
7. Wax PM, Becker CE, Curry SC. Unexpected "gas" casualties

in Moscow: a medical toxicology perspective. *Ann Emerg Med.* 2003;41(5):700–705.
8. CBRNE—Chemical detection equipment. 2006. Available at: http://www.emedicine.com/emerg/topic924.htm. Accessed June 13, 2007.
9. Dunn MA, Hackley BE, Sidell FR. Pretreatment for nerve agent exposure. In: Sidell F, Takafuji E, Franz D, eds. *Medical Aspects of Chemical and Biological Warfare.* Bethesda, MD: Office of the Surgeon General, U.S. Army; 1997:181–196.
10. Bobb AJ, Arfsten DP, Jederberg WW. N-Acetyl-L-cysteine as prophylaxis against sulfur mustard. *Mil Med.* 2005;170(1):52–56.
11. Darling RG, Catlett CL, Huebner KD, et al. Threats in bioterrorism. I: CDC category A agents. *Emerg Med Clin North Am.* 2002;20(2):273–309.
12. Gracia R, Shepherd G. Cyanide poisoning and its treatment. *Pharmacotherapy.* 2004;24(10):1358–1365.
13. McManus J, Huebner K. Vesicants. *Crit Care Clin.* 2005;21(4):707–718, vi.
14. Sidell FR. Nerve agents. In: Sidell F, Takafuji E, Franz D, eds. *Medical Aspects of Chemical and Biological Warfare.* Bethesda, MD: Office of the Surgeon General, U.S. Army; 1997:129–179.
15. Traub SJ, Hoffman RS, Nelson LS. Case report and literature review of chlorine gas toxicity. *Vet Hum Toxicol.* 2002;44(4):235–239.

Personal Protective Equipment for the Tactical Team

Greene Shepherd, Dorothy Lemecha, Jeffery C. Metzger, Phillip Carmona, and Robert Dickerson

OBJECTIVES

After reading this section, the reader will be able to:

1. Occupational Safety and Health Administration and National Institute of Occupational Safety and Health safety standards regarding personal protective equipment (PPE)
2. The history of PPE
3. Airway and dermal protection methods of PPE
4. What is necessary in a PPE program including medical screening
5. The pros and cons of the different levels of PPE

HISTORIC PERSONAL PROTECTIVE EQUIPMENT PERSPECTIVE

In today's world the threat of terrorism with chemical, biological, radiological, or nuclear weapons is higher than ever, prompting an increase in public/civil awareness and preparedness for these potential disasters. Public service agencies such as law enforcement, emergency medical services (EMS), and fire are among the first to respond to render care, establish order, and gather evidence in such an event. The tactical team is likely to be called on for operations when an unconventional weapon threat is known or suspected. Duties in such situations may include apprehension of suspects, hostage rescue operations, dignitary protection missions, or standoffs where the use of such weapons is threatened or used. In such operations, to avoid becoming casualties themselves, tactical teams must be appropriately trained and equipped with personal protective equipment (PPE), which protects the wearer from inhalation and dermal exposure from hazardous materials.

The Environmental Protection Agency (EPA) and Occupational Safety and Health Administration (OSHA) have defined four levels of PPE based on respiratory protection: Levels A to D (Table 40.1). The level of protection necessary for a given environment depends on the toxicity of the agent, the form it is in (gas, liquid or solid), the length of ex-

posure to the hazard, and the duties to be performed in the hazardous environment. It is critical for the tactical team to understand the benefits and limitations of each level of protection and select the appropriate type of PPE to allow the team to perform its mission as safely as possible.

The use of PPE in the workplace is regulated by OSHA, whose mission is assuring the safety and health of America's workers by setting and enforcing workplace standards; providing training, outreach, and education; establishing partnerships; and encouraging continual improvement in workplace safety and health (1). OSHA works in partnership with the Centers for Disease Control (CDC) and the National Institute of Occupational Safety and Health (NIOSH) to create national safety standards. These are augmented by state and local safety and health regulations. Regulations for PPE are found in hazardous waste operations and emergency response (HAZWOPER) standards 29 CFR 1910.120 and 29 CFR 1910.134 (2,3).

It is important to note that military PPE standards are not equivalent to OSHA's regulations (1–5). In the United States, law enforcement agencies are governed by OSHA regulations rather than military standards. This has been a source of confusion for the law enforcement community when selecting equipment and creating policies and procedures. However, there is an ongoing effort by NIOSH, law enforcement, and the U.S. military to establish clearer standards (1).

▶ **TABLE 40.1. Occupational Safety and Health Administration Personal Protective Equipment Levels and Respiratory Protection Utilized.**

Level	Description	Equipment	Pros	Cons
A	At the site of a CBNRE event or when atmosphere has <19.5% oxygen	Positive-pressure, full-face-piece, SCBA or positive pressure-supplied air respirator with escape SCBA, approved by NIOSH Totally encapsulating chemical-protective suit	Highest level of airway and skin protection	Communication in SCBA almost-nonexistent Very expensive Duration of use limited by air available Very bulky
B	At a CBRNE event or when <19.5% oxygen is available, but the highest level of skin protection is not necessary	Positive-pressure, full-face-piece SCBA or positive pressure-supplied air respirator with escape SCBA (NIOSH approved) High level of skin protection not required		Expensive Limited by air available Bulky and isolated
C	Concentration(s) and type(s) of airborne substance(s) known and criteria for using APRs met	APR/PAPR Splash- and vapor-resistant clothing	Not as much training involved If the battery dies in the PAPR unit the mask will revert to a negative-pressure respirator	PAPR: Hose connecting blower to filter provides an easy way for someone to pull the mask off the wearer. Hose can be crimped by equipment Blower is noisy, reducing the ability to communicate and making the mask unusable for stealth tactical operations
D	Normal work clothing A work uniform affording minimal protection: used for nuisance contamination only		Normal workwear	No respiratory protection.

NIOSH, National Institute for Occupational Safety and Health; CBRNE, chemical, biological, radiological, nuclear, and explosive; SCBA, self-contained breathing apparatus; APR, air-purifying respirator; PAPR, powered air-purifying respirator.

In this chapter, we review the four levels of OSHA-designated PPE and their various safety components, attributes, and limitations for the tactical team. Additionally, necessary medical monitoring and components of a PPE storage and maintenance program are also discussed. Note that although this chapter provides an overview of PPE, the authors strongly recommend that tactical teams and law enforcement agencies consult with an on-site expert when selecting and training with PPE. This consultant should make certain that team members can properly don and doff the equipment, perform maintenance, and understand the equipment's strengths and weaknesses for the various situations for which it may be used. PPE that is inappropriate, improperly worn, or poorly maintained can be more devastating to an officer's safety than no PPE at all (1).

There are three ways to be adversely affected by a chemical, biological, or radiological agent: inhalational, dermal, and gastrointestinal. Inhalation exposures have the fastest onset and can rapidly incapacitate personnel. It is because of this that OSHA defines PPE levels on respiratory protection (1). Although important in their own right, dermal and gastrointestinal routes of contamination can be protected against by wearing protective clothing and gloves and by not eating or drinking at the scene without being decontaminated first.

RESPIRATORY PROTECTION FOR PERSONAL PROTECTION EQUIPMENT

OSHA and NIOSH have specified respiratory protection levels based on concentrations of chemicals that would

▶ **TABLE 40.2.** Effects on the Body of an Oxygen-deficient Atmosphere.

Oxygen Concentration	Effect on Person in that Environment
19.5%	Minimum permissible level
15%–19%	Decreased manual dexterity
10%–12%	Cyanosis to lips, nails
8%–10%	Mental failure, unconsciousness
6%–8%	8 min: 100% fatal
4%–6%	40 s: coma, convulsions, death

Adapted from Clayton GD, Clayton FE, eds. *Patty's Industrial Hygiene and Toxicology.* 3rd. ed. New York: John Wiley & Sons; 1978; Arca VJ, Marshall SM, Lake WA, et al. *An Interim Summary Report for Law Enforcement, and Emergency Medical Services Protective Ensemble Testing.* Edgewood, MD: Abdereen Proving Ground, U.S. Army Soldier and Biological Command; 1999; and U.S. Occupational Safety and Health Administration. *OSHA Best Practices for Hospital Based First Receivers of Victims from Mass Casualty Incidents Involving the Release of Hazardous Substances.* Washington, DC: OSHA; 2005.

be immediately dangerous to life and health (IDLH) and permissible exposure limits (PEL) for chemicals and radiological entities. Additionally, the OSHA/EPA designations were created to describe the respiratory protection that employers must provide for workers.

In the tactical arena, a respiratory agent can incapacitate your team, so respiratory protection is very important. However, unless going into a confined space where known chemicals exist, you will be in ambient air, and a comprehensive filter should be adequate. If the concentration of breathable of oxygen is <19.5% or the available oxygen is displaced by other gases, team members must bring in their own breathable atmosphere (2).

There are two general categories of respiratory protection: the *air-supplied respirator*, which is broken down into two types—the self-contained breathing apparatus (SCBA) and the supplied-air respirator (SAR); and the *air-purifying respirator* (APR), which filters the air but does not supply any supplemental oxygen. The two categories of respirators provide varying degrees of protection against airborne toxic hazards, such as an oxygen-depleted atmosphere, which would impair judgment and cause death (e.g., carbon monoxide or halogen) (Table 40.2). Per OSHA regulations 29 CFR 1910.134, if an agency is using a face-fitting mask for respiratory protection the supervisory agency and wearer need to comply with the following basic regulations.

- Medical evaluations prior to allowing the tactical member to participate
- Fit testing procedures provided by an OSHA-approved person
- Annual fit tests for the mask
- Procedures for proper use of the equipment
- Procedures for maintaining masks and filters
- Training requirements for tactical members who will be wearing respiratory protection

Self-contained Breathing Apparatus

The SCBA offers the highest level of respiratory protection available because wearers carry their own air supplies and wear full face masks. An example of this is what firefighters wear for respiratory protection when they go into a smoke-filled building. The SCBA includes a tank that supplies compressed air through a hose to a well-sealed face mask. This system is used in areas of low oxygen concentration, when the concentration of the hazardous agent is unknown, or if the oxygen concentration is known to be <19.5% by volume. Oxygen deficiency may occur in confined spaces, which include, but are not limited to, storage tanks, process vessels, towers, drums, tank cars, bins, sewers, septic tanks, underground utility tunnels, manholes, and pits.

Although SCBAs offer the highest level of respiratory protection, their tank capacity and size limit their usefulness in tactical situations. Wearers are limited to the amount of air they can carry on their backs. The length of time that the tanks will last is typically <1 h, though this is affected by the ambient temperature, the amount of physical exertion required, and the physical fitness of the wearer, which can make the length of time on air 20 min. Although the SCBA affords the highest level of airway protection, it is costly, the training involved is very intensive, and equipment upkeep can be time-consuming. It can also be dangerous if struck by a bullet or shrapnel, as it is a gas under pressure. The drawbacks mentioned above often preclude the use of SCBA in the law enforcement environment. However, some specially trained law enforcement agencies use SCBA regularly when serving warrants at dangerous locations such as methamphetamine laboratories. These officers know that they are going into a hazardous respiratory environment likely to contain anhydrous ammonia, Freon, acetone, hydriodic acid, toluene, and other hazardous and toxic chemicals.

Supplied-air Respirator

The SAR (Fig. 40.1) is a full face mask or a hood connected by an air hose to a remote air source. When it is a sealed mask, its requirements for use are under the purview of OSHA and its regulations for safe use. It has the advantage of being less bulky than the SCBA and allows the wearer to remain in the contaminated area for longer periods of time, as the amount of air is "unlimited." Drawbacks include limited mobility due to the length of the hose, the requirement to exit from the point of entry, and, if there is hose damage, the risk of breathing contaminated air. Because of the dynamic nature of a tactical environment, SARs are rarely used in law enforcement or in dynamic hazardous material areas. Additionally, per OSHA standards, the wearer must have an escape bottle of air in case there is a problem with the hose.

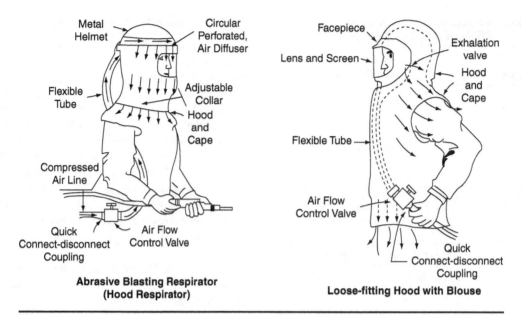

FIGURE 40.1. Air-supplied respirators. (From OSHA Technical Manual. Available at: www.osha.gov. Accessed March 27, 2007.)

Air-purifying Respirator

The concept of filtering atmosphere to make it less dangerous has been used to protect workers for many centuries; during Roman times Pliny (circa 23–79 A.D.) discussed the idea of using loose-fitting animal bladders in the mines to protect workers from the inhalation of red oxide of lead (6). World War I saw the advent of modern offensive chemical and biological weapons. Early in the war, soldiers had no respiratory protection, so they used urine-soaked handkerchiefs for primitive respiratory protection from the chlorine gas used. The Germans were the first to develop a mask that used pads soaked in bicarbonate and sodium thiosulfate, with some charcoal between the layers of gauze (7). By the end of the war, the basis of the modern "gas" mask had been developed and was used successfully for both soldiers and livestock.

APRs are classified and rated by how and what they filter. There are three types of APRs: *particulate, vapor,* and *combination.* Particulate filters, also known as mechanical filters, are nondiscriminating and are rated by the minimum size of particle they can filter. Early APRs used a mechanical filter with materials such as wool, glass, and/or cellulose to mechanically trap particles as air passes through. These are most useful for respiratory protection from biological infective agents, such as tuberculosis (N-95 respirator) and radiological particles. The thicker the filter and the finer the mesh, the more efficient it is at filtering-smaller sized particles. *Chemical filters* use sorbents and catalysts to remove gases and vapors from air drawn through the unit. The *combination* APR is a chemical filter with a particulate filter (2).

Respiratory protection is not new to the tactical team. During riots, respirators have been worn for protection from the riot control agents used to control crowds. However, the same cartridge that renders the wearer impervious to the effects of riot control agents will, with a high probability, not work for other chemicals such as nerve agents, blister agents, and HAZMAT chemicals. It is important to be sure that the filter cartridge not only fits your mask but also fits your needs for protection! There are many different chemical cartridges on the market and you should use only those that are NIOSH approved. Some of these approved cartridges are for very specific agents, such as riot control agents; others are more inclusive and will protect against chemical warfare agents such as nerve agents, cyanide, and vesicants. These filters may be used only if the ambient atmosphere has an oxygen concentration of no less than 19.5%. Additionally, if the cartridge is to be used in a chemical, biological, or radiological setting, it must meet NIOSH standards as described in 42 CFR, Part 84. It is important to understand the limitations of your equipment. Note that no canister/filter is rated for vapors or gases that have no odor, for example, carbon monoxide and carbon dioxide. The reason is that in the environment you are working in, if the canister is faulty and there is a leak, you will not be able to tell if you are being exposed to the gas or vapor.

Delivery System for Air-purifying Respirators

There are two types of delivery systems: *negative-pressure respirators* (Fig. 40.2), where the filtered air is supplied by the effort of the wearer's inhalation, like a standard gas mask; and the positive pressure *powered air-purifying respirator* (PAPR) (Fig. 40.3), which uses a motor to pull the ambient atmosphere through the filter and then blow the

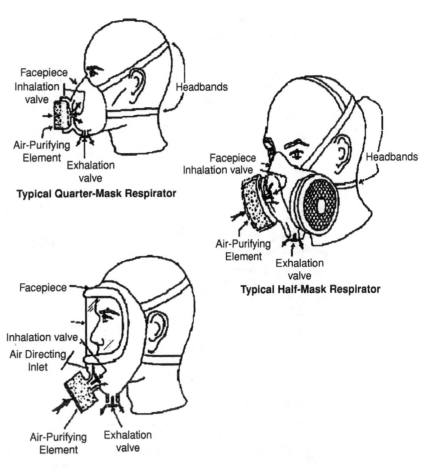

FIGURE 40.2. Full-face respirators. (From OSHA Technical Manual. Available at: www.osha.gov. Accessed March 27, 2007.)

filtered air into the wearer's face. The positive-pressure airway device can be used with both a mask and a hood, while the negative-pressure device may only be used with a form fitting mask. If a mask is used, you must follow OSHA's regulations for fit testing and training. The hooded device does not need to be fit tested and is adventitious for people with facial hair.

It is important to remember that since this type of respirator does not supply air, it cannot be used in oxygen-deficient atmospheres or some IDLH atmospheres where the gases or vapors present are at such high concentrations that the filters are quickly rendered useless. The filters can only be used for protection against the contaminants listed on the cartridge. Additionally, it is important that the wearer leave an area immediately if the smell of gas or vapor is detected inside the mask or if the breathing resistance increases.

Negative-pressure Air-purifying Respirators

One of the most important factors in selecting a mask is the fit and comfort for the tactical officer. As stated previously, all face-fitting respirators, per OSHA, must be fit tested annually. In addition, if wearers have undergone any

facial shape changes, that is, facial hair or weight loss or gain, they must also undergo a new fit test (1). If a mask is uncomfortable, the wearer may experience headaches or have leak points. Masks come in a full-face and a half-face configuration. For the tactical team the full-face type should be used and is recommended by the military and law enforcement experts. The face piece comes in three sizes: small, medium, and large. A drinking tube provides the ability to carry a canteen or other hydration device attachment when in a contaminated atmosphere for a prolonged period of time. Additionally, if the wearer needs to wear corrective lenses, there should be a removable spectacle kit for mounting corrective lenses inside the mask, as the tactical officer will not be able to wear normal glasses because the arms will break the mask seal.

Negative-pressure face pieces come in two styles: single and biocular lenses. The bi-ocular version, which the military uses, may limit the wearer's field of vision but offers better impact resistance for the mask. The single-lens mask offers a wider field of view with better peripheral vision. Regardless of the lens, it is important for the tactical team to make sure that there are mounting locations for the NIOSH-approved filter cartridge attachment point on both the right and the left sides, to allow the officer the

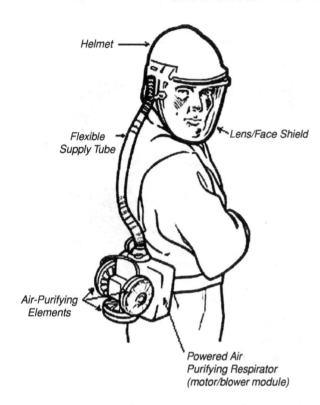

Loose-Fitting Facepiece

FIGURE 40.3. Powered air-purifying respirator, nonmedical. (From OSHA Technical Manual. Available at: www.osha.gov. Accessed March 27, 2007.)

ability to switch cartridge sides to facilitate shoulder firing of a weapon.

Positive-pressure Air-purifying Respirators

Another type of APR is the PAPR. This device filters ambient air and delivers it in a positive-pressure manner to the wearer. A battery-powered motor pulls air through filters and then blows it to the wearer via a hose connected to a face mask or hood. The motor and battery are typically worn on a belt or shoulder harness. Full-face mask-style PAPRs are better suited for tactical use. Hooded models are widely used in hospitals and in industry but are not practical for the tactical setting due to their impairment of vision and hearing.

With a PAPR the work required for breathing decreases and the inside of the mask is cooler compared to negative-pressure masks. As a safety feature, if the motor fails, the respirator reverts from a positive-pressure to a negative-pressure device, but because the air has to be "pulled" through a hose, the work required for breathing is greater than with a standard canister mask.

As this is a form-fitting mask, which can be used as a negative-pressure respirator mask, its use falls under normal OSHA guidelines for training and annual fit testing. Although the positive pressure created by the motor re-

duces heat buildup and decreases the work required for breathing, there are disadvantages for the tactical team.

- The hose from the blower to the filters provides a way for someone to pull the mask off.
- The hose can be crimped or cut and will then cut off the filtered air supply.
- The blower is noisy and is not suitable for stealth operations.
- The battery pack is heavy.

OTHER EQUIPMENT AND SAFETY CONSIDERATIONS: SUITS, BOOTS, AND GLOVES

Respirators provide the fundamental protection from inhaled threats but additional protective garments are needed. Such garments create a barrier between the skin and harmful materials. The most common and immediate danger from dermal contamination comes from strong acids or bases. Weapons with contact hazards such as lewisite, sulfur mustard, and T-2 mycotoxin should also be protected against. Barrier garments will also protect against radioactive contamination from alpha and beta particles, but will not effectively shield against ionizing radiation from gamma rays or neutrons. Fortunately, low-dose exposures such as would be expected with radiation dispersal devices (a.k.a. dirty bombs) or radioactive fallout are not considered to be IDLH. If the tactical team is responding to an incident with suspected radiological contamination, they should be issued dosimeters for medical monitoring, which should be worn inside protective clothing and close to the skin. Dermal absorption of chemicals with pharmacologic activity is uncommon but there are notable exceptions including nerve agents, pesticides, T-2 mycotoxin, and vesicants. Although, dermal exposure does not produce agent effects as rapidly as respiratory exposure, it can be just as debilitating or deadly. To protect the tactical team more completely, we must discuss suits, boots, and gloves. All of these are covered under OSHA requirements for PPE: OSHA standards 1910.132 (4).

Suits

It is important that all exposed areas of the body are protected. Even a mild contact irritant may cause tactical team members to lose focus or panic, causing them to remove gear or even respiratory protection. This tactic was first used in World War I when phosgene was dispersed with chlorine to "trick" soldiers into removing their gas masks (6).

Standard police tactical uniforms offer a degree of protection but are not adequate to ensure that mission objectives can be completed in an environment where hazardous materials are present (8). There are three categories of protective suits to be considered for the tactical environment: permeable, semipermeable, and nonpermeable. Suits are primarily rated on their permeability, degradation, and penetration of chemicals over time. OSHA has outlined the standards for protective suits in 29 CFR 1910.120 App B (5). In selecting protective suits, several factors must be considered: the substance the tactical officer will be exposed to; the concentration of the substance; and its physical form—solid, liquid, vapor, or gas. In addition, the team must look at the conditions they will be working in; the durability of the suit, including its ability to withstand crawling, lying on the ground, and moving through unconventional ingress/egress points; the noise factor of the suit; its fit, including the wearer's ability to manipulate weapons and equipment; and the costs associated with acquiring and training in the suit. Suit manufacturers must provide protection ratings and penetration times for specific chemicals if they are NIOSH approved.

Nonpermeable suits are normally used in Level A situations where the IDLH is high, the atmospheric risk is unknown, or the breathable atmosphere has an oxygen concentration of <19.5% (5). These suits are fully encapsulating, and wearers must supply their own oxygen (SCBA or SAR). They are waterproof, but the fabric is not quiet and most of these suits are for one-time use. Additionally, they do not dissipate heat well, and there is an increased risk of heat-related illness in warmer weather or climates. In the tactical environment, there is very little reason ever to wear this type of protection.

Semipermeable suits are used for Level B and C hazardous environments (Fig. 40.4). They are splash and vapor resistant (5). Depending on the chemical and the suit's degradation time and permeability factor for that chemical, these suits will do well in the "warm zone" (Table 40.3). They are not as expensive as Level A suits, however, the most common brands, Tyvek and Tychem, are loud and crinkly sounding. Additionally, these suits were not found to be rugged enough for the tactical environment. However, by contacting the manufacturer you can get the specifications for various suits, including figures on penetration, degradation, and permeation for a variety of chemicals.

Permeable suits consist of charcoal-lined or impregnated suits similar to military chemical protective gear. These air-permeable suits are designed to protect the wearer's skin from chemical vapor by filtering and reacting with chemical agents through absorption by the carbon-impregnated cloth. They are designed to trap vapors while allowing moisture to escape. These suits are cooler to wear, and they can be washed and reused if they have not been exposed to a chemical environment. They can be purchased in a variety of colors and are more durable to normal environmental stresses. The U.S. Army Soldier and Biological Chemical Command (SBCCOM) established a program to test some of these suits and the results are available for law enforcement and first responders (1). These suits are be-

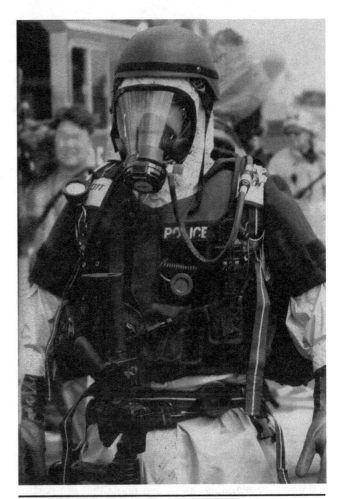

FIGURE 40.4. Level B suit. Note the full face mask and the hose over the left shoulder, connected to a self-contained breathing apparatus. (From Brockman K. 2007. *Police. The Law Enforcement Magazine*, August, p. 45, with permission.)

coming the garment of choice for general skin protection in the law enforcement realm when the tactical officer does not have to be in the "hot zone" or in the decontamination or warm zone.

Gloves

Various types of gloves are available, ranging from highly protective, very thick, and bulky (such as for Level A protection used by HAZMAT) to minimally protective latex gloves. In the tactical environment, the need to allow for manual dexterity to perform duties such as firing and reloading a firearm, handcuffing a suspect, and using other specialized tactical equipment is paramount. Similarly to the U.S. military, many law enforcement agencies are using cotton undergloves with butyl rubber gloves on top. When there is a need to maintain accuracy in firing a weapon, 7-mm butyl gloves are adequate. However, it was noted during testing that the glove's fingers can rip during pistol magazine reloading (1). Latex gloves are good protection

▶ **TABLE 40.3. HAZMAT Zones.**

Zone	Description	Level of PPE
Hot	At site of contamination	A/B
Warm	Area between site of contamination and noncontaminated areas	C
Cold	Area where there is no contamination hazard	D
Decontamination	Area where personnel, victims, and equipment are being cleaned	C with semipermeable suit

against bloodborne pathogens but provide little to no protection against chemical or radiological agents. Additionally, many people have an allergy to latex rubber, which can be limited to a contact dermatitis but can be severe enough to cause anaphylaxis. Because of this it is advisable to refrain from using latex gloves for Level C PPE.

Boots

Protection for the feet can range from paper-thin booties to thick, oversized PVC boots. The environment that a tactical officer is likely to encounter, such as liquid contamination and contaminated debris, should be considered when choosing footwear. It is important to try not to step into any contamination so as not to track it out of the area. Additionally, the ability of the tactical officer to move quickly and sure-footedly is equally important. There are three types of protective footwear: boots worn over shoes like galoshes, freestanding boots, and boots that are part of the protective suit. The thicker, more durable freestanding boots, although more expensive, will provide better protection in austere environments but may also limit mobility, as they are heavy and bulky. Additionally, if the wearer has larger calves, the standard boot cut may not fit. The other option for a work shoe covering is a rubber galosh; they are light and relatively inexpensive, and their sizing is general rather specific. They are often difficult to put on quickly and are not very sturdy for a rugged terrain. However, they are excellent for the radiological environment, where you want to be able to move quickly and have the protection of distance and shielding between your feet and the contamination. You should be aware that footies/booties sometimes come attached as a part of the protective suit. These do not have durable soles, so you should either cut them off or wear an overboot for better protection.

PUTTING IT ALL TOGETHER FOR THE TACTICAL TEAM: EQUIPMENT, MEDICAL MONITORING, AND TRAINING

Training and asking the right questions about the scenario (Table 40.4) are as important as the PPE worn. Once an

appropriate level of protection has been chosen, tactical team members should have ample training in donning and doffing, as well as performing their expected tasks while wearing, the equipment. PPE is significantly more cumbersome and bulky than the daily uniform a tactical officer usually wears. Issues such as wearing the ballistic vest and duty belt on the outside of the PPE must be addressed well before an incident takes place. The ability to maneuver and to accomplish the mission without adverse outcomes is the ultimate goal, and an effective training program is essential to its achievement. In the tactical environment, a respiratory threat can almost instantaneously incapacitate the team, so wearing the appropriate respiratory protection is important. In most situations that will mean that you will be wearing Level C protection.

■ Respiratory protection: negative-pressure APR or PAPR
■ Suit: permeable charcoal-lined, two-piece with a hood
■ Gloves: cotton undergloves with 7-mm butyl rubber overgloves
■ Boots: booties or regular rubber, hard-soled boots, dependings on the terrain and the hazard

A word of caution: Negative-pressure masks are very expensive, and there are many army and navy surplus stores

▶ **TABLE 40.4. Questions to Ask when Purchasing Personal Protective Equipment for the Tactical Team.**

1. Does the PPE provide the best protection for the specific agent?
2. Are the respirators well fitted, and do they create a good seal around the face?
3. Can a fully suited operator spend an adequate length of time in the contaminated area before being either exposed to the agent at large or adversely affected by the heat from wearing the suit?
4. Are the suits comfortable, and do they allow ease of movement sufficient to carry out the mission?
5. Do the masks allow wearers to see the environment without difficulty?
6. Can the operator wear tactical vests, operate weapons and other tactical equipment, and move with very little noise?
7. Do the gloves provide protection appropriate to the level of PPE but still allow an officer sufficient dexterity to operate weapons and other tactical equipment? Can the operator reload a weapon without tearing the gloves?

as well as Internet sites that sell surplus equipment for a fraction of the cost charged by established companies and suppliers. Buyers should beware, as not all filter canisters will fit on the older masks or they may not be NIOSH approved. Additionally, the protective mask's integrity will deteriorate over time and will reduce the protective qualities of the mask. It is important that you check the age of your mask and the availability of filters for it. The M17 mask, which has been phased out by the U.S. military, is used by many law enforcement groups, as these can purchased inexpensively or obtained for free; but it is important to realize that these masks are now more than 20 years old, and they will not provide adequate respiratory protection to the tactical team wearer.

Finally, a medical monitoring program is essential. OSHA regulations require at least annual medical evaluations for personnel who are expected to use PPE (2). This examination should include a general physical exam and respiratory testing. Immediately before and after operations where PPE use is expected, team members' general health status and vital signs should be monitored. It is also advisable to perform a follow-up health check either in person or by telephone the next day. A sample pre- and postevent health monitoring form is shown in Fig. 40.5.

TAKE-HOME POINTS

1. It is important to understand how your PPE works. Limitations can cause deaths or serious disruption of a mission.
2. PPE must be maintained in good condition and must follow manufacturers' recommendations for maintenance and upkeep.
3. All tactical team members who will be wearing PPE must have annual physicals and fit tests for fitted facemasks.
4. All tactical team members must have medical clearance vitals pre- and postdeployment.

SUMMARY

The use of PPE and medical monitoring is incredibly important for the safety of the individual and of the tactical team. However, wearing the wrong equipment or wearing the correct equipment but using it in the wrong way can have deadly consequences for the tactical team member wearing PPE. It is important that the tactical team understands the limitations of the equipment and trains with it so as to be able to use it appropriately and effectively.

GLOSSARY

Adsorb: To gather (gas, liquid, or dissolved substance) on a surface in a condensed layer (charcoal is an adsorbent

Air-purifying respirator: A respirator with an air-purifying filter, cartridge, or canister that removes specific air contaminants.

Degradation: A reduction in one or more physical properties of a protective material due to contact with a chemical

Filter cartridge: A container with a simple particle filter, sorbent, or catalyst, or a combination of these items, which removes specific contaminants from the ambient air

Fit protection rating (FPR): A multiple of the permissible exposure limit (a powered air-purifying respirator's FPR is 1,000)

HEPA filter: A high-efficiency particulate air filter, that is, a filter that is at least 99.97% efficient in removing monodisperse particles 0.3 μm in diameter. Good for infectious biological agents or radiological particles. Equivalent NIOSH 42 CFR 84 particulate filters: the N100, R100, and P100 filters

IDLH (immediately dangerous to life and health): An atmosphere that poses an immediate threat to life, would cause irreversible adverse health effects, or would impair an individual's ability to escape from a dangerous atmosphere. In most cases, egress from a particular worksite occurs in much less than 30 min, but as a safety margin, IDLH values are based on the effects that might occur as a consequence of a 30-min exposure.

OSHA 29 CFR 1910.120: Hazardous waste operations and emergency response standards set forth by the Department of Labor and OSHA

Penetration: The flow of a chemical through zippers, stitched seams, pores, or imperfections in materials

Permeation: The process by which a chemical moves through protective materials on a molecular level

Permissible exposure limit (PEL): Regulatory limits established to avoid adverse health effects from exposures, based on an 8-h workday/40-h workweek

Powered air-purifying respirator (PAPR): An air-purifying respiratory that uses a blower to force ambient air though filters; may be considered a positive-pressure device

Primary contamination: Direct contact to victim

Secondary contamination: Transfer of material from victim to personnel or equipment

Sorbent: A surface that causes absorption, adsorption, or a combination of the two processes

ON-SITE MEDICAL MONITORING (ENTRY TEAM)

NAME: _____

CASE: _____

CASE NO.: _____

DATE: _____ EXPOSURE RISK: HIGH / MED / LOW

PROTECTIVE EQUIPMENT: _____

SUBSTANCE(S) INVOLVED: _____

CONCENTRATION/LENGTH OF EXPOSURE: _____

MEDICAL TESTING: _____

COMMENTS:

****

**********PRE-ENTRY MEDICAL MONITORING:

WEIGHT: _____

TEMPERATURE: _____

METHOD: _____

PULSE: _____ BP: SYSTOLIC_____/DIASTOLIC_____

METHOD: _____ MONITORING CONDUCTED

BY: _____

****

********** POST-ENTRY MEDICAL MONITORING:

WEIGHT: _____ TEMPERATURE: _____

METHOD: _____ PULSE: _____

BP: SYSTOLIC_____/DIASTOLIC_____ METHOD: _____

MONITORING CONDUCTED BY: _____

COMMENTS:

FIGURE 40.5. Sample pre- and postevent medical monitoring form. (From U.S. Occupational Safety and Health Administration. *OSHA Best Practices for Hospital Based First Receivers of Victims from Mass Casualty Incidents Involving the Release of Hazardous Substances.* Washington, DC: OSHA; 2005.)

Vapor pressure: The pressure (expressed as millimeters of mercury; mm Hg) of a vapor in equilibrium with its liquid or solid form at a given temperature. The higher the vapor pressure, the greater the amount of chemical existing in the vapor phase. If >760 mm Hg at room temperature, the chemical exists as a gas.

Vesicant: A chemical agent used during warfare to produce blisters on the skin; developed for use during World War I and used in multiple conflicts since then. (Italy vs. Ethiopia, Iran–Iraq war)

REFERENCES

1. USASBC. *Guidelines for Use of Personal Protective Equipment by Law Enforcement Personnel During a Terrorist Chemical Agent Incident.* Edgewood, MD: U.S. Army Soldier and Biological Command; 2003.
2. Occupational Safety and Health Administration. OSHA respiratory standards 29.1910.134. Code of Federal Register. Available at: athttp://www.osha.gov/pls/oshaweb/owadisp.show_document?p_table =STANDARDS&p_id=12716. Accessed March 25, 2007.
3. HAZWOPER standards 29.1910.120. Code of Federal Register. Available at: http://www.osha.gov/pls/oshaweb/owadisp.show_document?p_table=STANDARDS&p_id=9765. Accessed March 25, 2007.
4. Occupational Safety and Health Administration. OSHA personal protective equipment standards 29.1910.132. Code of Federal Register. Available at: http://www.osha.gov/pls/oshaweb/owadisp.show_document?p_table=STANDARDS&p_id=9777.) Accessed March 27, 2007.
5. HAZWOPER standards Appendix B 29.1910.120. Code of Federal Register. Available at: http://www.osha.gov/pls/oshaweb/owadisp.show_document?p_table=STANDARDS&p_id=9767. Accessed March 25, 2007.
6. Smart JK. History of chemical and biological warfare: an American perspective. In: Sidell F, Takafuji E, Franz D, eds. *Medical Aspects of Chemical and Biological Warfare.* Bethesda, MD: Office of the Surgeon General, U.S. Department of the Army; 1997:11–47.
7. Clayton GD, Clayton FE, eds. *Patty's Industrial Hygiene and Toxicology.* 3rd. ed. New York: John Wiley & Sons; 1978.
8. Arca VJ, Marshall SM, Lake WA, et al. *An Interim Summary Report for Law Enforcement, and Emergency Medical Services Protective Ensemble Testing.* Edgewood, MD: Abdereen Proving Ground, U.S. Army Soldier and Biological Command; 1999.
9. U.S. Occupational Safety and Health Administration. *OSHA Best Practices for Hospital Based First Receivers of Victims from Mass Casualty Incidents Involving the Release of Hazardous Substances.* Washington, DC: OSHA; 2005.

Chapter 41

Decontamination for Tactical Teams

Kelly R. Klein, Paul T. Mayer, Greene Shepherd, Richard V. King, and Matthew Ratliff

OBJECTIVES

After reading this section, the reader will be able to:

1. Decontamination operations for casualties of chemical or radiological contamination.
2. Decontamination procedures for tactical team members in protective equipment exiting areas with suspected chemical or radiological contamination.
3. Unique features of likely contaminants with respect to decontamination.

Tactical law enforcement (TLE) is frequently dispatched to execute missions in potentially contaminated environments. Tactical teams should be trained in the use of personal protective equipment (PPE) and decontamination procedures for such situations. Most of these events will involve chemical, biological, or radiological (CBR) substances from occupational or industrial sources. Release of these substances can occur for a number of reasons: (i) natural disasters (hurricanes, tornadoes, floods, tsunamis, and earthquakes), (ii) industrial accidents (e.g., 3 Mile Island, Chernobyl, and Bhopal, India), and (iii) intentional acts of terror (chlorine tanker explosions, Iraq; sarin releases, Japan). In this chapter we discuss decontamination principles and procedures for removing chemical and radiological contamination.

Contaminants can be in any state of matter, that is, solid (particles), liquid, and gas/vapor. Gases and most vapors, by nature, are an inhalation risk rather than a contamination risk but some vapors *are* a contamination risk, as are solids and liquids. Depending on their properties, gases and vapors may cause problems downwind from the incident, and therefore their hazard zone areas may be elliptical and longer on one side, depending on the wind direction.

In general, there are two types of contamination.

- *Primary*: Direct transfer of contamination from the source to a person or the person's equipment
- *Secondary*: Transfer of contamination from a victim, or a victim's clothing or equipment, to another person or object

Primary contamination is most likely to occur during missions that put the team in direct proximity to the contaminant source, such as a methamphetamine lab or the site of an explosion or dispersal as it is occurring. If the TLE team is providing perimeter security for a casualty decontamination site, then secondary contamination is more likely to occur from the victims and from equipment. In this chapter we discuss various facets of decontamination in general and the particulars of TLE team decontamination for both officers and equipment.

DECONTAMINATION BASICS

Decontamination can be defined as the removal or neutralization of harmful substances. For discussion purposes, there are two categories of decontamination.

- *Dry decontamination*: Removal of contamination from skin and equipment without the use of water. Generally this means the removal of clothing for casualties. Specialized foams and powders are available for equipment.
- *Wet decontamination*: Use of water, soap, or bleach to deactivate or wash off contamination from skin and equipment. Use of bleach is ONLY for equipment. It should not be used for skin decontamination except in extraordinary circumstances (e.g., where there is no water supply or in military operations). If bleach needs to be used, it must be a 10:1 dilution of 5% household bleach and it must be made up fresh everyday. For contaminated people, washing with copious amounts of soapy water only is recommended.

There are three main purposes for victim decontamination: (i) removal of contaminant from the victims, (ii) prevention of secondary contamination of others, and (iii) psychological comfort of the victims. Depending on the time of year and how much clothing a person is wearing when contamination occurs, disrobine may remove up to 70%–90% of the contaminant from the victim. The rest of the contamination will be on the parts of the body not covered by clothing: hair, face, hands, and other exposed skin areas.

It depends on the event at hand, but plans in most areas call for mass civilian decontamination at the scene to be handled by the fire department, with assistance from emergency medical services (EMS) and other assigned agencies. Decontamination at a health-care facility that will be receiving patients should be handled by hospital decontamination, with support if possible from EMS or fire. Unless the product is known to be nontoxic and not a respiratory threat, personnel performing victim decontamination should wear at least Level C respiratory protection and a water-repellent suit. Zones will be established indicating levels or risk for contaminant exposure (Fig. 41.1). The postdecontamination zone (or cold zone) is uphill of water runoff and upwind of the site (Fig. 41.2).

It is important to remember that regardless of the air temperature, victims who have been contaminated should first perform dry decontamination by getting undressed and then undergo wet decontamination with generous amounts of flowing water (Fig. 41.3). This is to prevent further insult to the victim from the agent, but also to prevent secondary contamination of rescue workers and first receivers at the hospital. After wet

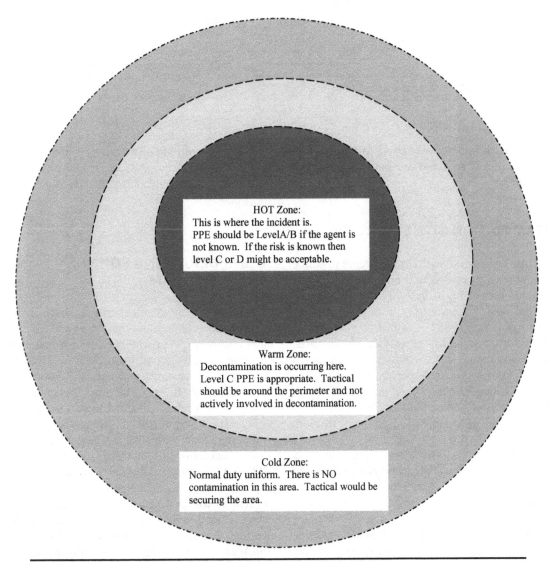

FIGURE 41.1. HAZMAT zones. These are fluid areas. Depending on the type of agent, terrain, and atmospheric conditions, the size and dimensions of the zones may change.

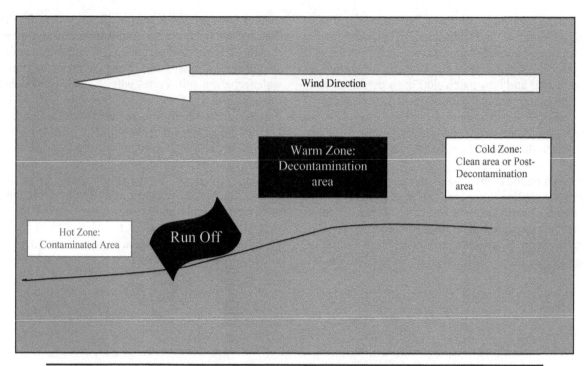

FIGURE 41.2. Decontamination zone. It must be uphill from the clean area but needs to be upwind of the HAZMAT site if there is an airborne risk.

decontamination it is imperative to cover patients, to conserve body heat, as well as to retriage patients for further medical assistance.

DECONTAMINATION SITE SELECTION

- *Location*: An area removed from the general public, preferably with easily controllable entry and exit points, should be selected. It must be upwind and upstream of the actual event. There must be a clearly delineated warm and cold zone.
- *Shower*: Warm water and no-tears soap are essential. There are many manufactured showers, which vary in cost (Fig. 41.4). However, a simple alternative is a PVC construction, which is simple to put up and take down. Runoff does not need to be contained. However, if possible, it should not be permitted to go into a drinking water supply.
- *Logistics*: Water source, electricity, lights, heating or cooling sources, clothes to change into, towels, an M291 kit (a carbonaceous adsorbent, a polystyrene polymeric, and ion exchange resins) for spot decontamination are necessary.
- *Security*: A plan for securing contaminated weapons must be in place (this must be predetermined in your local jurisdiction).
- *Decontamination of equipment*: Weapons and metal objects can be decontaminated either with soap and

water or with appropriately prepared bleach solutions (5% hypochlorite). All leather and certain fabrics cannot be efficiently decontaminated so must be disposed of properly.

CONSIDERATIONS FOR THE TACTICAL TEAM

Although law enforcement will not have a direct role in victim decontamination, their presence will be necessary, at a minimum, to provide security perimeters and ensure civilian compliance with instructions (Table 41.1). These duties are more consistent with the responsibilities of a general patrol officer but tactical team members are more likely to be pretrained and knowledgeable in the use of PPE, so they may be tasked with these duties. Law enforcement personnel providing security for victim decontamination operations in the warm zone should wear Level C PPE but different styles of respirators and suits are needed for security operations (see Chapter 40). In general this ensemble will include a face mask-style respirator, rather than a hood, and a military-style charcoal-impregnated cotton suit rather than a plastic suit. In situations where the team is performing offensive tactical operations in contaminated areas, members may need to wear higher levels of PPE but need to be trained in their use. Spot decontamination kits (e.g., the M291 kit) may be used in the field

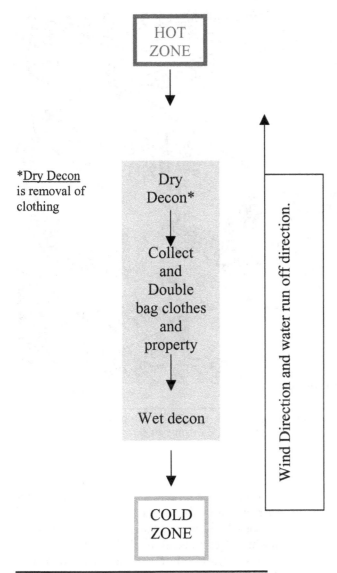

HOT ZONE

*Dry Decon is removal of clothing

Dry Decon*

Collect and Double bag clothes and property

Wet decon

COLD ZONE

Wind Direction and water run off direction.

FIGURE 41.3. Victim decontamination schematic.

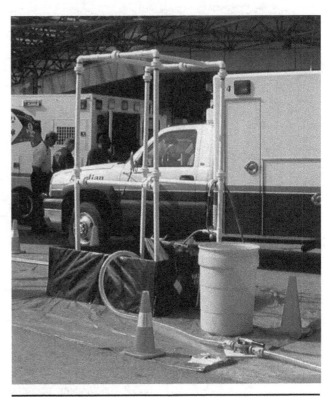

FIGURE 41.4. PVC decontamination shower. (Personal collection, Kenner, LA, 2005.)

ment is aware of the team's need for wet decontamination and will be prepared to provide it. Therefore, it is important that the tactical team coordinate with fire Incident Command for the decontamination of tactical team members and their equipment. If there is a high concern about the provision of wet decontamination for the TLE team, it might be prudent to invest in a small, portable wet decontamination system for the team's use only. The team must become self-sufficient if it is going to properly drill

to remove obvious contaminants from the exterior of garments or from the skin if the suit breaches. If team members become compromised during an operation before respiratory protection is removed and decontamination is attempted, they should be evacuated to a strategically safer area.

Upon exiting contaminated areas the tactical team must undergo a process known as technical decontamination. In this process they wash off the outside of their PPE and remove it in a safe manner. Also, during this process their weapons and equipment should be cleaned and reclaimed or secured. This process is very similar to the military field decontamination procedure shown in Fig. 41.5. Such decontamination operations can require a large number of personnel (Table 41.2) and a lot of equipment. If the tactical team does not have its own wet decontamination capabilities, it should not be assumed that the fire depart-

> **TABLE 41.1. Potential Areas for Tactical Law Enforcement Support in a Decontamination Situation.**

Crowd control and perimeter security along the perimeter of the warm zone

Security for personal property

Security of the decontamination corridor: personal equipment, crowds, etc.

Security of law enforcement equipment

Processing of evidence out of the warm zone

Investigators' processing of a crime scene at a CBR event

Bomb technicians' operations in a contaminated area or defusing of a suspected chemical explosive devise

Tactical operations in a known or suspected chemical agent environment

Takedown of a person who is contaminated with a CBR agent

CBR, chemical, biological, or radiological.

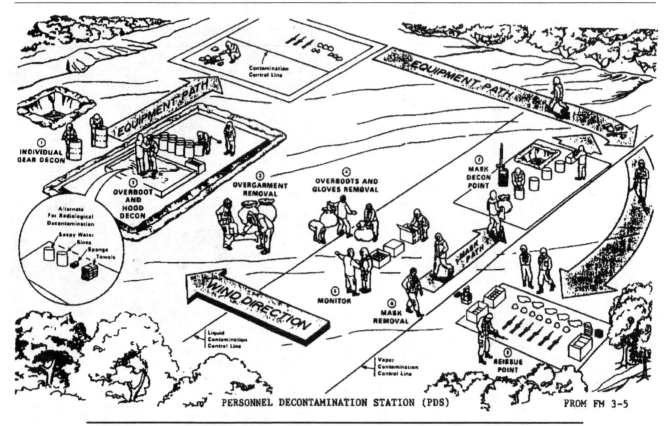

FIGURE 41.5. Diagram of decontamination for tactical team. (From U.S. Department of the Army. *Field Manual 3-5 NBC Decontamination*. Bethesda, MD: U.S. Department of the Army; 2000.)

and respond to a chemical or radiological event. This has been commented on in after-action reports from multiple drills where the fire department has taken down the decontamination facilities before law enforcement who were still in the warm/hot zone processing personal effects and performing perimeter control were decontaminated (1).

The most probable scenarios for the tactical team include industrial exposures and accidents and contact with hazardous components found in illicit methamphetamine labs. However, in the tactical scenario, a terrorist or crim-

inal might disperse and lay down a persistent chemical to form a perimeter or might use hazardous materials as offensive weapons. In these cases the risk of team contamination is quite high. Nerve agents, like VX, and blister agents, like sulfur mustard, are both very persistent in the environment and pose both a primary and a secondary contamination threat. Secondary contamination can be a major problem, as evidenced during the Tokyo subway incident, where secondary contamination affected health-care workers at hospitals taking care of the sarin-contaminated patients (2–5).

▶ **TABLE 41.2.** **The Initial People Needed in a Decontamination Incident: They will Need to Be Replaced Regularly Depending on Ambient Temperatures and Conditions.**

Decontamination Team Personnel	Small Incident	Large Incident
Safety officer	1	1
Security officer (law enforcement)	1	1–4
Triage officer	1	2–5
Litterbearers/escorts	4	14
Decontaminators (personal protective equipment)	4	8

There are five major properties of chemicals affecting decontamination.

- *pH*: A numeric measure of the acidic or basic nature of a substance and its potential for causing chemical burns: 1= strongest acid, 7= neutral, and 14 = strongest base.
- *Persistence*: The duration for which a contaminant stays in the environment and is a skin risk. Lipophyllic substances are usually more persistent than water-soluble ones.
- *Volatility*: The opposite of persistence, which involves evaporation. Perfume is volatile. Volatility depends on ambient temperatures. The more volatile, the more respiratory risk but the less need for decontamination.
- *Boiling point*: The temperature at which a chemical's vapor pressure is equal to the atmospheric pressure. A boiling point at or below room temperature means that the chemical is in its gaseous state at room temperature.
- *Pharmacologic effects*: Possible toxic effects caused by inhalation or dermal absorption of the chemical.

SPECIFIC HAZARDS

Chapter 39 describes the clinical presentation and treatment of various chemical weapons and radiation exposures. This section evaluates unique features of decontamination relating to specific agents.

Nerve Agents

Nerve agents are all liquid under common weather conditions but there is significant variability among agents in terms of viscosity and volatility (6). Delivery is typically achieved by pressurizing the liquid for aerosolized dispersal. Exposure is most often through inhaled vapor, but nerve agents are also well absorbed topically so they also represent a contact hazard. Secondary contamination is a significant risk with nerve agents (2). Anyone suspected of exposure should undergo thorough wet decontamination. The physical characteristics that allow dermal absorption also cause these chemicals to penetrate many common porous materials, leather, in particular, in a manner that renders common decontamination techniques ineffective. Therefore, such materials should be containerized or destroyed.

Blood Agents

Many different cyanide compounds are oral poisons but hydrogen cyanide and cyanogen chloride represent inhalational threats if aerosolized or offgassed in a fire. Gaseous forms of cyanide are typically released during a reaction between a cyanide salt (e.g., potassium cyanide) and an acid. Both hydrogen cyanide and cyanogen chloride are gasses in warm climates but may be liquids in colder areas. Fortunately, under warm conditions both forms will dissipate within a few minutes (7). Even in liquid form these highly reactive chemicals degrade quickly.

Blister Agents

Blister agents include sulfur mustard, lewisite, and phosgene oxime. Decontamination within 1 or 2 min after exposure is the only effective means of preventing or decreasing tissue damage from mustard. Unfortunately, most victims will not recognize the exposure until the window of opportunity has passed. Secondary transfer is of significant concern since these agents are highly persistent (8).

The physical properties of these agents will change dramatically between 10° and 38°C (50°–100°F) (8). When cool they will be very thick liquids or possibly solids, which are highly persistent, while at temperatures above 38°C they will be almost exclusively vapor hazards, which are much easier to decontaminate. These agents can be mixed with solvent chemicals to increase their volatility under cooler conditions.

Pulmonary Agents

Pulmonary agents represent a number of gasses and highly volatile liquids that combine with water to form acids and bases that result in effects ranging from mild irritation to severe burns. They are primarily a respiratory hazard but, at high concentrations, can cause irritation of mucous membranes or even the skin (9). For these agents evacuation to a safe area and dry decontamination will be appropriate for the majority of victims.

Radiological Contamination

Radioactive contamination, which is most prevalently in the form of dust or particles, is a threat in any stage of matter. Contamination effects are difficult to assess, since radioactivity is unlikely to cause acute effects and cannot be detected without special monitoring equipment. However, the decontamination procedures are essentially the same as for nonradioactive or radiostable chemicals (10). The main difference for decontamination staff is the need for team members to be monitored with a survey meter before entering the clean zone to ensure that all of the radioactive contaminant had been removed. Although dry decontamination can remove a significant portion of surface contamination, anyone with suspected radioactive contamination should undergo wet decontamination, remembering to provide protection from inhalation or ingestion of radiological particles.

TAKE-HOME POINTS

1. There are two types of contamination: primary—direct transfer from the source to persons or their equipment; and secondary—transfer of contamination from victims, their clothing, or their equipment to another person or object.
2. There are three main purposes for victim decontamination: (a) removal of contaminant from the victims, (b) prevention of secondary contamination of others, and (c) psychological comfort of the victims.
3. Dry decontamination methods such as simply disrobing may remove up to 70%–90% of the contaminant from the victim.

SUMMARY

The modern reality is that the tactical responder may have to perform missions in contaminated environments. Preplanning, training, and education are critical in preparing tactical responders for dealing with these realities. In the event of the need for mass civilian decontamination, TLE should have their own decontamination site setup, removed from the general population's decontamination site. This setup should be precoordinated with Incident Command, and as stated before, TLE should not assume that anyone else will take care of their decontamination needs.

GLOSSARY

Adsorb: To gather (gas, liquid, or dissolved substance) on a surface in a condensed layer (charcoal is an adsorbent

Air purifying respirator: Respirator with an air purifying filter, cartridge, or canister that removes specific air contaminants.

Degradation: The reduction in one or more physical properties of a protective material due to contact with a chemical

Filter cartridge: A container with a simple particle filter, sorbent, or catalyst or a combination of these items, which removes specific contaminants from the ambient air.

Fit Protection Rating: Multiple of the permissible exposure limit (PAPR's FPR is 1,000)

HEPA filter: High efficiency particulate air filter. It is a filter that is at least 99.97% efficient in removing monodisperse particles of 0.3 micrometers in diameter. Good for infectious biological agents or radiological

particles. The equivalent NIOSH 42 CFR 84 particulate filters are the N100, R100, and P100 filters.

IDLH: (Immediately dangerous to life and health). An atmosphere that poses an immediate threat to life, would cause irreversible adverse health effects, or would impair an individual's ability to escape from a dangerous atmosphere. Although in most cases, egress from a particular worksite could occur in much less than 30 minutes, as a safety margin, IDLHs were based on the effects that might occur as a consequence of a 30-minute exposure.

OSHA 29 CFR 1910.120: Hazardous waste operations and emergency response standards set forth by the Department of Labor and OSHA.

PEL: Permissible exposure limit. Regulatory limits established to avoid adverse health effects from exposures, based on an eight-hour workday/forty-hour workweek.

Penetration: The flow of a chemical through zippers, stitched seams, pores, or imperfections in materials

Permeation: The process by which a chemical moves through protective materials on a molecular level.

Power air purifying respirator (PAPR): An air purifying respiratory that uses a blower to forces the ambient air though filters. It may be considered a positive pressure device.

Primary contamination: Direct contact to victim.

Secondary contamination: Transfer of material from victim to personnel or equipment.

Sorbent: A surface which causes the absorption, adsorption or a combination of the two processes.

Vapor pressure: The pressure (expressed in mm of Hg) of a vapor in equilibrium with its liquid or solid form at a given temperature. The higher the vapor pressure, the greater the amount of chemical existing in the vapor phase. If greater than 760 mm Hg at room temp then the chemical exists as a gas.

Vesicant: A chemical agent used during warfare to produce blisters on the skin. Developed for use during WWI. It has been used in multiple conflicts since then. (Italy vs. Ethiopia, Iran-Iraq war used since WWI up to modern day).

REFERENCES

1. U.S. Army Soldier and Biological Command. *Guidelines for Use of Personal Protective Equipment by Law Enforcement Personnel during a Terrorist Chemical Agent Incident.* Revision 2, December. Washington, DC: USASBC; 2003.
2. Ohbu S, Yamashina A, Takasu N, et al. Sarin poisoning on Tokyo subway. *South Med J.* 1997;90:587–593.

3. Smart JK. History of chemical and biological warfare: an American perspective. In: Sidell FR, Takafuki ET, Franz DR, eds. *Medical Aspects of Chemical and Biological Warfare.* Textbook of Military Medicine series. Bethesda, MD: Office of the Surgeon General; 1997:11–47.

4. Kaidver H, Adams SC. Treatment of chemical and biological warfare injuries: insights derived from the 1984 Iraqi attack on Majnoon Island. *Milit Med.* 1991;15:171–177.

5. U.S. Department of the Army. *Field Manual 3-5 NBC Decontamination.* Bethesda, MD: U.S. Department of the Army; 2000.

6. Sidell FR. Nerve agents. In: Sidell F, Takafuji E, Franz D, eds. *Medical Aspects of Chemical and Biological Warfare.* Bethesda, MD: Office of the Surgeon General, U.S. Department of the Army; 1997:129–179.

7. Baskin SI, Brewer TG. Cyanide poisoning. In: Sidell F, Takafuji E,

Franz D, eds. *Medical Aspects of Chemical and Biological Warfare.* Bethesda, MD: Office of the Surgeon General, U.S. Department of the Army; 1997:277.

8. Sidell FR, Urbanetti JS, Smith WJ, et al. Vesicants. In: Zajtchuk R, ed. *Medical Aspects of Chemical and Biological Warfare.* Bethesda, MD: Office of the Surgeon General, U.S. Department of the Army; 1997:197–228.

9. Urbanetti JS. Toxic inhalational injury. In: Sidell F, Takafuji E, Franz D, eds. *Medical Aspects of Chemical and Biological Warfare.* Bethesda, MD: Office of the Surgeon General, U.S. Department of the Army; 1997:247–270.

10. Alt LA, Forcino CD, Walker RI. Nuclear events and thier consequences. In: Walker RI, Cerveny TJ, eds. *Medical Consequences of Nuclear Warfare.* Bethesda, MD: Office of the Surgeon General, U.S. Department of the Army; 1989:197–228.

Training Programs and Scenarios

Section Editor: RAYMOND L. FOWLER

Chapter 4 2

Tactical Training and Continuous Education for the Tactical Provider

Raymond L. Fowler, Alexander L. Eastman, Brian Krakover, Jeffery C. Metzger, and Troy Johnson

OBJECTIVES

After reading this section, the reader will be able to:

1. Discuss the necessity of a TEMS traing program.
2. Define the necessary elements of a TEMS training program.
3. Discuss the application of scenario based training in TEMS education.

This chapter presents key features in the initial training and continuous education of the tactical medical provider. A principal consideration in this work is that each individual assigned to participate in a tactical incident bears medical responsibilities of some type, thus requiring appropriate training to be able to carry out those responsibilities. Therefore it may be said that the tactical medical provider represents a key link in a continuum of safety and care

This work identifies key areas of training for those offering the spectrum of medical care in the tactical environment. In many areas reference is made to areas in which specific training should be sought, rather than covering the specifics of the training in these procedures, for example, endotracheal intubation (ETI) and needle decompression of the thorax. Ample references in the medical literature are available to the tactical provider that provide this training in detail. Rather, this chapter provides the margins and material comprising the spectrum of training for those involved in tactical emergency medical support.

Medical needs during a tactical event cover a broad realm. Injuries can be as minor as simple lacerations or minor burns and as serious as penetrating wounds that may be immediately life-threatening or even fatal. All personnel assigned to a tactical scenario must have been trained in basic assessment techniques that allow for identification of acute injury or illness on the part of any member of the team (1). In a dangerous setting such as being under fire, the first medical help will most likely come from another member of the tactical team before the tactical paramedic or physician becomes available to initiate further evaluation and treatment (1).

The most essential link in the chain of field survival is not the fully trained and certified medic. Knowing how to apply "self-aid" and "buddy aid"—teaching fighters to take care of themselves and those on their right and left—will allow initial assessment and treatment to occur much sooner than the care that will come later from medics, in many circumstances. Whether the mission is one of running a combat logistics patrol on a highway, running dismounted combat patrols in a military theater, or delivering a warrant to a suspected drug haven, the number of shooters will often outnumber the available medics.

In this regard, training should be focused substantially on the individual who will provide initial care. This care is not definitive but rather is stabilizing and temporizing. Medical providers will step forward later with advanced skills and patient sustainment efforts. Instructors and trainees in these initial skills must fully embrace the well-documented understanding that when skills are not used regularly, proficiency will decline. Thus, the authors believe that the teaching of a smaller skill set with frequent refresher training will achieve better results than the teaching of a large initial skill set with only yearly refresher training.

The type of training needed for tactical emergency medical support has been a subject of some debate. National experts in the field indeed have stated that "law enforcement agencies who attempt to apprehend dangerous, heavily armed criminals with a special operations team that lacks the expertise to treat the medical consequences that may arise from such a confrontation may be negligent of deliberate indifference" (1).

Specific points of the initial training for the tactical emergency medical provider include that the course (a) must be hands-on and based on the experience of the provider and (b) must include physician responders and minimal training to allow physicians to become members of the special weapons and tactics (SWAT) efforts.

Finally, recognizing the growing need for standardized education for the tactical emergency medicine provider. An initiative is currently underway to standardize this training. This initiative is being lead by academia and industry (2).

ESSENTIAL GENERAL PRINCIPLES

- Safety is key.
- Skills to be learned must be taught and trained in a tough, realistic environment. For example, if medics are

being trained to treat casualties from an Improvised Explosive Device, then these providers will best learn their skills if the actual training requires them to carry out their responsibilities while explosions are occurring. Gaining experience in sensory deprivation, stress management, and management of a scene involving a vehicle crash is vital as well.

- The tactical medical provider must be trained using the actual gear and matériel that will be available in a future scene.
- Feedback must be sought from experienced operators to keep tactics, techniques, and procedures current and useful.
- Trainers have to have real-world experience to offer optimum benefit to trainees. Absence of "real-world training" limits the scope of insight and applicability of the trainer.
- Many different products and devices, offered by a myriad of salespeople, are now active and available in the tactical casualty care world. Training should be focused on principles and processes so that people will still know what to do when their equipment fails or they are presented with a scenario for which they did not train.

SPECIFIC TRAINING STANDARDS FOR THE TACTICAL EMERGENCY MEDICAL PROVIDER

Assessment of Illness or Injury

- Evidence of acute injury or illness, such as penetrating injury or chemical contamination
- Abnormal mental status
- Abnormal sounds, such as snoring or gasping
- Obvious airway problems upon inspection, such as trauma or hemorrhage
- Elevated or depressed respirations
- External hemorrhage
- Obvious alterations body habitus, such as extremity angulation as well as abnormal posture or position

Airway Assessment and Management

Assessment

All members of the tactical team should be trained in basic airway assessment and management. A compromised airway can rapidly result in injury or death due to airway obstruction and/or to bodily fluids contaminating the lungs.

Training for airway assessment begins at the level of the individual being trained. Personnel without medical backgrounds must be trained to recognize an individual who appears to have some abnormality of the mouth or neck that interferes with normal airflow.

- Trauma to the mouth, for example, can obstruct the flow of air.
- Snoring sounds from a previously well airway likely indicates soft tissue obstruction of the airway.
- Blood, other fluids, or debris seen in the airway may well present a hazard to the safe movement of air into the lungs.
- The recognition of obvious breathing difficulty must be a standard of training for all responders. Such difficulty includes all of the above findings plus obvious struggling by the victim to move air, elevated or diminished rates of breathing, and indication by the victim that difficulty breathing is occurring, for example, clutching the throat to suggest airway obstruction.

Basic Management

Standard airway management maneuvers should be taught to all personnel. These maneuvers include the following.

- Training in basic cardiopulmonary resuscitation (3)
- Manual clearing of the oropharynx
- Suctioning of the oropharynx and hypopharynx
- Positioning of the mandible and neck (if neck positioning is permitted by condition) to facilitate air exchange, including jaw thrust and hyperextension
- Insertion of an oral airway, if available, indicated, and permitted by the scenario
- Insertion of a nasopharyngeal airway, if available, indicated, and permitted by the scenario
- Assistance of ventilation with pocket mask or bag-valve-mask

Invasive Management

Advanced airway management maneuvers should be available to trained, qualified personnel. These maneuvers include:

- Insertion of a supraglottic airway, which may include the Esophageal-Tracheal Combitube, Easy Tube, Laryngeal Mask Airway, King Airway, or Cobra Airway: The provider must be trained in both insertion of the device and ventilation of the patient utilizing the device.
- ETI, including the following techniques:
  Standard ETI utilizing a laryngoscope
  Digital intubation
- Transtracheal jet insufflation

- Surgical cricothyrotomy *or* utilization of an approved transcricothyroid membrane ventilatory device, such as the Melkor or QuickTrach

Ventilatory Assessment and Management

Assessment

All members of the tactical team should be trained in basic assessment of respiratory status. Specific signs of ventilatory assessment include:

- Training in the appearance of normal breathing
- Training in elevated and depressed rates of breathing
- Training in assessment for increased work of breathing
- Training in appearance of the use of accessory ventilatory muscles
- Training in assessment of normal skin color and cyanosis
- Training that conditions of elevated respiratory rate may be associated with conditions producing shock, such as hemorrhage, tension pneumothorax, or cardiac tamponade

Management

All members of the tactical team should be trained in basic management techniques for respiratory emergencies:

- Application of face masks, including simple masks as well as non-rebreathers
- Assistance with ventilation utilizing mouth-to-mouth respiration
- Assistance with ventilation utilizing a pocket mask
- Assistance with ventilation utilizing a bag-valve-mask with and without either an oral airway or a nasopharyngeal airway in place
- Assistance with ventilation utilizing a supraglottic airway
- Assistance with ventilation utilizing an endotracheal tube
- Assistance with ventilation via a transtracheal route

Point of Caution

Training in ventilatory management for tactical medical providers must include information regarding avoidance of "overzealous ventilations" of injured victims who may be in shock for any reason. Training should include that overzealous ventilation may involve either rate or tidal volume. Important causes of shock include diminished venous return (tension pneumothorax or cardiac tamponade) and hypovolemia (hemorrhagic shock). In these clinical scenarios, positive pressure ventilation may decrease venous return and worsen shock.

Hemorrhage Assessment and Management

Assessment

All members of the tactical team should be trained in basic assessment of a possible hemorrhagic condition. Tactical providers must be carefully oriented to the two general types of hemorrhage: external and internal. Specific training in the signs of shock must include:

- Training in the appearance of external bleeding
- Training in the appearance, moisture, and temperature of normal skin
- Training in the appearance of skin in patients in shock
- Training in wounds that may be associated with internal hemorrhage
- Training in complaints by the injured person that may be associated with internal hemorrhage

Management

All members of the tactical team should be trained in basic management techniques for emergencies that may involve hemorrhagic shock. The techniques include:

- Rapid identification of the individual at risk of hemorrhage
- Rapid application of direct pressure on sites of external bleeding
- Technique of tourniquet application to involved extremities
- Placing the patient in the shock position
- Rapid determination of means of evacuation of patient at risk for hemorrhage

Point of Caution

Training in management of the victim with hemorrhagic conditions for tactical medical providers must emphasize that it may not be obvious that injured victims may have uncontrolled internal bleeding.

Intravascular Access

Some experienced members of the tactical team may be instructed in basic techniques of accessing the vascular space for the purpose of rendering fluids and medications to the injured victim. Specific training standards that must be taught to these providers include the type of device, the location of the access site, and techniques of use of approved intravenous fluids and medications for resuscitation and treatment.

- Intravenous access: preferred puncture sites and techniques (4–6)
- Intraosseous access: approved sites, techniques, and available devices (7,8)

- Use of intravenous fluids (4–6)
- Use of low-volume resuscitation intravenous flow rates in the setting of uncontrolled hemorrhage (4)
- Use of standard-volume resuscitation intravenous flow rates in the setting of victims with controlled hemorrhage

Splinting

Tactical emergency medicine providers must have basic training in application of splints to injured areas. Broken bones have sharp edges that may lacerate internal structures including blood vessels and nerves. Disrupted connective tissues like ligaments can cause instabilities that may be dangerous to the victim, including in the neck and back. Important splinting techniques include (4–6):

- Placement of a cervical collar
- Application of a triangular bandage to an upper extremity
- Splinting of potential forearm fractures in a position of comfort using available splints or bulky material
- Splinting of injured lower extremities using the opposite extremity and wrapping material to hold them together
- Application of a long spine board for both patient stabilization and transport
- Note: Specific mention of standard long-leg traction splints is de-emphasized *unless* frequent retraining is maintained, due to the loss of skills

Management of the Victim in Pain

Many conditions cause pain, ranging from mild to severe. These conditions can be as relatively straightforward as the fracture of an arm to as complex as an abdominal gunshot wound. Training considerations for pain control include:

- Placement of injured victims in positions of comfort (e.g., avoiding movement of injured extremities)
- Use of verbal counseling for victim reassurance
- Use of intravenous, intramuscular, or intraosseous morphine for pain control, with appropriate precautions regarding using lower dosages in a serial manner

Management of the Acutely Agitated Victim

Head injuries, hysteria, drug-induced intoxications (such as the anticholinergic effects of BZ), acute psychosis, and other conditions may result in a victim's becoming extremely agitated, possibly to the point of violent delirium. Training for this scenario may include:

- Application of safe "take-down" techniques
- Application of restraints
- Use of a TASER to control the victim's activity

■ Chemical restraints through intramuscular, intravenous, or intranasal/buccal routes (e.g., midazolam, where authorized)

Rendering Care in Hazardous Situations: Assessment and Management

All members of the tactical team should be trained in what basic assessment must be conducted during a hazardous situation of any type. Training must include techniques in recognition of a victim in distress. Tactical providers must be carefully oriented to limiting assessment during times of extreme hazard and instead opting to remove victims to safe zones. Specific areas of training must include:

■ Carry maneuvers for victims with potential spinal injuries
■ Carry maneuvers for victims with potential airway compromise, including bleeding and vomit threatening the airway
■ Carry maneuvers utilizing multiple rescuers
■ Airway management during transport of the victim
■ Training in management of airway, ventilation, and hemorrhagic conditions in scenarios during which victims cannot be moved due to hazards

CONTINUOUS EDUCATION FOR THE TACTICAL EMERGENCY MEDICINE PROVIDER

Skills that are not refreshed through experience and retraining deteriorate over time (9). This is a cognitive and technical breakdown that has been studied and documented for more than a generation (10). As discussed, skills for the tactical emergency medical provider run the gamut from assessing airways to decompressing a tension pneumothorax. However, many of these skills may be seldom, if ever, utilized. Skills requiring the most technical knowledge break down fastest, and despite frequent use, basic skills also may be lost. Increased time since initial training has been shown to be associated with the greatest loss of skills among trained paramedics (10).

At this juncture in the history of emergency medicine, a critical focus is being placed on many aspects of emergency care. One example is the use of ETI by prehospital emergency medical providers. Recent research has shown a worrisome association between the application of prehospital ETI and an increase in the risk of death from traumatic brain injury (11). The effect of such research should be to revisit in what circumstances such devices or techniques are utilized and to seek alternative, safer treatments when possible. A useful example that is on point to the cited study is the utilization of "alternative" or

"rescue" airways where possible—such as the King airway or the Combitube—instead of ETI.

Continuous education should be provided in all of the skills mentioned in the initial training section, from patient assessment through all of the procedures. When the cycles of education should occur for each assessment technique or procedure is less clear. As mentioned, assessment skills have been shown to deteriorate, and thus these skills should be refreshed periodically. Likewise, procedure skills such as starting intravenous lines must be maintained through active practice and timely remediation where indicated.

Some method of continuous quality improvement (CQI) is appropriate to provide remediation to medical staff members who may show suboptimal performance in some area. Indeed, recognizing the need for CQI processes to assess the skill sets of providers, the National Registry of Emergency Medical Technicians allows for as many as a third of continuing education hours to be generated through needs identified in the CQI process (12). The technique of CQI might be as specific as a medical record that may be generated for the care rendered and may be reviewed by a supervisor. A handwritten EMS patient care report is an example of one such record that might be generated. Self-reporting by staff members should be encouraged to initiate the continuing education process as well.

The methods of providing continuous and remedial education are broad. Distributive learning through the Internet has become an extremely versatile method of bringing both the spoken and the written word to students worldwide (13). Many programs offer accredited continuing education in this manner. Specific skills, though, such as placement of intravenous lines and airway management techniques, require hands-on training.

Continuous Education Cycles for the Tactical Emergency Medical Provider

Assessment Skills

Techniques of patient assessment should be reviewed periodically. The authors suggest a minimum of annually. The specific assessment skills to be addressed mirror the initial training, though they need not be as comprehensive. Specific areas of training must include:

■ Injury and illness assessment, including looking for alterations in level of consciousness
■ Airway assessment
■ Ventilatory assessment
■ Circulatory and hemorrhage assessment
■ Assessment for fractures

Management Skills

Specific management skills relative to each of the above areas must be addressed in continuous education. The authors suggest a maximum period that should be allowed between refresher training periods. Specific areas of training must include:

- Basic airway maneuvers: 1 year
- Advanced airway maneuvers including advanced airway placement: 6 months
- Ventilatory assistance: 1 year
- Hemorrhage control: 1 year
- Intravenous, intraosseous, and intramuscular access: 6 months
- Application of splints: 1 year
- Pain management: 1 year
- Agitated patient control: 1 year

Finally, a useful reference site to locate training programs relative to tactical medicine is the Texas Tactical Police Officers Association Web site (14).

A SUGGESTED MINIMUM TRAINING CURRICULUM FOR A TACTICAL MEDIC INTENSIVE COURSE

1. History and development of tactical emergency medical services (TEMS)
2. General history, development, and operation of SWAT units
3. General operational philosophy/model of armed versus unarmed SWAT medics
4. Legal/ethical issues related to SWAT and TEMS
5. Funding and interagency cooperation of TEMS units
6. Basic SWAT operations/tactics and intervention strategies
7. Patient movement in the tactical environment
8. Weapons familiarization/make safe issues
9. Medical threat assessments
10. Medicine "across the barricade"
11. Patient assessment in austere environments
12. Advanced airway management
13. Operational planning/extended operations mitigation
14. Chemical agents/less-lethal devices overview and treatment modalities
15. TEMS units equipment carry considerations
16. Team health/team sustainment issues
17. Advanced trauma management
18. Other TEMS-pertinent subjects

TACTICAL TRAINING SCENARIOS

Scenario 1: Injured Undercover Officer

Setup

During an undercover narcotics buy, a suspect shot and wounded the undercover officer. The officer was able to move behind a concrete retaining wall and nearby patrol elements surrounded the house and have exchanged fire with the suspect. SWAT was called in to assist.

Assignment

1. Develop a medical threat assessment, including priorities for assessing the undercover officer's injuries and assessing if the suspect is wounded, and develop a rescue plan for extricating the officer from the location.
2. What treatment is necessary at the current location (self-aid vs. medic treatment) and how can the officer be moved from the current location (self-extraction vs. team extraction)?
3. How thorough an exam can be done once the officer is removed to the warm zone?
4. What treatments can be rendered in the warm zone?

Scenario 2: Mass Casualty

Setup

A man has taken a city bus hostage. Approximately 25 civilians are onboard. After an intense standoff, the suspect becomes enraged and begins stabbing the hostages. The snipers take a shot, and the entry team storms in. Once the suspect has been secured, the team calls up the medic.

Upon entry you see multiple hostages with stab wounds and various levels of bleeding. The suspect has been shot in the head through the mouth, and he is bleeding profusely. He is not making purposeful movements, but he has a pulse and is breathing. He seems to be choking on blood.

Assignments

1. Develop a method to triage the patients.
2. Do you use other officers to assist in triage?
3. Where does the suspect fall in the triage system?
4. Do you treat minor injuries sustained by the hostages before treating the suspect?
5. How do you arrange transport for multiple casualties?
6. What other services do you have available?
7. Do you allow other medics into the crime scene?

Scenario 3: Warrant Service

Setup

The team is serving a high-risk warrant on a drug dealer known to have high-powered rifles and other weapons. As the entry team is setting the breaching device, shots ring out through the front door and wall. The first three officers in the stack are struck by rounds.

- The first officer goes down and is not moving.
- The other two officers are able to move to the corner of the building and take cover.
- The rest of the team either stays with the two officers on the corner or retreats to the armored vehicle.
- No further shots are being fired.

Assignment

1. Develop a plan to rescue the injured officers.
2. Do you go to the house to begin treating the officers or use other teammates (or the vehicle) to extricate them?
3. The first officer in the stack is not moving and not responding to verbal commands. The officer appears to have been struck in the head. At what point do you attempt a rescue versus presume the officer is dead and stay back? What tools might help in making that decision?
4. How do you direct treatment for the other officers while next to the house and what treatments are necessary prior to evacuation?
5. Once in a cold zone, do you go to the hospital with the officers as they are transported, or do you stay on the scene?

Scenario 4: Murder/Suicide

Setup

The team is called to a hostage situation that began as a domestic disturbance. A man is holding his wife hostage with a revolver. After tense negations, the man shoots his wife in the head and then shoots himself. The team makes entry and secures the weapon. They call the medic for assistance. Upon entry:

- The woman has a wound from the back of her head through her anterior neck, with obvious brain matter exposed.
- The suspect has a wound behind both eyes. He has gasping respirations, at a rate of approximately four per minute, and a barely palpable pulse of 30.

Assignment

1. How aggressively do you treat the suspect?
2. Do you attempt resuscitation?
3. Can you declare him dead?

Scenario 5: Bank Robbery

Setup

During a bank robbery, several suspects barricade themselves inside the bank and hold the customers and staff hostage. A security guard has been shot in the arm. During negotiations, the suspects tell the negotiator that there is a lady who claims to be diabetic and is beginning to feel lightheaded, sweaty, and like her heart is racing.

Assignment

1. How do you get information regarding the severity of the injured security guard and the woman's medical illness?
2. How do you instruct a person with no medical background what to look for and how to treat these problems?
3. What diagnostic tools may be available (such as a glucometer)?
4. At what point do you recommend to command that negotiations should be directed toward the release of these injured or ill hostages?

REFERENCES

1. Rinnert K, Hall W. Tactical emergency medical support. *Emerg Med Clin North Am.* 2002;20(4):929–952.
2. www.toccourse.com
3. American Heart Association. *American Heart Association Basic Life Support Manual.* Dallas, TX: American Heart Association; 2005.
4. Deparment of Defense. *Emergency War Surgery.* 3rd U.S. ed. Washington, DC: Department of Defense; 2004.
5. Fowler R, Pepe P, Stevens J. The evaluation and management of shock. In: *International Trauma Life Support Manual.* Oakbrook Terrace, IL: International Trauma Life Support; 2007.
6. Prehospital trauma life support. Available at: http://www.naemt.org/PHTLS/aboutPHTLS/.
7. National Association of EMS Physicians Position Paper on Intraosseous Vascular Access in the Out-of-Hospital Setting. *Prehosp Emerg Care.* 2007; Jan-Mar; 11(1):62.
8. Fowler R, et al. The role of intraosseous vascular access in the out-of-hospital environment. *Prehosp Emerg Care.* 2007;11(1):63–66.
9. Wolfram R, Warren C, Doyle C, et al. Retention of Pediatric Advanced Life Support (PALS) course concepts. *J Emerg Med.* 2003;25(4):475–479.
10. Skelton M, McSwain N. A study of cognitive and technical skill deterioration among trained paramedics. *JACEP.* 1977;6(10):436–438.
11. Wang H, Peitzman A, Cassidy L, et al. Out-of-hospital endotracheal intubation and outcome after traumatic brain injury. *Ann Emerg Med.* 2004;44(5):439–450.
12. The Flexible Core Content represents education over topics identified by EMTs to have both high potential for harm and high frequency of delivery. NREMT-Intermediate 85/99s, NREMT-Paramedics, states, or employers may choose which patient assessment and care tasks they wish to review based upon individual, system or state needs assessments. *Natl Registry EMTs Newslett.* Spring 2004. Available at: www.nremt.org.
13. The interested reader should access the site www.utsw.ws for examples of online lectures provided to EMS personnel at the University of Texas Southwestern School of Allied Health.
14. Texas Tactical Police Officers Association; www.ttpoa.org.